CLINICAL RESEARCHES

ON

DISEASE IN INDIA

CLINICAL RESEARCHES

ON

DISEASE IN INDIA

CHARLES MOREHEAD, M.D.

GYAN

Published by

Gyan Publishing House
5, Ansari Road
Daryaganj, New Delhi-110002
Phone: 011-47034999, 9811692060
E-mail: books@gyanbooks.com

Distribution Network
gyanbooks.com
India, USA, Canada, UK, Australia, France

ISBN: 978-81-212-9408-9 (PB)
First Published, 1856

2nd Impression 2023

Printed at: Gyan Press, Delhi.

CLINICAL RESEARCHES ON DISEASE IN INDIA

AUTHOR: CHARLES MOREHEAD

DISEASE IN INDIA

CLINICAL RESEARCHES

ON

DISEASE IN INDIA

BY

CHARLES MOREHEAD, M.D.

FELLOW OF THE ROYAL COLLEGE OF PHYSICIANS : PRINCIPAL OF GRANT MEDICAL COLLEGE : PROFESSOR OF THE PRINCIPLES AND PRACTICE OF MEDICINE AND OF CLINICAL MEDICINE : SURGEON TO THE JAMSETJEE JEJEEBHOY HOSPITAL, AND FORMERLY ASSISTANT-SURGEON TO THE EUROPEAN GENERAL HOSPITAL, AT BOMBAY

SECOND EDITION

LONDON

LONGMAN, GREEN, LONGMAN, AND ROBERTS

1860

TO

JOHN M^cLENNAN, M.D.

FELLOW OF THE ROYAL COLLEGE OF PHYSICIANS, LATE PHYSICIAN-GENERAL OF THE ARMY, AND MEMBER OF THE BOARD OF EDUCATION, OF THE PRESIDENCY OF BOMBAY,

CONSPICUOUS THROUGHOUT A LENGTHENED PERIOD OF PUBLIC SERVICE

FOR PROFESSIONAL ATTAINMENTS, ADMINISTRATIVE ABILITY,

AND GENEROUS PHILANTHROPY,

COMMEMORATED, ON HIS DEPARTURE FROM INDIA,

BY THE UNITED TESTIMONY OF THE GOVERNMENT AND ALL CLASSES OF THE COMMUNITY,

THIS WORK IS DEDICATED,

WITH THE ADMIRATION AND REGARD WHICH LONG FRIENDSHIP HAS INSPIRED.

PREFACE

TO

THE SECOND EDITION.

The haste inseparable from the circumstances in which this work was originally prepared and published, led to numerous defects of arrangement and execution, which I have endeavoured to amend in the present edition. While the size of the book has been much reduced by the adoption of a smaller type, a more careful selection of cases, and a thorough revision of the text,—full use has been made of three years' additional experience in India, partly as Professor of Clinical Medicine, and partly as Superintending Surgeon of the Poona division of the Bombay army.

My matured opinions on the therapeutic value of quinine and of arsenic, and on the best methods of using these medicines in malarious fevers, have been explained. The occasional occurrence of Typhoid—Enteric—fever in India has been acknowledged; and chapters on Sun-Stroke and on the Hill Sanitaria of the Deccan have been added.

London, August, 1860.

PREFACE

TO

THE FIRST EDITION.

THE desire which I have long entertained of contributing to the resources of practical medicine in India, has been realised at the present time, in obedience to the wishes of the Honourable Court of Directors of the East India Company, originating in the following minute, which was submitted on the 15th May, 1854, by Dr. Mc-Lennan, Physician-General of the Bombay Army, to his colleagues in the Board of Education, approved by them and by the Government of Bombay:—

MINUTE.

"I now beg to submit to my colleagues the proposition to which I lately adverted, when treating of the approaching departure of Dr. Morehead on sick leave. My own impression was, that in all probability eighteen months would be necessary for the purpose of recruiting his health; but in consideration of the special nature of the leave applied for, the Medical Board restricted their recommendation to a period about which there could be no doubt, and, therefore, mentioned twelve months only as the time deemed requisite for his restoration to health and efficiency.

"I would now submit, that the Board of Education make a suggestion to Government, in view to its transmission to the Honourable Court of Directors, that at the end of that period Dr. Morehead be requested to occupy himself in advancing the cause of Indian Medical Education by the preparation of a work on the Diseases of India, calculated, not only for the Students educated in Indian Medical Colleges and for Indian Graduates, but also for Medical Commissioned Officers of the Honourable Company's Service on first arrival in India, and till such time as they have acquired that experience which years of service alone supply. The period necessary to bring out such a work, with the materials already accumulated by Dr. Morehead, would probably not exceed another year, and thus the whole term of absence, both on account of health and duty, would not exceed that for which leave within the limits on the old Furlough Rules has hitherto been given.

"It may be well that I should say something of the grounds on which I venture to make this recommendation, and here I would say that Dr. Morehead's experience has been varied and extensive. On first arrival in India he served for two years with European, and for as many years with native troops, at different stations. He was then for two years in charge of the sanatory station of Mahableshwur; — thereafter, for more than six years, resident Assistant Surgeon of the European General Hospital, Bombay — an institution in which the inmates are of very varied circumstances as to habits, position in life, nature of duties, and length of residence in India, &c. In that hospital are accommodated the newly arrived European and the old servant of many years' Indian residence — the seamen of the Royal, Indian, and Mercantile navies — the soldiers of all arms and both services, Queen's and Company's — the townsman — mechanic — clerk — male and female — adult and child — from most classes of life, and many stations in the interior. The opportunity for seeing variety of disease, therefore, under great diversity of circumstance, is considerable.

"Dr. Morehead was likewise for six years Surgeon of the Byculla Schools. In parts of 1843 and 1844 he was in Sinde, and had an opportunity of observing the state of health of Europeans and Natives after the sickly season of 1843.

"He has been for nearly nine years Surgeon of the Jamsetjee Jejeebhoy Hospital, and for six years has been engaged in teaching Medicine and Clinical Medicine in the Grant Medical College; and the records of the Clinical Wards have been carefully preserved during the whole of this period.

"He has been twelve years Secretary to the Medical and Physical Society, during which time there has been afforded him by the Medical Board the opportunity of becoming acquainted with the tenor of the medical reports and cases from all parts of the Presidency.

"In 1833, and again in 1853, Dr. Morehead had the opportunity of observing some of the hospitals and medical institutions in Madras, Calcutta, Colombo, &c. &c.

"Very numerous papers on Dysentery — Dracunculus — Diseases of the Abdominal Viscera — Intermittent and Remittent Fevers — Delirium Tremens — Diseases of the Brain — Hepatitis and Cholera — Measles in the Byculla Schools, &c. &c., have been inserted by him in the Edinburgh Medical and Surgical Journal, Transactions of the Medical and Physical Society of Calcutta, and Transactions of the Medical and Physical Society of Bombay.

"In the last work, too, at a comparatively recent date, five papers, based on observations chiefly made in the Clinical Wards of the Jamsetjee Jejeebhoy Hospital, on the important subjects of Smallpox — Bright's Disease of the Kidney — Diseases of the Heart — Pneumonia — and Beriberi — have been contributed, and there are records from which to make the same kind of observations in respect to other important diseases treated in the same wards, such as Hepatic Abscess — Dysentery — Fevers — Phthisis Pulmonalis — Paralytic Affections, &c. &c.

"Having thus detailed the sources from which Dr. Morehead's experience and fitness for the task which I have ventured to suggest have been derived, I may now add a few words as to the nature of that want which I propose he should supply; and here I honestly give it as my opinion, that till some work of the kind I suggest be brought forth, the efforts of Indian Governments and their servants in medical education will be incomplete. At present, Graduates and Students of Indian Medical Colleges are without any book on practice in Indian Disease, as now generally followed, or as requiring modifications to meet peculiarities of native habit and constitution.

"The duties of the Clinical Wards in the Grant Medical College have been so carried on, and so recorded, as to constitute an important collection of facts and practice, which may be brought to bear on this want. The labour of collecting, digesting, and condensing for such a work will be considerable, and, as it is valuable for Indian purposes, it should (it seems to me) receive support and encouragement from the Indian Government, which Dr. Morehead has so zealously and usefully served.

"I, therefore, trust my colleagues will support my proposition, and recommend, that after the expiration of the leave lately granted, Dr. Morehead may have, for the above purpose, another year in England on Indian allowances, and to count as service, with the right of returning to that place in the Grant Medical College, over which he has so beneficially presided." *

In performing this duty I have endeavoured to embody my experience in a connected form, and to illustrate my opinions by cases which have passed under my immediate observation† and care; while, at the same time, I have not been inattentive to the views of other inquirers.

My clinical researches have been directed to disease, as occurring both in Europeans and in the Natives of India. I have aimed not merely to increase practical knowledge of the diseases usually termed tropical, as malarious fever, hepatitis, dysentery; but, also to show that affections—pneumonia, phthisis pulmonalis, pericarditis, Bright's disease—familiar to European observers, are sufficiently common in India, more particularly in some classes of the native community.

Cases have been introduced chiefly with the object of elucidating the Symptomatology and Pathology of disease. They have been used freely in the form of summaries, which have in every instance been carefully prepared by myself. The graduates of the Indian Medical Colleges, for whose benefit I have chiefly written, may often, for many years yet to come, be placed in positions remote from their professional brethren, and in circumstances ill adapted for the prosecution of pathological research. The recollection of this fact has removed any hesitation which I might otherwise have felt relative to the expediency of inserting so many illustrative details. But, at the same time, I have been careful so to arrange the text of the work, that it may be readily perused independent of the cases; and so to classify and indicate the cases, that they may be referred to without difficulty by those who may be engaged in the close investigation of the diseases to which they relate.

* Report of the Board of Education, Bombay, from May 1, 1854, to April 30, 1855, p. 144.

† The few cases not observed by myself which have been inserted, are indicated by an asterisk.

In my remarks on the treatment of disease I have invariably endeavoured to explain fully the principles, and to state the means by which they may be best applied. Cases illustrative of treatment have been sparingly used by me, because practical conclusions arrived at, after a lengthened course of experience, are grounded partly on cases successfully treated, partly on those which have proved fatal, and partly on the observation of different methods in the hands of others. Therefore the physician, on looking back to the records of his practice through a long series of years, is not likely to meet with many cases calculated to illustrate at all points his matured therapeutic opinions.

Making exception, then, of the few cases which have been detailed in explanation of treatment, I would request the reader to refer exclusively to the text for my views on this important part of my subject. Doubtless the principles inculcated by me will be found applied in the management of many of the cases which have been narrated with a different object; but, on the other hand, I am very sensible that some of them may be fairly open to criticism.

It was my desire to have concluded this work with a chapter on the Diseases of Females and of Children, but the time at my command has come to a close. In respect to some of the diseases of which I have treated, reference has been made to their occurrence in females, and in the early periods of life; and a little reflection will readily suggest the modifications of the pathological and therapeutic principles, which I have endeavoured to enforce, to the circumstances of difference of sex and of age. Still, the subject is of much interest and importance, and I would indulge the hope that I may be permitted, at some future time, to supply the omission which at present I have been unable to avoid.

London, May, 1856.

CONTENTS.

	PAGE
Preface to Second Edition	vii
Preface to First Edition	ix

CHAPTER I.

Introduction. — General Remarks on the Causes, Pathology, and Treatment of Disease in India 1

CHAPTER II.

Remarks on the Statistics of the European General Hospital, and of the Jamsetjee Jejeebhoy Hospital at Bombay 11

CHAPTER III.

General Remarks on Fevers in India 16

CHAPTER IV.

ON INTERMITTENT FEVER.

Section I. — Different Types of Intermittent Fever 17

Section II. —Simple Intermittent Fever. — Symptoms, Pathology, and Treatment 20

Section III. — Intermittent Fever complicated with Enlargement of the Spleen. — Symptoms. — Pathology. — Treatment 36

Section IV. — Intermittent Fever with Hepatic Complication. — Symptoms. — Pathology. — Treatment 43

Section V. — Intermittent Fever complicated with Jaundice, or Affections of the Stomach or Bowels 47

Section VI. — Intermittent Fever complicated with Cerebral Affection . 49

Section VII. — Intermittent Fever complicated with Bronchitis, Pneumonia, Rheumatism, Scorbutus, Pericarditis, Asthma 52

CHAPTER V.

ON REMITTENT FEVER.

PAGE

SECTION I. — The Diagnosis of Remittent Fever, from Intermittent Fever and ardent Continued Fever. — Division into Simple and Complicated . . 56

SECTION II. — Symptoms of Remittent Fever. — Ordinary, Inflammatory, Adynamic, Congestive, Badly developed, with unexpected Collapse, with peculiar Features. — Also complicated with Cerebral Affection, Irritability of Stomach, Jaundice, Bronchitis, Pneumonia. — Diagnosis from Hectic and Symptomatic Fever 58

SECTION III. — Pathology. — Mortality from Remittent Fever. — Relation of Type to Diathesis and previously existing Structural Lesions. — Complication with Cerebral Affection and Consideration of the Pathological Import of Cranial Serous Effusion. — Complication with Gastric Irritability, Affection of the Bowels. — Hepatitis, Jaundice, Parotitis, and Pneumonia . . 75

SECTION IV. — Treatment. — Contrast of the Principles of Treatment of Malarious Remittent Fever, and the Zymotic Continued Fevers of Cold Climates. — Treatment of Ordinary, Inflammatory, Congestive, Adynamic, and Irregular Types of Remittent Fever. — Then of those complicated with Cerebral Affection, Gastric Irritability, Jaundice, Hepatitis 105

SECTION V. — Treatment further considered in Remarks on Blood-letting, Mercury, Cold Affusion and Wet Sheet Packing, Purgatives, Emetics, Blisters, Opiates, Quinine, Diet, and Change of Air 122

CHAPTER VI.

ON CERTAIN OBSCURE PHENOMENA, PROBABLY RELATED TO MALARIA . . 153

CHAPTER VII.

ON ADYNAMIC REMITTENT FEVER OF SUSPECTED INFECTIOUS CHARACTER . 155

CHAPTER VIII.

ON TYPHOID FEVER 160

CHAPTER IX.

ON COMMON CONTINUED FEVER — FEBRICULA — AND ARDENT CONTINUED FEVER.

SECTION I. — General Remarks 162

SECTION II. — Common Continued Fever — Febricula 162

SECTION III. — Ardent Continued Fever 164

CHAPTER X.

ON THE FEBRILE AFFECTIONS OF CHILDREN IN INDIA. — FEBRICULA. — INTERMITTENT AND REMITTENT FEVER 168

CHAPTER XI.

STATISTICS OF FEVER IN THE EUROPEAN GENERAL HOSPITAL, THE JAMSETJEE JEJEEBHOY HOSPITAL, AND BYCULLA SCHOOLS, AT BOMBAY.

SECTION I. — European General Hospital. — Total Fevers . . . 170

SECTION II. — European General Hospital. — Intermittent Fever . . 172

PAGE

SECTION III. — Jamsetjee Jejeebhoy Hospital. — Total Fevers . . . 175

SECTION IV. — Jamsetjee Jejeebhoy Hospital. — Intermittent Fever . . 176

SECTION V. — European General Hospital. — Remittent Fever . . . 177

SECTION VI. — Jamsetjee Jejeebhoy Hospital. — Remittent Fever . . 179

SECTION VII. — Byculla Schools. — Intermittent and Remittent Fever . . 181

CHAPTER XII.

ON ERUPTIVE FEVERS.

SECTION I. —Prevalence in the Native Army 182

SECTION II. — Small-pox, as observed in Bombay. — Prevalence. — Prevention by Vaccination 182

SECTION III. — On Measles in Bombay and the Deccan . . . 194

SECTION IV. — Scarlatina. — Erysipelas. — Varicella. — Hooping Cough. — Cynanche Parotidea 199

CHAPTER XIII.

ON EPIDEMIC CHOLERA.

SECTION I. — Remarks on the Seasons of Prevalence and on the Causes of Cholera 202

SECTION II. — Symptoms considered in reference to their degrees of severity. — Diagnosis from Bilious Cholera, Irritant Poisoning, and Collapse of Remittent Fever 208

SECTION III. — The General Rate of Mortality. — Its Relation to Age, Period of Epidemic, and Duration before Admission considered. — General Pathology shortly noticed. — Morbid Anatomy described 215

SECTION IV. — Treatment in the different degrees and stages of the disease.— Recapitulation 221

SECTION V. — Statistical Tables relative to Epidemic Cholera in European General Hospital, the Jamsetjee Jejeebhoy Hospital and the Byculla Schools at Bombay 233

CHAPTER XIV.

ON DYSENTERY.

SECTION I.—The Importance of Dysentery in India.—Order in which the subject will be treated 236

SECTION II.—Pathology.—Detailed Statement of the Morbid Anatomy . 237

SECTION III. — Etiology of Dysentery. — Importance of distinguishing exciting and predisposing Causes. — Exciting Causes. — Cold, Food. — Predisposing Causes.—Cachectic States.—Action of Malaria discussed . . . 273

SECTION IV.—Symptoms of Dysentery 280

SECTION V. — Treatment. — General Principles and Indications. — Detailed Remarks on Blood-letting, general and local, Calomel, Mercurial Influence, Ipecacuanha, Purgatives, Diaphoretics, Opium, Chloroform, Astringents, Tonics, Fomentations, Blisters, Enemata, Diet, and Change of Climate . 288

PAGE

SECTION VI.—Dysentery in Children in India 314

SECTION VII.—On Gastro-Enteritis 316

SECTION VIII.—On Diarrhœa 316

SECTION IX.—Statistics of Dysentery in the European Hospital, and of Dysentery and Diarrhœa in the Jamsetjee Jejeebhoy Hospital and Byculla Schools at Bombay 318

CHAPTER XV.

ON HEPATITIS.

SECTION I.—Comparative Prevalence of Hepatitis 321

SECTION II.—Preliminary Remarks on the nature of the Symptoms of Hepatic Disease.—Arrangement of the Subject 323

SECTION III.—Pathology.—Preliminary Remarks on the General Pathology of Hepatitis.—Morbid Anatomy of Stage of Vascular Turgescence, of Exudation of Lymph, and Formation of Abscess explained.—The several Courses and Situations of Rupture of Hepatic Abscess.—Abscess Absorption.—Secondary Peritonitis and Formation of circumscribed Purulent Sacs.—Secondary Pleuritis, circumscribed and general Empyema.—Secondary Pericarditis.—General Secondary Peritonitis.—Colour of Pus in Hepatic Abscess . . 325

SECTION IV.—Etiology of Hepatitis.—Exciting Causes.—External Cold, elevated Temperature, Intemperance, Mechanical Causes.—Importance of Predisposing Causes stated.—The Complication of Hepatic Abscess and Dysentery considered in reference to the Pyœmic Theory of the Causation of Hepatic Abscess 361

SECTION V.—Symptoms of Hepatitis.—Early Stages.—Pain, Respiratory Movements.—Physical Signs.—Altered Secretion, Jaundice.—Constitutional Disturbance.—Suppuration.—Course of Hepatic Abscess 370

SECTION VI.—Treatment of Early Stages.—Blood-letting, general and local.—Mercurial and other Purgatives.—Mercurial Influence.—Blisters.—Treatment when Abscess is forming and is perfected.—Question of Puncture considered.—Change of Climate 384

SECTION VII.—Hepatitis in Females and in Children 415

SECTION VIII.—Occasional Difficulties and Errors of Diagnosis . . 416

SECTION IX.—Statistics of Hepatitis in the European General Hospital and the Jamsetjee Jejeebhoy Hospital, at Bombay 417

CHAPTER XVI.

ON CIRRHOSIS, CONGESTION, LARDACEOUS AND FATTY ENLARGEMENT, CANCER AND HYDATID OF THE LIVER.—AFFECTIONS OF THE BILIARY DUCTS AND GALL-BLADDER.—BILIARY CALCULI.—JAUNDICE.—INCREASED AND DEFECTIVE SECRETION OF BILE.

SECTION I.—Cirrhosis.—Pathology.—Symptoms.—Treatment.—Complication with Hepatic Abscess 421

SECTION II.—Congestion of the Liver.—Œdema 426

SECTION III.—Lardaceous and Fatty Liver.—Cancer, and Hydatid Formations 428

SECTION IV.—Inflammation of the Gall-Bladder and Biliary Ducts.—Distention of the Gall-Bladder.—Biliary Calculi 431

SECTION V.—Jaundice.—Pathology.—Causes.—Treatment 433

SECTION VI.—On Increased and Defective Secretion of Bile 440

CHAPTER XVII.

ON PERITONITIS, ILEUS AND COLIC.

PAGE

SECTION I. — Peritonitis. — Pathology. — Plastic and sero-puriform Exudations related to Diathesis.—Chronic Tubercular.—Chronic not Tubercular, and not Consecutive on Acute.—Treatment 443

SECTION II.—Ileus and Colic 453

CHAPTER XVIII.

AFFECTIONS OF THE STOMACH.

SECTION I.—Gastritis, Acute and Chronic 458

SECTION II.—Glossitis 461

SECTION III.— Dyspepsia. — General reflections on Pathology and Principles of Treatment 462

CHAPTER XIX.

ON BRIGHT'S DISEASE OF THE KIDNEY AND ALBUMINOUS URINE.

SECTION I.—Prevalence of Bright's Disease in the Hospital-frequenting classes of the Natives of India 465

SECTION II.—The Relation of Bright's Disease to Albuminous Urine stated.—The Morbid Anatomy and Pathology of the Fluids.—Pathology of the Secondary Affections.—The Uræmic Theory.—The Proximate Cause of Albumen in the Urine 466

SECTION III.—Etiology.—Scarlatina not influential in India.—Relation to Caste, Age, Occupation, Habits, Season.—Cold an exciting Cause sometimes of the Kidney Disease, generally of the Secondary Affections 487

SECTION IV.—Symptoms.—Referable to the Kidney.—Condition of the Urine.—Treatment.—Of the Kidney Disease.—Of the Secondary Affections, chiefly the Dropsical Effusions 491

CHAPTER XX.

ON ABNORMAL STATES OF THE URINE.

SECTION I. — Preliminary Pathological Remark. — A want of Information in respect to the Normal Condition of the Urine in India 497

SECTION II.—Chylo-serous Urine.—Short Notice of its Pathology and Treatment 498

SECTION III.—Saccharine Diabetes.—Infrequent in India.—Diuresis . . 502

SECTION IV.—Uric, Oxalic, and Phosphatic Diathesis 505

CHAPTER XXI.

ON PNEUMONIA.

SECTION I. — Pneumonia. — Rare in Europeans in Bombay. — Asthenic Form common in Natives 508

SECTION II.—Etiology.—Relation to Sex, Age, Caste, Habits, Constitution, and Season 509

PAGE

Section III.—Pathology.—Preliminary Question relative to the Affected Capillaries.—Rate of Mortality.—Duration of Illness before Admission.—Stage of the Disease.—Which Lung most frequently Affected.—Period of Residence in Hospital.—State of the Lung on Discharge.—Morbid Anatomy . . 512

Section IV.—Symptoms.—Fever, Pain, Dyspnœa, Cough, Delirium, Character of the Sputa.—Physical Signs 527

Section V.—Treatment.—General and Local Blood-letting, Tartar Emetic, Mercury, Blisters, Quinine, Liquor Potassæ, Stimulants.—Concluding Remarks 534

Section VI.—Statistics of Pneumonia 547

CHAPTER XXII.

ON PLEURITIS, BRONCHITIS, AND ASTHMA.

Section I.—Pleuritis.—Symptoms, Causes, Pathology, Treatment . . 548

Section II.—Bronchitis.—Asthma 552

Section III.—Statistics of Bronchitis 553

CHAPTER XXIII.

ON PHTHISIS PULMONALIS.

Section I.—Causes, Symptoms, Pathology, and Treatment . . . 554

Section II.—Statistics of Phthisis Pulmonalis 560

CHAPTER XXIV.

ON PERICARDITIS AND ENDOCARDITIS.

Section I.—Introductory Remarks 561

Section II.—Causes, Symptoms, and Treatment 562

CHAPTER XXV.

ON ORGANIC DISEASE OF THE HEART AND AORTA.

Section I.—In Natives of India 581

Section II.—In Europeans in India 600

CHAPTER XXVI.

On Sun-stroke 603

CHAPTER XXVII.

ON DELIRIUM TREMENS.

Section I.—On the Symptoms and Treatment of Delirium Tremens in the European General Hospital at Bombay 624

Section II.—On the Pathology, the Principles of Treatment, and Diagnosis . 641

Section III.—Delirium Tremens in the Natives of India . . . 645

Section IV.—Statistics of Delirium Tremens 646

CHAPTER XXVIII.

ON CEREBRAL DISEASE AND PARALYSIS.

PAGE

SECTION I.—General Preliminary Remarks on the Pathology and Treatment of Cerebral Disease 648

SECTION II.—Apoplexy.—Meningitis.—Acute and Chronic Hydrocephalus.—Morbid Growths within the Cranium.—Paroxysmal Headache . . . 650

SECTION III. — Paralysis.—Hemiplegia. —Myelitis.—Paraplegia.—Paralysis from Arsenic.—Facial Palsy 658

SECTION IV. Statistics of Paralysis 671

CHAPTER XXIX.

ON TETANUS.

SECTION I.—The prevalence of Tetanus in certain classes of the community in India 672

SECTION II.—Pathology.—Nature of the Deranged Action with reference to the Physiology of the Spinal Cord.—Division into Idiopathic and Traumatic, Acute and Chronic.—Morbid Anatomy 673

SECTION III.—Etiology.—Diathesis, Cold, Entozoa?—External Injuries . 678

SECTION IV.—Symptoms.—Muscular Rigidity and Spasms.—Respiration.—Pulse.—Febrile Disturbance, &c. 680

SECTION V.—Treatment of Tetanus 683

SECTION VI.—Statistics of Tetanus 688

CHAPTER XXX.

ON HYDROPHOBIA.

SECTION I.—Short allusion to Symptoms and Pathology.—Illustrative Cases detailed 689

CHAPTER XXXI.

ON BLOOD DISEASES.

SECTION I.—Object of the Chapter explained 692

SECTION II.—Pyœmia.—Short notice of Symptoms and Pathology.—Illustrative Cases. 692

SECTION III.—Leprosy.—Tubercular and Anæsthetic.—Short account of the Symptoms and Pathology 695

SECTION IV.—Elephantiasis.—Symptoms.—Pathology.—Causes.—Treatment . 698

SECTION V.—Scurvy.—Prevalence in India.—Short Practical Remarks . . 701

SECTION VI.—General Dropsy.—Beriberi.—Symptoms.—Pathology.—Treatment.—Illustrative Cases 704

SECTION VII.—Rheumatism.—Prevalence in India 715

SECTION VIII.—On Snake Bite 716

CHAPTER XXXII.

ON DRACUNCULUS.

PAGE

SECTION I. — Prevalence of, in Bombay Presidency. — Relation to Season. — Allusion to Theories respecting its mode of origin. — Short notice of Symptoms and Treatment 720

SECTION II. — Statistics of Dracunculus 725

CHAPTER XXXIII.

ON THE HILL SANITARIA OF THE DECCAN 728

APPENDIX.

A. — On the Meteorology of Bombay 741

B. — Sanitarium at Poorundhur 747

LIST OF CASES 753

LIST OF STATISTICAL AND METEOROLOGICAL TABLES 765

INDEX 769

ON

DISEASE IN INDIA.

CHAPTER I.

INTRODUCTION. — GENERAL REMARKS ON THE CAUSES, PATHOLOGY, AND TREATMENT OF DISEASE IN INDIA.

CLINICAL research is the study of Pathology and Therapeutics, by careful observation and comparison of numerous instances of disease; and in conducting it, the truth soon becomes evident that the course and treatment of all forms of disease are modified by previously existing habits of the body, congenital, or acquired in one of the three following ways:—

1. By the neglect of a right condition of the agencies termed vital stimuli, which are as essential to the physiological performance of function as organic integrity: they are food, water, atmospheric air, heat, light, electricity, exercise and repose of body and mind. 2. By undue discharges from the blood. 3. By the reception into the blood of external injurious agencies—poisons; or by the retention of excretions.

Under these heads may be classed—(*a*) States unduly plethoric or sthenic; (*b*) Asthenia and cachexia, from insufficient food, struma, scurvy, vitiated atmosphere, elevated temperature, etiolation, depressing mental affections, bodily fatigue, prolonged lactation, hæmorrhages, exhausting medical treatment—excessive in degree or too long continued, malaria, syphilis, carcinoma, mercury, arsenic, lead, alcohol, albuminuria, rheumatism, &c. Though in these cachexiæ there may be peculiarities special to each, still there are features common to all. The vital actions of the system are defective, the nutrition of the blood and of the tissues is impaired, secretion is diminished and deranged, nervous influence and muscular irritability are imperfect, and the generation of animal heat is lowered in degree.

In my clinical remarks on the different forms of disease, frequent reference will be made to these states under the terms Asthenic and Cachectic: by the first is meant only a low degree of function; but by the second, a defect in quality as well as in degree.

It is very probable that an essential condition of all cachectic states is an altered quality of the blood, and that our present ignorance of the alterations peculiar to each may be removed by future pathological research.

In directing medical treatment, the physician is constantly reminded of the obstacles which asthenic or cachectic states interpose to the success of his remedies, and of the necessity which exists of making the removal of these states a leading indication in the management of all forms of disease. Thus two important practical lessons are enforced:—

1. Though the details of sanitary science and art are not within the province of clinical instruction, yet the great importance to the public health, and to the successful treatment of disease, of a well-organised sanitary system, is a prominent inference from clinical research.

2. The advantage derived in practice by the removal of the sick from the influence of the causes productive of cachexiæ serves to substantiate this truth: that a rational system of medicine is one which includes a careful adjustment of the vital stimuli and the removal of lædentia, as well as the use of medicines; and that when the cachectic condition is very marked, then the two first therapeutic principles are the most essential.

These doctrines will be frequently adverted to in my remarks on different diseases.

The necessity of carefully considering the general condition of the body, in the treatment of disease, is universally true; but when investigation has reference to a particular country, then the preliminary question arises whether, as regards this field of observation, there are special causes exercising an influence on the constitution of man.

In applying this rule to India, it may be stated that, on comparing tropical with temperate climates, we find, 1st, that the heat of the summer season of the former readily acts as the exciting cause of serious forms of disease in the recently arrived plethoric and sthenic natives of the latter; 2nd, that in tropical countries, not much elevated above the level of the sea, there are two special causes of asthenia and cachexia, more or less prevailing — the influence of long-continued and frequently repeated high temperature, and the action of malaria.

The effect of elevated temperature on the European constitution, in increasing and deranging the biliary secretion, has been a constant theme with a succession of able writers on the diseases of Europeans in tropical climates. Though the observations made on the recently arrived, on which these opinions mainly rest, are correct, still they are erroneous when applied to the far more numerous class of established residents; in them the secretion of bile is not habitually increased.

One consequence of high atmospheric temperature on the animal system is a diminished necessity for animal heat: hence there is less demand for food, less metamorphosis of tissue, and less excretion. This truth is made manifest by the asthenic condition of the residents in warm climates, compared with the sthenic state of the inhabitants of colder latitudes.

The European soldier or sailor, on arrival in India, does not appreciate, and therefore does not readily adopt, the alteration in habits of life necessary to the maintenance of health under the circumstances of a warmer climate; consequently the excesses, which in the cold climate might be unattended by disorder, are, under the predisposition caused by the action of increased heat, followed by derangement. Ardent continued fever or febricula, bilious cholera or diarrhœa, are under these circumstances very apt to occur. The increased metamorphosis of tissue, or of constituents of the blood, related to diathesis, or consequent on food taken in excess of the normal requirements of animal heat, may in part explain the proclivity to these forms of febrile disease. The theory usually conceived of the biliary derangements may be correct: viz. that the decreased elimination of hydro-carbon by the lungs, resulting from the less demand for animal heat, is liable to lead to the office of eliminating the excess of these elements present in the system, being transferred to the liver. But it by no means follows, that when there is the just relation between the quantity and kind of food consumed and excretion, which is implied in the habits of every prudent resident in a hot climate, there exists a greater degree of action of the liver vicarious of that of the lungs in the one climate than in the other.

Questions relative to the proportion of ingesta to excreta, and of the various excreta to each other, under varying circumstances of the animal system, can only be satisfactorily determined by careful observation and experiment. Inquiry of this kind, on an extensive scale, is still amongst the desiderata of physiological science; and, in the absence of the requisite data, all that can be safely affirmed in reference to India and other tropical countries is, that in the normal state of the system, all the solid* excreta are considerably less in amount than in the colder climates of Europe. The evidence that the biliary excretion is not increased, rests on the fact, that in the natives of India, and in Europeans whose habits of living have become adapted to the climate, derangement of this kind is very rarely observed.†

Malaria is the exciting cause of the intermittent and remittent types of fever. It also induces cachexia, either in consequence of frequent febrile recurrences, or by the exercise of a slow and gradual influence, irrespective of distinct paroxysms of fever. To the terrestrial miasm, whatever it may be, which is believed to produce these and other allied effects, the term Malaria will be restricted throughout this work, and will never be used in that more general sense, not unfrequently adopted by modern writers, and which it may be feared is leading to needless confusion, and obscurity in our views on the causes of disease.

The subject of Malaria is well and fully discussed by our best systematic writers, and it will therefore be sufficient to state, very shortly, the leading facts which are generally accepted relative to the generation and action of this morbific cause.

1. The presence of malaria is determined by the occurrence of certain derangements of health attributed to its influence, for as yet all other means of investigation have failed in detecting it.

2. A certain degree of heat acting on the earth's surface, previously soaked with water, is essential to the production of

* I use the term solid, to exclude that water which has been received and eliminated without resolution into its elements.

† When this statement was written in the first edition of this work, I was not aware that a similar opinion had been expressed by Dr. Henry Marshall, in his work on the diseases of Ceylon. Confirmed by the previous observation of this distinguished medical officer, it is now repeated with assured confidence. Dr. Marshall thus writes:—"It is, I believe, a very common opinion, that an excessive secretion of bile is general in warm climates. Upon what foundation is this opinion assumed? With regard to Europeans in health, I have not been able to observe any remarkable difference between the secretory functions of the liver in a tropical climate from that of the same organ in high latitudes; and with respect to the indigenous inhabitants of inter-tropical regions, I am not convinced that the biliary secretion is unusually copious."—*Notes on the Medical Topography and Prevailing Diseases of Ceylon*, p. 145.

malaria. It is more certainly generated while the process of drying is going on—when aeriform emanations exist, in degree proportionate to the rapidity with which the desiccation is effected. Hence malaria is most abundant in marshy grounds after the quantity of water has been reduced by evaporation to that condition when the drying of the surface of the ground begins, and while the atmospheric temperature is still high. It is then, after the heats of summer have passed, and the autumnal season has set in,—the months September and October,—that in marshy countries malarious fevers chiefly prevail.

3. In those tropical regions, in which there are periodical rains associated with elevated temperature, the generation of malaria coexists with the periods when the heavy falls have ceased and the drying of the earth's surface is going on. Consequent on the rains of the south-west monsoon, which commence about May and terminate in September, malarious fevers are prevalent sometimes in July, but generally most extensively in October. But there may be variations in respect to the particular months in different years. The necessary conditions are such relation between the rain-fall and the temperature as shall cause the rapid drying of a surface previously soaked with moisture.

4. There are districts of countries, chiefly in the warmer climates, subject to the periodical inundation of large rivers; and, should the subsidence of the waters coexist with elevated temperature, then the generation of malaria, as evidenced by the prevalence of intermittent and remittent fever, takes place. The Ganges, the Indus, the Euphrates, and the Nile, are rivers of this kind. Consequent on the melting of the snows in the mountain regions, at the sources of these rivers, the supply of water is increased. They begin to rise about the month of March, and attain their greatest elevation, overflowing their banks and covering extensive tracts of country, in the month of September. Then they gradually fall; and, as the surface of the inundated tracts becomes exposed, rapid drying commences. It is under these circumstances that malarious fevers appear in these districts in their most aggravated form.

It would seem that, whether in tracts habitually swampy, or regions wetted by periodical rains, or the overflow of large rivers, still the autumnal season is that in which malarious fevers are most prevalent.

5. Malaria seems to show a preference for low levels, and

the surface of the ground, compared with elevated sites and higher atmospheric strata.

6. It often coexists with decaying vegetation, but not unfrequently occurs, independent of it, in situations where the surface is sandy, dry, and bare, and where the drying—that essential condition in the generation of malaria—must be going on in the damp subsoil.

7. Its influence on the system is more surely experienced at night, and near to the surface of the ground.

8. Malaria may be wafted by currents of air from the spot where it has been produced, and thus infect adjacent localities; or by the same power, combined with the tendency to remain near the surface of the earth, it may be carried up the slope of a mountain, just as fogs are.

9. Malaria is believed to lose its noxious properties by passing over a surface of water even of small extent. It is attracted by the foliage of trees, and thus accumulates around them, and between them and the surface of the ground, rendering jungly tracts in tropical countries very dangerous at the malarious season of the year. This property of the foliage of trees, however, may be made subservient to the protection of tracts of country, when belts of wood are interposed between them and malarious localities.

10. Malaria is lessened by cultivation and adequate population, but becomes rapidly increased when lands have been deserted and allowed to run waste.*

* Such general statements as these, relative to the generation and action of malaria, rest upon evidence which may be found in the Medical Statistical Reports of the British Army, and in the medical histories of military or naval expeditions to the coasts of Africa and Arracan, to Burmah, Java, the peninsula of Spain, and to other countries. They are, moreover, amply confirmed by observations made in my own field of research, or in districts adjacent to it. The fevers which occur in the months of September and October in the provinces of Guzerat, Candeish, and Scinde, illustrate the relation of malaria to elevated temperature and rapid drying of the earth's surface. In the Deccan, and at Hursole, in Guzerat, there is evidence of malaria without vegetable decomposition; while at Deesa they have occurred in association together. The history of a fever which prevailed among the marines of her Majesty's frigate "Endymion," in the dockyard at Bombay (to be more particularly alluded to in the Chapter on Remittent Fever), affords a striking proof of the greater influence of malaria by night than by day. At Tatta and at Hyderabad, in Scinde, the malaria generated in the adjacent lowlands was carried by the prevailing winds up the hill slopes on which the troops were stationed. That malaria is attracted by, and accumulates about, trees has been in too many instances painfully proved by the history of detachments of troops injudiciously marched, at unseasonable periods, through the extensive tracts of jungle which intervene between the provinces of Candeish and Guzerat. In the fallen condition of the city of Ahmedabad, and in

Exciting Causes of Disease.—Reference has been made to asthenic and cachectic states as predisposing to disease of all kinds, and the importance of a right appreciation of their influence in causing and modifying disease in India will be frequently inculcated in various parts of this work. Malaria has also been regarded as a predisposing and exciting cause, and the other ordinary exciting causes of disease in India must now be shortly alluded to. Of these, external cold is the most common. In judging of the facility with which the temperature of the surface of the body becomes reduced in India, we must bear in mind the diminished power of generating animal heat characteristic of warm climates and asthenic states; and that consequently, in these circumstances, the surface of the body may become lowered in temperature by an amount of external cold inadequate to produce this effect in colder climates or stronger constitutions.

In order to form a just estimate of this exciting cause of disease, it is very necessary to study carefully, in respect to the sphere in which we practise, the physical features of the country, and the characters of the different seasons of the year; more particularly those conditions of the atmosphere which favour the abstraction of heat, such as absolute lowness of temperature, diurnal range, moisture, direction, duration, and force of the winds.* It is further of importance to consider these atmospheric states in reference to the presence or not of pre-existing causes of asthenia or cachexia, as malaria, scarcity, elevated temperature, syphilis, &c. For it is well known that cold, as well as other exciting causes of disease, acts very readily on debilitated persons; and if this fundamental doctrine in etiology—the influence of predisposition—be neglected, we shall often be unable satisfactorily to explain the prevalence of disease,—as types of fever, diarrhœa, dysentery, rheumatism, perhaps cholera,—in localities usually healthy, and

the state of health of the troops at Hyderabad immediately after the battle of Meanee and the capture of Scinde, we have illustrations of the statement that the production of malaria is favoured when districts are deserted, and previously cultivated lands are left waste. The references made to the dockyard in Bombay, and to Tatta and Hyderabad, in Scinde, rest on my own observation and inquiry; those relative to Guzerat, the Deccan, and Candeish, on two very instructive and interesting descriptions of the provinces of Guzerat and the Deccan, by Mr. Gibson, published in the first and second numbers of the "Transactions of the Medical and Physical Society of Bombay;" also a "Report on Candeish Fever," by Dr. Graham, in the fourth number; and one by Dr. Brown, on the "Diseases of the Horse Artillery at Deesa," in the first number of the "Transactions" of the same Society.

* See Appendix.

further be unable to account for the want of success attending our treatment.

Though the elevated temperature of an Indian climate is chiefly influential as a predisposing cause of disease, yet it is not to be doubted that heat sometimes acts as an exciting cause in some forms of fever, in some affections of the nervous system, and perhaps in hepatitis, as will be explained more fully when these diseases are treated of.

The exclusive observation of disease in unacclimatised sthenic Europeans by a succession of writers on tropical diseases, and the rapid course sometimes followed by bad forms of malarious fever and of dysentery in such subjects, have created an impression that inflammatory disease in India, compared with colder climates, is characterised by speedy progress and excessive vascular action. When, however, investigation is extended beyond the limited circle of this class, we find that this opinion is erroneous. It has been already stated that the common type of disease in India, both in Europeans and natives, is asthenic; and the law in respect to this type, verified in other countries, may be also safely affirmed of disease in India, viz. that inflammations in asthenic and cachectic habits are generally distinguished by an obscurity of symptoms and a slowness of progress, in proportion to the degree of asthenia or cachexia.

These features of asthenic disease often lead in India to neglect of application for relief till disorganization of structure has well advanced; and they, moreover, sometimes tend to mislead the practitioner in respect to the stage, and thus create the erroneous impression that the morbid changes have been rapidly effected.

This belief in the severity of inflammatory disease in India, originating in the manner just explained, naturally gave rise to the opinion that disease in India generally required to be met by a freer use of active antiphlogistic remedies. But, if the statement made relative to the frequency of asthenic forms of disease be correct, then it follows that blood-letting, mercury, purgatives, and all other depressing antiphlogistic remedies, should as a general rule be used with greater caution, not with more freedom, in India than in colder climates.

The pathological doctrines now generally current on blood-diseases, and on various forms of degeneration of tissue consequent on defective or perverted nutrition, are very valuable in the study of disease in India, and demand the careful attention of pathologists in that country.* They, moreover, serve to enforce additional caution in respect to the abuse of antiphlogistic remedies, to

* Since this passage was written, a paper has been published by Mr. Macnamara, in the third volume of the "Indian Annals of Medical Science," the object of which is to show that fatty degeneration of the liver and other organs is the chief cause of the high rate of mortality among European troops in Bengal. The arguments are—1. The statement that in twenty-four post-mortem examinations of men of the 1st European Bengal Fusiliers, made by the author, fatty degeneration existed in all, with one exception, in the liver, the kidneys, the heart, and coats of the large blood-vessels. 2nd. The diet ration is excessive, as regards both nitrogenous and carbonaceous principles. 3rd. The elevated temperature, close barracks, and indolent habits of the soldier in India, are unfavourable to the pulmonary elimination of hydro-carbon; and as these elements are rarely deposited in India in the form of adipose tissue, their only remaining outlet is by fatty degeneration,—hence the great frequency of this structural change supposed by Mr. Macnamara to exist in India. The statements and the reasoning are not convincing, because,—1st, A succinct clinical history and description of the post-mortem appearances of not one of the cases is given; therefore, though they may satisfy the observer himself, it does not follow that they will convince others; 2nd. Though the ration may be excesssive,—though there may be instances of gluttony and great indolence in the barrack-room as well as elsewhere,—it does not follow that all the food placed on a barrack mess-table is uniformly eaten, any more than it is at the officers' mess-table; 3rd. That in the hot season of India the soldier is little disposed for active exercise in the heat of the day, and that there is great necessity for enlargement of barrack-rooms, and covered workshops and buildings for in-door recreation, is very true; still this is not the habit of the European soldier in the cold season in India, or when active exercise is likely to be beneficial; 4. It does not accord with my observation to say that the formation of adipose tissue is rare in India. Fat Europeans and natives are common enough.

I still believe that, as a rule, there is no increase of elimination of hydro-carbon by the liver to substitute a supposed deficiency of that by the lungs, because the appetite soon brings about the just harmony between assimilation and general excretion, which must render vicarious action unnecessary. I do not look for fatty and other degeneration in India as a consequence of excesses in food, but as the result of the lowered nutrition of the system, proceeding from the continuance of climatic and other debilitating influences.

The different transient effects produced on the portal blood or its secretion by different kinds of food, during the passage of those constituents which pass by this channel, not by the lacteals, are not here adverted to.

In Dr. Budd's work, fatty liver, consequent on fatty food, removable by change of diet and active exercise, is sufficiently explained; and Frerichs, in his late work, "Klinik der Leberkrankheiten," has added further to our knowledge by experiments, which show that in dogs receiving in their daily food from half an ounce to one ounce of oil, the following changes take place in the hepatic cells:—After twenty-four hours there is an increase of molecular contents; after three days, numerous fat globules are apparent; and, after eight days, the hepatic cells are almost completely filled with larger and smaller fat globules. The fatty contents of the cells disappear after some time, when the diet is changed; probably a part, as supposed by Frerichs, returns to the blood as fat; and another, according to the functional design of the liver, is expended in the formation of bile. This, however, is not fatty degeneration of the liver, but the normal condition of the organ when certain articles of food are used. Mr. Macnamara seems to confound this normal fatty state with fatty degeneration. It is very

enhance the importance of the judicious use of tonic regimen* and medicines, and to suggest further inquiry into the therapeutic value and rational use of eliminants and alteratives.

likely that the former existed in some of his cases; but when it is stated that not only was there fatty degeneration of the liver in twenty-four cases, but also fatty degeneration of the heart, kidneys, and blood-vessels, then some fallacy in the observations may be suspected; and the absence of careful clinical histories, and descriptions of the post-mortem appearances, must be felt as decisive against the acceptance of these cases as authority on this question.

* I use the term to signify those just arrangements of food, atmospheric air, exercise and repose of body and mind, and of water as regards the functions of the skin, and its tonic action when cold, which conduce to the maintenance of health and favour the elevation of the animal system from a state of debility to one of strength.

CHAP. II.

REMARKS ON THE STATISTICS OF THE EUROPEAN GENERAL HOSPITAL, AND OF THE JAMSETJEE JEJEEBHOY HOSPITAL AT BOMBAY.

In the clinical remarks on the various forms of disease treated in this work, frequent reference will be made to the European General Hospital and to the Jamsetjee Jejeebhoy Hospital at Bombay, because much of my practical acquaintance with disease in India has been acquired in these institutions.

The first-named hospital has accommodation for 120 sick. The inmates are Europeans, partly military, partly sailors, and partly the poorer classes of the civil community. The wives and children of these classes are also received. I was the Resident Assistant-Surgeon in this hospital for a period of six years, — from June, 1838, to October, 1844.

The Jamsetjee Jejeebhoy Hospital has 300 beds: of these 240 are for males, and 60 for females. It is for the reception of native sick of all castes and countries (Europe excepted). A large proportion of the inmates belong to the poorer classes of the civil population, and many of them are received into the hospital in a very destitute condition. A smaller proportion consists of sick labourers, artificers, lascars, and watchmen who are in the employment of Government. The hospital is open for the free admission, on application, of the sick of those numerous classes for whose relief it is intended. I discharged the duties of principal Medical Officer of this hospital for a period of nine years, — from 1845 to 1854, and again for a year and a half between 1856 and 1859.

During the period of my service in the European General Hospital, 9303 admissions took place: and during that in the Jamsetjee Jejeebhoy Hospital 34,719 in-patients, and about 90,000 out-patients were treated.*

These statements are made with the view of showing a part of the extent and kind of clinical experience, on the faith of which I have ventured to express myself with some degree of con-

* The admissions during my service in this hospital subsequent to the publication of the First Edition of this work are not included.

fidence on several points of pathology and therapeutics. The Tables hereto appended are inserted with a similar object, as well as with reference to the few practical inferences which may be deduced from them; and as affording data necessary to the calculations in the tabular statements of particular diseases which will be found in different parts of this work.

Tables I. and IV. relate to periods of my own service in these hospitals: Tables II. and III. have been supplied to me by the kindness of Dr. Stovell, when surgeon of the European General Hospital.

The inferences which may be drawn from these Tables, relative to the proportion of sickness and death in Bombay in different seasons of the year, are not to be received as absolutely correct; because the classes of the community, both European and native, whose sick resort to these hospitals, are a fluctuating body, of whose varying numbers at different seasons of the year there is as yet no accurate census. Still the inferences, such as they are, may be stated here.

In the fifteen years from 1838 to 1853, the admissions into the European General Hospital amounted to 20,146, and the average mortality to 6·3 per cent. Of these admissions 10,495 took place in the half-year from June to November*, and 9653 in that from December to May; being an excess of 840 in favour of the first period. But the mortality in the first stated half-year was 5·7 per cent, and that in the second 6·9; being an excess of 1·2 in favour of the latter.

In the six years from 1848 to 1853 the admissions (Table IV.) into the Jamsetjee Jejeebhoy Hospital were 25,190, and the average mortality 16·3 † per cent. Of these admissions 12,465 took place in the half-year from June to November, and 12,725 in that from December to May; being an excess of 259 in favour of the latter. But the mortality in the first-stated period was 15·4

* I divide the year in this manner, because in Bombay from June to November includes the rainy season and that immediately succeeding it, and, therefore, the season in which malaria is chiefly generated. From December to May in Bombay includes the cold and hot months, and, therefore, the seasons in which both cold and heat, as exciting causes of disease, are influential.

† The statistical inquirer, possessing no other information respecting these hospitals than that supplied by the figures, would conclude either that disease is more fatal to natives than to Europeans in Bombay, or that treatment was less judicious in the Jamsetjee Jejeebhoy Hospital than in the European Hospital. Both inferences would be erroneous. The explanation is simply this, that a large proportion of the inmates of the Jamsetjee Jejeebhoy Hospital is admitted in a destitute state, and in far advanced stages of disease; hence the high mortality.

per cent, and that in the second 17·1; being an excess of 1·7 in favour of the latter.

I learn from Mr. Leith's Mortuary Returns of Bombay, that the deaths in five years, from 1848 to 1853, amounted to 68,423; of these, 29,667 took place in the half-year from June to November, and 38,756 from December to May: being an excess of 9089 in favour of the latter period.

These Returns, however, enable us further to divide this mortality into that proceeeding from all causes except epidemics (52,450), and that proceeding from epidemic causes, viz. cholera, small-pox, measles (15,973), and to show that in the half-year from December to May there is of the first class (all causes) an excess in the mortality of 2300; and of the second (epidemic) an excess of 6789.

Though the half-year from December to May is that in which the fluctuating population of Bombay is most numerous, still I think it may be fairly inferred from these several statements, that the period which includes the monsoon and succeeding season is that of the greatest amount of sickness not epidemic; but that the half-year which includes the cold and hot months is that of the greatest mortality both from general and epidemic causes.

TABLE I.*—*Admissions and Deaths, with Per-centage, from all Diseases, in the European General Hospital at Bombay for the Five Years from July*, 1838, *to July*, 1843.

	July, 1838, to July, 1843.		Monthly Average.
	Admissions.	Deaths.	Per Centage of Deaths on Admissions.
January	549	43	7·6
February	411	32	7·7
March	506	33	6·5
April	581	41	7·
May	860	80	9·3
June	781	51	6·6
July	718	37	5·1
August	607	35	5.7
September	546	52	9·5
October	722	27	3·7
November	685	47	6·8
December	613	66	10·7
Total	7579	544	7·1

* In this Table, and in all the others throughout the work, the figured details of each year were given in the First Edition, but it is now considered convenient to omit them.

Table II.—*Admissions and Deaths, with Per-centage, from all Diseases, in the European General Hospital at Bombay for the Five Years from* 1844 *to* 1848.

	1844 to 1848.		Monthly Average.
	Admissions.	Deaths.	Per Centage of Deaths on Admissions.
January	617	46	7·4
February	516	35	6·8
March	485	30	6·2
April	509	31	6·0
May	583	30	5·1
June	714	33	4·6
July	679	36	5 3
August	549	15	2·7
September	458	22	4·8
October	605	38	6·3
November	559	31	5·5
December	522	40	7·6
Total	6796	387	5·7

Table III.—*Admissions and Deaths, with Per-centage, from all Diseases, in the European General Hospital at Bombay for the Five Years from* 1849 *to* 1853.

	1849 to 1853.		Monthly Average.
	Admissions.	Deaths.	Per Centage of Deaths on Admissions.
January	450	39	8·7
February	369	18	4·9
March	440	34	7·7
April	517	25	4·8
May	518	24	4·6
June	572	29	5·1
July	529	33	6·2
August	494	38	7·7
September	356	25	7·0
October	395	23	5·8
November	524	30	5·7
December	608	40	6·6
Total	5772	358	6·2

TABLE IV.—*Admissions and Deaths, with Per-centage, from all Diseases, in the Jamsetjee Jejeebhoy Hospital at Bombay for the Six Years from* 1848 *to* 1853.

	1848 to 1853.		Monthly Average.
	Admissions.	Deaths.	Per Centage of Deaths on Admissions.
January	2090	450	21·5
February	1894	319	16·8
March	2149	386	17·9
April	2105	343	16·3
May	2183	287	13·1
June	2083	307	14·7
July	2020	306	15·1
August	1999	328	16·4
September	2062	311	15.1
October	2134	339	15·9
November	2167	331	15·2
December	2304	397	17·2
Total	25190	4104	16·3

CHAP. III.

GENERAL REMARKS ON FEVERS IN INDIA.

IDIOPATHIC fevers constitute a very important class of disease in India, as is apparent from the following statement* which exhibits the per-centage of admissions and mortality from fevers in the European and Native troops of the three Presidencies: —

Presidency.	Europeans.		Natives.	
	Per-centage of Admissions to Strength.	Per-centage of Deaths to Strength.	Per-centage of Admissions to Strength.	Per-centage of Deaths to Strength.
Bengal . . .	72·64	1·99	48·50	·528
Bombay . . .	61·93	1·37	41·20	·57
Madras . . .	31·62	0·37	25·04	·30

When attention is directed to the Native civil population, abundant evidence of the importance of this class of disease also appears. In the Island of Bombay, the deaths from fever, in five years, amounted to 27,212 †, which is in the ratio of 40·26 per cent of the total mortality.

Exclusive of the eruptive forms, they are limited to intermittent and remittent fever, caused by malaria; and to ardent continued fever, and febricula (ephemeral, common continued fever), excited by ordinary causes.

The occurrence of typhoid fever ‡, in some parts of India, has also been lately established.

The plague, yellow fever, maculated typhus, and relapsing fever, are as yet unknown in India.

* "Vital Statistics of the Armies in India." By J. Ewart, M.D.

† "Deaths in Bombay." By A. H. Leith.

‡ The term typhoid throughout this work is restricted to the sense in which it is used by Dr. Jenner, as signifying the enteric or intestinal form of zymotic continued fever.

CHAP IV.

ON INTERMITTENT FEVER.

SECTION I.—*Different Types of Intermittent Fever.*

I SHALL restrict my remarks to the three principal types of intermittent fever,—quotidian, tertian and quartan. The further varieties — double and duplicated tertian and quartan — doubtless occur, but they are practically unimportant: indeed, when the object of treatment from the very commencement of an attack is to prevent the recurrence of the paroxysm by antiperiodic remedies, the character not only of these varieties, but also of the leading types, is liable to be modified, and the opportunity of studying the natural course of the disease is lost.

It has been generally stated by systematic writers that, of the three leading forms, the tertian is the most frequent, then the quotidian, and lastly the quartan.

The statement, relative to the quartan type, will be generally accepted. Of 243 cases of intermittent fever in Natives of different castes in Bombay, selected for the purpose of clinical instruction, there was not a single instance of the quartan form. Of 1344 cases of intermittent fever treated during the period of my service in the European General Hospital, the quartans, if any, were very few in number.

That tertians are more common than quotidians, is not confirmed by my experience, and is opposed to that of observers in India generally. Of the 243 clinical cases, 211 were quotidians and 27 tertians, and of 5 the type has not been recorded. In the European General Hospital the greater prevalence of the quotidian type, more particularly during the malarious months, in first attacks, in seamen, the military staff of the garrison and the poorer classes of the fixed resident European community, has also been noted by me. Nor has my observation on this point been confined to the Island of Bombay. At an earlier period of my service, while doing duty with Her Majesty's 4th Light

Dragoons, at Kirkee in the Deccan, the same fact respecting intermittent fever in that regiment during the monsoon season was noticed by me.

Though the quotidian is the most common form in India*, still the tertian is also of frequent occurrence. Nor is it difficult to explain the different circumstances in which these types respectively occur.

Quotidians will be found to prevail most generally at those seasons of the year when the generation of malaria is supposed to be actively going on; and they may probably be viewed as affording evidence of the recent action of the morbific cause. It is the type which the disease for the most part assumes in first attacks.

Tertians, on the other hand, usually occur in individuals who have suffered on previous occasions, and in whom the fresh attack is often traceable to ordinary and recently applied exciting causes, as sudden alternations of temperature, atmospheric moisture, fatigue, debauch, &c. The occurrence of this type may generally be regarded, not as the evidence of the recent introduction of malaria into the system, but as that of a pre-existing abiding influence, sometime dormant, now re-excited into action by an ordinary cause.

If these views be correct, quotidians may be looked for chiefly from May to October in districts within the range of the rains of the S. W. monsoon, in November and December in those subject to the influence of the N. E. monsoon, and from August to October in tracts exposed to river-inundation and recession. Tertians, on the other hand, may be expected in the colder months of the year, December, January, and February; also in the course of the monsoon season on the occurrence of sudden changes of atmospheric temperature or moisture.

Moreover, if it be true that the tertian type implies a pre-existing malarious influence, then we may generally expect it to appear in individuals who have been resident in malarious localities, and to be frequently complicated with splenic enlargement. Of the 27 clinical cases of tertian fever, the atmospheric

* Though the quotidian is the most common type in India, and in other countries also, it does not follow that this is the proportion observed in all countries in which intermittent fevers prevail. It appears in the Statistical Report of the army of the United States of America, that in the Northern Division, north of 40° N., the Middle Division, between 35° and 40° N., and the Southern Division, between 30° and 35°, tertians predominate; but that in Florida, Texas, and California, quotidians preponderate.

vicissitudes of the monsoon season were influential on 18: of these, 16 were dockyard peons*, and in 14 splenic enlargement was present. In the European General Hospital, the tertian type was present most generally in individuals who had suffered from the more obstinate intermittents of the autumnal months of other localities; and who had been either sent to Bombay, with the view of deriving benefit from change of climate, or who had arrived there at certain seasons in the course of their professional duties. They consisted chiefly of European seamen, who had acquired the disease while serving in the Persian Gulf, the Red Sea, on the Coast of China†, or in the steam flotilla of the river Indus. They arrived in Bombay usually after the opening of the season subsequent to the monsoon, viz., in November, December, and January; and, under exposure to the atmospheric vicissitudes of these months, became liable to tertian attacks. A cachectic state and an enlarged spleen were also frequently present in this class of seamen.

These opinions on the causes of the relative prevalence of the

* Of the 243 clinical cases, 85 were dockyard peons; many of them, however, readmissions, as the period extends to six years. I was previously familiar with the dockyard at Bombay as a malarious locality, from my experience in the European General Hospital, to which I shall have to allude in connection with remittent fever. The frequent admission of these peons into the Jamsetjee Jejeebhoy Hospital, confirmed my former impressions, and I requested Dr. Bhawoo Dajee, at the time one of my clinical clerks, to ascertain from one of the peons the leading facts connected with their service. The following is a summary of the information thus obligingly obtained for me:—

There are fifty dockyard peons. They wear a blue woollen dress, which they may lay aside for a cooler material in the hot weather. Their pay is sufficient to supply them with the food of good quality and adequate quantity used by their class. About one-half are Hindoos, the other Mussulmans. They live within the precincts of the dockyard. Their place of sleeping varies according to the duty of the day. They sleep in the open air in the dry season; in a shed during the monsoon, but are still liable to be exposed to air currents. They are on duty four hours in the day and four in the night. These periods are respectively divided into a service of two hours, and an interval of rest for four hours; for example, a peon serving from 6 A.M. to 8 A.M. returns at noon, precisely, to serve two hours more—12 till 2 P.M. The same order is observed in respect to the four hours' night duty. While on duty they are walking about as guards of the stores, &c. In the day many use an umbrella to protect themselves from the heat of the sun, but many do not. They do not get wet in the monsoon, for they resort to guard-rooms and sheds for shelter. The sickness from fever, which they are aware is considerable, and chiefly in the rains, is attributed by them to the air and water of the place. There is no complaint of want of attention to cleanliness, nor are they annoyed by disagreeable odours. The water they use is not brackish.

† This was at a time when military operations were being carried on in China.

quotidian and tertian types*, might be readily strengthened by a reference to other sources; but they are not brought forward with any claim to novelty, nor with any desire to enforce them. They have seemed to me to suggest a generalisation practical in its tendency, and probably the best which at present can be offered.

Section II.—*Simple Intermittent Fever.—Symptoms, Pathology, and Treatment.*

Symptoms.—The intervals of twenty-four, forty-eight, and seventy-two hours, which distinguish the quotidian, tertian, and quartan types of intermittent fever, are so fully set forth in systematic treatises on disease that it is unnecessary further to describe them. The not unfrequent transition, however, of one type into another, is a circumstance of practical importance. The quotidian may become tertian in its character before it finally ceases, and this change in type is an indication that the disease is in progress towards recovery. On the other hand, the tertian (and it is occasionally observed in the quartan also,) may pass into the quotidian type, or the quotidian may assume the remittent form: these occurrences evince an aggravation of the disease, and careful inquiry will sometimes show that this has been coincident with the access of inflammation in an important internal organ.

It is generally stated, that the period of attack of the quotidian is the morning, of the tertian about noon, and of the quartan the afternoon. Of the 243 clinical cases of which 211 were quotidian, 27 tertian, and none quartan, the period is noted in respect of 155 cases: of these it was between 6 A.M. and 2 P.M. in 74, and after 2 P.M. in 81. This statement, then, does not accord with that of systematic writers, but their accu-

* The discrepancy in respect to the relative prevalence of tertians and quotidians is also in part probably due to the very general sense in which the term tertian was used by the old writers. Cleghorn, in his "Observations on the Epidemical Diseases in Minorca from 1744 to 1749," uses the term in a generic sense, and includes under it intermittents and remittents of various types and severity. It would seem that the word tertian suggested to these writers the doctrine of the odd days of Hippocrates, and by such phrases as simple, double, triple, and semi-tertian, they are made to accord with it. Cleghorn describes a tendency in these fevers gradually to lessen and to terminate on the odd days, as the 5th, 7th, 9th, and 11th; also the occasional tendency of simple tertians to become double, then remittent, and ultimately continued.

racy is not, therefore, to be called in question, for it has been already explained that the treatment of the disease by the early exhibition of antiperiodics tends to destroy its natural characters, by either preventing or postponing the recurrence of the paroxysm.

The division of the febrile paroxysm into cold, hot, and sweating stages, the greater duration of the cold in tertians and quartans, and that of the hot stage and indeed of the entire paroxysm in quotidians are well known facts. It is assumed that the clinical student is already acquainted with the phenomena characteristic of these several stages; but there are facts in respect to each which it is important to impress upon him.*

First, of the *cold stage* it should be recollected that the action of the heart is depressed from the sedative influence of the morbific cause, and that the blood in consequence tends to circulate languidly and to accumulate in important internal organs. Sometimes the congestion is present in unusual degree in particular organs: giving rise in the brain to undue drowsiness and sense of weight in the head, ringing in the ears, and various undefinable sensations; occasioning, when in the lungs, the heart, and great vessels, a sense of great præcordial oppression, a respiration unusually hurried and sighing, and a pulse very feeble and depressed. Or the undue congestion may exist in the stomach and liver, and lead to much retching and vomiting, and derangement of the biliary secretion; or it may be to the mucous membrane of the intestinal canal, and be attended with copious intestinal discharges. It should be further remembered that, associated with these several local phenomena, there will be present some degree of the general depressed state of the circulation characteristic of the cold stage, indicated by a feeble pulse, a pale skin and features more or less contracted. When these undue local congestions occur, the duration of the cold stage is generally prolonged, and the hot and sweating stages are sometimes so slight as readily to escape notice.

These exceptional cases are important, not so much from being generally attended with immediate danger to life, for such is not usually the case; but from their nature being very often misunderstood. They are apt to be regarded as instances of congestion

* If the reader has not these details present in his mind, he should refer to some systematic treatise; otherwise the occasional facts to which allusion is chiefly made in the text may assume undue prominence in his estimation.

or other derangement, independent of malarious influence, and thus to suggest needless alarm, and prompt to injurious and unsuccessful treatment. The right diagnosis can only be established by a careful consideration of all the circumstances of each particular instance; such as the existence or absence of previous attacks of malarious fever, or of exposure to malarious season or locality, and the periodicity or persistence of the phenomena. Inquiry on these points, coupled with due attention to the habits of the individual, and a careful scrutiny into the physical condition and functional state of all important organs, will generally conduct to a satisfactory conclusion.

The kind of phenomena just alluded to have frequently been described under the name of "*Masked Intermittent.*" But as they are evidently more related to one stage than to the entire paroxysm, there is a practical advantage in noticing them in connection with that stage.*

Hot Stage. — The degree of febrile reaction varies in the different types of the disease, and is also related to the character of the constitution of the individual affected. The excited circulation, the increased heat of the surface, the diminished secretions, the thirst, the coated tongue, the restlessness, and the headache are present in greater degree in the quotidian than in the tertian type; and in the sthenic constitution of youthful Europeans lately arrived in India, than in the more or less asthenic condition of the old resident European and of the different classes of the native population.

The state of the tongue is in many respects a useful practical guide. It is frequently more coated in attacks of ephemeral fever than in true intermittents: while in the latter the degree of fur is not only related to the duration of the hot stage of each paroxysm, but also to the state of the patient's system. The tongue is more coated in the quotidian type and in sthenic habits, than in the tertian type and in asthenic constitutions: indeed, it frequently happens in tertians, sometimes even in quotidians, in asthenic natives that the tongue is nearly quite clean throughout the paroxysm as well as the intermission. Again, in tertian fevers on the morning of the day of the paroxysm we are occasionally, by the coated or clean

* The occasional occurrence of great and dangerous congestive phenomena at the outset of malarious fevers will be noticed in connection with the remittent type of fever.

state of the tongue, enabled to judge of the probability of the attack.

It is useful to bear these facts in mind, but in order to appreciate them truly it is necessary to recollect another important fact, viz., that by the undue use, in fever, of mercurial and other purgatives, and of preparations of antimony we may increase and maintain a coated state of the tongue, and thus not only do positive harm, but also vitiate the indications of a valuable symptom.

Sweating Stage. — The disappearance of the febrile phenomena, after more or less sweating, and the succession of a complete intermission is the usual course observed in this disease. When the subject of remittent fever comes under consideration, it will be explained that occasionally, instead of the usual remission of the febrile reaction, a state of dangerous — it may be fatal — collapse unexpectedly occurs. Though an event of this kind is unusual after a paroxysm of intermittent fever, still there are circumstances under which it is necessary carefully to guard against it: in all instances of intermittent fever in very asthenic individuals, whether Europeans or natives, the degree of exhaustion which attends the close of the paroxysm must be attentively watched. If this precaution be neglected we shall assuredly, from time to time, experience the painful surprise of learning that our patient has died suddenly, and to us unexpectedly, with perhaps merely symptoms of general exhaustion, or it may be with some degree of diarrhœa, or tendency to coma. If in these cases we are satisfied with judging of the progress of the disease by the amount of the hot stage, a very serious error will often be committed; for it not unfrequently happens that a diminution in the degree of febrile reaction precedes death by exhaustion. Indeed, a failing pulse, increasing emaciation, and decreasing heat, ought to lead us to anticipate early and rapid sinking at the close of a paroxysm, and to provide against it by assiduous care in the use of appropriate stimulants and nourishment. My attention was first directed to these clinical facts in respect to natives in the year 1831, when in medical charge of detachments on field service, at Sassoor in the Deccan; then in January 1844, while serving at Hyderabad in Scinde, with the 15th Regiment Native Infantry; and latterly in the clinical and other wards of the Jamsetjee Jejeebhoy Hospital at Bombay. As regards Europeans, the most striking instance which occurs to me is that of an officer of the 15th Regiment at Gharra in Scinde, who had suffered some months previously from several attacks of intermittent fever while at Hyderabad. I saw this officer during a recurrence of the disease at Gharra, and then the single paroxysm was succeeded by a state of alarming collapse, requiring the free use of alcoholic stimulants for its removal. My further experience in India, subsequent to the publication of the first edition of this work, not only in my own practice, but also in that of others known to me, when officiating as superintending surgeon at Poona, has again impressed upon me the importance of watching for indications of exhaustion in intermittent fever in asthenic subjects. Several fatal cases of this nature were reported to me in the Poona division, and in all of them the medical officers were unaware of the true explanation of the unlooked-for event.

Pathology.—Mortality from Simple Intermittent Fever. That in the cold stage of intermittent fever there is a sedative influence exercised by the morbific cause on the heart, and a tendency in the blood to circulate languidly and to accumulate in the capillary system of important internal organs, may be very safely affirmed. But whether this influence first acts on the blood, and through it on the fibre of the heart, or intermediately on the nervous system, or in any of the other various ways which the imagination may suggest; and what the nature of the changes effected in the blood may be, are questions which have been much discussed, without as yet having led to a satisfactory solution of the difficulties with which the subject is beset.

Into these speculations I shall not enter. They are foreign to the spirit of safe and useful clinical instruction.

The *mortality* in India, resulting directly from simple intermittent fever, is not great; but it is not accurately known, nor can it be determined by ordinary hospital returns. During my service in the European Hospital, the returns show a mortality of 1·33 per cent. from intermittent fever. But the complicated cases are also included; and, from the greater number of deaths having taken place in December, February, March, and April, it is evident that the fatal result must have arisen from the sequelæ of the disease.

Though the immediate risk to life from a paroxysm of intermittent fever is slight, still the mortality to which the disease indirectly leads is very great, though not expressed in statistical tables as at present framed.

Continued exposure to malaria or frequent recurrences of intermittent fever engender, as is well known, a cachectic state of the system; in which the nutritive processes of the tissues and of the blood are defective and perverted, and in which splenic, hepatic, and other local congestions, tend to occur. This cachexia not unfrequently terminates in death by exhaustion. But it is not in this manner that the indirect mortality from intermittent fever chiefly arises. It takes place because the cachexia caused by the fever is a state in which the system becomes very predisposed to local inflammation or congestion under the influence of external cold. The structure most liable to be thus affected is the mucous lining of the intestinal canal; and the diseases induced are classed, in hospital returns, under the heads diarrhœa and dysentery. There can be no question that much of the mortality attributed in India to "bowel complaints" is, though indirectly, yet fairly chargeable to the account of malarious fevers. The principal season of malarious fever, excited by the direct action of malaria, and consequently the chief season during which this deterioration of the system occurs may, in general terms, be said to range from June to the end of November. Then follow December, January, February, and March, with their lower absolute temperature, their greater range, their frequent chilling winds; and it is in these months that the asthenic constitution is liable to suffer from dysentery and diarrhœa.

Further, if the malarious season be preceded by one of exhausting heat, and succeeded by one of considerable reduction and alternations of temperature, whether from great diurnal range, varying humidity, or chilling winds, then we have conditions of climate which lead to much mortality, from the consequences of intermittent fever, unless it be prevented or lessened by judicious sanitary measures.

It would be easy to accumulate illustrations of this pathological law, but it will be sufficient to refer to the most striking which have passed under my own observation. After the conquest of the province of Scinde, in the spring of the year 1843, troops were stationed in the fort and town of Hyderabad, and in many of the adjacent villages. In July, the canals were sensibly filling with the water of the Indus; and during the latter part of that month, as well as in August, the inundation was at its height: the subsidence commenced in September and continued during October.

The 15th Regiment, Native Infantry, was stationed during June, July, August, and part of September in a small village close to the west bank of the Indus, surrounded by broken ground, water-cuts, and cultivated fields interspersed with trees and covered with underwood. It was then moved to another position not less malarious, and finally located in the fort of Hyderabad, where I assumed medical charge of this corps at the end of December, continued with it at Hyderabad throughout the greater part of January, and accompanied it down the Indus to Tatta, thence to Gharra (where we were detained about fifteen days), and finally by Kurrachee to Bombay, which we reached towards the end of February.

The following statement shows the strength of this regiment, with the numbers ill from fever, and the *total* mortality during the greater part of the period above adverted to:—

15th Regiment Bombay Native Infantry.

1843.	Strength.	Fevers.	Total Deaths.
June	887	97	1
July	958	44	4
August	1012	153	3
September	1046	580	6
October	1024	973	6
November	998	1095	32
December	948	896	25

The great increase of fever in September and October is well shown; and of the cases under treatment in November and December, a large proportion remained from the admissions of the two preceding months, proving the obstinacy of the disease, and the frequent occurrence of its sequelæ.

In November the temperature at Hyderabad begins to fall, and continues to decline in December and January. North-easterly winds also commence, and are frequently fresh and chilling. The comparison of the mortality of November and December with that of the months preceding is very striking: the great increase was caused chiefly by dysentery. The precise number* of deaths in January and February is unknown to me; but the great mortality from bowel complaints

* The numbers given above, and those stated in Mr. Carter's paper on the prevalence of intermittent fever, &c., in Sindh (Transactions, Bombay Medical and Physical Society, No. 8, p. 32), will be observed to be the same. Both are taken from the same source, my MS. notes.

continued, and frequent bronchitic and occasional pneumonic complications, with in some instances death, apparently from œdema of the lungs, also occurred.

During part of the year 1843 the Bombay 2nd European Regiment was divided. One wing was moved to Kurrachee in Scinde in May, was healthy, and lost few men; the other wing was stationed at Bhooj in the province of Cutch during the monsoon and suffered much, chiefly in September, from intermittent and remittent fever. The sick of this wing were sent to Mandavie, on the coast of the province, with a view to their transport to Bombay, but they were delayed there about a month, badly supplied with quinine and other necessaries; and then, instead of being sent to Bombay, were shipped to Kurrachee, and arrived there in November. About the middle of December, through the kindness of Mr. Cahill, the surgeon of the regiment, I was permitted to visit the hospital at Kurrachee. It contained 237 sick, chiefly men from Cutch, and there were still upwards of 100 sick left behind at Mandavie. In many the spleen was enlarged, and some were anasarcous; and 40 deaths, chiefly from dysentery, had taken place between the beginning of November and the period of my visit.

During the monsoon of 1841, Her Majesty's 17th Regiment was stationed in the barracks at Colaba, in the island of Bombay. This season of that year was generally unhealthy in the island, and the following admissions of malarious fever took place in this regiment:—

Month	Admissions	Month	Admissions
In June	55	In November	180
July	136	December	180
August	165	January	50
September	187	February	38
October	375		

Dr. A. S. Thomson, from whose report * this statement is taken, thus writes :—" In October a few cases of dysentery occurred; but when the cold nights of November and December came, dysentery became more prevalent, and 130 cases were admitted during these two months, and 23 died.".

During the month of October, 100 fever cases of the 17th Regiment were treated in the European General Hospital; all came under my observation, and many under my immediate care.

* Transactions, Medical and Physical Society of Bombay, No. 5, p. 84.

I had, therefore, a personal knowledge of the character of the fever and of the condition of the men.

Treatment of Simple Intermittent Fever.—The treatment must be considered with reference to the several stages of the paroxysm and to the intermission.

If the *cold stage* merely threatens, if it be the first or second paroxysm, if the tongue be coated, expanded and not florid, and the constitution of the individual be good, and evacuant remedies have not been previously exhibited, then an emetic of ipecacuanha may be given with advantage. If, on the other hand, the circumstances which indicate the use of an emetic are not present, a moderate opiate may be substituted. But when the cold stage has fairly formed, all that can be done is to lessen the discomfort of the patient by additional covering, the use of external heat to the extremities and the exhibition of warm diluents. It may occasionally happen, when the depression is very great, that the use of ammoniated and other stimulants is indicated; but this is seldom necessary in Indian intermittents, except in very asthenic individuals.

In the *hot stage* there is excess of vascular action, and the indication is to carry the patient on to the sweating stage with as little of this excess of action or of derangement of other functions as can be safely effected. To prevent this stage or materially to shorten it is beyond our power, but by judicious management the general discomfort and the amount of derangement of particular functions may be considerably mitigated.

In youthful sthenic Europeans at the commencement of first attacks, when febrile excitement runs high with headache and much flushing of the face and a pulse full and firm, then general blood-letting, to the extent of sixteen or twenty ounces, may occasionally be an expedient and useful proceeding; but when carried beyond this or used at more advanced periods or in other states of constitution, it is not only unnecessary but becomes positively injurious: it accelerates the cachectic condition, and not only does not check the progress of the attack, but tends to protract it.

Under the usual circumstances of intermittent fever in India, it is sufficient to allay the vascular excitement by light clothing, the removal of all lædentia, sponging the surface of the body repeatedly with tepid water, cold applications to the head, suitable drinks, and the use of antimonials, ipecacuanha, aqua acetatis ammoniæ, or nitrate of potash, in moderate doses. In cases in which headache is much complained of, and no contra-indication exists*, leeches may be applied with advantage in the first or second paroxysms. If the tongue be coated, expanded, not florid at the tip and edges, the bowels confined, and the stomach not irritable, and the paroxysm be the first or second, and not far advanced, then an emetic of ipecacuanha, followed by a mild purgative should be had recourse to. These evacuant remedies are adopted partly with the view of lessening vascular excitement, but chiefly with that of preparing the system for the fullest influence of the means of cure appropriate to the intermission.

During the *sweating stage*, under ordinary circumstances, there is little to be done. The surface must be protected by adequate coverings from the risks of too rapid evaporation on the one hand, while on the other the excess of sweating which will result from too much covering must be avoided. While these principles are sufficient for the ordinary management of this stage, still what has been already stated in respect to the occasional occurrence of great and unlooked-for exhaustion must be carefully remembered. When this event is indicated, then no suitable means of strengthening the patient must be left untried, and towards the close of the paroxysm stimulants and animal broths must be freely given.

It has been stated, that the treatment during the paroxysm is palliative, and should be as little debilitating as possible; but nothing so certainly debilitates the system and accelerates cachexia, with all its attendant evils, as a frequent recurrence of the febrile paroxysm. Therefore, to prevent this is the leading indication in the management of the *intermission*, and, it may be added, in the treatment of this disease. This object is to be effected by the exhibition of antiperiodic remedies; and the earliest intermission should, with this view, be taken advantage of. *Quinine* is the only certain and generally appropriate medicine of this class. There has been much discussion in respect to the best method of using quinine; but it will be sufficient for me to state the opinions which I have myself formed from clinical experiment and the study of the written observations of others:—

1. The quantity of quinine sufficient to prevent the paroxysm

* In recommending the use of leeches in India, it is impossible to be precise in regard to the number. The leech varies much in size in different parts of the country. The number must further depend on the state of the constitution and the degree of local vascular derangement. I would, however, express my belief that local blood-letting should, as a rule, not be carried to the degree of very sensibly depressing the general action of the heart, but be used chiefly with a view to its local derivative action.

varies according to the severity of the attack, or, in other words, the intensity of the malarious influence.

2. It should be given during the intermission in such manner as to ensure the whole quantity being taken at least three hours before the expected paroxysm, so that it may be absorbed and assimilated.

3. In Indian intermittents, from twelve to thirty grains are in general sufficient. In more intense intermittents it may be necessary to give sixty grains and upwards, but of these larger quantities I have no personal experience. The selection of the quantity in the first intermission will depend on the circumstances of the case, indicating the probability of much or little malarious influence; and correct judgment in this particular can only be acquired by careful clinical observation.

4. According to Briquet, quinine in doses of from two and a half to four and a half grains stimulates the circulation, respiration, and nutrition; but in doses of from nine grains and upwards it exercises a disturbing and sedative influence on the nervous system, the circulation and general muscular system, which, when present in great degree, may endanger life. These are the effects of quinine on the system in a normal state; but in intermittent fever there is a tolerance of this agent, by which is meant that these characteristic symptoms of depression (cinchonism) require a larger quantity for their production; therefore, generally speaking, there will be tolerance of that quantity which, in particular cases, is required to prevent the access of the paroxysm. Consequently this quantity may be given in one dose with perfect safety. On this point, however, my own experience does not extend beyond doses of twenty grains.* But, in applying this rule, it is necessary to remember that an exhausted state of the system diminishes the tolerance for quinine; and that, therefore, even when there is evidence of much malarious influence, large doses are unsafe in states of exhaustion and collapse. From this it follows, that where there is much sweating and debility at the close of the paroxysm, the quantity of quinine allotted for the intermission should be given at intervals, — in four or five-grain doses, — accompanied with suitable stimulants and nourishment.

5. The practice of giving the whole quantity at once, or in

* The exclusive exhibition of quinine in scruple or half-drachm doses, instead of smaller ones frequently repeated, first followed by French and American physicians, has been chiefly advocated in the treatment of Indian intermittents by Drs. Corbyn, Mackinnon, Mactier, and C. Murchison ("Indian Annals of Medical Science," No. 1, and "Edinburgh Medical and Surgical Journal for April, 1855").

divided doses, should vary in different cases. Assuming that the quantity has been correctly determined with reference to the tolerance, it will, in the great proportion of cases, be effective in quotidians at whatever period of the intermission it is given, provided this be at least three hours before the expected paroxysm; and as the quantity in each case is supposed to be regulated with reference to the tolerance, it may be given in one dose with safety, and when there is not time for divided doses, it is best thus to use it.

6. When there is doubt in respect to the quantity likely to be required, when there is sufficient time, when there is an exhausted state of the system, and when the type is tertian or quartan, then quinine is most advantageously given at suitable intervals in from three to six-grain doses, between the cessation of one paroxysm and three hours from the expected period of the next.

7. It is unnecessary to give quinine till symptoms of cinchonism begin to appear; for this is to overstep the tolerance, in pursuit of a guide which the experienced physician does not require.

8. Though the full quantity of quinine given in one dose in the sweating stage is sufficient to prevent the accession in an ordinary quotidian, still the conclusion, from my own clinical experience, is, that its power is greatest when given nearer to the period of expected paroxysm, provided time is allowed for absorption and assimilation.

9. The idea that quinine has a diaphoretic action would seem to have arisen from inattention to the fact that a checked, but not prevented, paroxysm may be evidenced merely by a sweating stage unpreceded by a hot one; and this may suggest the belief of diaphoresis from the quinine, when in fact the quantity had been sufficient merely to modify, but not to prevent the return.

10. The efficiency of quinine is most certain when exhibited in perfect solution.

11. When large doses of quinine are necessary, when it is of much moment to ensure its fullest therapeutic effect, and an idiosyncrasy adverse to its action is supposed to exist, it is of great importance that the patient, after taking the quinine, should be kept very quiet; that his senses should be little acted on by light, sound, or other external influences; and that the excitement of trains of thought, by reading, or conversation, should be avoided as much as possible.*

* I am indebted to Dr. McLennan for having called my attention to the great advantage resulting from these precautions. He informs me that, by observing them,

12. After the recurrence of the paroxysm has been prevented, quinine should be continued in decreasing quantities for the three or four succeeding days.

Arsenic, in the form of arsenious acid, is the antiperiodic remedy next in power to quinine; but it is not so generally appropriate, and requires the exercise of much caution and the careful selection of cases to insure its safe administration.

The results of my clinical experience* of this remedy are arranged under the following heads:—

1. The principles relative to the exhibition of quinine during the intermission, and a tolerance proportionate to the intensity of the malarious influence, equally apply to arsenious acid.

2. In Indian intermittents, an eighth to a fourth of a grain —that is fifteen to thirty minims of liquor potassæ arsenitis—given in the intermission, has no evident antiperiodic power.

3. Half-a-grain—one drachm of liquor potassæ arsenitis—given so as to be all taken two hours before the expected period of paroxysm,

he had on several occasions been enabled to give quinine with excellent effect to patients with whom it had been previously believed to disagree, and that he is satisfied that much of the utility of this essential agent in the treatment of malarious fever is often lost from their neglect. Further, he is of opinion that this benefit derived from mental repose may often be readily secured in practice by selecting, when the intermission or remission corresponds, the stillness and darkness of night for the period of exhibition.

* These statements relative to the anti-periodic power of arsenic differ materially from those in the first edition. They consist, not of a correction of previous error so much as of the results of an extended experience. When passing through Paris, on my return to India, I was fortunate enough to meet M. Boudin in his hospital. The use of arsénic in intermittent fever came under discussion. My unfavourable results were stated. M. Boudin not only kindly showed me cases under treatment, but favoured me with the subjoined memorandum on his method of using arsenic—

"Acide arsénieux, un gramme; eau distillée, mille grammes: *faire bouiller* pendant un quart d'heure. Ajoutez vin blanc, mille grammes.

"Cent grammes de cette liqueur réprésentent cinq centigrammes, ou *un grain* d'acide arsénieux. On donne à Paris en moyenne un demi-grain par jour, dans l'intervalle des accès. Mais on peut donner plus. Il importe de fractionner la dose totale le plus possible. La tolérance pour l'arsénic baisse en général avec la disposition de la fièvre. Le premier signe d'intolérance est l'eau à la bouche. Il faut profiter de la tolérance pour saturer le malade. Il faut continuer plus ou moins longtemps après la cessation de la fièvre. Opposer à la diathèse paludienne un diathèse arsénicale; voilà le but qui je me propose.

"BOUDIN.

"Paris, le 14 Juillet, 1856."

I have since carefully read M. Boudin's paper on intermittent fever in the supplement to the "Dictionnaire des Dictionnaires de Médicine," also the article at p. 530 of the 2nd volume of the "Traité de Géographie et de Statisques Médicales," by the same author. To these works I would refer the clinical student for full information on this interesting and important subject.

is sufficient to prevent the recurrence in mild intermittents in India. It may be exhibited with safety in this quantity in cases in which there is no tendency to gastric or intestinal irritation, and most advantageously in repeated doses of ten minims or less, sometimes combined with a few minims of tincture of opium.

4. Half a grain of arsenious acid has seemed to me to be about equivalent in power to fifteen grains of quinine. It may, therefore, be easily understood why the quantity—an eighth to a fourth of a grain—usually given, has no sensible effect in intermittent fever in India. Three grains and a half to seven grains of quinine would be equally inefficacious.

5. As fifteen grains of quinine are insufficient to prevent the accession of the severer and greater number of Indian intermittents, half a grain of arsenious acid is equally so; but we may, in many cases, without incurring the risk of larger doses of arsenic, economise quinine by preventing the recurrence in the first place by an adequate quantity of quinine, and then trusting to arsenious acid for the completion of the cure.

6. My experience is limited to the quantity of half a grain in the intermission; but the practical question remains, whether in intermittent fever in India, uncomplicated with gastric or intestinal irritation, arsenic can with safety be given to the extent of one grain and a half and upwards, as by M. Boudin, and thus suffice for the cure of all cases? The answer may probably be thus stated:—M. Boudin has shown that by divided doses, enemata, &c., the full effect of arsenious acid may be obtained; just as former physicians, by pharmaceutic skill, achieved more with the crude cinchona than is ever now attempted. Used with the skill and precaution observed by M. Boudin, arsenious acid may be adequate for the effective cure of Indian intermittents; but the treatment of a disease so common cannot be safely left to the contingency of great experience and tact.

My practical knowledge of other anti-periodic remedies* is con-

* The subject of febrifuge remedies has been fully discussed in the 3rd, 4th, and 5th volumes of the "Indian Annals of Medical Science," by Falconer, Cleghorn, Macpherson, Cornish, and Waring.

There are questions of special therapeutic interest to the medical inquirer in India: —(1.) To substitute cheap and common indigenous articles of materia medica for the rarer and more expensive products of other countries is very expedient, as a measure of convenience and economy. (2.) To strengthen the materia medica by the removal of inert drugs and the addition of others of undoubted efficacy, is very essential to the character and usefulness of practical medicine. The Indian Government and

fined to the *sulphate of bebeerine, muriate of narcotine, chiretta, cæsalpinia bonducella, berberry,* and *atees* (Aconitum heterophyllum). These in my hands have proved unequal to preventing the paroxysm of ordinary intermittents; and in estimating the value of remedies of this class, it should be remembered that they are of little value unless they produce this effect. The tendency of a large proportion of cases, more particularly quotidians, at the commencement of the rainy season, in climates in which the rain-fall is not great, is to terminate spontaneously after from the fifth to the ninth paroxysm: therefore there is no proof of a febrifuge effect from remedies in fevers which have followed this course.

The extent to which *mercurial* and other *purgatives* should be given in the treatment of intermittent fever, depends upon the state of the constitution, the duration of the attack, the appearance of the tongue, the character and amount of the alvine discharges, and the co-existence or not of hepatic or splenic congestion. When the system is asthenic, when the disease has continued for some time, and purgative remedies have not been neglected in the early stages of treatment; then it matters not what may be the state of the tongue, or of the alvine excretions, or what the condition of the liver or of the spleen, the period for further evacuation* by purgatives or other means has passed; for, if now had recourse to, it will favour the development of cachexia, the recurrence of the paroxysm, and the persistence of the attack. Purgatives, moreover, under

Medical Boards have evinced a laudable desire to advance these objects; but the means usually adopted have been insufficient, and have generally failed of success. They have consisted of casual and hasty experiments, without reference to the practical qualifications of the experimenters or regard to the adequacy or appropriateness of the conditions of the experiment. The result is that medical literature has become oppressed with feeble and trifling reports, and practical medicine invested with a character of vacillating imbecility, which forms no part of its scientific pursuit. To test and determine the properties of medicines is a work which can only be safely entrusted to physicians of large clinical experience, and of calm and matured judgment, familiar with an enlightened pathology, and acquainted with the natural history of disease, and the action of existing medicines. It may be that these qualities are rare; but it is, nevertheless, true, that it is only by these qualities that therapeutic science can be advanced and entitled to confidence and respect.

* The careful reader will not understand this passage as implying that in these conditions of intermittent fever, the purification of the blood by excretion is to be neglected. It must be remembered that this important function may be in very useful action without very evident evacuation, by attention to the purity and temperature of the atmosphere, suitable ablution and clothing, well-arranged food and drinks, and the use of appropriate tonic and alterative medicines. The influence of tonics and alteratives — regimen and medicines — necessarily involves increased excretion.

these circumstances, are apt, by irritating the intestinal mucous lining, to excite dysentery.

The use of purgatives in the hot stage, with the view of lessening vascular excitement, and preparing the system for the full benefit of anti-periodic remedies during the intermission, has been already adverted to. Purgatives, however, act with more certainty during the intermission, and when the object is merely to obviate constipation, they are given with most advantage in this stage, either in combination with quinine, or towards the end of the paroxysm, so as to take effect early in the intermission; but they should never be used in such manner as to interfere with the administration of the anti-periodic remedy. Further precautions are also necessary. The *free* action of a purgative towards the end of a paroxysm should be avoided; for it may induce dangerous exhaustion: it is also apt, in the intermission and during convalescence, to re-excite the paroxysm.*

Attention to the *diet* of those suffering from intermittent fever is of very great importance. In sthenic subjects, with deranged alvine secretions, the food during the two or three first days should be spare, and the strength be chiefly sustained by moderation in treating the hot stage, and by the adequate use of quinine during the intermission. In asthenic subjects, from the commencement, and in all constitutions in the advanced stages, support by suitable alimentation, and occasional stimulants, is a leading indication of treatment. The intermissions are the periods when these means should be most assiduously used. It is by the careful observance of this rule that the occasional occurrence of the unlooked-for, and sometimes fatal, exhaustion at the close of a paroxysm, already alluded to, can alone be prevented. This precaution, necessary in the management of intermittent fever in all asthenic individuals, is very essential in the asthenic natives of India; for I have in many instances seen reason to attribute death to its neglect.

* It would be easy to confirm this latter observation by references to established authorities. For example, Cullen writes: "But I can say that Sydenham and many other practitioners have observed that we are in danger of bringing back intermittent fevers if we employ purgative medicines soon after we have stopped them with bark; and we have the same observation in De Haen."—*The Works of Cullen*, Edited by John Thomson, M.D. vol. i. p. 642.

SECTION III.—*Intermittent Fever complicated with Enlargement of the Spleen.—Symptoms.—Pathology.—Treatment.*

Symptoms.—Enlargement of the spleen is the most common complication of intermittent fever.* It does not usually occur in first attacks, but after several recurrences of the quotidian or the tertian type. If a first attack, however, has been badly managed, and several paroxysms have taken place, then in it also splenic enlargement may be looked for.†

This condition of the spleen is always associated with some degree of cachexia; and a dingy appearance of the conjunctivæ, with anæmic pallor of the surface and of the tongue, may serve to excite suspicion and to direct inquiry. The enlargement may range from the degree which can only be determined by careful percussion to that which causes an abdominal tumour reaching to the crest of the ilium and inwards beyond the mesial line.

The co-existence of systolic cardiac murmur with enlargement of the spleen is occasionally observed; and when this occurs without any other physical sign of cardiac disease, there should be no hesitation in relating the murmur to the altered condition of the blood, which so generally attends splenic cachexia. But it is of importance further to be aware, that enlargement of the spleen may cause abnormal præcordial dulness, and that cardiac murmur may be associated with it. This dulness may be produced partly by displacement of the heart upwards, and partly by the enlarged spleen preventing the free descent of the diaphragm, and the full expansion of the lung, with complete overlapping of the left side and base of the heart by its thin edge. The following cases will illustrate this clinical observation:—

1. *Abnormal Præcordial Dulness from Enlarged Spleen.*—Abdoola Ibrahim, a Mussulman labourer, eighteen years of age, had for upwards of a year been the subject of frequent attacks of intermittent fever. He was admitted into hospital on the 23rd of June, 1851, enfeebled and reduced by disease. The spleen was much enlarged; a line drawn transversely from the cartilage of the

---

* As evidence of its frequency I find that out of 243 clinical cases of intermittent fever, enlargement of the spleen was present in 91. It is unnecessary to collect further proof of so familiar a fact.

† Enlargement of the spleen is generally classed under "Splenitis" in Indian Hospital Returns; but this is very inaccurate. Inflammation of the spleen is very rare; abscess I have never seen. The only appearance probably related to inflammation which I have witnessed, was a thickened, almost cartilaginous, state of the capsule.

left sixth rib to the vertebral column marked its upper limit, and a curved line from the same cartilage to the umbilicus, and thence to about an inch above the crest of the ilium, marked the lower limit. The apex of the heart beat between the third and fourth ribs; and the præcordial dulness was confined to the third and fourth left costal cartilages and the interspace between the second and third, and at the outer lower limit was almost continuous with the splenic dulness.

2. *Abnormal Præcordial Dulness from Enlarged Spleen associated with Systolic Murmur.*—Hurreem Adamjee, twenty-three years of age, a Mussulman, native of Ahmedabad, and frequently suffering from intermittent fever, was admitted into the Jamsetjee Jejeebhoy Hospital on the 9th August, 1852. He was pale and anæmic. The spleen was much enlarged, extending downwards almost to the crest of the ilium, internally beyond the umbilicus; and its upper limit, as indicated by percussion, reached to the sixth left intercostal space. The præcordial dulness commenced at the left second intercostal space, and became continuous with the splenic dulness. At the level of the third intercostal cartilage it reached transversely from the middle of the sternum almost to the nipple. The apex beat between the fourth and fifth ribs internal to the nipple. A faint but distinct systolic murmur was heard at the left second intercostal space, close to the sternum, but was not audible at the apex, where the sounds of the heart were both distinct. There was no increased impulse. A distinct venous murmur was heard at the junction of the jugular and subclavian veins of the left side.

3. *Abnormal Præcordial Dulness from Splenic Enlargement.—Systolic Murmur present.*—Abdul Cadur, fifteen years of age, a Mussulman peon, the subject of quotidian intermittent fever for thirteen days before admission into hospital on the 16th July, 1851. The spleen was not felt below the ribs; but, as ascertained by percussion, its upper limit was as high as the eighth rib, and its internal one was a vertical line half an inch external to the nipple. Præcordial dulness extended from the third to the fifth rib, and between the nipple and the sternum. There was a distinct systolic murmur not louder at the base than at the apex of the heart. On the 2nd August, the internal limit of the splenic dulness was a vertical line an inch external to the nipple; the upper limit was unchanged. The upper limit of the præcordial dulness was the upper margin of the fourth costal cartilage. The cardiac murmur was disappearing.

4. *Abnormal Præcordial Dulness from Enlargement of the Spleen.— Systolic Murmur present.*—Francisco Antonio, twenty years of age, an inhabitant of Lisbon, of stout and well-proportioned frame, the subject of tertian intermittent fever for fifteen days, was admitted into hospital on the 25th July, 1851. The pulse was of moderate volume, and somewhat jerking. The indurated edge of the spleen was felt below the margin of the left ribs. Its upper limit was the ninth rib; its internal limit a vertical line about an inch external to the nipple. The præcordial dulness extended from the lower border of the third rib to the lower border of the fifth rib, and externally to about half an inch internal to the nipple. There was a distinct systolic aortic murmur. The recurrences of fever were prevented; and on the 2nd August, the internal limit of the splenic dulness was a vertical line from the posterior fold of the axilla. The upper limit of the præcordial dulness was the interspace of the third and fourth ribs; and the external limit was a vertical line an inch internal to the nipple. The systolic murmur had altogether disappeared.

These cases prove that disease of the heart is not necessarily present when abnormal præcordial dulness, with or without cardiac murmur, is associated with enlargement of the spleen. The abnormal dulness has been attributed to the mechanical influence of the enlarged spleen on the heart, and on the expansion of the lungs. But there is more than this. The præcordial dulness and murmur may exist in very anæmic states, without splenic enlargement, in consequence of the incomplete expansion of the lungs, from the limited respiratory function, which necessarily attends on a great degree of anæmia.*

The following case is illustrative of this last statement.

5. *Extended Præcordial Dulness, with Systolic and Venous Murmurs, without Splenic Enlargement.*—Antonio Domingo, a native of Goa, and following the occupation of a shepherd. Had been out of health for some months, suffering from palpitation, præcordial uneasiness, occasional dry cough, œdematous feet, and febrile accessions coming on towards evening without distinct chills. He had never suffered from rheumatism. He was admitted into hospital on the 1st January, 1854, presenting a very anæmic appearance. The pulse was small, jerking, and somewhat frequent. The præcordial dulness was bounded superiorly by the third rib, internally by the median line, and externally by a vertical line drawn a quarter of an inch external to the nipple, and below by the sixth rib. A blowing systolic murmur was audible over the third left costal cartilage, increasing in the line of the aorta upwards, loudest at the top of the sternum, and decreasing in the direction of the apex, which beat in the intercostal space between the fifth and sixth ribs, an inch and a half below and half an inch external to the nipple. There was a venous murmur on the left side of the neck. The abdomen was slightly full. There was slight enlargement of the liver, as indicated by a distinct indurated edge felt below the right ribs. There was no enlargement of the spleen. He continued under treatment till the 15th February. During this time the febrile accessions frequently returned. The urine was often examined; it was of low density, but gave no traces of albumen.

When discharged, he had lost much of his anæmic appearance. The jerking character of the pulse was no longer observed, and the cardiac and venous murmurs had almost ceased. The last note of the præcordial dulness was on the 15th January; and it gives, as the external limit, a vertical line drawn over the nipple.

Pathology.—In the cold stage of intermittent fever, the blood is determined from the surface of the body to internal parts, and is liable to accumulate in such venous arrangements as those of the spleen, and the portal system of the liver; and when stagnating in the splenetic capillaries, its transfer, in undue quantity, into the pulpy parenchyma of the organ, readily takes place. Under recurrences of the cold stage, these events are repeated, and the bulk of the spleen necessarily increases.

* Since these observations were written, I have had the advantage of referring to Dr. Sibson's very valuable and instructive work on Medical Anatomy. In the first fasciculus this extension of præcordial dulness, by shrinking of the lungs, is pointed out. I leave the text as originally written, for I find nothing at variance with it in Dr. Sibson's remarks.

The density of the enlarged spleen bears relation to the quantity and quality of the blood present in the vascular system of the organ, as well as on the increase and the condition of the parenchymatous pulp; as whether any of the fibrinous or albuminous constituent has become converted into tissue of low organization. When this change of part of the fibrine or albumen into tissue takes place, then some degree of enlargement will become permanent; but when the enlargement depends merely on excess of blood in the vessels, or excess of unorganized pulp, it may be concluded that the organ may still be restored to its normal condition by a gradual, slow process of absorption and elimination.

This accumulation of blood in the spleen, being an abstraction of it from the purposes of the circulation, must derange that which remains in the general vascular system by reducing the proportion of corpuscles, of fibrine, and of albumen, and by increasing the proportion of watery constituent.

If enlargement of the spleen only occurred as a result of intermittent fever, the statement just made of its relation to the altered condition of the blood, viz., that the enlargement is the antecedent, the altered blood the sequence, might be sufficient. But when it is recollected that enlargement of the spleen and concomitant cachexia may take place from the influence of malaria, without the intervention of fever, then the belief must be entertained that malaria exercises a primary deteriorating influence on the blood; and that the altered state thus induced favours stagnation, and in some circumstances is the chief, if not the only proximate cause; but that in others, it merely co-operates with the favouring conditions of the cold stage. This view of the injurious influence of malaria may the more readily be assented to, when it is found that nothing so surely leads to removal of enlargement of the spleen as well-directed means for improving the state of the blood.*

* Frerichs—"Klinik der Leberkrankheiten"—endeavours to particularise the condition of the blood brought about by recurring paroxysms of fever, and which leads to general cachexia and structural change of organs, as the spleen, the liver, and kidneys, and brain. He believes that it proceeds from an excess of dark pigment in the blood; that the blood, stagnating in the splenic venous system, has the colouring matter of some of its corpuscles converted into black pigment; that thus the corpuscular constituent of the blood is diminished, and the pigment entering the circulation is conveyed to, and accumulates in, the capillaries of different organs, causing discoloration, with structural and functional derangement. The form of fever which he has found usually to precede and accompany these changes he describes as intermittent, generally quotidian or double tertian: of 51 cases, 38 proved fatal. In 28 of the 51 cases, severe cerebral disturbance—delirium, convulsions, coma—was present;

Treatment.—To prevent the paroxysms of intermittent fever, to remove the cachectic state by all means which tend directly to this end, and to avoid all measures which are calculated to increase asthenia, or still further to deteriorate the blood, are the leading indications of cure.

If the paroxysms still recur, they should be prevented by quinine. When this has been effected, the cachectic state will be removed more certainly by the continued use, for some time, of preparations of iron in moderate doses than by any other means. Sulphate of iron in combination with small doses of quinine, the citrate of iron and quinine, the tincture of the sesquichloride and the solution of the persesquinitrate are suitable preparations. The treatment which lessens the cachexia will also be the most successful in reducing the size of the spleen; for improvement of the general system and decrease of the splenic enlargement always progress together, independent of any special local appliances. Due attention must at the same time be given to all other measures which are necessary to the preservation of health and to its restoration when deranged,—as atmospheric purity, food suited to the power of digestion and assimilation, and the judicious regulation of the excretions. The state of the mind should also be carefully considered, and cheerful occupation be provided.

The treatment of enlarged spleen by the periodical application of leeches, and the daily use of moderate purgatives combined with tonics, as recommended by Mr. Twining *, has not proved efficacious in my hands. The abstraction of blood is opposed to the indications of cure, as already stated; and though a mild purgative, occasionally used when the alvine discharges are scanty and cachexia not far advanced, is beneficial, still it may confidently

in 20 there was albuminuria; and in 17 profuse diarrhœa. In all the fatal cases the liver was rich in pigment. In 30 the spleen was enlarged and contained pigment.

The diagnosis chiefly rested on the peculiar ash-grey colour of the skin, and the presence of numerous pigment particles in the blood when some drops were examined under the microscope.

On these statements of Frerichs I can only observe, that intermittent fever, with a mortality so large, and complications so various, acute, and severe, has not come under my observation in India; and I am not aware that this form of fever has been described by any writer on tropical disease. Nor does it accord with my impressions that the viscera, after death, in individuals who have suffered much from intermittent fever, present any peculiar discoloration; but to this remark I attach little importance, for it is the statement of a general impression, and not of the result of attentive observation directed to the question.

* "Clinical Illustrations of the most important Diseases of Bengal," vol. i. Second Edition.

be asserted, that when the cachexia is considerable, frequent purgatives increase it and are very apt to excite dysentery.

The internal use of preparations of *iodine* and *bromine* has been recommended. Experience does not enable me to speak with certainty on this question of practice. In the treatment of the disease among the better classes of Europeans, after benefit has ceased to result from the measures already advised, change of climate would be had recourse to as the most likely means of cure. In hospital practice the patient is generally so fully satisfied with the improvement of the general health and of the spleen by the use of quinine, preparations of iron, and general tonic management, that he is unwilling to continue longer under treatment. For these reasons the opportunity is not often afforded to the practitioner in India of testing the powers of iodine and bromine at the period appropriate for their use. I say appropriate for their use; for it would be a grievous practical error to turn to such remedies as iodine and bromine, and neglect the tonic principle of management, of which the efficacy has been well proved and the theory is so much in accordance with physiological and pathological doctrine. When this principle has been fairly applied and enlargement still remains, then preparations of iodine and bromine may, with propriety, be had recourse to, if no contra-indicating circumstance exists in the general state of the system, or the condition of the digestive organs. It may be urged that iodine or bromine may be used at the same time with preparations of iron, and tonic management. The objection to this course is its inexpediency, for it is impossible to estimate justly the value of subsidiary means applied at the same time with remedies of acknowledged efficacy; and nothing so injures the character of therapeutic science as desultory and inconclusive experiments.

To Mr. Twining * the merit is due of pointing out with clearness and force the evils which attend the use of *mercury* in enlargement of the spleen and its co-existing cachexia, viz.: the great susceptibility to, and the destructive effects from, its action. The changes effected in the blood by mercury are probably not very different from those caused by malaria; at all events both are favourable to degeneration and destruction of tissue, and unfavourable to restoration and repair. To the unbiassed judgment it seems a strange idea to endeavour to correct the evils of the one by the super-addition of the analogous evils of the

* "Clinical Illustrations of the most important Diseases of Bengal," vol. i. p. 452. Second Edition.

other. Mercurial preparations are unquestionably injurious in splenic enlargement and cachexia, and their use should be carefully abstained from.

The application of external remedies to the region of the spleen — as sinapisms, lotions with iodine or nitro-muriatic acid, &c.,— is sometimes useful in relieving local uneasiness; and the two last remedies may possibly exercise a deobstruent action; but as they are seldom used singly, it must be very difficult to isolate their therapeutic value. Applications which vesicate or cause pustular eruptions, should be avoided in a state of the system prone to destructive ulceration and sloughing. Mr. Twining's suggestion of passing long needles into the enlarged spleen is hardly in accordance with the spirit of rational medicine.

The means as yet described for the cure of splenic enlargement and cachexia very often prove inadequate, and then change to another locality in India, or to more temperate latitudes, is a measure essential to recovery. It is vain to expect much benefit from medical treatment in the hot and malarious seasons, — from March to the end of November,— in the alluvial and littoral plains and jungly tracts of India. Nor in these states of the system are the hill climates, from the middle of June to the beginning of March, more suitable: malaria may not be equally generated; but they are cold and wet, and therefore liable in malarious cachexia to excite tertian fever, diarrhœa, and dysentery.

The part of India least likely to be injurious in splenic cachexia in the malarious season, from the middle of June to the end of November, is the strip of the Deccan table-land, between 20° and 15° N. lat. and from 60 to 100 miles east of the Western Ghauts. There the fall of rain is inconsiderable, the temperature moderate, and, in well-selected localities, the generation of malaria is not great. In December, January, and February, the climate of the sea-coast, and from March to the middle of June, a hill station, with an elevation of from 4,000 to 6,000 feet, will prove the most conducive to recovery.

But when changes of climate such as these, and the use of suitable remedies, fail in reducing the spleen and removing the cachexia, then there should be no hesitation in recommending an early sea voyage, and a prolonged residence in a temperate climate. Care should be taken, when practicable, that the patient should arrive in the temperate climate early in summer, and thus avoid the winter and spring of the cold, and the summer and autumn of the hot latitudes. In all changes from warm to cold, and from dry to damp climates, great attention to clothing is necessary, in order that impressions of cold on the surface of the body, and consequent attacks of tertian fever, diarrhœa, and dysentery may be prevented. When the patient comes at first under observation in a state of confirmed malarious cachexia, and the season for removal to a temperate climate is suitable, time should not be lost in expectation of benefit from treatment and change of air in India. A change from India to Egypt in the winter, and to Syria in the summer and autumn, is sometimes had recourse to; but it is an inexpedient measure. In the year 1840, a medical officer of feeble constitution, who had suffered from malarious fever in Guzerat, Bombay, and the Deccan, left Bombay, on my recommendation, in the month of February, for Egypt. At Cairo, from the influence of the Kamsin wind, he suffered from congestion of the head and lungs; was attacked with remittent fever at Alexandria, and again in the month of May at Smyrna, and subsequently at Constantinople, where the attack proved fatal. Since the occurrence of this case, the history of four other Indian invalids (two of them medical men) have come to my knowledge, in which obstinate malarious fever was acquired in Egypt or Syria; and it is a curious circumstance that the febrile paroxysm was, in two of the cases, attended with severe strangury.

SECTION IV.—*Intermittent Fever with Hepatic Complication.—Symptoms.—Pathology.—Treatment.*

Hepatic inflammation or enlargement in intermittent fever has, in my experience, been of rare occurrence, both in Europeans and natives.

Of the 243 clinical cases of natives in the Jamsetjee Jejeebhoy Hospital, completion of hepatic affection was observed only in eighteen; in six, it was considered to be inflammatory; in twelve, to be passive enlargement. Two cases, one of inflammation and one of enlargement, are subjoined. The first is of interest, because death caused by cholera gave the opportunity of observing the appearances presented by the liver. The absence of fibrinous exudation is probably an illustration of the law established by Dr. Alison, that when inflammation complicates idiopathic fever it does not so readily pass on to its results, as when it is itself idiopathic. This pathological law, moreover, justifies caution in the mercurial treatment of hepatitis when it co-exists with intermittent fever:—

6. *Intermittent Fever complicated with Hepatitis.—Death from Cholera.—Liver in a state of vascular Turgescence.*—Mohedeen, a Mussulman sailor, of twenty years of age, a native of Cochin, and suffering there on two or three occasions from febrile attacks. While on a voyage from the Persian Gulf, he was wrecked on the coast adjoining the island of Bombay, and consequent upon exposure to wet he became affected with fever, which, preceded by chilliness, recurred in irregular paroxysms, and, after seven or eight days' duration, was accompanied with pain of the right side of the chest. He was admitted into hospital on the 17th June, 1851, ten days after the commencement of his illness. There was pain of the right side of the chest, increased by full inspiration and coughing; also pain below the margin of the right false ribs, increased by pressure. There was some degree of yellowness of the conjunctivæ; but no perceptible induration or dulness below either margin of the ribs. The febrile accession recurred twice in the twenty-four hours. He was treated with repeated four-grain doses of quinine during the intermission. Leeches were applied to the right side of the chest and to the margin of the ribs, followed by a small blister on the former. Blue pill and ipecacuanha, with an occasional laxative, were also given. The fever did not return after the 19th. On the 20th, the pain below the margin of the right ribs was gone, and that of the chest very much lessened. In this state he continued till 1 A.M. of the 27th, when he was attacked with cholera, and died at 3 P.M.

Inspection twenty-two hours after Death.—Both lungs collapsed freely, and were crepitating. The costal and pulmonary pleuræ of both sides were free of adhesions or traces of lymph exudation. They were healthy, with exception that the inferior-anterior part of the right costal pleura presented a slight blush of redness, which was not the case with the corresponding portion of the opposite side. The heart was somewhat flabby, but its size and structure were healthy. The peritoneum was healthy. The liver was much congested, and bled freely when cut into. The stomach contained a small quantity of thin whitish fluid, and its mucous membrane was pale. Peyer's glands in the ileum were slightly enlarged. The kidneys were flabby, but healthy in structure.

7. *Intermittent Fever with enlargement of the Liver.*—Saccaram, a Maratha labourer, of thirty-three years of age, addicted to the moderate use of spirits, was admitted into hospital on the 9th December, 1849. He was much emaciated, and had been for four or five years the subject of epigastric swelling, attributed to frequent attacks of fever. The irregular febrile accessions, generally preceded by chills, with increased epigastric fulness, for which he sought admission, had been present five days. The hepatic dulness reached to within an inch of the umbilicus, and midway between the tenth rib and crest of the ilium. There was sense of uneasiness and weight rather than distinct pain. He remained under treatment till the 13th January. There was no return of fever after the day subsequent to that of his admission. The urine was free, generally of low density, and showing no traces of albumen. He was treated with quinine, the external application of nitro-muriatic acid lotion, and latterly of an ointment containing iodine. He was discharged much improved in general health, but with little diminution of the size of the liver.

Pathology.—Enlargement of the liver, consequent upon intermittent fever or slow malarious influence, must be carefully distinguished from that depending upon chronic inflammation.* The diagnosis may be determined by the history of the case;

* It can hardly be necessary to suggest a caution against the possible error of mistaking enlargement of the liver from forming abscess, associated with hectic fever, for the enlargement now under consideration, associated with malarious febrile accessions.

and it is important, for the treatment of the two affections is very different.

The pathology of this enlargement resembles that of enlargement of the spleen. It may result from recurrences of the cold stage, or from a gradual malarious influence without the intervention of febrile disturbance; and may be assumed to arise from stagnation of deteriorated blood in the venous system of the organ.

The proximate cause of enlargement of the spleen was supposed to be vascular congestion, and addition to the splenic pulp and to the connecting fibrous tissue by low organisation of exuded fibrine and albumen. These three conditions, however, are not all necessarily present. The last is the one most frequently absent, and probably only occurs in cases of long persisting enlargement.

The same view may be taken of malarious hepatic enlargement, —that there is stagnation of blood in the portal and hepatic venous systems, addition to the contents of the hepatic cells, and perhaps exudation into the meshes in which the cells are placed. In cases of long standing, the connecting areolar tissue probably becomes hypertrophied by a low organising process.

The chief points which the microscope has still to determine are the degree and character of the additions made to the contents of the cells; also, whether there is deposit external to the cells or not, and if so, its nature.

Treatment.—If there be much that is common in the pathology of hepatic and splenic enlargement, it is reasonable to conclude that similar principles of treatment are applicable to both affections, though not necessarily to be carried out by the same means. It may be anticipated that enlargement, dependent on vascular congestion and excessive deposit in the cells, may in time be recovered from by processes of slow absorption and elimination.

If febrile accessions still recur, the first indication is to prevent them by the adequate exhibition of quinine, and the next is to lessen the cachexia by change of climate, attention to the general state of the excretions, and the use of small doses of quinine, the mineral acids, and extract of taraxacum. The diet should be carefully regulated with reference to the state of the digestive organs and the assimilating powers; and nitro-muriatic acid lotion, or preparations of iodine may be applied externally with advantage.

The preparations of iron, though very important in the allied affection of the spleen, have not been generally used, but they seem to me worthy of careful trial in small doses.

The reasoning relative to the exhibition of purgatives in splenic enlargement also applies to the present affection. It is true that derivation to the intestinal mucous surface reduces stagnation in the vascular system of the liver more directly and surely than that in the spleen, and that moderate purgatives may be used with advantage in the early stages of enlargement, while as yet there is little else than vascular congestion and only commencing cachexia. But when the enlargement has been of some duration, and there is probably more than mere congestion, and when the cachectic state is fully developed, then even more caution than in the instance of splenic enlargement must be observed, for the proclivity to dysentery and diarrhœa is greater. Under these circumstances the first indication is to mitigate the cachexia, and then, in addition, to have recourse to gentle aperients.*

The observations made on *iodine* and *bromine* in relation to the spleen may be repeated in reference to the liver, but with the injunction of still greater caution and reserve. Lastly, in respect to *mercury*. The milder preparations may be occasionally used in small doses with advantage to produce a gentle cholagogue action, but the constitutional influence of mercury is as injurious in malarious cachexia with co-existing hepatic enlargement as in that with co-existing enlargement of the spleen, and for the same reasons. That mercury acts on the secreting function of the liver in a manner which may be turned to good practical account in the treatment of various forms of disease is true; but that its constitutional influence has any effect on structural changes of the tissues of the liver, different from that which it exercises upon the analogous tissues of other organs, is, according to my belief, altogether without proof; yet it would not be difficult to show that an opposite opinion has affected injuriously the treatment of various forms of hepatic disease.

The occurrence of gastric or intestinal hæmorrhage as a consequence of enlargement of the liver or spleen and of the co-existing cachexia, is an occasional, but, judging from my own experience, a rare event. †

* It is after the cachectic condition has been materially lessened by change of climate that hepatic and splenic enlargement is often advantageously treated by the aperient natural waters of Germany and other spas; but it by no means follows that this kind of treatment is safe in the same condition of these organs while the patient is still in India, with a constitution unimproved by removal from malarious influence. On the contrary, it may be asserted with confidence, that a routine treatment by purgatives under these circumstances will frequently lead to a fatal result.

† Mr. Twining's experience in Bengal on this point was different. He says: "During the existence of diseases of the spleen attended with much enlargement of

SECTION V.—*Intermittent Fever complicated with Jaundice, or Affections of the Stomach or Bowels.*

Jaundice.—This complication is not common in intermittent fever. Of 243 clinical cases, it is noted only of three. Jaundice is much more frequently observed in remittent fever, and will be treated of in detail in connection with that type.

Affection of the Stomach and Bowels.—It is not my intention to consider, under this head, those affections of the intestinal canal which are produced in malarious cachexia by ordinary exciting causes, to which the attention of the reader has already been directed in my observations on the pathology of simple intermittents, and which ought to be borne carefully in mind when we estimate the direct and indirect mortality resulting from malarious fever. These forms of disease will be elsewhere more appropriately described.

My present inquiry relates to the complication of derangement of the stomach and bowels with recent attacks of intermittent fever.

In sthenic Europeans this form of fever is very rarely attended with diarrhœa or dysentery; and when gastric symptoms, as irritability of stomach, a tongue florid at the tip and edges, and some degree of epigastric uneasiness are present, then the habit of spirit drinking, or too much drugging with medicinal irritants may be suspected. At a very early period of my practice—first with natives at Sassoor,

the organ, hæmorrhages from the nose, lungs, or stomach, are very liable to occur." Dr. Graham reports a striking case of gastric hæmorrhage witnessed by him in the Native General Hospital in Bombay—the same field in which, for many years, my own observations have been made. ("Transactions, Medical and Physical Society, Bombay," No. 5, p. 29.) In my notes of sick officers, I find a case reported by Dr. Don of an officer at Poona under his care in 1842. This officer had been affected with enlarged spleen for fifteen years. He died on the 14th April. On the 10th he vomited two pints of blood, and on the 11th a similar quantity, and on the 13th a pint and a half; on the day of his death there was also a recurrence of the hæmorrhage.

In the year 1858-59, the 1st Bheel Corps was, consequent on the nature of the service required of it, more than usually exposed to the malaria of Kandeish. The number treated was 266; of these 19 were remittent, and 234 quotidian intermittent. Though a considerable number of the cases were adynamic, some with jaundice, vomiting, and much headache, others with dark, grumous, bloody discharges from the bowels, or obstinate epistaxis, yet no deaths occurred. These facts are extracted from the report of Mr. Burn, the medical officer in charge.

and then with European soldiers of the 4th Light Dragoons at Kirkee—I became convinced of the fact that irritability of stomach was not unfreqently caused and kept up in quotidian fever by the unnecessary use of calomel and purgatives during the hot stage.*

It is when intermittent fever attacks individuals of asthenic constitution that it is apt to be complicated by gastro-intestinal irritation. The proportion of cases will be influenced by the system of treatment; for, as already explained, diarrhœa and dysentery are in these states of constitution very readily excited by the injudicious use of purgatives.

Affection of the stomach or bowels was present in twenty-two of 243 clinical cases, under the form of dysentery in eleven, diarrhœa in seven, and gastric symptoms in one; and to mark the relation of this complication to diathesis, it further appears that, in seventeen of the cases, an asthenic state was present. The tongue is usually florid at the edges and tip, and not unfrequently is the first symptom to arouse suspicion of the existence of this complication. A florid tongue, however, may attend paroxysmal febrile phenomena in asthenic individuals unaccompanied with gastric irritability or diarrhœa; and its presence should always excite apprehension, for it not unfrequently exists in asthenic states in individuals affected with hectic fever consequent on inflammatory action of some important organ. The practical rule in all asthenic cases is to maintain a careful watch over all important organs, for their structures are apt to be invaded by processes of obscure degeneration and destruction.

When diarrhœa co-exists with intermittent fever, a tendency in the febrile accessions to alternate with the diarrhœa may occasionally be noticed; the one being present for three or four days, then ceasing, and being succeeded by the other. This feature of these cases has been observed by me in Scinde, as well as in the European General Hospital and the Jamsetjee Jejeebhoy Hospital at Bombay; but it is generally a character of old fever cases, not of recent ones. It was probably the observation of facts of this kind that led Sydenham to regard dysentery as fever turned in upon the bowels.

Treatment.—The treatment of gastro-intestinal derangement, to be explained in its appropriate place, should be applied with due regard to the asthenia generally present in these complications. But the

* This question of practice is more important in reference to remittent fever, and under that head will be again noticed.

important practical question is, whether, in consequence of these affections, quinine is to be withheld during the intermission. In reply, it may be affirmed that whatever the complication of an intermittent fever may be,—the use of quinine during the intermission is always a ruling indication of treatment; because the local derangement is sure to be aggravated during the paroxysm, and to be mitigated during the intermission. Gastro-intestinal irritation is the complication to which the applicability of this principle might be justly doubted; but it is no exception, as the following case illustrates:—

8. *Intermittent Fever with Gastric Irritation treated with Quinine.*—Dowlut Sabajee, a Maratha labourer, of twenty-nine years of age, frequently suffering from intermittent fever in his native place, but free of it for a year past, during his residence in Bombay. He was admitted into the hospital on the 26th October, 1849. He was a good deal reduced in strength, and indulged occasionally in the use of spirits. He had for eight days been suffering from daily accessions of intermittent fever, commencing with chills in the morning, and terminating with sweating towards evening. The febrile symptoms were accompanied with *frequent vomiting*, headache, soreness of limbs and slight cough, with tenderness of abdomen during the last three days. There was no diarrhœa on admission. The abdomen was retracted, resistent, and tender on pressure chiefly in the epigastric and left hypochondriac regions. The spleen was enlarged and reached nearly to the level of the umbilicus. The tongue was much coated, dryish, and rather florid at the tip and edges. The gums were spongy, and somewhat discoloured. The pulse was very feeble. The day subsequent to his admission was the single one of febrile recurrence. The only treatment used was the exhibition of quinine, first in four-grain doses in powder, repeated six times about the period of expected febrile accession, with intervals of two or three hours; then in five-grain doses in solution, with dilute sulphuric acid. The quinine was now gradually reduced to three and two-grain doses given four times in the twenty-four hours, and latterly was combined with half a grain of sulphate of iron. The only other means used were the application of one sinapism to the abdomen, and effervescing draughts on the day that the quinine was exhibited in powder. Under this treatment there was no recurrence of fever or of vomiting. The tongue became gradually cleaner and moister, and lost its florid tip and edges, and the patient was discharged on the 12th November in much improved condition, and with the spleen so decreased that it could no longer be felt under the false ribs.

SECTION VI.—*Intermittent Fever complicated with Cerebral Affection.*

Symptoms and Pathology.—Head symptoms—drowsiness, confusion of mind, suffusion of countenance—dependent on cerebral congestion and followed by imperfect reaction, are occasionally observed in the cold stage in sthenic habits. But somewhat similar symptoms may also occur, in all states of the constitution, from the direct sedative influence of the morbific cause on the nervous system, irrespective of local congestion, and may in general be recognised by the co-existence of a feeble pulse, pallid countenance, and low temperature of the general surface of the body.

During the hot stage in sthenic habits there may also be present such degree of headache as to call for special treatment; but there is seldom any considerable disturbance of the cerebral functions.

In the congestive cases there is merely a greater degree, as respects the head, of the kind of phenomena alluded to in my remarks on the cold stage of simple intermittents: they are, however, apt to be misunderstood, as is shown in the treatment of the following case:—

9. A gentleman, of stout habit, resident at Poona, on the 14th, 15th, and 16th July, 1837, suffered from pains of the limbs, lassitude, and furred tongue. On the 17th he experienced difficulty in articulating words, and numbness of the lower extremities. The countenance was suffused. He was bled and leeched freely. At noon on the 18th, 19th, and 20th, there was a slight recurrence of the same symptoms, followed by sweating. He was now sent to Bombay, and experienced there several febrile accessions ushered in with chills. In the treatment of this case quinine was very feebly given at Poona.*

After several paroxysms in asthenic habits, the hot stage may terminate with incoherence or delirium. This symptom, under these circumstances, is generally indicative of exhaustion, and is usually attended by other evidences of this condition. These cases are also liable to be misunderstood, and to be improperly treated.

Head symptoms in intermittent fever may likewise be related to organic lesion of the membranes of the brain. The two following cases illustrate this, and are otherwise instructive. They both show that though the symptoms were dependent on structural change, yet they were absent during the intermission, and only present during the period of febrile accession. They, therefore, verify the therapeutic principle of preventing a febrile recurrence, as a means of lessening a local derangement. The first is also an instance of death by unexpected collapse at the close of a paroxysm, favoured by the injudicious use of depletion at that period. The second exemplifies the curious fact that in com-

* Though I did not see this patient, yet I was in the neighbourhood of Poona at the time, and know that at first the nature of the case was not rightly understood. Had it been so, there would have been less depletion and a freer exhibition of quinine. This gentleman is now (1859) in good health, and has never, to my knowledge, been the subject of apoplectic threatenings.

plicated intermittent fever, the period of accession is occasionally characterised, not by febrile reaction, but only by symptoms of the local derangement.

10. *Intermittent Fever, with Chronic Meningitis.* — *Symptoms chiefly during Accession.* — *Death from unexpected Collapse.* — J. S., aged thirty-three, of stout habit, not long resident in Bombay, and latterly occupied in conducting an hotel, was admitted into the European General Hospital on the evening of the 24th September, 1840, at half-past 5 P.M. It was stated that for the five or six previous days he had been affected with fever of the quotidian or tertian type, and had suffered from a paroxysm ushered in with rigors at noon on the day of admission. When seen he had pyrexia with slight wandering, tongue pretty clean, pulse frequent and feeble, abdomen supple. An effervescing draught was ordered every second hour for three or four doses, and twenty-four leeches were applied to the temples and cold cloths to the head. A foot-bath was directed to be used at bedtime, and a draught, c. tinct. muriat. morphia one drachm, to be exhibited, should the headache cease and there be no delirium. Was reported to have had no headache or wandering after the application of the leeches, and the skin to have become cool. The draught was given about half-past 10 A.M. He was reported to have got up to make water when he fell down convulsed. The head was immediately shaved, and a blister was applied to the nucha. He died at 11 P.M.

Inspection fifteen hours after Death.—Body stout and loaded with fat. There were purple sugillations of the depending and posterior parts of the body. *Head.*—The sinuses and veins were turgid with blood, and there was a good deal of capillary vascularity of the pia mater over the entire convex surface of the brain. The arachnoid membrane was thickened and opaque, and in many places, chiefly at the dipping down between the hemispheres, there were patches and granules of lymph between the arachnoid and pia mater. The substance of the brain, when incised, showed numerous bloody points, but was tolerably firm in texture. There was an ounce of serum at the base of the skull, but not more than the usual quantity in the ventricles. *Chest.*—The lungs were healthy and very little congested. The cavities of the heart were moderately distended with blood. The inner lining of the aorta had a rosy tint, and there was a commencing white deposit, in spots and streaks. The muscular parietes of the heart were healthy. *Abdomen.*—The intestines and omentum were loaded with fat. The former, distended with air, pushed the liver up to the level of the fourth rib. The mucous coat of the stomach had a dusky leaden tint, and was slightly more tender in texture than natural. The kidneys were healthy, and there was no distension of the bladder. The spleen was considerably enlarged. The liver was of a greyish tint when incised, but was natural in texture.

11. *Intermittent Fever: some of the Paroxysms complicated with Convulsive Fits, one of which terminated fatally.—Thickening and Opacity of the Arachnoid Membrane.* —Richard Parkman, aged twenty-eight, seaman, Honourable Company's receiving ship *Hastings*, after having been ill with intermittent fever for two or three days, was admitted into the General Hospital on the 24th March, 1842. On that day he experienced a febrile paroxysm attended with headache. An emetic was exhibited, and followed by repeated doses of quinine. On the 25th, there was neither fever nor headache. On the evening of the 26th, he was seized with a convulsive fit, but denied having been ever subject to such attacks. On the morning of the 27th, he was free of fever or headache. Cold affusion to the head, with a hot foot-bath, was used twice; and the only complaint made that day was of a sense of constriction of the throat towards night. On the morning of the 28th, he was free of fever, and quinine was directed to be given. He had a convulsive fit in the course of the day.

and again at night. On the morning of the 29th he was free of complaint, and the skin and pulse were good. The liquor arsenicalis was directed to be given thrice, and cold affusion to be used to the head in the event of a recurrence of the fit. Towards evening there was a slight febrile accession, but he slept well; and, at the morning visit of the 30th, he was reported to have no headache, and to have had no return of the convulsions. The remedies used on the 29th were directed to be repeated. About half an hour after that report, he was seized with convulsions (reported to be not more severe than the former ones), and he died in about five minutes.

Inspection.—*Head.*—On the upper surface of the brain there was a thin veil of serum between the arachnoid and pia mater. The former membrane was opaquish in parts, with here and there deposit of distinct yellow points, but in no great number. The substance of the brain was healthy. There were about two ounces of serum at the base of the skull. *Chest.*—The right ventricle of the heart was distended with blood; but the other contents of the chest were in a healthy state. *Abdomen.*—Old adhesions bound the liver to the side. The viscera were otherwise healthy.

Treatment.—When cerebral congestion is present in the cold stage, general or local blood-letting, according to the state of the constitution, the pulse, and the urgency of the symptoms, must be had recourse to; but these measures are not to be used to the same extent as would be necessary if the congestion were independent of a transient influence. The application of heat to the extremities, and the use of purgatives, are also indicated. The important consideration, however, in such cases is, a careful diagnosis, and then prevention, by the adequate exhibition of quinine; for it is a serious error to neglect this, and to rest satisfied with endeavouring to remove the cerebral symptoms by the repeated use of evacuant remedies.

In asthenic states, when the nervous symptoms seem to depend on exhaustion, suitable nourishment and stimulants, with quinine during the intermission, are the means of cure. The restlessness and wandering may perhaps suggest a full opiate towards the close of the paroxysm; but this proceeding under these circumstances is very dangerous, as case 11 has already illustrated.

The use of opiates in the treatment of malarious fever is an important subject, and will be fully considered in connection with remittent fever.

Section VII.—*Intermittent Fever complicated with Bronchitis, Pneumonia, Rheumatism, Scorbutus, Pericarditis, Asthma.*

Bronchitis.—This complication is not common in Europeans in India; but in natives, next to splenic enlargement, is the most frequent. The cause of this difference between Europeans and natives is, probably, of easy explanation: the former are usually much better protected from cold and wet.

Bronchitis has been observed by me in the fevers of natives in the Deccan, Scinde, and in the Jamsetjee Jejeebhoy Hospital at Bombay. It is also common in Guzerat, and presumably throughout India generally, in places and at seasons when alternations of temperature are considerable, rain frequent, and winds chilling.

It is in the cold months, December, January, and February, and in June and July, — the months of commencing rain-fall in much of the tract of country subject to the influence of the south-west monsoon, — that this complication chiefly occurs.* It may be associated with the quotidians and tertians of those seasons; but it must be remembered that bronchitis with febricula is apt to be mistaken for the affection now under consideration.

Bronchitis is readily detected by the characteristic symptoms and physical signs, and is usually slight; for when it becomes extensive the fever tends to assume a remittent form. It was present in 36 of the 243 clinical cases.

Treatment. — Quinine, with small doses of tartarized-antimony, is in general sufficient for the cure.

Febricula with a periodic tendency, associated with bronchitis, may be confounded with intermittent fever; and this error is sometimes corrected by the results of treatment. Cases, supposed to be intermittents complicated with bronchitis, are occasionally met with in which quinine fails, and antimony proves successful. These have not, in all probability, been true intermittents, but rather instances of febrile and bronchitic phenomena excited by cold or wet in individuals in whom there lingers some degree of previous malarious taint, to which the intermittent character of the fever may be attributable. Whether the explanation now given be just or not, the therapeutic observation is correct and useful to remember.

Pneumonia. — Pneumonia was present in 5 of the 243 clinical cases of intermittent fever; but this complication is much more common in remittent fever, and will be considered in connection with that type.

Rheumatism. — In 4 of the cases a degree of pain of the joints coexisted with the paroxysmal febrile symptoms, sufficient to justify the inference that some amount of the rheumatic diathesis was present.

* In districts subject only to the north-east monsoon, the latter half of October and November probably take the place of June and July.

Scorbutus.—In 5 cases sponginess and discoloration of the gums indicated the presence of this taint. The fever was attended with more pain of the loins and limbs than is usual in this type; and in this and allied forms of cachexia, though observing distinct accessions and intermissions, it is usually characterised by a less amount of reaction, and the distinction into stages is often inappreciable: still, it is to be regarded as malarious, and as requiring anti-periodic remedies, combined with the appropriate means of correcting the cachexia.

Pericarditis.—This complication is rare, and the following is the only case which has come under my notice. It illustrates well the efficacy of that principle of treatment which combines remedies for the inflammation and for the fever. The pericarditis was accompanied with some degree of pneumonia of the right lung.

12.—*Intermittent Fever with Pericarditis and Pneumonia.—Recovery.*—Joaquim Manoel, an African sailor, of stout habit, and twenty-two years of age, was admitted into hospital on the 19th September, 1851, after four days' illness, which, attributed to exposure to wet, commenced with febrile symptoms ushered in with chills, and followed by præcordial uneasiness. On the succeeding days intervening between that of attack and admission into hospital, the febrile paroxysm returned daily, with chills, at 11 A.M., and ceased, with sweating, at 5 P.M. When first seen there was febrile excitement, with full pulse. The tongue was thinly coated, and was florid at the tip and edges. There was abnormal dulness and bronchial respiration in the right dorsal region. There was lancinating pain in the præcordial region, increased by cough and full inspiration. The præcordial dulness was bounded above by the third left rib, below by the sixth, internally by the left margin of the sternum, and externally by a line perpendicular from the nipple. A rough murmur, obscuring both sounds, was heard generally over the præcordial region; but it was most distinct an inch internal to and a little above the nipple. There was no induration or dulness below the margin of the false ribs of either side. He had never suffered from rheumatism. He indulged moderately in the use of spirits. Fifty leeches were applied to the præcordial region; and a pill of five grains of calomel, with ipecacuanha and opium, one grain each, was given. On the morning of the 2nd there was febrile intermission, the præcordial pain was much less, the murmur was not audible, and crepitus began to be heard in the right dorsal region. Quinine, in five-grain doses, was given in the usual way, a blister was applied to the præcordial region and warm turpentine to the right dorsal region, and the pill was repeated at bed-time. From this time there was no recurrence of fever, and there was gradual amendment of the signs of pericardial and pulmonic affection. The quinine was continued; the pill was repeated on the 21st; then discontinued. The quinine was subsequently given, in combination with Dover's powder. He was discharged on the 28th, when the præcordial dulness was bounded above by the fourth rib, below by the fifth, internally by the left sternal margin, and externally by a perpendicular line half an inch internal to the nipple. With exception of slight harshness of the first sound, nothing abnormal was heard. The dulness of the right dorsal region was nearly gone, and vesicular respiration was present. The urine was frequently examined. It was scanty at first; then became more abundant; the specific gravity ranged from 1019 to 1025; it gave no traces of albumen.

Asthma. — The following is the only instance of this complication: —

13. *Intermittent Fever complicated with Asthma.*—Chitim, a Hindoo drummer, of thirty years of age, of stout frame, and a native of Golconda, had suffered for about eight months from intermittent fever and asthma, which was liable to return at intervals of fifteen days. He was admitted into hospital on the 2nd August, 1850. The physical signs of emphysema of the lungs were present. The paroxysm of fever and of dyspnœa recurred together at night, and ceased towards the morning. He was treated with quinine in four-grain doses, at first uncombined, then with sulphate of iron (one grain) and dilute sulphuric acid. No treatment, except rubefacients to the chest, was specially directed against the asthmatic symptoms. On the first and second day after admission, the fever and asthma were much less: they ceased on the third day. He was discharged on the 8th August.

This case is interesting from its bearing on the therapeutic fact, that some cases of spasmodic asthma in India are most successfully treated with quinine and small doses of sulphate of iron during the absence of the paroxysm, and in these it is reasonable to infer that the asthmatic symptoms have been related to malaria as a cause. To determine the probability of a previous malarious influence, by inquiry into the history of the case and the condition of the spleen, constitutes an important part of the examination of asthmatic patients in India. If there be good reason for suspecting it, quinine and iron are indicated, and a more favourable prognosis than in asthma under other circumstances, provided the emphysema is not great, may be entertained.

Prevention of the paroxysm, by an anti-periodic remedy given during the intermission, has throughout these remarks been inculcated as the ruling therapeutic principle in the treatment of intermittent fever, simple and complicated; but means appropriate for the complications, when existing, are not therefore excluded. On the contrary, they are also to be adopted, in the modified manner suggested by the diathesis, and the fact of the control exercised by the prevention of the paroxysm.

CHAP. V.

ON REMITTENT FEVER.

SECTION I.—*The Diagnosis of Remittent Fever, from Intermittent Fever and ardent Continued Fever.—Division into Simple and Complicated.*

THE causes of remittent fever are the same as those of intermittent fever. The essential difference between the two types is, that in the remittent there is merely an abatement—a remission—of the febrile reaction; but in the intermittent, a complete cessation—an intermission. As in the remittent form there is a longer period of fever, it is necessarily a more serious disease; and its prevalence may be looked for when the causes are intense, or the state of predisposition is great.

The evidence that remittent and intermittent fever are different degrees of the same kind of derangement, is of the following nature:—

It is often observed that when the conditions of malaria exist in great degree, remittent fever prevails; but that when these lessen, the type becomes intermittent. It is not unusual for cases of fever, remittent at their commencement, to become intermittent before their close, or for cases that have been intermittent at the outset to pass into the remittent form in their advanced stages. Instances are also not unfrequently met with which seem to occupy an intermediate position, which by some would be classed as intermittents, by others as remittents,—cases in which there is an intermission of the pyrexia, but in which the tongue continues coated, the secretions more or less deranged, and the succeeding paroxysm comes on gradually without rigor.

In well-marked cases the diagnosis is easy; and in respect to the intermediate ones, it is not of much practical importance, for the principles of treatment are similar.

The *common continued fever* which occurs in many parts of India in the hot, dry months of the year, chiefly in April and May, in its most aggravated form in recently-arrived robust Europeans, often favoured by intemperance and fatigue, also requires to be distinguished from remittent fever.

This diagnosis is materially assisted by bearing in mind whether the season is one generally free from malaria or not, whether the temperature is high, and whether the sufferers have been previously exposed to malarious influence or not. The character of the febrile disturbance likewise assists us,—as whether reaction is great, whether there is much cerebral or gastric complication, and whether the remission is distinct.

If the attack be in a hot and non-malarious season, in a recently-arrived European, and the febrile excitement be high and continued, there need be no hesitation in considering the disease to be continued fever, not malarious remittent. The diagnosis is important, for, as will afterwards be explained, the principles of treatment are different; but unfortunately, it is not generally of this simple nature. High fever with cerebral and gastric disturbance may occur in lately-arrived sthenic intemperate Europeans in June, July, August, September, October, months in which, in many parts of India, elevated temperature and the conditions of malaria coexist; or fever in April or May (non-malarious months) may attack Europeans or others, who, though tainted by the malaria of a previous season, are still sthenic, perhaps intemperate, and frequently exposed to the sun: but the fever, if closely watched, will in both instances be found to be characterised by distinct, though perhaps short remissions. The simplest and most practical view of this last, and in European troops at some stations* in India, not infrequent form of fever, is to consider it as compound in its nature, the product partly of malaria, and partly of elevated temperature conjoined with other ordinary exciting causes, acting on sthenic constitutions. The principles of treatment will necessarily consist of a combination of those applicable to the unmixed continued and remittent forms.

Remittent fever may be divided into *simple* and *complicated.* In the first, the derangement of different functions is not greater than is usual in the severer forms of all fevers. In the second, there is present either a local inflammation, or an aggravated de-

* As in the plains of the Ganges and Indus and their tributaries, the Coromandel coast, and the table-lands of the Deccan and Malwa.

gree of some other kind of local derangement. It will be practical and convenient to treat of simple and complicated remittent fever under the separate heads of Symptoms, Pathology, and Treatment.

SECTION II.—*Symptoms of Remittent Fever.—Ordinary, Inflammatory, Adynamic, Congestive, Badly developed, with unexpected Collapse, with peculiar Features.—Also complicated with Cerebral Affection, Irritability of Stomach, Jaundice, Bronchitis, Pneumonia.—Diagnosis from Hectic and Symptomatic Fever.*

Ordinary Remittent Fever.—The first accession of remittent fever is generally preceded by a sense of chilliness, slight, however, in comparison with the rigor which usually ushers in an attack of the intermittent type. The chilliness is succeeded by heat of skin, headache, flushing of the face, frequency of pulse, occasional vomiting, furred tongue, thirst, pain of the loins and limbs, deficient, vitiated alvine secretions, and scanty, high-coloured urine. These symptoms continue for a period of varying duration, and are then followed by a stage of abatement or remission; when the pulse falls in frequency but does not return to the natural standard; the headache, with the pain of the loins and limbs, becomes less, but is not altogether removed; the temperature of the skin decreases, but does not fall to the normal degree; the skin becomes softer, with even a little moisture about the head and trunk; the thirst decreases, and the tongue becomes moister, though still coated.

This remission of the febrile symptoms continues for a time varying in different cases, or in different endemics; and then the exacerbation recurs, sometimes, but this is rare, with commencing chilliness, as on the first accession. Most commonly, however, there is no sense of coldness, but a gradual increase of the fever, till it again reaches its acmé.

In intermittent fever the duration of the paroxysm and of the intermission, and the periods of accession, may vary; and so may the duration and periods of the exacerbation and of the remission in remittent fever.

1. There are cases in which the exacerbation comes on about noon and declines before midnight. The remission continues during the night, and till the noon of the following day, when the exacerbation again recurs.

2. The exacerbation comes on about midnight and continues

till morning, when the remission takes place and remains till night. It is not improbable that in these cases it will be frequently found that the exacerbation has become postponed from the influence of quinine: but on this point I do not speak with confidence.

3. The exacerbation comes on about noon, and is succeeded towards evening by a remission which continues till midnight. Then an exacerbation again takes place, to be followed by a morning remission. This variety is by no means uncommon, and indicates a severe form of the disease,—one in which the fever shows a tendency to become continued, and in which adynamic symptoms are likely to arise.

4. It is sometimes observed that the exacerbation takes place at different hours on alternate days, being on one day earlier, on the other later. In this respect there is an analogy to the double tertian.*

Such are the variations in regard to the duration and periods of exacerbation and remission; but it is impossible to anticipate which of them a particular case will assume: nay more, the natural course of the disease may be changed by treatment, as happens in intermittent fever.

This uncertainty in regard to the periods of exacerbation and remission makes it necessary that the peculiarities, in this respect, of each case, should be ascertained by careful frequent observation.

It will not, however, fail to be remarked that there is one feature common to all,—the morning is the most certain period of remission.†

* No observer of tropical fevers has written with more accuracy on this and other points than Dr. Francis Balfour, in his collection of treatises on the effects of sol-lunar influence; but his labour has been in a great measure lost, in consequence of his practical researches being obscured by trifling theories and affected language. His statement respecting the periods of exacerbation and remission in remittent fever, divested of its peculiar phraseology, amounts to this. The day and night are divided into four periods. Two consist of seven hours each,—viz., from 8.30 A.M. to 3.30 P.M., and from 8.30 P.M. to 3.30 A.M. These are the times of exacerbation, and the latter or nocturnal one is that in which the paroxysms generally appear first, disturbing rest, obscure, often not recognised by the patient, or scarcely recollected after the slumber which succeeds it; and as the disease advances, the febrile symptoms are higher in it than in the diurnal period; and again, as the fever declines, the paroxysm often continues to recur in the nocturnal, after it has ceased to appear in the diurnal, period. The remaining two divisions consist of five hours each,—viz., from 3.30 to 8.30 P.M. and from 3.30 to 8.30 A.M. These are the periods of remission, and at the beginning of fever the first or evening one is distinct; but as the disease advances, and the febrile symptoms run high, it becomes so obscure as not to be observed. *The second or morning period of remission is, in all cases, more distinct, and is almost invariably present in some degree.*

† Hunter, in his observations on the diseases of the army in Jamaica (1779), states

These variations in the period of exacerbation and remission are not peculiar to the ordinary form of simple remittent fever, but are also observed in those other varieties which we shall find owe their peculiarities to an aggravated degree of the stage of exacerbation, or of that of the initiatory cold stage, or to a decreasing period of remission and an increasing duration of exacerbation; while there are others characterised by adynamic phenomena, or complicated by inflammation of an important organ, or other local derangement.

This description of the symptoms of ordinary remittent fever applies to the disease as observed in the European General Hospital at Bombay in seamen*, more or less habituated to a tropical

that the practice of visiting hospitals in the early morning originated in this being the usual period of remission in remittent fever; and it is very probable that the similar practice in India had a similar origin. It is essential to the successful treatment of remittent fever that this fact should not be overlooked, and that the tendency, which I have noticed in medical officers not acquainted with tropical disease, to visit their hospital at a later hour should be checked.

* In some—and these, in some instances, the worst cases—the fever was attributed to the malaria of the dockyard, a locality already alluded to by me.

At the time of my service in the European General Hospital, with the view of ascertaining to what extent the crews of ships undergoing repairs in the dockyard at Bombay were liable to be affected with fever, I obtained, through the kindness of Captain Ross, the Master Attendant, a list of ships of all kinds received into the dockyard during the period (viz., from 1st July, 1838, to 1st July, 1843), to which my notes on fever in the European General Hospital have reference, with the date of docking and undocking each ship. The number of ships amounted to 170. This list I compared with the Hospital Register, and noted opposite to the name of each ship the number of the crew admitted for fever into hospital during the time the vessel was in dock. The following is the result:—Of the steamer *Atalanta*, in dock from the 23rd October, 1839, to the 19th February, 1840, 9 fever cases; of the private ship *Orleana*, in dock from 13th October to 11th November, 1840, 12; of the ship *Herefordshire*, in dock from the 13th October to 10th November, 1840, 10; of the private ship *Morley*, in dock from the 22nd July to the 15th August, 1841, 10; of the remaining ships, 3 fever cases were admitted from one, 2 cases from three, and one case from ten, respectively. From the remaining 152 ships, there were not any admissions of fever during the time they were in the dockyard.

The fevers from the ships *Orleana* and *Herefordshire* I recollect very distinctly: I am in possession of a memorandum to the effect that, on the 8th November, 1840, there were 26 cases of fever in the hospital, of which there were 22 from these two ships, showing that the shipping in the harbour was comparatively free from the disease. The type was chiefly the mild remittent. The admissions from the ship *Morley* were of similar type; and during the time that the ship was in dock, H. M.'s frigate *Endymion* was also there, and part of her crew suffered severely from fever of a very adynamic type. There were not more than 3 or 4 cases admitted into the General Hospital from the *Endymion;* but the following facts have been extracted by me from official records to which I have been allowed to refer.

The *Endymion* was in dock from the 19th July to the 19th August, 1841. On the 28th July, the first cases of fever among the marines took place; from that date to the 12th August, 27 cases occurred; and to the 23rd, 11 more, and 2 additional

climate, and usually seeking admission into hospital, after having been ill three or four days: it also applies to the disease as occurring in natives of good constitution.

Inflammatory Remittent Fever.—It was stated, in reference to intermittent fever, that the amount of febrile reaction in the hot stage had relation to the sthenic or asthenic state of the constitution: so it is also in remittent fever. In robust Europeans, lately arrived in India, exposed to malarious influence, and neglectful of the ordinary means of preserving health, remittent fever, with severe exacerbations, is likely to occur, attended with much headache, pain of limbs, restlessness, flushing of the face, perhaps delirium. The skin is hot and pungent, and the pulse full and frequent. A sense of oppression is experienced at the epigastrium, accompanied by nausea and frequent vomiting. The tongue is much coated, and its edges and tip are often florid. Thirst is urgent, and the excretions are scanty and vitiated. The remissions are well marked, but they are proportionate to the severity of the exacerbation, so that the febrile state in them may almost equal in degree that of the exacerbation in the ordinary mild form of the disease. The term inflammatory, as applied to remittent fever, is not to be understood as implying the presence of local inflammation: it is used merely to express a high degree of febrile reaction.

If to this variety of remittent fever, as now described, the influence of exposure to elevated temperature, or of excesses in drinking be added, then that compound form to which I have already alluded,—in which the exacerbation is of longer, and the remission of shorter duration, and in respect to the classification of which, as continued or remittent, there is often doubt,—will be produced.

cases were subsequently admitted, making altogether 40 marines affected with fever in one month, all of whom had slept on board in the tour of their duty during the time the *Endymion* was in dock; and in addition to these 40, there were only 2 others who slept on board. Thus of 42 who slept on board occasionally, 40 were affected with remittent fever; and to mark the severity of the type, up to the 30th of August 14 had died, and 10, several of whom were in a doubtful state, remained in hospital. Whilst such was the extreme suffering of the marines of the *Endymion*, whose duty as sentries over stores led to their exposure to the noxious night air of the dockyard, the following was the condition of the seamen. From the 24th June, the date of the arrival of the *Endymion* in Bombay, to the 30th August, there were 95 seamen (blue-jackets) ill with fever. In none of these did the type resemble that of the marines, and none proved fatal; and it is distinctly noticed that the carpenters employed *during the day* upon the repairs of the bottom of the vessel, with one exception, escaped any severe attack, and several of them were not attacked at all.

It is a rule of the dockyard that the crews shall not sleep on board whilst the ship is undergoing repairs there; and the statements which have been just made show the salutary operation of this very necessary regulation.

Remittent Fever tending to become continued, then adynamic in character.—It has been stated that sometimes in ordinary remittent fever the exacerbations are double,—one in the day, another in the night. Such cases are generally severe, because the hours of exacerbation are increased in number; and it often happens that after the first or second day of the double exacerbation, or it may be from the very commencement of the attack, the remissions are so slight as to be hardly observed: the fever becomes almost continued in character.* This may proceed from the intensity of the malaria acting on an ordinary constitution, or from a less degree of malaria acting on an asthenic constitution, or (and this is probably a very frequent cause) from the early exacerbations not having been judiciously managed—from neglect of the withdrawal of causes of irritation or excitement, or by the application of means of cure too depressant. Finally, the continued form may be favoured by the access of local inflammation.

When remittent fevers, which have thus passed into the almost continued form, do not prove fatal in the early stages from sudden depression of the vital actions of the nervous system or of the heart, or from congestion, or inflammation of some important organ, but continue beyond the eighth day, or earlier when the asthenia has been great, then a new train of symptoms begins to appear. The pulse becomes more frequent and feeble, the tongue dry, brown and unsteadily protruded. The hands are tremulous, with tendency to subsultus tendinum. There is more or less muttering delirium and drowsiness, and death takes place from exhaustion or coma. In other words, the remittent fever has assumed an adynamic character. With this form of the disease in Europeans I became familiar in the General Hospital at Bombay; and in natives not only in the Jamsetjee Jejeebhoy Hospital, but also in all the other various circumstances in which I have had the opportunity of observing their diseases.

When these phenomena of depressed vital action are present in their most aggravated degree, petechial spots may show themselves

* The term "continued" having been already applied to a different set of circumstances from that in which it is here used, it would have been well, to prevent the risk of confusion, to substitute another term; but I am not prepared to suggest departure from usage. It can only be a very careless reader who will confound the *common* or *ardent continued* fever of the hot months, occurring in sthenic individuals, with fever generally remittent at the beginning, then becoming continued, occurring at malarious seasons, in constitutions asthenic at the outset, or made so by the intensity of the cause or injudicious treatment in the early stages.

on the surface of the body, or there may be oozing of blood about the gums and lips, or epistaxis, or vomiting of blood or of dark-coloured grumous-looking fluid; or mælæna or hæmaturia may be present. These symptoms prove that the chemical and vital conditions of the blood have become signally deranged. To remittent fever thus characterised by petechiæ and hæmorrhages, the term *malignant* has been applied. In its aggravated form it is seldom observed in Bombay; but in its slighter degree it occasionally occurs.

To what are these adynamic symptoms to be attributed? To the intensity of the cause, to the greater amount of febrile excitement consequent upon the fever having become continued, to the previous influence of predisposing causes, as insufficient food, lengthened exposure to hot weather, intemperance, depressing passions, bodily fatigue, or previous disease: or they may arise from medical treatment having been neglected at the commencement, or from its having been too depressing in character, — too much general blood-letting, leeching, antimony, calomel, catharsis, and the neglect of quinine and nourishment.*

When several of these conditions co-exist, — as intense malaria, predisposition, and injudicious medical treatment, — then are combined the conditions most calculated to produce a fever of a highly adynamic and malignant character.

* FEVER, with an unusual proportion of adynamic cases, and consequent mortality, prevailed in the gaol at Sattara from October 1858, to May 1859. A short account of the leading facts will serve to illustrate some of the statements in the text.

The gaol is very faulty in construction, and badly situated; but, generally speaking, has not been unhealthy. The system of dieting and general management has for the most part been good. On the 4th of August, 1858, the dietary was modified by the Assistant-Judge in such a manner as to create general discontent, and affect the comfort and health of the prisoners; but the original system was reverted to on the 2nd of October. The prisoners had also been imperfectly clothed during the greater part of the monsoon and the commencement of the cold season.

A new gaol, distant about a quarter of a mile from the old one, was being built by the prisoners. All, without reference to their previous occupations, were, after a slight meal, marched daily at 6 A.M. to work at the new building, and continued so engaged till 3 P.M., when the labour of the day was finished, and the prisoners returned to the gaol for their principal meal. Consequent on the increase of fever, and the discovery that some of the drains in the gaol were foul, the prisoners were removed on the 23rd of December to the fort of Sattara, placed on a hill 1200 feet above the city, nearly 4000 feet above the sea, and about a mile and a half distant from the new gaol. Thus the prisoners were exposed to greater fatigue in going to and from work, and to greater cold from elevation. The fever and mortality increased, work was intermitted for a time, and the prisoners returned to the old gaol, which had been thoroughly cleaned and whitewashed, on the 15th February, 1859.

The admissions and deaths from fever were as follows: —

Congestive Remittent Fever.—The term congestive is used in the sense in which it has been generally applied by late writers*

	Admissions.	Deaths.
October	10	1
November	16	3
December	24	1
January	34	4
February	42	5
March	37	5
April	15	5
	178	24

With the view of determining the characters of the fever, I examined 93 diaries of recovered cases, and made the following classification with reference to month of admission and type:—

	Intermittent.	Remittent.	Febricula.
November	11	0	0
December and January	10	2	0
February	24	4	9
March	13	5	7
April	6	0	2
	64	11	18

The 75 intermittents and remittents presented no peculiarity; they were the ordinary types which prevail in the Deccan, more or less, every year from October to February. Slight jaundice was present in 16, delirium in 5, and epistaxis in 2. The cases of febricula were also of the type usually prevailing in the Deccan in February, March, and April, more or less, according as the ordinary exciting causes —heat, exposure, fatigue, vicissitudes of temperature—and the predisposition from a plethoric or debilitated state, are present. They occurred in greater proportion among lately arrived ramosees, goldsmiths, writers, and shopkeepers,—classes whom the out-door labour of the gaol system was likely to affect injuriously. They were mostly a few days under treatment, and there was nothing in their origin, type, and course to justify a suspicion (which the gaol authorities were disposed to entertain) that infection from old fever cases acting on new arrivals was the cause.

The notes of 21 fatal cases are before me. They are all remittent, with, in some, a commencement as intermittent. Death was caused by prostration, in some coming on quickly, in others after the lapse of several days. There was jaundice in 7. Six of the fatal cases were under two months' residence, and their ages were, of two 32, and one 35, 48, 65, and 80.

Of the recovered and fatal cases, 4 were stated to have been in attendance on the sick when taken ill. Two recovered; one an ordinary intermittent, the other a mild

* "Outlines of Physiology and Pathology." By Dr. Alison, p. 485.

to a state of depressed action of the vascular and nervous systems in the early stage of fever; the former characterised by a feeble pulse, a cold often damp skin, sighing respiration, and defective secretions; the latter by languor and drowsiness. This condition is probably correctly attributed to the intensity of the malarious poison. Death may take place speedily in the stage of congestion without distinct febrile excitement; or reaction may follow, and the remittent character become well marked and the disease under careful management terminate successfully; or the remissions may be indistinct, the fever almost continued in type, and adynamic symptoms early evolved. There is, as has been remarked by Dr. Alison *, considerable analogy between the symptoms of this form of fever and those of cholera. The collapse of cholera resembles in many features the stage of congestion, and when secondary fever occurs, it is not unlike the reaction which sometimes attends the congestive form of remittent fever. The secondary fever of cholera is, however, apt to run a longer course, and to be complicated with subacute inflammation of important organs. Congestive remittent fever is occasionally observed in the European General Hospital, as well as in Europeans elsewhere

remittent. Two died; one, æt. 41, after one year and six months in the gaol, and one month's attendance on the sick; the other, æt. 52, after 15 years and six months in gaol, and three months' attendance on the sick. There is, therefore, nothing in these facts to justify the suspicion of infection, and it is further probable that these men were selected for this duty because unequal to hard labour. The symptoms and course of the fatal cases—the prostration, the attendant jaundice—in no respect differed from those usually observed in adynamic cases of remittent fever in India, when occurring in persons previously debilitated and out of health.

The medical treatment was faulty: it favoured the duration of the attacks, and the change of type from intermittent to remittent, and from the latter to continued, with development of adynamic phenomena. The defects were, 1. Too active treatment of the stage of reaction by leeches, antimony, calomel, and purgatives. 2. The inadequate use of quinine during the remission: it was often too long delayed, the period was not watchfully selected, and the quantity was insufficient. 3. Insufficient support by frequently repeated suitable nourishment and stimulants chiefly during the remissions. 4. The neglect of an improved and appropriate diet to restore strength before discharge from hospital and return to the system and work of the gaol; hence relapses, with increasing adynamia in each. Several cases were said to be free of fever, but they sank from exhaustion, or, to express it more distinctly, from inanition. In this record there is illustrated—1. The influence of temporary errors in dieting and clothing, of fatigue, and of vitiated atmosphere, in creating a predisposition to be acted on by the malaria of the locality, and the reduced temperature of season and of elevation—thus increasing the quantity of fever. 2. The effect of the predisposition thus engendered, and of ill-directed medical treatment and management in aggravating the type and augmenting the mortality.

* "Outlines of Physiology and Pathology," loc. citat.

in Bombay, chiefly in the malarious season of the year: it has also been noticed by me in the cold season in asthenic natives, who had been badly fed and clothed, and exposed to inclement weather.*

Remittent Fever with badly-developed Symptoms.—In intermittent fever in asthenic individuals, there is not unfrequently, as already explained, an irregularity in the characteristic stages of the paroxysm. Instances of remittent fever similar in kind may also occur: it is a form of disease little calculated to arrest attention. The exacerbation is badly marked, is attended by little heat of skin or vascular excitement; indeed, these symptoms of fever may be absent, but instead of them, there may be some degree of undue restlessness or fretfulness, or incoherence of mind, with tremulous hands, and a tongue coated in the centre; or nausea with tendency to vomit or to diarrhœa may be present. The remission is distinct, but the nights are generally restless. With each recurring exacerbation, the pulse loses strength, the tongue becomes drier and tremulous, tremor of the hands increases, the slight wandering passes into muttering delirium, and perhaps unexpectedly, about the tenth or twelfth day or earlier, the delirium lapses into coma; or the exacerbation terminates with extreme collapse and death.

Mr. Twining's "Insidious Congestive Fever of the Cold Season," † is, it seems to me, of this nature. But this form of fever

* A greater degree of these congestive phenomena, in very malarious districts, has been described by authors. The term has, however, been applied by English writers to other forms of febrile disease. This is much to be regretted. Mr. Twining's "insidious congestive fever of the cold season" is different, and relates to sets of symptoms, some of which I have already alluded to under the head of adynamic remittent fever, and others of which I shall subsequently have to advert to; but none of Mr. Twining's descriptions express merely an undue degree and continuance of the phenomena characteristic of the cold stage. This seems to me the sense in which we should apply the term congestive fever, and, while we thus use it, it by no means follows that we are subscribing to any particular pathological doctrine, as, for example, that which attributes the phenomena of failing heart and nervous system to antecedent congestion of blood; on the contrary, all the phenomena seem to me to be coincident and sequences of the influence of the morbific cause.

Again, the term congestive has been used, as in Reports of the 4th Dragoons, in my possession, in the sense of remittent fever, with marked congestion of the mucous membrane of the stomach or bowels, or of the liver. This is also a faulty use of the term.

† Dr. Edward Goodeve, in a clinical lecture on typhoid fever, published in No. XI. of the "Indian Annals of Medical Science," suggests that Mr. Twining's "insidious congestive fever of the cold season" is that form of continued fever now designated "typhoid;" and much consideration is due to the opinion of this accurate and experienced physician. Though the view taken in the text of similarity between

is not peculiar to this season, for I have witnessed it in Europeans in June and July. The last case which came under my notice was that of an old officer about to leave India, who, in his journey to the coast, sustained a severe fracture of the fore-arm. The injury with other causes of anxiety and long service in India had impaired his constitution. He became affected by the obscure symptoms just described, — restlessness, slight incoherence, then delirium, tremor of the hands, tongue coated and tremulous. The exacerbations and remissions were well marked, and death took place by coma.

This form of disease is important, and liable to be overlooked. It requires careful treatment and close watching. If there be much prostration, increasing from day to day, without any very evident cause, it may be assumed that at some time or other in the twenty-four hours a febrile exacerbation takes place, and the period should be ascertained without delay. If the tongue tends to become coated in the centre, then brown and dry, the existence of a febrile period becomes certain.

This variety of fever may be apprehended in persons whose constitutions have become deteriorated by exposure for successive seasons to elevated temperature, anxiety of mind, intemperance, the causes of scurvy, secondary syphilis, the abuse of mercury, the influence of malaria; and it is not unlikely that in some instances it may depend on previously existing structural disease. But to this latter condition further allusion will be made under the head Pathology.

Remittent Fever with unexpected Collapse. — It was stated that in asthenic individuals the third stage of intermittent fever is sometimes attended by so much exhaustion as to require the assiduous use of stimulants and nourishment. The same feature, is much more frequently observed in remittent fever; and there is no practical fact of greater importance to remember in the management of this disease, than the marked tendency to great collapse so often evinced towards the close of an exacerbation — collapse not unfrequently terminating in death.*

We have learnt that from malaria, habit of body, and continuance

Twining's insidious congestive fever and the varieties described by me as adynamic, remittent fever with badly developed symptoms may be incorrect; still I retain the conviction that none of the forms of fever described in this chapter are of the nature of true "typhoid."

* It is probably to the occurrence of this collapse early in the disease, that the term Algide has been applied by Dr. Haspel and other writers on the diseases of Algeria.

of febrile excitement, there takes place, sooner or later, in all protracted cases of fever, a marked depression of vital action, chiefly of the heart and nervous system. In remittent fever, when this state supervenes, it generally first appears at the commencement of a remission, or just as the exacerbation is passing into it. Therefore, under these circumstances, it is necessary that towards the close of the exacerbation, all agencies — leeches, purgatives, antimonials, — calculated to hurry on and increase the depression, should be carefully avoided; for it is by the injudicious employment of such means that unlooked-for collapse — thready pulse, shrunken features, a cold and damp skin — is apt to occur.* Hence the practical lesson, that in all remittents after the 7th or 8th day, or earlier if the pulse has been feeble, or the hands and tongue tremulous, or the mind wandering, or any other symptom of debility present, we should be careful to avoid depressant means of treatment, more especially towards the close of the exacerbations, and to give suitable nourishment and stimulants assiduously during the remission. At the close of a paroxysm symptoms of exhaustion should be carefully watched for, and should they threaten, then stimulants and nourishment, as ammonia, wine, and strong animal broths, must be liberally administered. Cases of remittent fever have, to my knowledge, been lost, from want of forethought and preparation to carry out these very evident indications of treatment. The following is an instance of unlooked-for collapse terminating fatally.

14.—*Remittent Fever fatal from unexpected Collapse.*—A gentleman of about fifty years of age, of sallow complexion, who had lived several years at different times in tropical climates, and had experienced his share of the cares of life, became, in Bombay, the subject of remittent fever. After the illness had continued four or five days, his medical attendant, not satisfied with the state of his patient, yet not anxious in regard to his safety, wrote to me at one of his evening visits a note requesting me to meet him the following morning. The note was not to be delivered till the early morning, but it was sent at midnight, accompanied with an urgent verbal

* It was in Mr. Twining's writings that I first became acquainted with the full importance of this truth, and it is among the most valuable of his many excellent clinical lessons. It is now upwards of twenty-five years since this accurate observer published his "Clinical Illustrations," yet I am satisfied, from personal observation and the perusal of the diaries of cases, that this important feature of remittent fever is not yet generally understood and appreciated by medical men in India. It is still not uncommon to hear of "anomalous" cases of fever terminating fatally, unexpectedly, "notwithstanding the usual treatment having been actively followed,"— the marvel being, not the occurrence of death, but the want of knowledge of the disease, the consequent surprise at the result, and the neglect of the means of its prevention.

message, begging me to come immediately. The house was in my neighbourhood, and I was there in a very short space of time, but I found that the patient had just died. The evening febrile exacerbation had terminated in unexpected and fatal collapse.

In Dr. A. S. Thomson's report * on fever in Her Majesty's 17th Regiment, at Colaba, in the year 1841, an epidemic to which I have already alluded in the chapter on intermittent fever, there is the following case: —

15.* *Great Collapse in the course of Remittent Fever.—Recovery by Stimulants.*—"Private W. S., aged twenty-two years, in India three years, sanguine habit. Admitted on the 1st July, 1840, complaining of general debility, &c. A vein was opened; but he fainted before many ounces slowly came, and no more could be got; had an emetic and purgative; he afterwards complained of headache and had sixty leeches applied to the head, and a diaphoretic mixture constantly given. 2nd of July: Pulse 84, skin hot and moist, no pain. Continued the diaphoretic mixture. At night occasional delirium, skin moist and hot bowels open, eyes wild, pulse 124, soft; complains of abdominal pain. A blister was applied to the neck and head, and a draught composed of wine, tinct. morph. muriat. and tartar emetic given; the head to be rubbed over with strong tartar emetic ointment.

3rd. Slept a little after draught; pulse 120, skin moist, bowels open, much irregularity in his manner. Diaphoretic mixture and wine every second hour, with forty drops of tinct. muriate of morphia at night.

4th. Pulse 79: skin moist; eruption on head from antimony; slept none; bowels open; occasional delirium. The wine and diaphoretic mixture continued; at night five grains of calomel and five of hyoscyamus.

5th. Slept well last night, no fever; pulse 76. Six grains of quinine every third hour. *Vespere.* Calomel, antimony, and hyoscyamus.

6th. Fever with delirium came on yesterday at noon, and has continued since; had sixty leeches to the head, and this morning pulse 109; skin hot and dry; head warm and temples throbbing; thirty leeches applied to the head and diaphoretic mixture given.

7th. The most fearful collapse followed the application of the leeches and the fever; skin covered with cold perspiration and pulse scarcely felt. Brandy and carbonate of ammonia given every ten minutes. Had forty drops of tincture of morphia last night and slept well. Pulse 106 this morning; skin cold and clammy; no pain; the brandy and carbonate of ammonia to be continued.

8th. Strength impaired; pulse 120; skin hot. Diaphoretic mixture to be given with wine; bowels open.

9th. Pulse 96; skin hot and moist; no pain; occasional delirium.

It is useless to detail this case further. No violent paroxysm of fever occurred again, although there was occasional slight increase of fever. He was convalescent on the 31st of July, but was not fit for duty until the 11th of September, 1840."

It is almost a corollary from the feature of remittent fever which has just been considered, that the period of death in protracted fatal cases will be not the exacerbation but the remission.

Certain other occasional Features of Remittent Fever. — 1. It occasionally happens that cases of remittent fever which ultimately

* "Transactions of the Medical and Physical Society of Bombay," No. 5, p. 84.

prove severe, have not this character at the commencement; but assume it after two or three slight exacerbations. This is best explained by supposing that at first the incubation is not perfected, and that its completion is followed by the aggravation. It may be further suggested that, if this explanation be true, we can readily understand how treatment, unduly depressing in the early days, may intensify the action of the malaria and advance its incubation.

2. In remittent fever in asthenic constitutions there may be a decreasing degree of the febrile exacerbations, but, if this be attended with marked increasing asthenia in the remissions, we must be careful not to interpret favourably the lessening exacerbation: it is generally otherwise — the febrile excitement has merely diminished in consequence of the sinking power of the vital actions. Such cases if misunderstood, and not very carefully watched and treated, are apt to terminate fatally by collapse at the close of an exacerbation.

3. In remittent fever a state of great exhaustion sometimes takes the place of the period of exacerbation; and if such cases do well, the recurrence of febrile reaction at the period of exacerbation is probably of favourable import. I quote a fatal case in which this feature was observed.

16. *Exhaustion taking the place of Exacerbation in Remittent Fever.*—A gentleman, some years resident in India, living freely, and suffering from occasional attacks of intermittent fever with irritability of stomach in the malarious season of the year consulted me for irritability of stomach, which soon ceased, but left complete disinclination for food. Some nights he slept badly, others well; sometimes from a morphia draught, sometimes without one. He complained only of great languor, and looked very exhausted. Three or four glasses of wine, with beef-tea and jellies, were taken daily. He continued for three or four days to attend to his avocations, till one afternooon febrile heat of the skin was for the first time noticed; it was present during the night and the following morning, but then in less degree. Eight-grain doses of quinine and nourishment were given. At noon there was exacerbation, but towards the after part of the day he became very feeble and exhausted. Wine and nourishment were freely given. He rallied towards night, and passed the night quietly. On the following morning he was free of all fever, and much less exhausted than on the previous day. The quinine was resumed, and beef-tea and wine were freely given. At 1 P.M. there was rather more exhaustion, but no fever. The wine was more frequently given, and the quinine and nourishment continued, but without effect. The exhaustion increased towards evening. Brandy was substituted for the wine. He continued quite collected till midnight, when he became somewhat drowsy, and died at four o'clock of the following morning. In this case there was no vomiting. The wine and nourishment were retained. There was no diarrhœa.

Complicated with Cerebral Symptoms.— Under this head are included cases of remittent fever in which there is evident derangement of the cerebral functions, as delirium, drowsiness, convulsion.

Delirium occurs under two sets of circumstances. It may come on in the early exacerbations attended with much headache, flushing of the face, vascularity of the conjunctivæ, and may be more or less active: this is its usual character in sthenic constitutions, and at the commencement it is unattended with failing action of the heart. In less sthenic individuals there is incoherent rambling, with less headache and flushing; and though there may be no distinct adynamic phenomena, the pulse is deficient in power. Delirium is present chiefly in the exacerbations; and when not altogether absent in the remissions, is generally much moderated. Should medical treatment fail in checking the fever and removing these head symptoms, then, after a time, varying in different cases, the delirium gradually passes into drowsiness, coma, and death. This change is generally first observable towards the termination of an exacerbation, and is always attended with failing action of the heart. When these symptoms occur under the circumstances just described, they may be regarded as depending upon the co-existence of inflammation or undue determination of blood to the brain and its membranes.

Delirium, however, may commence at a more advanced stage of the fever, as after the eighth or tenth day, or later when the constitution has been good, and earlier when it has been bad. It is low and muttering, without headache or flushing of the face; and is attended with commencing adynamic symptoms, as tremor of the hands, twitching of the fingers, a tongue tremulous and dryish, and a pulse of increasing frequency and decreasing strength. Should amendment not take place, the delirium will after a time pass into drowsiness, and death by coma will succeed, unless this event has been anticipated by collapse at an earlier period before the stage of coma has arrived. Symptoms of deranged and failing cerebral function, in adynamic fever, merely express the concurrence of the brain in the general failure of vital actions.

From this description of delirium in fever, it would seem that the difference between that from adynamia and from active determination to the brain, is the co-existence, in the former, of tremors of the tongue and hands, and twitching movements of the fingers. Too much importance, however, may be attached to these deranged muscular actions as diagnostic of merely an adynamic state; for they are not unfrequently met with in association with subacute cerebral inflammation, either idiopathic or complicating fever, and are to be regarded as indicative of adynamic derangement of the nervous system, only when the other phenomena of adynamia are well marked, and the history of the case distinctly points to the same conclusion.

It has been stated that the delirium when continued passes into drowsiness.* This symptom, when thus arising, is of most unfavourable prognosis. But drowsiness occasionally appears in remittent fever, unpreceded by delirium, generally in the earlier stages and usually associated with a slow pulse and other congestive phenomena. Drowsiness under these circumstances is by no means so dangerous a symptom as when it follows delirium; care should be taken not to confound these two conditions. The first is probably dependent on passive congestion; the second on commencing serous effusion. Lastly, there are occasional cases with delirium or tendency to drowsiness coming on early in the disease, towards the end of a paroxysm in fevers of bad type, accompanied with signs of general collapse and dependent on enfeebled nervous energy.

In the chapter on Intermittent Fever a case is narrated in which only the period of paroxysm was marked by cerebral derangement. This feature may also occur in remittent fever. In asthenic cases with cerebral symptoms the period of exacerbation is sometimes indicated by increase of delirium or of drowsiness, rather than by distinct aggravation of febrile excitement.

In some cases convulsion comes on intermediately between delirium and coma. This event may generally be referred to excesses in drinking, to derangement of excretion from structural or other causes, or to inflammatory action of the membranes or substance of the brain.

Complicated with Irritability of Stomach.—Occasional vomiting may be present in ordinary remittent fever, and may occur in greater degree in the inflammatory form of the disease; but under these circumstances it is merely one of the symptoms of an uncomplicated type.

But gastric irritability may be urgent, attended with uneasiness and tenseness of the epigastrium and a tongue florid at the tip or

* The liability to retention of urine in this state of the cerebral functions is so well known that it seems almost unnecessary to allude to it. Yet I have seen it overlooked sufficiently often to convince me that attention cannot be called too frequently to the fact.

edges. In this state there is probably some degree of gastritis, and it may exist in constitutions either sthenic or asthenic. Remittent fever thus complicated has been termed *Gastric Remittent.* At other times the vomiting is frequent, and the matters ejected are tinged with bile, and the tongue is covered with a yellow fur, but without florid edges and tip. This form of the disease is confined to sthenic constitutions, and has been termed *Bilious Remittent.*

Complicated with Jaundice.—This complication exists occasionally in Europeans, but still more frequently in natives. The notes of twenty-seven cases treated in the clinical ward are before me, and they will be particularly alluded to in the Section on the Pathology of the disease.

The presence of jaundice is easily recognised by the tint of the skin and conjunctivæ, the state of the urine, and the generally pale colour of the alvine discharges; and there is usually present some degree of tenderness below the margin of the right false ribs. Jaundice is rarely observed from the very commencement of the attack. It generally comes on after the fifth day, and has not, as a rule, in my experience, been attended with irritability of stomach. The tongue for the most part has a yellow slimy appearance, and general soreness of the body is not unfrequently complained of.

The few observations which I have to make on affections of the *bowels*, the *liver* and *spleen*, as complications of remittent fever, will be included under the head Pathology.

Complicated with Bronchitis and Pneumonia.—These affections do not frequently complicate remittent fever in Europeans in India; but we are told by Dr. R. H. Hunter*, in his interesting Medical History of the Queen's Royal Regiment in Affghanistan and Beloochistan, in 1838 and 1839, that in the colder climate of these countries, chiefly in the winter months, pneumonia was a frequent complication of remittent fever.

Bronchitis is a common accompaniment of remittent fever in natives of India; and in the Jamsetjee Jejeebhoy Hospital at Bombay pneumonia is the most usual of all the inflammatory complications in asthenic subjects. Indeed, so often is pneumonia present, that great risk is incurred of overlooking its existence in this class of patients, unless, in the management of all fever cases, we observe the rule of careful examination by percussion and

* "Transactions of the Medical and Physical Society of Bombay," No. 3, p. 183.

auscultation. But it is not only in hospital patients that this complication is met with. It occurs in all classes of the native community, and I have been consulted in not a few instances in which it had been previously overlooked, to the great hazard of life, merely because it had not been sought for.

The detailed consideration of this important subject will be included in the Chapter on Idiopathic Pneumonia.

Diagnosis of Remittent Fever from Hectic and Symptomatic Fevers.—The distinction of remittent from intermittent and continued fevers has already been noticed; but the further diagnosis will be more conveniently considered now. The frequent complication of inflammation of important internal organs with this type of fever has been stated. In a general hospital, into which patients are admitted often at advanced periods of disease, and in which a large proportion of the inmates are asthenic, affected with local inflammations characterised by great obscurity of symptoms, it may happen that hectic may be confounded by the superficial observer with remittent fever.* Careful inquiry into the previous history of the case and scrutiny into the state of all important organs ought to prevent an error of this kind.

When an abiding malarious influence is present, febrile disturbance excited by ordinary causes generally assumes more or less of a periodic character; and when an individual thus tainted with malaria becomes affected with idiopathic inflammation of an important organ, the symptomatic fever is also often characterised by periodicity: it may, indeed, be distinctly remittent.†

It is in individuals who have been long resident in tropical climates that this tendency of symptomatic febrile disturbance to become remittent is chiefly observed; and consequently when local inflammation and remittent fever co-exist in such subjects, it may be often doubtful whether the fever is idiopathic and complicated with an inflammation, or the inflammation idiopathic and the fever symptomatic. In determining this question the history of the attack affords material assistance. The inflammatory complications of remittent fever do not generally arise till several days after the commencement of the fever; whereas the symptoms of idiopathic inflammation and the febrile disturbance are nearly coincident. Moreover, in idiopathic fever, the febrile phenomena are greater in

* The diagnosis between remittent fever and the adynamic febrile disturbance of pyœmia will be considered in the Section on Pyœmia in the Chapter on Blood Diseases.

† The same fact is often observed in surgical practice, when individuals of this kind of constitution become the subjects of serious injuries.

proportion to the inflammatory action, and are attended by a greater amount of general derangement of function than usually obtains in symptomatic fever. Notwithstanding attention to these considerations, the diagnosis is often uncertain, for in hospital practice the history of disease is generally imperfect. It is fortunate, however, that the doubt which may thus arise does not affect the treatment; for the same therapeutic principles are in a great measure applicable to both forms of disease.

Section III.—*Pathology.—Mortality from Remittent Fever.—Relation of Type to Diathesis and previously existing Structural Lesions.—Complication with Cerebral Affection and Consideration of the Pathological Import of Cranial Serous Effusion.—Complication with Gastric Irritability, Affection of the Bowels.—Hepatitis, Jaundice, Parotitis, and Pneumonia.*

When the effects of malaria are compared with those of the special causes of the zymotic continued fevers of colder climates, this striking difference is observable: in the former, there are daily suspensions of the influence with a return more or less complete to normal action; in the latter, the influence is continuous for many successive days. On this distinction centres the difference in the principles of treatment.

The rate of mortality from remittent fever depends upon the type of the disease. I am not acquainted with any data which give the mortality of ordinary remittents separated from the other forms: it is doubtless very small. The inflammatory, congestive, adynamic and complicated varieties occasion the chief mortality; and in general hospitals the frequent lateness of the period of admission tends to increase it.

In 113 selected clinical cases of natives, 19 deaths occurred. Nine of these were complicated with jaundice, 3 with cerebral affection, 3 with pneumonia*, 2 with bronchitis, 1 with dysentery, and 1 with splenic enlargement. In 7 of the 19 fatal cases the fever was adynamic, viz. in the 3 with cerebral affection, the 2 with bronchitis, 1 with pneumonia, and 1 with jaundice.

Through the courtesy of the Medical Board of Bombay, the opportunity has been afforded me of referring to the fatal cases of European officers in the Bombay army and civil service; and

* These are distinct from the cases which I shall have to notice when considering idiopathic pneumonia.

also to the cases of those recommended for change of climate, from the year 1829 to 1848. They amounted to 1699. Notes were made of the recovered cases of chief interest: they were 372 in number, and 49 were of remittent fever. I have also notes of 311 fatal cases which constitute nearly the whole mortality of the period: of these there were 90 deaths from remittent fever, that is, 28·7 per cent. of the total mortality. On inquiring into the character of the fever in these 90 fatal cases, it appears that in 33 death took place by coma preceded by delirium, with intermediate convulsion in some. In a considerable proportion irritability of stomach was present: in 6 it was the most prominent symptom. Death occurred from early and speedy collapse in 12 cases, and in the greater number of them the influence of depressant remedies, pushed too far in the exacerbation, was very apparent. Adynamic symptoms were present in 8, and congestive phenomena also in 8. Jaundice complicated, 7, and hepatic inflammation, 2.*

Before proceeding to the consideration of the pathology of the several varieties of remittent fever, it is desirable that attention should be directed to two general observations which are applicable to all.

Inattention to the diathesis and habits of the affected, and to the intensity of the morbific cause, has led to needless confusion in the pathology, and to serious errors in the treatment of remittent fever. The discrepancy of opinion on these points, between the writers on tropical diseases towards the end of the 18th century and those of a later period, is best explained by this oversight. The first class observed the disease in individuals tainted with scurvy, and excited by intense malaria; the second, in persons of sthenic constitution, and excited by a less degree of the morbific cause. The one trusted to bark and stimulants for the cure; the other, to bloodletting, mercury, and purgatives. Both were in extremes. The truth lies between.

2. In my report† on remittent fever in the European General Hospital in Bombay, published in 1843, there is the following remark: "In regard to the character of the subjects in whom these congestive symptoms are likely to appear, my impression is that they will be found to occur most frequently in persons who have passed the meridian of life, and in whom there exists more or less

* I shall return to the mortality from remittent fever in Chap. VI.

† "Transactions of the Medical and Physical Society of Bombay," No. 4, p. 186.

long-standing organic disease of the heart, the liver, or the kidneys." Subsequent experience has confirmed the importance of this suggestion, not only as regards congestive symptoms, but also all other phenomena of depressed action, as well as some of the complications, particularly the cerebral.

Indeed it is very evident that we cannot fully comprehend any case of fever, or direct its treatment with advantage, unless by close inquiry into the previous history and careful scrutiny of the state of all important organs, we have determined whether it is an idiopathic fever in a system previously sound, or in one generally deteriorated or the subject of structural imperfection of an important organ.

Haspel *, in his treatise on the diseases of the French troops in Algeria, expresses the same idea, when he suggests that the phenomena of Algide fever are probably related to a structurally feeble heart.

In my notes on the fatal cases of sick officers, there are three of remittent fever in which after death Bright's disease of the kidney was found; but in only one is the character of the febrile symptoms noted, they were obscure, the stomach was irritable, and death took place by coma.

The five following cases †, illustrative of these remarks, were observed by me in the European General Hospital, and in the Jamsetjee Jejeebhoy Hospital.

17. *Remittent Fever.—Death by coma.—Bright's disease of both kidneys.*—John Robinson, aged thirty-seven a stout sailor of intemperate habits, was in the European General Hospital from June 28th to July 1st, 1838, affected with anasarcous swelling of the feet and legs. He was discharged and had returned to his duty on board one of the steam-vessels. He was again brought to the hospital on the 12th July in a drowsy state. The pulse was frequent and small and the skin warm. The tongue had a yellow fur at the sides, but was florid in the centre. It appeared from his own statement that he had suffered from fever since the 8th, with vomiting and diarrhœa, but that he had not been ashore since he left the hospital on the 1st instant. The head was shaved, a blister was applied to the neck, and ten grains of calomel were given. At 6 P.M. the drowsiness had increased, the skin was moist and cold, the pulse frequent and feeble, and the bowels had not been opened. A turpentine injection was exhibited, sinapisms were applied to the feet, and a blister to the epigastrium, and a draught with camphor mixture, carbonate of ammonia, and nitrous ether, was given every third hour. On the 13th, the bowels had been freely moved, there was less drowsiness, and the pulse was 100, small and sharp. The draughts were directed

* "Maladies de l'Algérie," vol. ii. p. 320.

† These cases are quoted merely as illustrative of febrile phenomena in individuals with old structural disease of important organs. I do not stop to inquire whether the treatment might have been better or not.

to be continued, with the addition to each of fifteen minims of colchicum wine, and a scruple of calomel was given at bed-time. The drowsiness recurred, and increased to coma, the pulse sank, and he died at 4 A.M. of the 14th.

Inspection four hours after death.—The body was stout and muscular. *Head.*—The membranes and substance of the brain were congested.—*Chest.* The lungs did not collapse fully, and there were costal adhesions of the right one. The heart was soft, flabby, and contained fibrinous coagula. *Abdomen.*—The liver was pale, and parts of its surface were marked with cicatrices, as if from former abscesses. The mucous coat of the stomach was of dark red colour and softened. That of the colon and rectum also was of dark red tint. Both kidneys were enlarged to double their natural size, and had undergone yellow degeneration.

18. *Remittent Fever with adynamic symptoms.—Serum underneath the arachnoid and at the base of the cranium.—No coma.—The liver much enlarged.—Dark rosy tint of the mucous coat of the stomach.*—John Martin, aged fifty-eight, cook of the ship *Herefordshire*, was admitted into hospital on the 31st October, 1840. He stated that for two days he had suffered from vomiting, purging, headache, and sense of oppression at the lower part of the sternum, attributed to exposure to the sun whilst the ship was undergoing repairs in dock. On admission, the face was flushed, there was anxiety and oppression; the pulse was 120, jerking and easily compressed, abdomen full, tongue dryish and florid, and the skin hot and dry. He was freely leeched on the epigastrium and blistered, was cupped on the nucha, and subsequently blistered. He took two or three ten-grain doses of calomel, and one of a scruple. The symptoms altered little. There was much restlessness and moaning, oppressed breathing, frequent vomiting, dejections of dirty light grey colour and watery, tongue dry and florid, pulse frequent and compressible, skin dry and generally above the natural temperature, and the abdomen full. He continued quite sensible, and died in the forenoon of the 2nd November.

Inspection five hours after death.—Head. There was a thin veil of serum under the arachnoid membrane on the convex surface of the brain, and an ounce at the base of the skull. On incising the substance of the brain, more than the usual number of bloody points were observable. *Chest.*—There were old adhesions of the right lung. Both were moderately collapsed, and there was no congestion of the posterior parts. The cavities of the right side of the heart were full of blood, and there was commencing disease of the aortic valves and beginning of the aorta. *Abdomen.*—The omentum was loaded with fat, and the intestines, both great and small, were collapsed. The liver enlarged reached to the crest of the os ilium and to the umbilicus, was of pale yellow colour, and, when incised, did not give out much blood. The gall-bladder was rather flaccid. The spleen was soft and pulpy. The mucous coat of the stomach had a dark rosy tint throughout, with dark brown patches, but the texture was not softened. The kidneys were somewhat lobulated and rather small, but there was no well-marked disease of their structure.

19. *Remittent Fever with irregular symptoms in an intemperate man of very corpulent habit, and in whose head, heart, liver, and kidneys there was extensive old organic disease.*—Thomas Moss, aged thirty-seven, an engineer of the steam department, of full and corpulent habit, who had served ten years in the West Indies and ten months in Bombay, was admitted into the European General Hospital on the 5th April, 1841. The abdomen was full and uneasy but not very tender on pressure, the skin was dry and of the natural temperature, the pulse 100 and sharp, and the tongue pretty clean. He stated that since the previous day he had suffered from pain of abdomen with occasional bilious vomiting and purging. He was bled to twenty ounces, and some leeches were applied to the abdomen, a warm bath used, and fifteen grains of calomel, one grain of ipecacuanha, and two grains of opium given at bed-time. He passed a restless night, and on the morning of the 6th the breathing was

hurried and oppressed. The abdomen was full, with dulness on percussion for two or three inches beyond the margin of the right ribs and extending across the epigastrium to the left hypochondrium, and between the last left false ribs and the os ilium. The pulse was 120, easily compressed but wiry, the action of the heart and the sounds were confused, tongue coated, bowels not opened, no vomiting, and the conjunctivæ were yellowish. He was cupped on the cardiac region, a scruple of calomel was given, and afterwards a purgative draught. The bowels were freely moved, but the symptoms were unchanged, with exception that the pulse on the evening of the 5th was feeble. It was now reported that he had been a man of intemperate habits. A blister was applied over the cardiac region, and diuretics with gin were given repeatedly. The symptoms continued with failing pulse and coldish skin, and on the morning of the 7th, commencing coma: he died at 10 A.M. of that day.

Inspection five hours after death.—The body was extremely corpulent; there was a layer of fat fully two inches thick in the abdominal parietes. *Head.*—Much blood flowed on separating the scalp from the cranium. All over the convex surface of the hemispheres the arachnoid was pearly, and in many places much thickened; and underneath it there was a layer of serum veiling in many places the interspaces of the convolutions. There were about three drachms of serum in the lateral ventricles, and two ounces at the base of the skull. In the coats of the basilar artery and of those of the vessels forming the circle of Willis, and given off from it, there was much thickening from white deposit, in places, almost ossific in character: in these vessels there was a small coagulum of blood moulded to their shape. *Chest.*—Adhesions connected both lungs to the costal pleuræ. The greater part of the lower lobe of the right lung was in a state of red hepatisation, and when cut serum streamed from it. The left lung was œdematous posteriorly, but not hepatised. The heart was the size of a bullock's chiefly from hypertrophy with dilatation of the left ventricle, the right ventricle was rather small, the right auricle was dilated and filled, as well as the ventricle, by a firm yellow fibrinous coagulum. There was commencing yellow deposit on the inner surface of the aorta, but it had proceeded to no great extent. *Abdomen.*—The contents of the abdomen ascended to the level of the fourth rib, and thus encroached on the capacity of the chest. The omentum was much loaded with fat, the mesentery consisted of a layer of fat fully a quarter of an inch thick, and the intestines were in general contracted and looked like a fringe to the more conspicuous mesentery. The liver was much enlarged, of bright yellow colour externally and internally, and the incised surface had a small granular aspect. Spleen healthy. Both kidneys were considerably enlarged, with cysts from the size of a pea to a filbert standing in relief from the surface. The substance of the kidneys was also occupied by similar cysts; and the contents of some consisted of a dark grey grumous fluid, while that of others was straw-coloured serum. In one of the kidneys there was also a good deal of yellow degeneration.

20. *Remittent fever in a person of very intemperate habits, with symptoms in some respects resembling delirium tremens.—Death by coma.—Three ounces of serum at the base of the skull; Liver much enlarged.—Commencing degeneration of the kidney.—Mucous coat of the colon softened with here and there red patches, with a mucous follicle in the centre of each discoloration.—Softening of the mucous coat of the stomach.*—Thomas Chittenden, aged thirty-four, an engineer of the steam department, of intemperate habits, and frequently in hospital suffering from febrile attacks, was admitted on the 30th of August, 1839. He stated that for eight or nine days he had been affected with febrile symtoms attended with irritability of stomach. On admission he complained much of headache, and the bowels were relaxed and the tongue yellow. Thirty-six leeches were applied to the temples, and six grains of calomel, one grain of ipecacuanha and one of opium were given. At the evening visit it was reported that he had vomited frequently and been affected with general tremors which con-

tinued. The tongue was tremulous and yellow, the abdomen was somewhat full and tender on pressure at the epigastrium and right ribs, there was much headache, the skin was covered with moisture, and the pulse was compressible. The bowels had not been opened. A purgative enema was ordered, blisters were directed to the epigastrium and to the nucha, and ten grains of calomel and two of opium were given at bedtime. The blister acted well, and on the morning of the 31st (full moon) the headache was lessened, the pulse 90, and the tongue not so tremulous. He was ordered saline mixture with tartar emetic and tincture of hyoscyamus. He slept for two hours during the day and his bowels were freely moved. During the night, there was no sleep, and on the morning of the 1st of September the tongue and hands were tremulous, the countenance flushed, the pupils dilated, and the pulse 96. Cold affusion was ordered to the head, and saline mixture with two drachms of tincture of hyoscyamus every second hour for three doses. At the evening visit he was still tremulous, his manner was startled, and he muttered to himself, the pulse was feeble and the skin moist. One dark-coloured dejection had been passed. Cold affusion to the head. Camphor mixture one ounce and a half, antimonial mixture four drachms, tincture of hyoscyamus two drachms every second hour till he sleeps; brandy one ounce every hour for three doses, and then every second hour, and calomel eight grains, opium one grain h. s. The pills were taken, also four ounces of brandy and the draught three times, but he continued agitated, talking incoherently and tearing the dressings from the blister, and at midnight there was constant inarticulate muttering, spasmodic action of the muscles of the face, pupils dilated and insensible to light, skin hot, and the pulse rapid and feeble. Cold affusion was directed to be used to the head every hour while the scalp continued hot, sinapisms were placed on the feet and the other remedies omitted. He became comatose and died at 6 A.M.

Inspection nine hours after death. — The body stout, and the external surface tinged deeply yellow. *Head.* — The dura mater was faintly tinged yellow. The vessels of the membranes were moderately congested. The convolutions of the convex surface of the depending parts of the hemispheres were veiled with serum effused beneath the arachnoid membrane, and there were between two and three ounces at the base of the skull. *Chest.* — The lungs were emphysematous and only partially collapsed. The heart was healthy. The cavity of the chest was encroached on by the liver which on the right side reached to the fourth rib and coursed obliquely across to the seventh rib of the left side. *Abdomen.* — Omentum loaded with fat. The liver weighed seven and a half pounds, was externally mottled chocolate and buff, and admitted of a ready separation of the peritoneal coat; the incised surface was of yellow colour, mottled and softened. The gall-bladder contained about an ounce of thin bile. The mucous coat of the cardiac end of the stomach was of dark-marbled red colour, somewhat thinned and somewhat softened, of the pyloric end pale and mammillated. There was vascularity of the commencement of the mucous coat of the duodenum but the texture was sound. The large intestine was distended throughout but there was no thickening of its walls, the mucous coat was tinged yellow, thinned, and generally softened, the mucous follicles were in many places apparent but not prominent; and throughout the colon there were red patches here and there, mostly the size of a split pea, some larger, with a follicle in the centre of many of them, and in these places the mucous coat was thin, soft, and pulpy, and after its removal the areolar tissue underneath presented in some instances a vascular patch. The bowel was filled with thin yellow feculence. The spleen was of natural size. The kidneys were nearly natural, with perhaps commencing yellow degeneration of the cortical substance, evinced by buff streaks.

21. *Remittent Fever with adynamic symptoms.* — *Obscure pneumonia.* — *Death without coma.* — *Bright's disease of both kidneys.* — Crooshnah Sutooa, aged twenty-six, a Maratha labourer, was brought to the Jamsetjee Jejeebhoy Hospital on the 5th

of July, 1852, being the first day of his illness, with febrile symptoms. There was slight jaundice, and he was reported to have been delirious during the night. There were irregular exacerbations and remissions, and the pulse was frequently badly developed. He had uneasiness at the margin of the right ribs. There was not much delirium, neither brownness nor dryness of tongue. The breathing was hurried, but no signs of pneumonia were noted before the 13th, when there was slight dulness of the right dorsal region which, however, did not increase, and on the 20th occasional crepitus was detected in the right lateral region. He had occasional cough. On the evening of the 20th there was commencing erysipelatous inflammation of the back, with large bullæ resting on a dark base. On the 21st the pulse became feeble, the breathing more hurried, and he died without coma on the 23rd. The state of the urine had not been inquired into.

Inspection eighteen hours after death. — *Chest.* There were old adhesions of the third lobe of the right lung to the parietes and to the diaphragm, and slight serous effusion in the sac of the right pleura. There was increased redness of the substance, and considerable œdema of the right lung, with hepatised nodules here and there in the upper and third lobes. Of the left lung there were slight adhesions, slight œdema with increased redness, and here and there hepatised nodules. The heart was healthy. *Abdomen.* — The stomach and intestines were distended with flatus. The liver was slightly enlarged, flabby, and of pale yellow colour. The kidneys were both enlarged, the right weighed seven ounces, the left six and a half. On removing the capsule from the right kidney the surface was observed to be mottled dark red and yellow, and the cortical substance was of dark red colour and encroached on the tubular portion which was hardly distinguishable. The left kidney was externally mottled yellow and red; the cortical portion internally was of fatty appearance and yellow colour and was considerably increased in size, with merely traces of the tubular part here and there.

This case was treated and reported by Mr. S. Carvalho. The treatment consisted of quinine, diaphoretics, and stimulants. The wet sheet was twice used with removal of the febrile heat; but it seemed to me that it increased the internal congestions.

Complicated Remittent Fever. — Cerebral Complication. — The pathology of this complication is very important; for fully one third of the fatal cases of remittent fever in European officers in the Bombay Presidency is of this nature, and it is probable that the proportion is still greater in the remittents of sthenic European soldiers. But the cerebral affection is not, in all cases, attributable to malaria alone, but is often caused by undue exposure to the sun, or intemperance. The influence of mental anxiety ought also to be regarded; and, in natives, the habit of opium eating and ganja smoking must not be lost sight of.

When describing the symptoms of this complication, I stated that they might depend on different conditions of the brain.

1. Headache, flushing of the countenance, delirium occurring early in the attack — due to the direct influence of the causes, and not merely to that of frequently recurring exacerbations — depend, for the most part, on active determination of blood to the membranes and substance of the brain which, unless re-

moved or prevented by treatment, is likely to terminate in serous effusion.

The following six cases are illustrative of cerebral symptoms appearing under these circumstances, and in four of them the influence of intemperance is apparent.

22. *Remittent Fever—Death by convulsion and coma.—Vascular congestion of the vessels of the pia mater.—Rosy tint of the substance of the brain.—One ounce of serum at the base of the skull.—The heart dilated and its tissue pale and flabby.—Partial redness, thinning, and softening of the mucous coat of the stomach.—Peyer's glands enlarged.—The spleen enlarged and softened, and the kidneys congested.*—Laurence Fearon, aged thirty-seven, an engineer of the steam department, and of full habit. During the four months of his residence in Bombay, he had been several times in hospital ill with fever, attended with gastric irritability. He was again admitted on the evening of the 2nd of September, 1839, having been ill with fever for about a week before admission. There was headache with pain at the margin of the right false ribs, diarrhœa, thirst, febrile heat, pulse 108, full. He was bled to sixteen ounces, the head was shaved and cold cloths applied, a warm bath was ordered at bed-time, and six grains of calomel and one grain of opium with ipecacuanha. On the morning of the 3rd there was no headache, and the epigastric uneasiness was removed, the skin was covered with moisture, but the bowels had not been opened. An ounce of castor oil was given. At the evening visit the pulse was 96, there was no local pain, the bowels had been moved, and the evacuations were bilious. A warm bath was directed at bed-time, and two grains of quinine early the following morning, and to be repeated every second hour for three doses. On the morning of the 4th general uneasiness of the upper part of the head was complained of, the pulse was upwards of 100, and the urine scanty. The quinine was omitted, and rhubarb and magnesia with colchicum wine given. At the evening visit the bowels had not been moved, and at noon there had been rigors followed by pyrexia; the pulse was 116, the epigastrium tender, the pupils slightly dilated, and some confusion of thought and slight tremors of the muscles were present. A purgative enema was exhibited, thirty leeches were applied to the temples, and fifty to the hypochondrium, and a blister was placed between the scapulæ. At midnight he had a convulsive fit, and about twenty minutes afterwards, was found with dilated pupils, breathing heavily, and passing into coma; the skin was covered with sweat, and the pulse was full; the bowels had not been opened. He was cupped on the temples to ten ounces, a purgative enema with turpentine oil was exhibited, fifteen grains of calomel were given, and after two hours, four ounces of haust. cathart. were directed to be taken. About an hour afterwards he was again much convulsed; the bowels had not been moved. A foot-bath at temp. 110° was ordered, and a blister to the epigastrium. At 2 A.M. he had passed into perfect coma, with stertorous breathing and convulsive movement of the arms and legs; surface hot. He died at 1 P.M. of the 5th.

Inspection twenty-three hours after death.—Body stout. *Head.*—There was a general bright red blush of the smaller vascular ramifications of the pia mater, and the medullary substance presented a pale rosy tint. There was about an ounce of serum at the base of the skull, but none elsewhere. *Chest.*—The lungs were emphysematous anteriorly, and adhered freely to the costal pleuræ; there was very little congestion posteriorly. The heart was about twice the size of the fist; all its cavities were dilated, but chiefly the left ventricle, the walls of which were somewhat thinner than natural. The muscular tissue of the heart was pale and flabby, there was a fibrinous coagulum in the left ventricle, but the cavity was not distended with blood. The lining membrane of the commencement of the aorta had a deep rosy colour (imbibition), and the surface was roughened by cartilaginous deposit. The aortic and the auriculo-ventricular valves were healthy. *Abdomen.*—The stomach was dilated. The liver reached about two inches below the right false ribs, extended to the left of the mesial line about four inches, adhered closely to the diaphragm, and was natural in texture but of greenish olive tint. The stomach contained about half a pint of dark green fluid, and at the cardiac end there was a dark red patch, and the mucous coat was thinned and pulpy; elsewhere the coat was of natural thickness, of leaden grey colour, and generally somewhat softer than natural. At the end of the ileum the solitary glands were prominent. The mucous coat of the colon was of grey tint, but of natural texture, with the follicles not distinguishable. The spleen was considerably enlarged and softened. The kidneys were considerably congested, chiefly in their tubular part.

23. *Remittent Fever in a man of intemperate habits.—Fatal with convulsion, coma, and tumultuous action of the heart.—Considerable effusion of serum in the head.—Streaked redness and softening of the mucous membrance of the stomach.—Deep red tint of the endocardium and muscular tissue of the heart.*—James Riley, aged twenty, a boiler maker of stout habit and a few months resident in India, was admitted into the European General Hospital on the 2nd of July, 1838, affected with mild febrile symptoms. He stated that for several days previously he had suffered from a sense of oppression of the chest which he had attributed to cold but which did not prevent him from following his occupation of boiler-maker. It was subsequently ascertained that he was a man of intemperate habits, and that he had been drinking to excess before his present illness. On the morning of the 3rd, after a restless night, the skin was warm and soft, pulse soft and of natural frequency, tongue slightly furred in streaks, thirst considerable, no uneasiness of the chest or fulness of abdomen. About six P.M. there was tenderness of the epigastrium, pulse frequent, hard, and sharp, manner excited and skin hot. He was bled, but fainted after the loss of sixteen ounces of blood. Ten grains of calomel with quarter of a grain of tartar emetic and a similar quantity of opium were given. During the night the bowels were frequently moved and the evacuations were green and watery. On the morning of the 4th the skin was warm and soft, pulse 80 and firm, tongue moist and little furred, no excitement of manner. Five grains of calomel and twelve grains of Dover's powder were given. At the evening visit he felt better, the bowels had been twice moved, and the evacuations were dark and bilious. He was ordered a warm bath and a powder of chalk and mercury with Dover's powder. The night was passed without sleep; skin cool. Cold affusion was used, and he took during the daytime two doses of antimonial mixture with one drachm of tincture of opium. Sleep did not result, and after the evening visit the cold affusion was again used, and a draught with one drachm and a half of tincture of opium was given. He slept for several hours, but on the morning of the 6th he continued nervous and agitated, and the action of the heart and of the carotids was strong. He was directed to be cupped on the cardiac region; but whilst the operation was being performed he was seized with convulsions, and died comatose after about an hour.

Inspection six hours after death.—Much of the external integuments was of purple tint. *Head.*—There was considerable effusion of serum at the base of the skull and between the membranes of the brain. *Chest.*—There were old costal adhesions and considerable infiltration of the lungs. The lining membrane of the heart and also the muscular tissue were of a deep red tint: The valves were healthy. *Abdomen.*—The substance of the liver was paler than natural and variegated here and there with large spots of dark red. The mucous coat of the stomach was streaked dark red and softened. The spleen was soft and large; and the kidneys were normal.

24. *Remittent Fever in a man of intemperate habits.—Death by coma.—Increased vascularity of the membranes of the brain and considerable effusion of serum.*—

Softening and vascularity of the mucous coat of the stomach and large intestine.—Commencing degeneration of the kidneys.—The commander of a merchant brig, aged forty-seven, of intemperate habits, was brought to the European General Hospital on the 13th July, 1838. It was stated that he had been feverish for some days, and had been drinking to excess. On admission he laboured under mental illusions, but when his attention was kept fixed on one subject he answered questions rationally regarding it. There was no tremor either of the hands or tongue. After cold affusion and a draught with a drachm of tincture of opium and a third of a grain of tartar emetic he became composed but did not sleep. The tongue was clean and the pulse frequent towards night. The bowels were freely moved, but the pulse became feeble. Stimulants were substituted for the antimonial, and after the second dose he slept several hours. On the morning of the 14th, the hands and tongue were tremulous, skin natural, pulse 96, full and soft. Camphor mixture with diffusible stimulants was directed to be given every second hour. Towards noon, the skin became hot, the pulse increased in frequency, the tongue became dryish and more tremulous, and the delirium and general tremors increased. Twenty-four leeches were applied to the temples, and at 8 P.M. a blister to the back of the neck, and a draught with two drachms of tincture of opium was given. An hour afterwards he fell asleep. In the middle of the night the pulse became thready. He was roused with difficulty, then became completely comatose, and died at 10 A.M. of the 15th.

Inspection five hours after death. Head.—There was much vascular congestion of the pia mater, with considerable effusion of serum between that membrane and the arachnoid, and also into the ventricles. *Chest.*—The lungs did not collapse. The heart was flabby, and filled with fluid blood. *Abdomen.*—The liver was of dark grey colour and softened. The mucous coat of the stomach and large intestines was vascular and softened. The spleen was enlarged and reduced to a bloody pulp. In both kidneys the distinction between the tubular and cortical substance was ill defined.

25. *Remittent Fever.—Simulating delirium tremens.—Pia mater very vascular, with bullæ of air between the arachnoid and pia mater and in the vessels.*—William ——, aged twenty-nine, a conductor in the Ordnance Department, of slight frame and frequently affected with febrile attacks in which the head was more or less implicated. On the 11th May, 1839, he was admitted into the General Hospital, suffering from diarrhœa for which chalk mixture and calomel with opium were given. On the morning of the 13th (new moon), his skin was hot, he was excited, talked incoherently, and had been walking about the ward a great part of the night. The pulse was frequent and the tongue rather furred in the centre. Cold affusion was used, and antimonial mixture with tincture of hyoscyamus was directed every two hours. At the evening visit the skin continued hot, and he had not been asleep. The cold affusion was repeated, and calomel four grains, tart. antimon. quarter of a grain, opium two grains were directed to be given at bed-time, and ol. ricini. four drachms the following morning. Towards midnight he became troublesome and excited, and the scalp was hot. Cold lotion was applied to the head, and a blister to the nucha. About 5 A.M. of the 14th he became comatose with sinking pulse and aboured respiration. Green-coloured dejections were passed in bed. He died at 8 A.M.*

Inspection five hours after death.—Examination of the head was only permitted. The vessels of the pia mater were generally turgid with dark-coloured blood to their

* In these three cases the influence of intemperate habits is well marked. In all the full opiate was injudiciously given. In the two first the remissions were well marked, but no advantage was taken of them in the treatment.

minute ramifications, and there were bullæ of air here and there in the vessels and also between the pia mater and arachnoid membrane. The sinuses were filled with blood which was coagulated in some of them. There was about half an ounce of serum in the ventricles, and an ounce at the base of the skull. The substance of the brain was natural, and did not present many bloody points.

26. *Remittent Fever proving fatal by collapse and coma at the close of an exacerbation.—No serous effusion in the head.—Dotted redness and softening of the mucous membrane of the stomach.—Enlargement of the mucous follicles of the colon and of Peyer's glands.—Lumbrici in the small intestine.*—George Castor, aged twenty, a seaman of stout habit, was admitted into the European General Hospital on the 23rd of June, 1838. He stated that he had been ill with fever for five days, during which time there had been headache and occasional vomiting. On admission his manner was sluggish, skin hot, pulse 120, full, but compressible, tongue furred and expanded. Six dozen leeches were applied to the temples, and pills of extract of colocynth, calomel, and tartar emetic were given. On the 24th the head, though relieved, was still uneasy, the skin was cool and moist, pulse 120 and feeble, the abdomen was soft, and during the night there had been seven watery bilious evacuations. A blister was applied to the back of the neck, which rose well, but caused strangury. At the evening visit there was less sluggishness, the skin was cool, pulse 120, soft, the bowels had been freely moved, and the tongue was cleaner. Draughts with nitrous ether were ordered, and pills of blue pill and ipecacuanha. The night was passed without sleep. On the 25th questions were answered freely, but giddiness was complained of. There was also uneasiness across the umbilicus, and there had been several ineffectual calls to stool, thirst moderate, tongue more furred and expanded. Compound powder of jalap was given with ether and camphor mixture. At the evening visit it was reported that he had slept, the skin was cool and moist, and no medicine was given. During the early part of the succeeding night he rested well, but towards morning there was a return of slight headache, increased by motion, with some intolerance of light, and flushing of the face. The skin was cool but dry, pulse 100, soft and of good strength, bowels freely opened, the tongue less furred, but somewhat florid at the edges. Six dozen leeches were applied to the temples, and a diaphoretic draught given every three hours. At the evening visit the head was easier, and the skin cool and moist. The succeeding night was passed without sleep, and at 3 P.M. of the 27th, there was a febrile exacerbation followed by much collapse in the night time. He became comatose and died at 7 A.M. of the 28th.

Inspection five hours after death.—Head. There was no increased vascularity of the membranes, or substance of the brain. There was about one drachm of serum in the left lateral ventricles, and about half an ounce at the base of the skull. *Chest.*—With the exception of some old costal adhesions, the thoracic viscera were healthy. *Abdomen.*—The liver was healthy and the gall-ducts free. The mucous lining of the cardiac end of the stomach for a space larger than the hand was of dark red colour, dotted, marbled, and its texture softened: towards the pyloric end the colour was natural, but the tissue was softened. The small intestines were filled with lumbrici. The aggregated glands of Peyer were enlarged. The mucous coat of the cœcum and colon was of dark grey colour, and studded throughout with dark points (enlarged follicles).*

* This case will be again alluded to as the single instance in my notes of head symptoms during life, without morbid appearances in the head after death. The treatment was defective in the neglect of quinine during the remissions, and too much depletion in the exacerbations. The appearance of the mucous lining of the large intestines indicated an undue use of irritants.

27. *Remittent Fever.—Drowsiness and coma.—Considerable quantity of serum effused in the head.—Vascularity and thickening of the mucous membrane of the stomach.*—Mary Anne Moor, aged forty-seven, a native of India, a fat corpulent woman of intemperate habits, was admitted into the European General Hospital on the 8th October. She stated that she had suffered from fever for five or six days. The skin, on admission, was hot, but soft, pulse 112 of good strength. The abdomen was distended but without pain. On the 9th there was slight delirium, and her hands were tremulous. This state continued till the 11th, when she was roused with difficulty, and when so, moaned and muttered to herself, the tongue was dryish, and the central part furred. This state continued with little alteration — the skin was dry but not often above the natural temperature, the pulse frequent and becoming feebler — till the 15th, when the drowsiness had increased and on the morning of the 16th had passed into coma. She died at 10 A.M. The treatment consisted in shaving the head, applying blisters to the nucha and scalp, free purging, and the use of antimonials with small doses of tincture of opium. Quinine and calomel were given in combination on occasions when there appeared a remission in the symptoms.

Inspection eight hours after Death. Head.—There was a considerable quantity of serum effused between the layers of the arachnoid membrane, and into the ventricles. The brain was firm in substance. *Abdomen.*—The integuments were loaded with fat. The mucous coat of the stomach was thickened and vascular, with abrasions here and there.

In the section on symptoms it was stated that delirium with tendency to drowsiness, associated with signs of general collapse and dependent on enfeebled nervous energy, was apt to come on early in fevers of bad type towards the end of a paroxysm. Head symptoms very similar in character sometimes occur, after the fifth or sixth day, in cases in which the treatment of the remissions has been neglected and that of the exacerbations has been injudiciously depressant.

In my notes on the cases of sick officers there are several which seem to have been of this nature, and it is of importance to bear them in recollection, for it would be a serious error to treat head symptoms thus arising in the same manner as those caused by cerebral determination. The following may be received as an illustration.

28. *Remittent Fever.—Coma from exhaustion.*—A gentlemen in the public service became affected with febrile symptoms at Tauna on the 4th of September. No treatment was adopted. He went to Bombay, and remained there also without treatment, experiencing febrile accessions till the 8th, when he returned to Tauna. He had rigors in the boat two hours before landing. On the morning of the 9th there was remission, and towards evening an exacerbation, for which an emetic and a purgative of calomel were given. On the 10th, at 4 P.M., there was again an exacerbation, with sense of swimming in the head. Eight dozen leeches were applied to the temples. There were rigors at midnight, followed by coma and death at 8 A.M. of the 11th.

2. Cerebral symptoms depending on inflammation of the membranes or substance of the brain also occur in the course of remittent fever; but this event is rare compared with determi-

nation of blood. Among the fatal cases of sick officers there are only two of this nature. The following three illustrations are taken from my own observations.

29. *Remittent Fever.—Meningitis.—Effusion of serum in the cavity of the arachnoid and sub-arachnoid space.—Opacity and thickening of the arachnoid membrane.*—William Woodward, aged seven, an Indo-Briton, was admitted into the sick ward of the Byculla Schools on the 6th June, 1838. He was affected with febrile symptoms, which did not attract much attention till the 10th, when there was increased heat of skin, and frequency of pulse, with a tendency to drowsiness. Twenty-four leeches were applied to the temples, a blister to the nucha, and the bowels were freely acted upon. During the two succeeding days the skin continued hot, the pulse was about 120, and the drowsiness remained unabated. An attempt was made to affect the system with mercury, the bowels were kept free, and a blister was applied to the scalp. On the 13th, there was frequent screaming and moaning, there was strabismus with dilated pupils, and the head was frequently raised from the pillow and moved slowly about, as if in search of some object. The symptoms progressed; the pulse continued frequent, and became feeble, the coma became more complete, and death resulted at midnight of the 14th.

Inspection twelve hours after death.—Head. There was more than usual vascularity of the pia mater, where it dips down between the convolutions of the brain. There was a considerable quantity of serum effused between the arachnoid membrane and the pia mater, chiefly on the superior and posterior parts of the hemispheres, and in these situations the arachnoid membrane was milky, firm, and thickened. There were adhesions between the arachnoid membrane and the falx, caused by small granules of lymph. There was also a considerable quantity of serum at the base of the skull, and more than the natural quantity in the ventricles. There were bloody points apparent on slicing the substance of the brain. The viscera of the thorax and abdomen were healthy.

30. *Remittent Fever admitted after a week's illness.—Head symptoms chiefly marked by unsteadiness of manner, and latterly drowsiness.—Arachnoid membrane opaque and thickened.—Increased serous effusion.*—William Subbeter, aged sixteen, after having been ill for a week with headache and fever, was admitted into the General Hospital on the 9th May, 1842. There was heat of skin, flushed countenance, undecided manner. The tongue was yellow in the centre and florid at the tip, and the epigastrium was tender. Twenty-four leeches were applied to the temples, and thirty-six to the epigastrium, the head was shaved, cold applications were used, sponging of the general surface had recourse to, effervescing draughts were exhibited from time to time, and some blue bill and ipecacuanha given at bed-time. On the morning of the 10th there was still heat and dryness of of skin, but in other respects the symptoms were improved. In the evening there was a distinct febrile exacerbation. Sponging, cold applications, and effervescing draughts were continued, and the blue bill and ipecacuanha were repeated. On the morning of the 11th, still pyrexia, pulse 92, tongue slimy and tremulous, bowels rather relaxed, and manner unsteady. The remedies were continued, with addition of spirit. æther. nit. to the effervescing draughts, and the application of a blister to the nucha. On the 12th, febrile heat and other symptoms continued, accompanied with slight subsultus. Camphor mixture c. spirit. æther. nit. was given every third hour, also chicken soup. On the 13th, pulse 104, four dejections feculent. In other respects as on the 12th. Sago and milk morning and evening, chicken soup for dinner, and the camphor mixture continued. On the morning of the 14th there was a distinct remission, and quinine and blue pill were ordered every second hour, with effervescing draughts. The evening accession was milder. On the 15th and 16th, the febrile exacerbation seemed to be

somewhat checked under the use of the quinine; but on the 17th the symptoms were all again aggravated. On the 18th he vomited several times, and passed three copious watery evacuations, followed by sunken features, feeble pulse, and damp skin. These symptoms continued, with the addition of drowsiness on the 21st; and death took place on the morning of the 24th.

Inspection eight hours after death. — *Head.* The arachnoid membrane over the convex surface of the brain was opaque and thickened with here and there small rounded granules of lymph, the size of a pin's head. There was about an ounce of serum in the lateral ventricles, and about an ounce and a half at the base of the skull. The substance of the brain was firm. *Chest.* — Old adhesions connected the right lung to the pleura; but the substance of the lungs was crepitating. Heart healthy. *Abdomen.* — The liver was healthy. The colon distended, but its mucous coat healthy. The mucous coat of the stomach was of dark grey tint with dark red streaks, but was sound in texture.

31. *Remittent Fever admitted in an advanced stage.* — *Death by coma.* — *Extensive lymph and serous effusion in the sub-arachnoid space.* — *Hepatisation of both lungs.* —Bappoo Mahomed, forty years of age, a Mussulman sailor, was admitted after twenty days' illness with fever on the 10th September, 1849, into the clinical ward of the Jamsetjee Jejeebhoy Hospital. There was trembling of the whole body and frequent twitching of the muscles of the forearms. He was affected with low muttering, delirium and drowsiness, the skin was above the natural temperature and dry, the pulse was frequent and feeble, he could not protrude the tongue, and the respiration was short and hurried. Anteriorly and laterally on the right side of the chest there was dulness on percussion and absence of breath sounds. He died on the afternoon of the 11th.

Inspection seventeen hours after death. — Between the pia mater and the arachnoid over the entire convex surface of both hemispheres of the brain, but greatest in degree on the left side and depending parts, there was effusion of lymph and serum, to such extent as to give a yellow opaque appearance to the surface. Similar effusion also existed over the cerebellum and in a slight degree over the pons varolii and medulla oblongata, but not elsewhere at the base of the brain. The surface of the convolutions of the brain was of natural appearance and consistence, and the substance of the brain elsewhere was also quite healthy. There were from six drachms to an ounce of serous fluid in the lateral ventricles, and about two ounces at the base of the skull.

The whole of the upper lobe of the right lung, except about half an inch of the apex, and also the whole of the middle lobe, were in a state of red hepatisation, having, when incised, a granular appearance with considerable oozing of frothy serum on pressure, and readily breaking down under the finger. The rest of the lungs was crepitating. The free anterior border of the lobe of the left lung, for about three inches, was in a state of red induration; the rest was healthy. The heart and pericardium were healthy. The large and small intestines were distended with air. The liver was of natural size and consistence, but was congested. The kidneys were not examined.

3. When delirium, drowsiness, and coma come on in the more advanced stages of remittent fever, associated with adynamic phenomena, then more or less increased serous effusion in the cavity of the cranium, unattended, however, with any great degree of vascular turgescence, is generally found after death. But it is very doubtful, for reasons presently to be particularly alluded to, whether, in a large majority of cases of this kind there is any

relation between the head symptoms and the increased effusion. The following are cases of adynamic remittent fever fatal with coma.

32. *Remittent Fever with adynamic symptoms.* — *Slight vascularity of the membranes of the brain with air in the vessels and beneath the arachnoid.* — *Turgescence and ulceration of Peyer's glands at the end of the ileum.* * — John Steptoe, private of her Majesty's 15th Hussars, two months resident in Bombay, was admitted into hospital on the 6th February, 1840, and died on the 15th. He had been ill before admission. The following were the leading features of the disease. Pyrexia almost constant with an occasional remission in the middle of the day, hands tremulous, pulse from 100 to 120, and compressible, tongue coated and dry in the centre, florid at the tip, sordes about the teeth, thirst, and more or less diarrhœa. On one occasion there was pain between the right ribs and crest of the os ilium. The eyes were suffused. At first there was wandering delirium at nights, and on the latter days drowsiness not amounting to coma.

Inspection. — *Head.* There was moderate turgescence of the vessels of the membranes of the brain, with numerous globules of air in the vessels or underneath the arachnoid. More than the usual number of bloody points in the brain, and an ounce of serum at the base of the skull. *Abdomen.* — The liver was quite healthy. The mucous coat of the cardiac end of the stomach was dotted dark red, but without softening. The mucous coat of the end of the ileum was of dark red colour, the patches of Peyer's glands were red, turgid, and prominent, and several of them were in different stages of ulceration. Close to the ileo-colic valve there was an ulcerated patch the size of a rupee. The mucous coat of the cœcum was of dark red colour, but not ulcerated. The rest of the large intestine was healthy.

33. *Remittent Fever.* — *Symptoms adynamic and badly-developed.* — *Serous effusion and slight vascular congestion in the head, also air in the vessels.* — *The colon distended and in part displaced.* — Neil Wallace, aged twenty-eight, seaman of the ship *Samuel*, was admitted into the European General Hospital, on the 21st October, 1841. He stated that for a fortnight past he had experienced a sense of weight at the centre of the chest, for which he had taken much medicine. On admission he inspired freely, and there was neither pain of chest nor cough, the skin was dry and above the natural temperature, the pulse frequent and of moderate strength, and the tongue florid. It was supposed that he had been living freely for some days. On the 22nd and 23rd the abdomen was full, the pulse from 88 to 92 and feeble, and on the latter day his manner and expression were dull and heavy. He was blistered on the nucha, a full dose of calomel (ten grains) was given, followed by castor oil, and on the morning of the 24th he was more alert. The bowels had been opened twice, the skin was moist, and the pulse 92 and feeble. Port wine and sago were given. At the evening visit the pulse still feeble, but there was febrile heat of skin, the tongue was florid, and the sluggishness of manner had increased. The head was shaved, cold applied, and a nitro-muriatic acid foot-bath used. He continued to lose ground, there was generally a morning remission and evening exacerbation of fever, the pulse became feebler, the hands tremulous and with subsultus tendinum, the tongue dry, the drowsiness increased, and at last passed almost into complete coma. He died on the 31st October.

Inspection fourteen hours after death.—*Head.* A thin veil of serum was effused between the convolutions on the convex surface of the brain. The small vessels

* While retaining this case in its original position I must admit that recent inquiry may suggest that it was true typhoid, not adynamic remittent.

of the pia mater were in part injected with blood and the larger ramifications contained air. No increased quantity of serum in the ventricles or at the base of the skull. *Chest.*—The lungs did not collapse freely. Heart healthy. *Abdomen.*—The liver was healthy. The colon was much distended with air and the sigmoid flexure thrown across the small intestines was applied to the inner aspect of the ascending colon. The large intestine was sound in texture.

When, as in the first* series of cases, we find head symptoms coming on early in the disease, and after death more or less vascular turgescence with increased serous effusion in the cranium, or, as in the second, head symptoms with opacity of the membranes or with lymph and serous exudations, there need be no hesitation in relating the morbid appearances found after death to the symptoms present during life.

But when, as in the last set of cases, the head symptoms which indicate failing function of the brain have been coincident with failure of other vital actions then it is very doubtful whether a relation between these symptoms and increased cranial serous effusion can be viewed as a probable inference. This so-called morbid appearance may, in adynamic states, be otherwise explained.

Thus, on carefully examining the reports of 205 fatal cases of disease observed by me in the European General Hospital at Bombay, it appears that while, on the one hand, of 59 cases in which head symptoms during life were well marked there is only one in which there was an absence of morbid appearances after death †, there are, on the other hand, 50 cases in which there were no head symptoms during life, but in which appearances in the contents of the cranium generally considered morbid were observed after death.

Of these 50 cases, the ages of the individuals were as follows: —

Between 10 and 15 years, inclusive	2
16 „ 20 „	4
21 „ 25 „	14
26 „ 30 „	7
31 „ 35 „	7
36 „ 40 „	2
41 „ 50 „	7
51 „ 60 „	4
61 „ 70 „	1
Ages not given	2
	50

* With one exception, No. 26.

† No. 26.

The deaths took place in the following months: —

January	4	July	3
February	5	August	4
March	6	September	4
April	5	October	1
May	6	November	2
June	2	December	4
	28		18
Months not stated			4

Of these 50 cases, the deaths were occasioned by the following diseases: —

Tubercular Phthisis	7
Pleuritis	1
Disease of the Heart	1
Hepatic Abscess	8
Dysentery	11
Peritonitis	4
Scurvy	3
Spasmodic Cholera	14
Rupture of the Spleen	1
	50

In 4 of the 50 cases the morbid appearance consisted of increased vascularity of the membranes of the brain. These were all instances of epidemic cholera.

In 19 cases both increased vascularity and increased serous effusion within the cranium were present. Death took place from the following diseases: —

Epidemic Cholera	9
Disease of the Heart	1
Dysentery	4
Peritonitis	2
Hepatic Abscess	2
Gastro-enteritis	1
	19

In 27 cases there was increased serous effusion within the cranium without increased vascularity.

Death in these instances was caused by the following diseases:—

Tubercular Phthisis	7
Hepatic Abscess	6
Dysentery	6
Peritonitis	2
Epidemic Cholera	1
Pleuritis	1
Rupture of the Spleen	1
Scurvy	2
Rheumatism (Scorbutic)	1
	27

In regard to the facts which have just been stated, it may be observed.

1. They do not show any relation between absence of head symptoms, associated with increased vascularity and serous effusion within the cranium, and particular age or season.

2. They show a relation between the absence of head symptoms, associated with increased vascularity with or without increased serous effusion within the cranium, and a state of general venous congestion dependent upon a feebly acting heart.

3. They show a relation between absence of head symptoms, associated with increased serous effusion without increased vascularity within the cranium, and death taking place by gradual asthenia. When death takes place after this manner, serous transudations from serous linings and into areolar tissue are familiar events: the cerebral serous effusion now referred to is analogous to these.

4. The increased vascularity in these cases is of congestion, not of inflammation. The increased serous effusion is not the result of inflammation, but of congestion and of those conditions of the tissue and of the *blood* which are believed to favour serous transudation.

They confirm therefore the opinion of Dr. Abercrombie,—that the head symptoms of acute hydrocephalus do not depend upon the presence of serous effusion within the cranium, so much as on the deranged capillary circulation (inflammation) of which the serous effusion is the consequence.

The serous effusion in the cases of which I now treat was not the result of *this* deranged state of the capillary circulation (inflammation); hence, though present within the cranium, head symptoms were not necessarily induced by it.

5. It should be borne in mind that increased vascularity and serous effusion within the cranium, found after death, does not necessarily prove their presence there during life. They may have taken place in some instances during the agony of death, or after the fatal event.

6. These facts which show a want of relation between increased vascularity and serous effusion within the cranium found after death and the proximate cause of the fatal result should be remembered in judicial inquiries on bodies found dead, and of the previous history of which nothing is known. *In such cases, if there be present within the cranium only increased vascularity or increased serous effusion separately or associated together, we can never*

be justified in attributing death to these conditions. These statements have been entered into not only from their relation to the similar after-death appearances in fatal cases of adynamic remittent fever, but also because they tend to confirm observations of a like tenor in the writings of Louis*, Abercrombie†, and Bright‡; and because facts of this kind are of much importance in reference to the pathology of the brain.

Gastric Irritability.—I pass over the occurrence of occasional vomiting as one of the deranged actions of the febrile state and here direct attention to those greater degrees of irritability of the stomach which depend upon local disease.

In the severe forms of remittent fever in sthenic Europeans cerebral symptoms and gastric irritability are very frequently combined. This was the case in the remittent fevers from which her Majesty's 4th Light Dragoons suffered so much at Kaira. In these it was very common to find after death increased vascularity of the vessels of the brain with some degree of increased serous effusion, and at the same time a deeply reddened state of the mucous membrane of the stomach and sometimes of the intestinal canal. It is very probable that the deranged capillary circulation was similar in both organs,—not inflammatory but rather passive congestion or active determination. In other instances the gastric complication is the principal: this occurred in 6 of the 90 fatal cases of officers formerly alluded to.

As respects the pathology of that form of remittent fever called *bilious*, I cannot view it in any other light than as a coincidence of the state now under consideration and the presence of a considerable quantity of bile in the gall-bladder and in the biliary ducts,—hence the notable admixture of bile in the ejected matters.§ The term has been too frequently and too vaguely used by writers on tropical fevers, and will not be repeated in this work.

Irritability of stomach also occurs in the course of remittent fever, both in sthenic and asthenic constitutions, developing itself somewhat more gradually, generally with distinct epigastric uneasiness, and a tongue more or less florid at the tip and edges and depending on inflammation of the mucous membrane. Evidence

* "Researches on Phthisis."

† "On Diseases of the Brain."

‡ "Reports of Medical Cases."

§ I am aware that there may also co-exist a similarly deranged capillary condition of the liver; but that this, during the presence of the febrile state, leads to increased hepatic secretion is very doubtful. It is more likely that the secretion is antecedent and in excess in the biliary passages and reservoirs at the onset of the fever.

of this will be found in cases 17, 18, 20, 22, 30, quoted in this chapter.

In 114 selected clinical cases of natives, gastric irritability is noted of 2 only.

Habits of intemperance as an auxiliary cause of head symptoms have already been adverted to. The same remark applies still more forcibly to irritability of stomach, whether of the nature first noticed, or that depending on gastric inflammation.

When treating of intermittent fever I expressed my conviction that irritability of stomach was not unfrequently caused and kept up in the quotidian type by the unnecessary use of calomel and purgatives in the hot stage; and this belief is still stronger in respect to remittent fever, because in it these means have been abused in still greater degree. The practitioner who uses these medicines guardedly, and with a clear apprehension of their evils as well as of their advantages, will find vomiting a less frequent symptom of remittent fever than it has usually been represented to be. This impression, left on my mind from a careful review of the whole subject, is sustained by the fact that in 357 cases of fever intermittent and remittent treated by me in natives in the clinical ward gastric irritability was present only in 6.

Affection of the Bowels.—The occurrence of dysentery in the early or advanced stages of remittent fever in sthenic or asthenic constitutions has been a rare event in my experience. From the writings of Mr Twining, and more lately from those of Mr. Hare*, it would appear that this complication has been more frequently observed in Bengal, and that the type of the fever has generally tended to be congestive or adynamic and the dysentery to be hæmorrhagic in character. It may be also inferred from Haspel's work on the diseases of Algeria and Bleeker's report on the dysentery of Batavia† that the co-existence of dysentery and of remittent fever is not unusual in these countries. It is in localities in which the period of the production of malaria is coincident with much atmospheric moisture and vicissitude that dysentery occurs, combined or contemporaneous with remittent fever. Since the doctrine that malaria is the exciting cause of intermittent and remittent fever became established, the co-operating and modifying action of ordinary causes—cold, wet, heat, intemperance—has been too much overlooked, and our knowledge of the etiology of the different forms and varieties of fever has in consequence been impaired.

* "Indian Annals of Medical Science," No. 2.

† Ibid. No. I.

Diarrhœa is, according to my observation, a more frequent complication of remittent fever, and is sometimes accompanied with gastric irritability; but it cannot be said to be common, for it was present in only 6 of 114 clinical cases in natives.

In fatal cases in which increased alvine discharges have been present during life we may expect to find evidence of inflammation having existed in the mucous membrane of the end of the ileum or of the large intestine. Cases 17, 26, 32, illustrate this observation, and the two following are further confirmatory of it.

34. *Remittent Fever, with head and gastro-enteric symptoms; two or three ounces of serum in the cranium. — Firm granular exudation on the mucous surface of the colon. — Dark redness of the end of the ileum. — The subject of a large hydrocele.* — John Daniel, aged fifty, a person of colour, born in Ceylon, of feeble and emaciated habit, was sent to the hospital on the 5th September, 1839, having been found in a state of destitution on the road. He was unable to give any account of himself, his tongue was dry and covered with a yellow crust, pulse 116, skin not of increased temperature. He was also the subject of a large hydrocele. He died on the 16th September. The leading symptoms during his residence in hospital were frequent hiccup and incoherent muttering, pulse generally about 100 and feeble, tongue crusted in the centre, and florid at the tip, the skin generally not above the natural temperature, two or three evacuations daily, passed in bed, feculent and containing lumbrici. Little food was taken. The treatment consisted of quinine with small doses of calomel, a blister to the epigastrium, wine and light nourishing food; and on one occasion an enema with ol. terebinth.

Inspection eight hours after death. — Body much emaciated, the skin and fibrous tissues deeply tinged yellow. *Head.*—The convex surface of the brain was partially veiled with serum; and there were between two or three ounces of it effused at the base of the skull. *Chest.*— Both lungs adhered to the costal pleuræ, but their substance was healthy. In both sides of the heart there were fibrinous polypi, entwining round the cords of the auriculo-ventricular valves. *Abdomen.*—The intestines externally had a dark greenish tint. The liver was of dark green colour and the gall-bladder was nearly empty. The stomach was contracted, and much of its mucous lining was mammillated, and thickened, — this was chiefly in the body and at the pyloric end. The mucous coat of the colon had a general dark grey tint, and in the cœcum, the descending colon, and the rectum there were extensive patches of lymph effused in detached pieces, presenting a roughened surface like shagreen. This lymph adhered firmly to the mucous coat which underneath presented a dark dotted red appearance, was firm and somewhat thickened with the submucous tissue more fibrous than is natural. At the end of the ileum there was much dark vascularity of the mucous coat. There was one lumbricus in the colon and one in that part of the small intestine which was opened. The kidneys were healthy. There were about ten pints of dark red turbid fluid, in the tunica vaginalis which was thickened, cartilaginous, and presented an inner surface of dark red tint roughened by closely adherent fragments of very firm lymph.

35. *Remittent Fever. — Peyer's glands enlarged and ulcerated. — Head symptoms with moderate turgescence of the vessels.* — Caroline Smith, an Indo-Briton, aged nine. On the 7th July, 1839, after having been in the sick ward for two or three days with mild febrile symptoms was observed to be affected with slight drowsiness and heat of head, for which twelve leeches were applied to the temples, and the bowels freely acted on with calomel, followed by senna mixture. On the 8th there was still heat of skin and of the head. The head was shaved and cold applications used. On the 9th she

seemed drowsy and the scalp was hot and the pulse frequent, the tongue was more florid than natural, she had vomited several times, and the bowels were open. Six leeches were applied to the temples and six to the epigastrium, cold applications were continued to the head, a blister was applied to the back of the neck, and effervescing draughts were given every fourth hour. She passed an uncomfortable night with frequent moaning. On the morning of the 10th there was a good deal of heat of scalp, and the general surface was above the natural temperature; the pupils contracted freely, but she lay with her eyes shut as if annoyed by the light, there was tenderness on pressure of the epigastrium; and the bowels had been opened during the night. Six leeches were applied to the margin of the right ribs, cold wash continued to the head, and an enema directed at noon. At the evening visit she was reported to have been cool and more lively at noon, but there was again a febrile exacerbation, bowels moved once. Calomel grs. iii. pulv. jalap grs. vi. to be taken at bedtime. She vomited the powder but passed the night quietly. On the morning of the 11th, bowels not opened, abdomen full, tongue pretty clean, skin cool but dry, pulse rather frequent, and she was still sluggish. A domestic enema, with turpentine oil, was directed to be used, and the following pills prescribed:—quinine sulph. and pil. hydrarg. aa. grs. iv. ipecac. gr. iss. tere bene ft. pil. iii., one to be taken every second hour, for four doses, should there be no fever, also chicken soup. She vomited several times during the day, and at the evening visit the pulse was 104, slight heat of skin and less drowsiness, and abdomen still full; the bowels had been opened by the enema but not otherwise, tongue not furred, and tolerably moist. Repet. enema c. ol. terebinth, and give an effervescing draught every fourth hour. During the night time, she vomited frequently, and was purged four or five times. Sinapisms were applied to the stomach, and a powder with hydrarg. c. cret. given. At half-past 7 A.M., of the 12th, the skin was cold, the pulse thready, and the tongue not coated. Recipe: quinine grs. vi. opii. gr. half, confect. aromat. q. s. at. ft. pil. iv. one to be given every third hour, and sago with wine or brandy occasionally. She vomited the sago and brandy. There was no recurrence of purging. At noon the pulse was hardly perceptible. Liquor lyttæ was applied to the epigastrium, and the remedies continued. The vomiting of ingesta continued, and she died about 10 P.M.

Inspection ten hours after death.—*Head.* There was moderate vascular turgescence of the membranes of the brain, and dotted points on incising its substance, and about an ounce and a half of serum at the base of the skull. *Chest.*—The lungs, partially collapsed, were somewhat emphysematous, and without congestion of their posterior part. *Abdomen.*—The liver was healthy. The stomach was contracted, and its mucous coat normal. At the end of the ileum the glands of Peyer were distinct, and there were three or four round ulcers, each the size of a split pea; cicatrization had commenced. In the colon the follicles were distinct, but the mucous coat was healthy. The mesenteric glands ranged in size from a pea to a horse bean, but were not tubercular.

The observation made in reference to affection of the bowels in intermittent fever, viz., that its frequency will be found to bear relation to the injudicious use of purgatives, is equally applicable to remittent fever.

Hepatic Affections.—Hepatitis has been, in my field of practice, an unusual feature of remittent fever. It was so in the European General Hospital and in 138 cases of remittent fever in European officers it is noted only of 7, and of these 5 were recoveries. In 114 clinical cases in natives, hepatitis was present in 3. The liver may be enlarged in the early stages of remittent fever from congestion, and this enlargement may also be an occasional sequence of the remittent just as it frequently is of the intermittent type.

Splenic enlargement existed in 20 of the clinical cases, and when occurring in remittent fever it may generally be viewed as indicative of former attacks of the intermittent form. This lesion has been already so fully considered in connection with intermittent fever, that further notice here would be superfluous.

Jaundice was present in 28 of 114 selected clinical cases of natives, and 10 of them proved fatal. Of the 90 fatal cases of remittent fever in European officers 7 were of this complication; and though it was not a common occurrence in the European General Hospital at Bombay, yet a season seldom passed without a few instances being met with. It varies in frequency, however, in different years: it was more common in 1848 in the clinical ward than in any of the five following years.

As the pathology of jaundice is not yet well understood, the narration of the 10 fatal cases will be useful. When these are compared with the recoveries it appears that the average duration of illness of the former before admission has been about eleven days, and that of the latter about eight, a difference of three days.

Mr. Twining believed that jaundice was sometimes caused by the mechanical pressure of enlarged lymphatic glands situated near the entrance of the common biliary duct into the duodenum, and the confirmation or correction of this opinion is important. With this view the state of these glands is generally noticed in the reports of the fatal cases: they were considered to be enlarged in 6 of the 10, but, with one exception, there was no reason to think that they had pressed on the duct; and in this case (39) the pressure was caused rather by the head of the pancreas than by the enlarged glands. In one of the 6 cases the hepatic and common ducts were obstructed by an impacted lumbricus; and in 2 there was constriction of the cystic duct but it was independent of glandular enlargement, and in both the gall-bladder was full of bile.

Traces of inflammation of the mucous membrane of the duodenum and stomach were observed in 6 cases, and in 3 of them the lymphatic glands were also enlarged, but in 2 of the remaining 3 the glands were not enlarged, and in one their condition was not noted. Of the remaining 4 of the 10 fatal cases, in one the state of the duodenum was not noticed, in one there was obstruction of the ducts from a lumbricus, in one neither enlarged glands nor gastro-duodenitis, and in one enlarged glands and pancreas without gastro-duodenitis.

These data are not sufficient to justify a positive opinion, but they cannot be regarded as confirmatory of Mr. Twining's views. When it is recollected that jaundice seldom comes on before the fifth day of the fever and is almost invariably attended with tenderness below the margins of the seventh, eighth, and ninth right ribs, it is probable that its most important relation is to inflammation of the mucous membrane of the duodenum. This conclusion is supported by the fact that remittent fever complicated with jaundice is best treated by the moderate use of leeches, small blisters, mild alterative aperients and quinine in the remissions, and is sure to be aggravated by the injudicious use of calomel and purgatives. As vomiting is frequently absent, the symptoms appear to be referable rather to the inflammatory condition of the duodenum than to the gastritis which generally co-exists.

These cases do not indicate a frequent dependence of jaundice on inflammation of the mucous lining of the ducts, for it was not observed in any of them. They are defective in that the microscope was used only in three, but in these the hepatic cells presented no abnormal appearance. None of these cases, however, had the characters of the yellow atrophy of Rokitansky in which head symptoms are prominent and the course rapid from probable direct destruction of the vitality of the cells by the influence of the morbific cause.*

36. *Remittent Fever with jaundice.—Drowsiness.—Biliary congestion of the liver. Enlarged lymphathic glands in the course of the common duct.—Slight dilatation of the hepatic duct.—Gastro-duodenitis.—Granular exudation on the mucous surface of the ileum and colon.—Nodules of pulmonary apoplexy, one softened into a cavity.*—Nuthagee, a Hindoo labourer of twenty-five years of age, was admitted into hospital, after ten days' illness with fever, on the 14th of September, 1848. The pulse was feeble, the skin was coldish, the bowels relaxed, the tongue coated and slimy, hiccup was present and the conjunctivæ were yellow. He was somewhat drowsy, but pointed to the right side as the seat of pain. The symptoms continued with little change till the 18th, when he became more drowsy and died, having expectorated some bloody serous fluid about ten hours before death. He was treated with quinine and Dover's powder, light nourishment and stimulants, and a blister was applied to the right side.

Inspection fourteen hours after death.—Abdomen. The liver, somewhat enlarged, was connected to the diaphragm by old adhesions, and was of olive-green tint when

* I shall again return to the Pathology of Jaundice in connection with the diseases of the liver.

incised. The gall-bladder was full, but not distended. Just beyond the junction of the cystic and hepatic ducts there commenced a chain of lymphatic glands, which surrounded and accompanied the common duct to its point of entrance into the duodenum. The thickness of the chain of glands was equal to that of a swan's quill. The hepatic duct was somewhat dilated. There was no redness of the mucous lining of the biliary ducts. The mucous lining of the duodenum presented a surface of bright red patches covered with adhesive mucus, but the tissue was not softened: similar patches were observed at the commencement of the jejunum. About two feet of the end of the ileum and the cœcum were laid open. The inner surface of the ileum was bright red in patches, which followed the transverse folds of the membrane, and were covered with granular lymph; in scraping off the lymph no softening of the membrane was found. Similar red patches, but without the granular effusion, occupied the mucous surface of the cœcum and commencement of the colon. There was not a trace of ulceration, and the groups of Peyer's glands at the end of the ileum were free of disease. The mucous surface of the stomach presented patches of redness at its cardiac end. *Chest.*—Lungs did not collapse. In both, but chiefly in the left, there were several black nodules from extravasated blood (pulmonary apoplexy); in one the texture of the lung had been broken down, and cavities had formed, the smallest was the size of a pea, the largest that of a pigeon's egg. There was also a good deal of œdema of the lungs. The heart was healthy.

37. *Remittent Fever with jaundice.* — *Tenderness at margin of right ribs.* — *Coma.* — *Gastro-duodenitis.* — *Enlarged lymphatic glands in the course of the common Duct.* — *Biliary congestion of the liver.* — Meerza Khan, a Mussulman peon of twenty-six years of age, a native of Peshawur, was, after eight days' illness, admitted into hospital, on the 21st of October, 1848. The surface of the body and the conjunctivæ were tinged of a deep yellow colour. He complained of pain, much increased by pressure at the margin of the right false ribs, and there was some fulness there. The tongue was much coated and dryish in the centre, and the bowels were reported to be confined. The pulse was quick, full, and soft. No heat of skin. He continued in hospital till the 26th, when he died. The exacerbations were marked by excitement of manner, not by increased heat of skin. The alvine and renal excretions were scanty. The pulse lost strength. The jaundice continued. He became drowsy on the 25th, then comatose. He was treated with twenty-four leeches to the margin of the right ribs, followed by a small blister. Mercurial purgatives were given, also quinine in two or three-grain doses with an equal quantity of blue pill, every third or fourth hour. As the pulse failed, wine and ammonia were given, and attention was paid to suitable nourishment. On the 25th a blister was applied to the nucha.

Inspection five hours after death. — All the tissues were deeply tinged yellow. *Chest.*—The lungs did not collapse freely, but were otherwise free of disease. The right side of the heart was distended with blood. The ascending aorta was a good deal dilated, and part of its inner surface was irregular. *Abdomen.* — The liver was not enlarged, but was of olive-green tint. The mucous membrane of the stomach and duodenum was dotted red, but sound in texture. The lining of the ileum was also reddened, but neither softened nor ulcerated. Lymphatic glands the size of a small bean embraced the common biliary duct near to its termination in the duodenum. On the external surface of both kidneys there were puckered cicatrices, which gave a lobulated appearance to the organ. In the left kidney, situated in a calyx, and branching into others, there was a calculus. The spleen adhered closely and firmly to the stomach and diaphragm. The head was not examined.

38. *Fever with jaundice.* — *Tenderness at the margin of the right ribs.* — *Drowsiness.* — *Biliary congestion of the liver.* — *Obstruction of the hepatic duct by a lumbricus, of which there were many in the duodenum and stomach.* — *No gastro-duodenitis.* — *Enlargement of the lymphatic glands in the course of the common duct.* —

Hepatic cells distinct. — Chottoo Ram, a Hindoo peon of twenty-five years of age, was, after ten days' illness, admitted into hospital on the 2nd February, 1849. He was much exhausted, there was heat of skin, a feeble pulse, yellow conjunctivæ, tenderness at the margin of the right ribs, and some degree of drowsiness. He died on the 4th, two days after admission.

Inspection twelve hours after death. — The tissues were tinged deeply yellow. The viscera of the chest healthy. *Abdomen.*—There was no peritonitic inflammation. The colon and cœcum were distended with air. The stomach contained greenish viscid mucus, and five or six lumbrici, and the contents of the duodenum were similar, with four or five lumbrici; the mucous coat of both was healthy. *Liver.* — The substance was of very yellow tint in places. The hepatic cells were seen distinctly under the microscope. The gall-bladder, not distended, was, however, full of dark thick bile. The hepatic duct was distended by a lumbricus, the sharp end of which extended into the common duct for about an inch beyond the junction of the cystic duct. The lumbricus was traced in the duct beyond its division, for about three inches into the substance of the liver, and in following the branch of the duct had been subjected to considerable curvature; but it was not traced to its end in the liver, for it had been accidentally cut across. There was no redness of the mucous membrane of the duct. The chain of glands along the lower side of the common duct equalled a swan's quill in thickness.

39. *Remittent Fever with jaundice. — Tenderness at the margin of the right ribs. — Drowsiness. — Enlarged lymphatic glands. — Enlarged head of the pancreas. — No duodenitis. — Biliary congestion of the liver.* — Balloo, a Hindoo labourer of thirty-five years of age, after suffering for fifteen days from fever characterised by evening exacerbations and morning remissions, was admitted into hospital in a reduced state on the 11th June, 1849. He had been jaundiced for six days. The tongue was streaked yellow, and somewhat florid at the tip and edges. There was tenderness, with resistance, below the margin of the right false ribs, and the edge of the spleen was perceptible under the left. During his stay in hospital the evening exacerbation was well marked, but frequently the remission in the morning was very slight. The jaundice persisted, the urine was of a deep brown colour, generally about twenty ounces in the twenty-four hours. The alvine discharges were of a pale colour, and there was no vomiting. He was quite collected on admission, but on the 20th June muttering delirium was first noticed. The pulse became feebler. There was subsultus on the 25th, and bleeding from the gums on the 26th. He became drowsy on the 28th, and died on the 5th of July, but without complete coma. The treatment consisted of twenty-four leeches to the margin of the right ribs, followed by a small blister, mercurial and other purgatives, quinine in three and-four grain doses, with blue bill and ipecacuanha during the remissions, frequent sponging of the surface of the body with tepid water, saline diuretics, sago and chicken broth.

Examination eight hours after death. — All the tissues were tinged yellow. *Chest.*— Left lung was collapsed, crepitating, and healthy. The right lung adhered by tender bands to the costal pleura, but was crepitating and healthy. *Abdomen.*—The intestines both small and large were contracted. The liver was somewhat enlarged, yellowish in colour, but natural in consistence. The gall-bladder contained some bile, but it was not distended. The common duct was surrounded in three fourths of its circumference by the head of the pancreas, which seemed somewhat indurated, and larger than natural, and there the duct was somewhat contracted. On the other side of the duct, in contact with it, was an enlarged lymphatic gland, about an inch and a half in length and a quarter of an inch thick. The common, hepatic, and cystic ducts were permeable. The mucous membrane of the duodenum was healthy, and covered with bile.

40. *Remittent Fever with jaundice. — Tenderness at the margin of the right ribs.*

Death from exhaustion. — Enlargement and biliary congestion of the liver. — Gastro-duodenitis. — Hepatic cells distinct. — Sutwa Purojee, a Hindoo rope-maker of twenty-seven years of age, and stout habit of body, after suffering for twelve days from febrile symptoms, without, as reported, distinct remissions, was admitted into hospital on the 7th August, 1849. The abdomen was full, without induration, but with tenderness at the margin of the right ribs. He had occasional vomiting, and the tongue was coated. The bowels were reported to be regular. He admitted that he made occasional use of spirits. Thirty-six leeches were applied to the epigastrium, quinine in four-grain doses, with blue bill and ipecacuanha, was given during the remission. There was not much heat of skin on the 9th and 10th, the pain was relieved, and the vomiting had ceased. Some compound powder of jalap was given on the 10th. On that evening there was a febrile exacerbation, which continued on the 11th (there having been shivering at midnight), with increase of tenderness at the epigastrium and margin of right ribs, dulness to within an inch and a half of the umbilicus, and commencing jaundice. Respiration short and hurried, pulse frequent and small, and tongue dry, with dark fur. Fifty leeches were applied to the margin of the ribs, and ten grains of calomel, with four of compound extract of colocynth, were given. At noon, the skin was cool, the pulse feeble, and one pale evacuation had been passed. The side was said to be easier, but the breathing continued hurried, and he died about an hour after the report.*

Inspection three hours after death. — The body was not much reduced, and the tissues were tinged deeply yellow. *Chest.*—The lungs were crepitating, but somewhat inflated. There were no adhesions between the pulmonary and costal pleuræ. The heart was healthy. *Abdomen.*—The liver was much enlarged, and reached beyond the margin of the false ribs, from the tenth rib of the right side to within an inch and a half of the umbilicus, and thence to the most prominent part of the seventh left rib. No adhesions existed between it and the surrounding parts. When incised, the surfaces were of a mixed red and olive-green tint, and the substance was softer than natural throughout. The gall-bladder contained serous-looking bile. The stomach was full of half digested food, and its mucous membrane was of a uniform rose colour except in a few places where there was a deeper dotted redness with some degree of softening. The inner surface of the duodenum was tinged with bile, and its mucous membrane, as well as that of the large intestine, was of a redder colour than natural. The kidneys were large, and of a dark (almost black) red colour throughout, evidently from congestion of blood. The spleen was not enlarged. The head was not examined. — A small portion of the glandular substance of the liver was examined under the microscope, and exhibited the hepatic cells distinct.

41. *Remittent Fever with jaundice in an opium-eater. — Tenderness at the epigastrium. — No coma. — Death from exhaustion. — Enlargement and biliary congestion of the liver. — No duodenitis. — No enlargement of the lymphatic glands.* — Synd Bux, a Mussulman, a native of Mooltan, sixty years of age and following the occupation of a Fakir, was in the habit of taking opium, but only he said to the extent of two grains daily. After twelve days' illness with fever and epigastric tenderness he was admitted into hospital on the 23rd January, 1850. There was tenderness on pressure at the epigastrium, and dulness for two inches and a half below the ensiform cartilage. The spleen was also enlarged. The pulse was frequent and feeble. The tongue dryish with a yellow central coat and florid tip and edges. The conjunctivæ were yellow. On the 23rd, 24th, and 25th there was a febrile exacerbation. The urine was high coloured, the alvine discharges scanty and pale. From the 26th to the

---

* In this case the fatal result was expedited by the injudicious use of depressants in the advanced state of fever; indeed, it is not improbable that the exacerbation on the 10th was favoured by the purgative then given.

1st of February, there was very little febrile disturbance and the jaundice seemed to lessen somewhat, but there was no improvement in the strength of the pulse, the emaciation rather increased, and the movements of the limbs were tremulous. On the 1st of February, his manner was sluggish, and from this time increase of the febrile disturbance and of the asthenia took place. He died on the 7th without coma.

The treatment consisted of a small blister to the epigastrium, an occasional laxative, and quinine in four-grain doses in solution combined with nitrate of potass and spiritus ætheris nitricus during the remission, also chicken soup and wine.

Inspection seventeen hours after death. — The tissues of the body, chiefly the adipose and areolar, were tinged yellow. On opening the chest the lungs remained slightly inflated. There were some old adhesions between the outer and back part of the right lung and the costal pleura. The substance of both lungs was crepitating. The walls of the heart generally were thin, but there was no structural change of the organ. *Abdomen.* — The liver was enlarged and extended across the epigastric region reaching on the right side to the ninth rib, and on the left to the cartilage of the eighth rib. The liver presented a uniform olive-green appearance, evidently from biliary congestion, but there was no structural change. The gall-bladder contained some bile. The common, hepatic, and cystic ducts were pervious. There was no enlargement of the lymphatic glands or of other structure about these ducts. The contents of the duodenum were tinged with bile and the mucous membrane was apparently healthy. The spleen was considerably enlarged, reaching from the sixth to the last rib. The stomach was somewhat contracted. The transverse colon was displaced, one portion of it forming an angle with another which was directed downwards. The kidneys were healthy.

42. *Remittent Fever with jaundice.* — *Tenderness at the margin of the right ribs.* — *Death from exhaustion.* — *Cirrhosis.* — *Gall-bladder distended.* — *Enlarged lymphatic glands around the common duct.* — *Duodenitis.* — *Granular exudation on the mucous membrane of the ileum and large intestine.* — Elaee Buccus, a Mussulman subsisting by begging, of sixty years of age and visiting Bombay on his way to Mecca, was admitted into hospital in a reduced state on the 10th July, 1850.* He stated that he had been ill with fever for about thirteen days. He was jaundiced. There was tenderness below the margin of the right ribs and dulness for the extent of two inches, enlargement of the spleen, increased heat of skin, tongue dry and coated in the centre, and florid at the tip and edges, and the bowels were reported to be slow. Calomel six grains with extract of colocynth eight grains were given, and on the following morning pulv. jalap. comp., one drachm, but with the effect of causing little action of the bowels. Twelve leeches were applied to the margin of the ribs followed by a small blister. On the 13th, quinine in four-grain doses was given and repeated daily, and from that time to the 24th there was no recurrence of fever. The abdominal tenderness and the jaundice also gradually disappeared, the urine was no longer tinged green by nitric acid, and the tongue cleaned and became moist; but there was little improvement in strength. On the 24th, abdominal uneasiness was complained of and a rhubarb draught was given, but it produced no effect. In the evening there was recurrence of febrile exacerbation, and on the 26th dysenteric discharges. Under these symptoms, but without return of jaundice, he continued losing strength till the 2nd August, when he died without coma.

Inspection ten hours after death.— The body was much emaciated. *Chest.*— The right lung collapsed freely and there were two or three large emphysematous bullæ at its anterior margin, but otherwise it was healthy. The left lung was connected to the

---

* In this case, as well as that which immediately precedes it, there was a check to the fever from the use of quinine, but no tendency to the recovery of strength, owing probably to the advanced age and asthenia of the subjects.

costal pleura by firm adhesions, also its base to the diaphragm and its anterior edge to the pericardium, but its substance was crepitating. The heart was healthy. *Abdomen.*—The liver consisted almost entirely of the right lobe. The gall-bladder distended, reached nearly to the centre of the epigastric region, and was situated over the gastro-hepatic omentum. The external surface of the liver was somewhat irregular, but the substance was not indurated, and though when incised the surface presented here and there white streaks apparently from hypertrophy of areolar tissue, there was however no distinct lobular appearance. The lymphatic glands about the common duct were about the size of an olive, but they did not press upon the duct, which seemed more dilated than usual: this duct, and the hepatic and cystic ducts, were permeable, and when laid open the mucous membrane presented the usual reticulated character, but not a trace of redness. The contents of the gall-bladder were dark green, and very adhesive from admixture of mucus. The mucous membrane of the stomach was very rugous, mottled red towards the pyloric end, but without softening. There was a good deal of dark redness of the mucous coat of the duodenum arranged in streaks and patches, and chiefly occupying the apices of the rugæ. Brunner's glands were distinct, numerous, and elevated, and the mucous lining of the duodenum was neither softened nor thickened. The inner surface of the lower end of the ileum,—about two feet of it—also of that of the cœcum, the ascending and transverse colon presented a dark red mottled appearance, with exception of the cœcum, where the redness was uniform. Here and there there was granular exudation on the surface, to a slight degree in the ileum, but more general on parts of the large intestine, and in places the exudation had a dark grey colour, and there was abrasion of portions of the mucous membrane, as if from superficial ulceration. In these situations the lining membrane was connected to the subjacent tunic more closely than natural. The spleen was somewhat enlarged (six inches in length), but apparently healthy in structure. The kidneys were healthy.

43. *Fever with jaundice.—Died exhausted.—Biliary congestion of the liver.—No enlargement of the lymphatic glands.—Contraction of the cystic duct.—Distension of the gall-bladder. Mucous membrane of gall-bladder and ducts normal, with exception of slight vascularity of common duct at point of entrance into duodenum.—Hepatic cells distinct.*—Sukeah, a Hindoo, of twenty-two years of age, was admitted into hospital after nine days' illness on the 28th of August, 1850. He was jaundiced, drowsy, and very exhausted. He died ten hours after admission.

Inspection ten hours after death.—All the structures were tinged yellow. *Abdomen.*—The liver projected about two inches below the ensiform cartilage and right false ribs; and its incised surface presented generally a yellowish appearance with natural consistence. On examination under the microscope the hepatic cells were distinctly seen. The hepatic and common ducts were of natural dimensions, not turgid with bile, and when laid open, the mucous surface presented its normal appearance, with the exception of slight vascularity at the termination of the common duct in the duodenum. The lymphatic glands around the common duct were not increased in size. The gall-bladder was distended with bile of a dark green (almost black) colour. The cystic duct was very much contracted, and there was some obstruction at its commencement which prevented the point of a probe from entering the gall-bladder, but the mucous lining was healthy. The mucous membrane of the duodenum presented a dark grey colour, with here and there streaks of redness, and the glands of Brunner were very turgid, but neither softening nor ulceration was detected. The stomach contained a few ounces of dark-coloured liquid, its mucous surface was of dark grey colour with patches of redness over the prominent rugæ, and two or three small projections apparently caused by some deposit, one (the largest) about the size of a pea, was covered with coagulated blood. There were also two or three small ulcerated spots on the mucous membrane of the stomach which could be easily peeled off from the subjacent tissue. The small intestines were rather contracted. The kidneys were natural in size and structure, but the substance was tinged yellow. The heart was healthy.

44. *Remittent Fever with Jaundice.—Drowsiness.—Enlarged lymphatic glands in course of common duct.—Constricted cystic duct.—Gall-bladder full.*—A Hindoo, about thirty years of age, was admitted into the hospital in February 1849, with fever, drowsiness, and jaundice, and died about twenty-four hours after admission.

Inspection thirty-three hours after death.—The gall-bladder was full of bile but not distended. Along the common duct for about two inches and reaching almost to the duodenum there were enlarged lymphatic glands, both below and above the duct, each about the size of a small olive, and when cut giving out a brown turbid fluid the result of decomposition. The hepatic duct was pervious, but the cystic duct above its junction was so constricted as not to admit the small end of the blow-pipe.

45. *Remittent Fever with jaundice.—No tenderness at margin of ribs.—Drowsiness.—No enlargement of lymphatic glands.—Dark redness of mucous membrane of duodenum.*—Syed Mohedeen, a Mussulman beggar of forty years of age and of feeble constitution, after suffering for twelve days from febrile symptoms coming on at irregular periods, preceded by chilliness and attended during the last eight days with looseness of the bowels, was admitted into hospital on the 28th August, 1850. He was jaundiced. There was no induration or dulness at the margins of the ribs and he made no complaint of pain. The pulse was feeble, and the tongue coated in the centre was florid at the tip and edges. He died on the 12th September. Whilst under observation the bowels were relaxed; the evacuations were generally of a yellowish colour, sometimes scanty and passed with straining, but not tinged with blood. From the 31st to the 5th there was improvement, the febrile disturbance lessened, the tongue became more natural, and the jaundice decreased; but from the 6th there was again aggravation with (on the 10th) tremulous hands, brown dry tongue, and drowsiness. The urine throughout was scanty and high-coloured, but showed no traces of albumen.

Examination thirteen hours after death.—Head. The vessels of the dura mater were found turgid with blood, and the tissue somewhat tinged yellow. The vessels of the pia mater were also congested. On the inferior surface of the posterior lobe of the right side, and extending into its sulci, there was some extravasation of blood into the meshes of the pia mater. The substance of the brain was free from structural change, but when incised it presented some bloody points here and there. There was no increased serous fluid found in the ventricles, and no extravasation of blood into the substance of the brain. *Chest.*—The upper lobe of the left lung and the thin anterior edge of the lower one were soft and crepitating, but the rest of the lower lobe was in a state of red hepatisation. The whole of the right lung was healthy, excepting the thin posterior margin of its lower part which was in a state of red engorgement. The structure of the heart was healthy, but its valves were tinged yellow. *Abdomen.*—The substance of the liver was healthy in structure. The stomach contained yellow brown mucous-like contents with several lumbrici, but its inner coat was healthy. The lining membrane of the duodenum presented dark red patches, and the glands of Brunner were more than usually prominent. No compression of the biliary ducts from enlarged glands was detected, and the common and hepatic ducts were found permeable. On the mucous membrane of the large intestines there were patches of red and grey discoloration, most marked in the ascending colon and cœcum, but no traces of ulceration nor change in the consistence of the tissue were observed. The mucous membrane of the ileum was healthy with the exception of patches of faint redness here and there and the glands of Peyer were normal. The spleen was much enlarged, measuring six inches by five, but was of natural structure, except at its convex surface, where there were two deposits of tubercular-like matter each the size of a small bean. The kidneys were healthy in structure, but tinged yellow.

Parotitis. — Considerable tumefaction, ending in suppuration, in the situation of one or both parotid glands is an occasional occurrence in remittent fever. I have witnessed it only in natives and always associated with febrile symptoms of marked adynamic character. The notes of three cases, the subjects of which recovered after a long and tedious illness are before me.

Pathology of Inflammatory, Adynamic, and Congestive Remittent Fever. — The pathology of these modifications of remittent fever has already been incidentally considered in connection with the symptoms: their relation to particular states of the constitution, degrees of the morbific cause, and previously existing structural disease are the leading facts which should be borne in mind.

Pneumonia. — This complication and idiopathic pneumonia will be treated of together.

SECTION IV. — *Treatment.* — *Contrast of the Principles of Treatment of Malarious Remittent Fever, and the Zymotic Continued Fevers of Cold Climates.* — *Treatment of Ordinary, Inflammatory, Congestive, Adynamic, and Irregular Types of Remittent Fever.* — *Then of those complicated with Cerebral Affection, Gastric Irritability, Jaundice, Hepatitis.*

It has been already stated that the essential difference between intermittent and remittent fever is that in the former a periodic cessation — intermission — of the febrile phenomena takes place, while in the latter there is only abatement — remission.

Both these forms of fever depend on different degrees of the same morbific cause — malaria, — a *materies morbi* generated without and received into the blood. Theory suggests that similar principles of treatment must apply to diseases so nearly allied, and clinical experience confirms the inference.

It may, therefore, be useful to preface the details of the treatment of remittent fever by recapitulating the leading principles which have already been inculcated in respect to intermittent fever, and then pointing out the general character of the modifications which the difference in degree of the morbid actions in the two types may require. When a paroxysm of intermittent fever has fairly commenced, a certain course which we are unable to check must be run before it comes to a close; and this fact of clinical observation is in harmony with the nature of the cause.

The susceptibility of enfeebled persons to attacks of intermittent fever and the tendency of the disease in them to be protracted, that is, to be liable to recurrences of the paroxysm — may be safely admitted. Clinical observation teaches us that if much debility be produced by treatment in intermittent fever, this greater liability to a protracted course becomes materially increased, and serves to illustrate the law that a morbific cause when in action is always more influential on the predisposed from debility, however induced.

If there co-exist with the febrile disturbance such derangement of the capillary circulation of important organs as is likely to injure their structures, or otherwise seriously to impair their functions, then the means appropriate for the removal of this complication must be had recourse to.

Though a paroxysm of intermittent fever cannot be stopped, yet the degree of vascular excitement may be modified in such manner as to lessen discomfort and mitigate local derangements when they exist. This object may be effected by ventilation, purity of atmosphere, reduction of the temperature of the surface of the body by the external application of cold, and attention to quietness and repose. These means do not abstract any of the constituents of the blood, and therefore do not debilitate. But the same end may be accomplished by blood-letting, purgatives or other evacuants, but agencies of this kind enfeeble, and they ought not to be used except in cases in which the necessity for decided and prompt reduction of vascular excitement or for free elimination is so pressing as to justify our disregarding for the time the lesser because the remoter evil.

Although a paroxysm of intermittent fever when once formed cannot be checked, yet after in its natural course it has ceased we have in quinine an effective means of preventing its return; and when we compare this statement with that of our inability to stop the paroxysm, it becomes evident that therapeutic force in this disease is confined to the period of intermission.

These general principles are equally applicable to the treatment of remittent fever, and it shall now be my endeavour to explain in what respect they require to be modified when applied to this type.

In intermittent fever there is for the most part little risk of injury to important organs during the stage of febrile reaction. A frequent recurrence of the paroxysm is not in general attended with immediate danger to life, but injures by deteriorating the constitution. In remittent fever, on the other hand, there is greater likelihood of harm from the increased vascular excitement of the exacerbation, and therefore recurrences of this stage are not unfrequently attended with immediate danger to life from lesion of important organs, or depression of vital actions. Hence, in the treatment of remittent fever, though there is often necessity for the reduction of febrile excitement in the exacerbation by depletory means, yet at the same time there is greater demand for the exercise of discriminating judgment, for the evils of the injudicious use of depressant remedies are more immediate, more certain, and more serious. If such are the dangers which may attend the exacerbation of remittent fever, then the prevention of its recurrence by the efficient use of quinine given during the remission is even more urgent than the same indication in the intermission of intermittent fever.

If it be true that at some periods of the exacerbation of remittent fever there may be risk of injury to important organs from excessive vascular action calling for control by depletion, and that, at other periods, there may be danger to life from exhaustion requiring the prompt use of stimulants and nourishment ; if it be also true that the time of exacerbation and remission is liable to vary in different cases, that it is most important to prevent the exacerbation, and that we are able to effect it; then it follows that there cannot be successful treatment of remittent fever, justice to the sick, or loyalty to the profession of medicine, unless our visits to the sick be frequent and our watching attentive and well-timed.*

* Since the publication of the first edition of this work, I have found in "Observations on the Diseases of the Army in Jamaica, by John Hunter, M.D., Physician to the Army, 1788," these principles inculcated with so much truth and force, that I here quote the passage for the instruction of the reader, and with the view of enforcing the analogous statement in the text:

"A surgeon that would do justice to the men under his care must be very frequent in his visits to the hospital; for unless he watch assiduously the remissions of the fever, and be ready to take immediate advantage of them, he will not be able to check the disease speedily, without which both the constitution and life of the patient will be in imminent danger. A man that has three or four fits of the fever is in greater danger of dying than one that has only one or two; but laying the risk of death out of the question, a man that has his fever stopped after the first or second fit, will generally be restored to health in a few days, whereas if he have four or five fits, it will often require as many weeks to recover the same degree of strength in the latter case as days in the former. It must, therefore, be obvious how much the diligence and attention of the surgeon importeth, of which a very striking proof occurred in a regiment which was strong and consisted of twelve companies. The regiment was pro-

At the opening of the section on the pathology of remittent fever it was stated that when remittent fever is compared with the zymotic continued fevers of the colder climates this striking difference is observable. In the former there are daily remissions of the fever, that is a return, more or less complete, to normal actions; but in the latter the fever is continuous and unabated for many successive days. This difference materially affects the principles of treatment. In both the febrile reaction is caused by a materies in the blood whose power when thus in operation we are unable to stop. In both, but more in remittent fever than in the others, there may be danger to important organs from deranged capillary circulation rendering necessary the adoption of means for lessening vascular excitement. In both there is danger to life from depression of vital actions—from the sedative influence of the cause, the continuance of the febrile disturbance, the previous condition of the subject, or of all combined—requiring stimulants and support.

In remittent fever there are periodic abatements of the febrile state, and there is an agent which, when effectively used in the remission, tends to prevent the recurrence of the exacerbation, and thus most materially to shorten the general course of the disease. On these circumstances our chief power in the treatment of remittent fever depends, but it has no place in that of the zymotic continued fevers. In these there is less frequently necessity for con-

vided with two hospitals and two surgeons, each of whom took charge of the sick of six companies. It was presently found that one hospital was much fuller than the other, which did not appear to proceed from a greater sickness among one division of the companies than the other, for there was no material difference in the number of sick sent from the several companies. In order to bring the sick in the two hospitals to an equality, a company was taken from one division and annexed to the other. The sick of the five companies were, however, still more numerous than that of the seven; and after a short trial, they were divided into four and eight companies, and then the sick in the two hospitals were nearly equal, and varied from forty to sixty in each. It may be supposed that so great a difference depended upon the method of treatment being entirely different in the two hospitals. That, however, was not the case; the general plan of treatment was nearly the same in both, and not materially different from what has been mentioned in speaking of the cure of the remittent fever. It was owing to the following circumstances: one surgeon visited his hospital four or five times a day, the other only twice a day; the first seldom allowed any remission to pass without taking advantage of it, the latter often; one was always at hand to palliate the untoward symptoms, as vomitings or purgings, proceeding either from the medicines or the disease; the other not. Add to these, that vigilance in the surgeon at the head of an hospital extends itself to the servants and nurses under him, and thence a greater degree of attention both in administering nourishment and medicines. The effect of all those causes was, that the men recovered in half the time in one hospital that they did in the other, and therefore the hospital for eight companies had no greater number of sick than that for four."

trolling local capillary derangements and little risk of sudden unexpected exhaustion. The course of the disease is, compared with that of remittent fever, steady and prolonged, and the main indication of cure is, by warding off undue prostration, to conduct the patient safely to its close. The treatment is, therefore, expectant and for several days in succession may be continued with little change. Contrast this with what has been already said of remittent fever, the changes from exacerbation to remission taking place within a few hours at varying periods, and requiring a decided modification of the remedies.

It was in order to point to this contrast in the principles of treatment that I have entered into this comparison between remittent and zymotic continued fever and have shown the invariable necessity of constant watching and action in the one, and the sufficiency, for the most part, of expectant principles in the other. It is well to fix attention on these doctrines, for observation has convinced me that medical men whose practical knowledge of fever has been acquired in hospitals in European countries do not quickly realise to themselves the frequent changes which take place from the very outset in remittent fever, the importance of watching them, and of regarding them in treatment. On the other hand, when we look back to the state of practice in fevers in India twenty years ago, it is evident that principles of treatment in the zymotic fevers of the colder climates which are equally applicable to remittent fever were lost sight of and neglected; principles which acknowledge our inability, in the present state of medical art, to cut short the febrile * disturbance of a zymotic cause, and which admit great danger to life from depression of vital actions, consequent on the persistence of the febrile state.

The treatment which is applicable to the different circumstances of remittent fever will be first described, and then a few observations will be offered on some of the principal remedies.

Ordinary Remittent Fever. —The description of the treatment of this form is chiefly derived from my experience in the European General Hospital at Bombay. The subjects were, in great part, seamen, and were admitted generally about the third day of the disease. In the exacerbation there was headache, with flushing of the countenance, and, in a small proportion of cases, vomiting, with some degree of epigastric tenderness. In the greater number the tongue was coated yellow in the centre, in some expanded, in others

* In applying this principle to remittent fever, I speak of the febrile disturbance of the stage of exacerbation.

contracted and pointed with florid edges and tip. The pulse was generally neither firm nor full, but frequent and moderate in strength. In a great many instances the secretions from the bowels were dark or greenish in colour, but became natural as the tongue cleaned. The remittent character of the fever was well marked.

In treating the exacerbation, general blood-letting was unnecessary. In cases in which there was much headache and flushing of the face, from thirty-six to sixty leeches to the temples, and cold applications to the head were required. In cases in which there was tenderness at the epigastrium, and a contracted tongue with florid edges and tip, there was necessity for more or less leeching of the epigastrium, the use of effervescing draughts, cold drinks in small quantity at a time, and the avoidance of emetics, antimonials, mercurials, and purgatives. When the headache was moderate, and gastric irritation was absent, then cold applications to the head, frequent tepid sponging of the surface of the body, antimony in small doses, or aqua acetatis ammoniæ, sufficed for reducing the febrile excitement.

Emetics were often useful at the commencement of the attack, but it was necessary to give them with much discrimination. In cases in which the tongue was foul and expanded but not florid, and in which there was nausea without vomiting or epigastric tenderness, twenty-five grains of ipecacuanha was the emetic which was generally used with advantage.

During the first two or three days of the attack, when the tongue was foul but not florid, the alvine excretions vitiated, the abdomen full and resisting, and the vascular excitement steady and without tendency to depression, it was an important part of the treatment to give a ten-grain dose of calomel, combined with a few grains of antimonial powder, and some hours afterwards an aperient, as the compound powder of jalap. The calomel was most generally administered at bed-time, and the compound powder of jalap in the morning. Calomel and purgatives, even to the extent now recommended, are seldom expedient after the third or fourth day of the disease, and they are unnecessary, even at an earlier period, if the abdomen be soft and without fullness, notwithstanding the presence of disordered alvine excretions and a coated tongue.

After the first or second exacerbation a full dose * of muriate of morphia was exhibited in many cases at bed-time with much bene-

* This recommendation must be carefully considered in connection with my subsequent remarks on the use of full opiates in remittent fever.

fit. When there is headache with great heat and dryness of skin and a full and frequent pulse, morphia is contra-indicated; but in most cases when there has been good management at the commencement — adequate leeching, the appropriate use of calomel and purgatives — there follows, on the succeeding night, slight pyrexia with restlessness, but without headache, a supple abdomen, a tongue still foul but moist, a pulse above the natural frequency but soft. In a case of this kind, calomel or blue pill, in a dose proportioned to the state of the tongue and the condition of the secretions in regard to quantity and quality, with a grain of ipecacuanha and one of muriate of morphia, preceded by a foot-bath, perhaps by a few leeches to the temples, will generally be succeeded by a quiet night, and a forenoon remission so distinct as to admit of quinine being freely exhibited. This method, moreover, tends to restore a natural state of the secretions with less risk of gastro-enteric irritation.

The remedial means as yet referred to are used with the view of decreasing the vascular excitement of the exacerbation, protecting organs important to life from harm by undue determination of blood, and correcting deranged functions. These are very important considerations, but they are subordinate to the main indication of cure in remittent fever, which assimilates in every respect to that already insisted upon in the intermittent type, viz. to take advantage of the earliest remission by adopting means to prevent a return of the exacerbation, or failing this to postpone its access or lessen its severity; and for this purpose quinine is as efficacious as in the intermission of intermittent fever. The same course should be observed in all subsequent remissions, irrespective of local complications, which may require special means for their removal, and which it is very important not to neglect, but which should not be allowed materially to interfere with the steady pursuit of the leading indication of cure as now stated.

The earliest remission should be regarded, and quinine be given in from four to six-grain doses every second or third hour, for four or five times. Should the exacerbation return the quinine is to be omitted, but should it not recur, the quinine is to be continued every third or fourth hour, till the febrile phenomena have disappeared, and the probability of return has ceased.

But in ordinary remittent fever derangement of functions often co-exists with the remission, and requires attention in the treatment. Though such derangements are most certainly and speedily corrected by the mere prevention of the exacerbation, yet advantage may often result from remedial means more especially directed against them. It may be acknowledged as a therapeutic principle in remittent fever, that all medicines not used merely to reduce excessive vascular action, are given, with less likelihood of harm and more probability of benefit, during the remission than during the exacerbation. Nor is it difficult to suggest the explanation. The less abnormal state of the general and capillary circulation, characteristic of remission, is more favourable to absorption and the other processes concerned in therapeutic actions. Thus it will sometimes be useful, when an aperient is indicated, to combine two drachms of sulphate of magnesia with the first and second doses of quinine, or when the bowels are slow and the tongue much coated, a grain or two of calomel or blue pill with aloes may be substituted for the salt. If there be tendency to diarrhœa, the quinine may be combined with appropriate opiates. If there be nausea, the use of effervescing draughts with the quinine is often beneficial. But while we act on these principles we must always remember that they are subordinate to the prevention of the exacerbation, and if their application at all interferes with this they ought for the time to be set aside.

These remarks on the treatment of ordinary remittent fever, though based on clinical observation in the European General Hospital, are equally applicable to this form of the disease in more sthenic Europeans and at earlier stages, with this addition, that at the outset of the attack a general blood-letting of from sixteen to twenty ounces may often be an expedient measure. They also apply to the same type of fever in natives of good constitution, with this exception, that in them there is less necessity for leeching, calomel, purgatives, and a full opiate used in the manner recommended.

In regard to diet. · In ordinary remittent fever so treated that there occurs no undue exhaustion from the injudicious use of depressant means, stimulants are unnecessary, and animal broths are not required till convalescence has fairly commenced.

On examining the diaries of sixteen well-marked cases of ordinary remittent fever treated in the European Hospital in accordance with these principles, it appears that from the commencement of the attack to the perfect cessation of all febrile symptoms, the average period was six days and a half: of these, two were passed before admission, and four and a half under treatment in hospital. The time occupied in the cure is an important consideration from its bearing on the degree of efficiency of the patient after recovery: this will always be in proportion to the judgment displayed in abstaining from unnecessary depressants in the exacerbations, and in the early prevention of exacerbations by the adequate use of quinine in the remissions. The stage of convalescence, moreover, will vary according to the nature of the treatment and the duration of the attack. If the management has been skilful, convalescence will be attended by little derangement of function, and will require only a moderate use of stimulants and special articles of diet; but if depletion, purgatives, and mercury have been used in excess, and quinine insufficiently in the remission, convalescence will be characterised by much debility, splenic enlargement, dyspepsia, palpitation, intermittent headache, and tendency to diarrhœa or dysentery; and stimulants and extras will be largely consumed.

When a body of men — a regiment — in India is not, or has not lately been very unfavourably placed, as respects locality and general sanitary conditions, and its hospital returns show a large proportion of dyspepsia and cardiac affections — palpitation — with a large consumption of wine and beer, the inference may be safely hazarded that its fevers have been unskilfully treated.

Inflammatory Remittent Fever. — In this form in sthenic Europeans recently arrived in India, in consequence of the greater febrile excitement, and cerebral and gastric derangement, depletion is more indicated in the exacerbation. There is more need for general and local blood-letting, and the assiduous application of cold to the head. In many cases in which the skin is dry and steadily hot, cold affusion may be used from time to time with great advantage; but emetics and antimonials are in general contra-indicated from the tendency to gastric irritability which usually exists.

Though to increase hepatic and intestinal excretion, with the view of lessening febrile reaction by evacuation and of removing the products of augmented metamorphosis of tissue, is a distinct indication, yet we are frequently obliged to be very cautious in the use of calomel and purgatives; for there is often present congestion of, or determination to, the gastro-intestinal lining, very apt to be increased or to pass into inflammation by the use of irritants, and thus to aggravate the fever. In this difficulty we must keep these opposing principles before us, and lean to one or other as our judgment may dictate in particular cases. We shall often succeed best by premising leeches to the epigastrium during the exacerbation, and deferring the one or two ten-grain doses of calomel which may be necessary till the period of remission, and then combining them with opium, while at the same time we exhibit quinine.

In the treatment of inflammatory remittent fever, freer depletion is required, but still it should be used with watching and caution, and the safest time is at the height, not the close, of an early exacerbation. Nor should we forget that evacuants are had recourse to, not in the hope of cutting short the attack, but merely of lessening the risk of injury from vascular excitement; and that they are being used in a disease which, if it persists, is sooner or later sure to terminate in signal depression of the vital actions. The best guide to the successful application of depletory remedies is the presence of a dry skin of steadily increased temperature, and a pulse frequent, firm, and of good volume, associated with hyperœmia of an important organ; but it must not be supposed, that a sthenic constitution, and an early stage of the attack, necessarily indicate the propriety of free depletion and other depressing means. It should be borne in mind that in all states of constitution, the sedative influence of malaria may be great at the very outset of the disease, and that then depressants are likely to be injurious. If then (it matters not what the constitution, or the duration of the attack may be) the pulse be badly developed and easily compressed, and the general surface of the body not steadily dry and of augmented temperature, we must be very cautious. I do not say that under these circumstances general blood-letting may never be had recourse to; but I am certain that we should be very watchful, that the finger should be on the pulse as the blood flows, and if the action of the heart does not speedily improve, which it seldom will, then the further abstraction of blood must be stopped.

Such then are the principles to be observed in the treatment of the exacerbation in inflammatory remittent fever. They must be considered in connection with what has previously been said on the management of the same stage of the ordinary form of the disease.

In the remission the principles advocated in ordinary remittents still more forcibly apply to the present form. Quinine in from five to eight-grain doses should be given every second hour, or it may be necessary, when the remission is very short, to give it every hour; and continue or intermit it in the manner already explained.

In the first section of this chapter, the diagnosis between remittent and common continued fever is stated, and it is remarked that under certain circumstances, in the plains of the Ganges and

Indus, the Coromandel coast and the table lands of the Deccan and Malwa, a compound type is occasionally met with, in which the remissions, though more marked than is usual in continued fever, are slighter than is commonly observed in the remittent form. This variety bears depletion better than pure remittents, because the sedative influence of malaria is less operative; and though quinine, in doses of from two to five grains, is necessary in the remission, a larger quantity is often badly borne, because the tolerance is less. It not unfrequently happens, in cases of doubtful diagnosis, that we are materially assisted by watching the effect of quinine.

Congestive Remittent Fever.—Having in the course of my remarks on the treatment of inflammatory remittent fever enjoined caution in the use of blood-letting, when the symptoms tend to be congestive, there need be no hesitation in condemning it when the congestive form is distinctly developed.

Viewing the internal congestion of blood, which doubtless exists in these cases as one of the conditions necessarily resulting from a depressed state of the vital actions of the vascular and nervous systems, general blood-letting has always seemed to me contra-indicated in theory; and my experience, so far as it has gone, has confirmed this opinion.

The treatment should consist of the judicious external use of stimulants, and the exhibition of calomel and quinine frequently repeated. The instance in which I have witnessed the most marked benefit from these remedies was in a seaman of the name of Crookberry, attacked with fever after exposure in the dockyard at Bombay, in October 1840. The skin was coldish and damp, the pulse frequent, compressible and becoming feeble, the manner heavy, with drowsiness and wandering delirium, and the secretions from the liver and intestines suppressed. He continued in this state for twenty-four hours, not improving under the use of free doses of calomel, a blister to the nucha, and wine. Quinine and calomel were then given in two-grain doses of each, and repeated at intervals.* The pulse and the skin improved, then followed two or three days of febrile exacerbation, succeeded by recovery.

When the symptoms of congestion cease and reaction follows, then the subsequent treatment should accord with the principles already inculcated in the ordinary and inflammatory forms, or with those which are about to be noticed in the continued and

* The quinine should certainly be given in larger doses than in this case.

adynamic types—as the one or the other happens to apply to the particular instance.

The suggestion made at the commencement of the pathological remarks on remittent fever—that congestive symptoms may in some cases be related to old-standing disease of the heart, the liver or kidneys—is an additional reason for observing great caution in the treatment of this form, more particularly in the use of depletion and other sedative remedies.

Remittent Fever tending to become continued, then adynamic in character.—In years and at seasons when the causes are intense or the predisposition great, remittent fever is frequently of an aggravated character, evinced not by assuming the inflammatory form, but by the remissions becoming less apparent, and the exacerbation, in the worst cases, putting on an almost continued form for two or three successive days. Cases of this kind are more difficult to cure, because quinine, in doses sufficiently large to make any great impression on the disease, is for a time often inappropriate; still even when the remission is very imperfect, it should be tried, and repeated, or not, in subsequent remissions, according to the effect.

When the evidence is good that quinine is not beneficial, all that can be done is to recollect the principles applicable to typhus and typhoid fever, and guide the patient through the attack, protecting important organs from undue determination of blood, and taking care that this indication is not effected by means which will too much depress the vital actions of the system, and favour the accession of adynamic symptoms; and then, so soon as a remission becomes marked, to have recourse to quinine. Though thus conceding that cases of remittent fever may occur in which, unfortunately, it is not admissible to use quinine very early in the disease, still I am convinced that the more closely such doubtful cases are watched, the more frequent the opportunities of exhibiting this remedy will be found to occur. This watchfulness should be enforced from the very commencement of the attack; for, as already stated, the tendency to a fair remission is very often greater during the two or three first days,—the continued character coming on as a subsequent event.

When remittent fevers have thus passed into the almost continued form, they are, after a time, as explained in my notice of the symptoms, liable to evince a train of adynamic phenomena, and then the only method of managing them is, to recollect the principles laid down by Cullen, that "fevers tend to cure themselves," and that the indication of cure is "to obviate the tendency to death."* In fact, all that can be aimed at in such cases is to reduce the increased temperature of the surface by tepid sponging; to sustain the pulse by light nourishment, wine and other stimulants; to attend to the excretions; and to apply cautiously small blisters over the organs which seem to be chiefly affected, taking care that they are not used to the degree of increasing febrile excitement, and recollecting that in the adynamic state of remittent fever, in the advanced stages, a tendency to run into gangrene is evinced equally as in European typhus.

Such are the resources to which we are restricted when adynamic symptoms co-exist with fever in which the remissions are not marked; but should a remission become distinct, dryness and brownness of the tongue offer no drawback to the use of quinine. I have seen cases, and of one the diary is before me, that of Penn, aged twenty-one, of her Majesty's ship *Endymion*, ill with dockyard fever, in which, after about ten days of almost continued febrile excitement, attended in the last days with brown dry tongue and other adynamic symptoms, a remission was taken advantage of and quinine was freely given and continued with marked benefit through each succeeding remission. The exacerbations decreased and quickly ceased, and, coincident with this result, the tongue became cleaner and moister,—because the dryness was but a sequence of the persistence of the febrile state, and one of the proofs of diminished secretion. Not only did the tongue in this instance become moist, but, for a similar reason, the secretions from the bowels became more regular, freer, and more natural in appearance.

We have every encouragement, under these circumstances, to persevere in the appropriate course of treatment; for, in young and previously healthy subjects, recovery not unfrequently takes place from an unfavourable train of adynamic symptoms, including more or less delirium, with well-marked tendency to drowsiness.

Remittent Fever with badly developed symptoms; with symptoms of unexpected collapse; with certain occasional features.—Under these heads, in the Section on Symptoms,

* Under these circumstances to attempt to affect the system with mercury, or to hope to control local inflammations by free leeching, or to correct the abdominal secretions by active purgatives, are measures so totally at variance with the indications of cure, and so destructive of the faint hope of recovery which it is useful to maintain, that were it not for the indiscriminate manner in which these means have been and still are frequently used it would be unnecessary to allude to them here.

phenomena are described, which all point to the tendency, in remittent fever, of vital actions to become depressed, and thus lead to death. In noticing these phenomena, with reference to treatment, all that can be said is, that they forcibly inculcate the necessity of familiarising ourselves with the principles which regulate the application of depressant remedies; and while they impress upon us the evils of the injudicious use of these means, they teach us to be prompt with those appliances — quinine, stimulants, and nourishment — which prevent prostration, or counteract it when present.

Remittent Fever with Cerebral Affection. — We have found that this complication is a frequent and fatal one in the remittent fevers of sthenic Europeans, and also in the adynamic forms of the disease. In order to understand the treatment, the remarks already made on the symptoms and pathology of this complication must be borne in mind. Headache, delirium, flushed countenance, with steady heat of surface, and a well-developed and firm pulse — present in sthenic Europeans — should be met during the exacerbation by detraction of blood, both general and local, the application of cold to the shaven head, free action of the bowels by mercurial purgatives, and the use of small doses of tartar emetic, when the state of the stomach will admit. But it is only in the very early exacerbations that we may hope to use these means with good effect. So soon as the pulse, still increasing in frequency, distinctly fails in strength, and the delirium becomes muttering and alternates with tendency to drowsiness, the stage for evacuants has passed, — their use will merely hasten the fatal issue. In bad remittents this state may come on as early as the fourth or fifth day of the attack, or earlier where the phenomena have been congestive at the commencement. Further, the remark made under the head Pathology, that undue depletion in the exacerbation sometimes leads to the development of head symptoms — muttering delirium, and tendency to drowsiness — at the close of a paroxysm, must be remembered.

These facts, which bring again before us the important truth of the marked tendency to prostration in remittent fever, and again point to the evils of undue depletion, are not, however, to be advanced as arguments against the use of evacuant means in appropriate circumstances. They teach us to be very watchful for the first symptoms of cerebral complication, and to be very prompt, but not rash, in the application of our remedies; to observe with care their effect on the cerebral symptoms and on the pulse; to be very assiduous in the application of cold to the head, and to enjoin great quietude, and the removal of all sources of excitement. It is by attention to principles such as these that we may hope to secure those advantages which depletory treatment, used with judgment and caution, is most certainly capable of conferring, and to avoid those evils which will as surely result from its abuse in unsuitable states of constitution and stages of disease.

When the period for local detraction of blood has passed, but head symptoms still continue and tend to drowsiness, a blister * may be applied to the nucha with advantage; and the time which should be selected is the commencement of a remission, not the height of an exacerbation.

Such, then, are the means of treatment when cerebral symptoms depend on determination or congestion. They must be viewed in connection with the principles elsewhere laid down for the treatment of the exacerbation in uncomplicated remittents.

Head symptoms, dependent on inflammation of the membranes of the brain passing on to effusion of lymph, are rare compared with those caused by other conditions. They are usually characterised by milder delirium, by less febrile reaction, by greater persistence of the symptoms during the remission, by agitated movements of the hands and fingers, and occasional convulsion; and are most likely to occur in the less sthenic states of constitution. They must be met by a judicious application of antiphlogistic therapeutic principles.

The muttering delirium and tendency to drowsiness coming on in more advanced stages of fever, and associated with adynamic phenomena, are to be controlled by means altogether different. The adynamia must be treated by appropriate stimulants and nourishment, and depressant remedies of all kinds must be abstained from. When, however, the tendency to drowsiness begins to appear, a small blister should be applied to the nucha, or, should that be inconvenient, to some part of the head. Under these means recovery not unfrequently takes place, particularly in youthful subjects.

Treatment of the pathological states of the brain, which cause head symptoms, by the induction of mercurial influence, has been practised, and the question of its propriety may be here discussed.

* The blistering preparation which I have generally used was introduced into hospitals in India on the recommendation of Dr. Donald Young in 1835, under the name of liquor lyttæ. It is considerably stronger than the acetum cantharidis of the Pharmacopœia. The latter preparation often fails.

Viewing the head symptoms apart from the fever which they complicate, mercurial action is clearly contra-indicated in the adynamic form, as well as in that depending on determination or congestion of blood, with threatening serous effusion: it is not sanctioned by any reasonable therapeutic doctrine. But in that train of head symptoms depending on inflammation tending to terminate in exudation of lymph, mercury may be proposed on theoretic grounds; and in occasional cases, in which the diagnosis is clear and the constitution suitable, it may be expedient to have recourse to it in the remission. Yet on the whole my judgment is opposed to this means as a rule of practice, for the following reasons. 1. Meningitis is rare, compared with other proximate causes of head symptoms in remittent fever, and it occurs more commonly in asthenic than sthenic constitutions. 2. It is often difficult to distinguish the symptoms depending on inflammation from those resulting from other pathological states, for which mercury is either unnecessary or injurious. 3. Mercurial influence and the process by which it is induced very generally prove injurious in that state — the fever — of which the meningitis is a complication; and it may be received as a pathological law, that whatever aggravates an idiopathic fever must aggravate the local derangement which complicates it.

The general question of the mercurial treatment of remittent fever will be considered in a subsequent part of my observations; and the use of opiates, which has also reference to the management of head symptoms, will likewise be afterwards discussed.

These remarks on the treatment of cerebral complication have hitherto referred to the stage of exacerbation. When explaining the treatment of the complicated forms of intermittent fever, I took the opportunity of stating my conviction that, whatever the complication might be, the adequate exhibition of quinine during the intermission was a ruling indication of cure. This rule of practice is equally true of remittent fever. It matters not what the nature of the cerebral symptoms may be, the sufficient use of quinine must never be neglected. There has, I am aware, been very often doubt and hesitation in giving quinine in the remissions of fever with head complication; not only is this unnecessary, but the suspicion may be entertained that part of the mortality from this complication has been due to the want of the remedial benefit of this agent. It is almost needless to add, that while we exhibit quinine we are not to neglect the other efficacious means which are also applicable to the stage of remission.

Remittent Fever with Gastric Irritability.—The observations made on the symptoms and pathology of this complication suggest the treatment. It should consist chiefly of local abstraction of blood from the epigastrium, followed by blisters when the further loss of blood is contra-indicated. As in the case of all inflammatory complications of remittent fever, the exacerbation is the appropriate period for leeching, the remission for blisters. The internal use of ice is also important.

We must be very guarded in giving mercurial preparations and purgatives, and should, on other grounds, the indication for their exhibition be pressing, then, after preliminary leeching in the exacerbation, they should be used in the remission rather than the exacerbation, and the calomel should be combined with opium. Quinine should be had recourse to in the remission, and it is important on this account so to manage the irritability of stomach during the exacerbation, as to render the rejection of the quinine in the remission less likely. Should this fail, it may be exhibited by enema.

Remittent Fever with Jaundice.—The co-existence of tenderness at the margin of the right ribs, with jaundice, suggests the presence of inflammatory action, and our pathological research has shown that the mucous membrane of the duodenum and of the stomach is frequently the seat of the inflammation. Observation has further taught us that jaundice generally does not appear till several days after the commencement of the fever. These facts inculcate watchfulness for the first indication of tenderness below the right ribs, and on its appearance, without reference to the presence or not of jaundice, the adoption of the remedies for inflammation appropriate to the particular case, as well as abstinence from the means likely to excite irritation of the mucous lining of the stomach and duodenum.

When jaundice is present, the treatment should consist of the application of leeches or small blisters to the tender part below the right ribs, and the use of quinine during the remission, combined with small doses of aloes and mild mercurials, or of some saline aperient.

Of the ten fatal cases which have been detailed by me (36 to 45), there are five in which, judging from the colour of the liver, biliary congestion was present; in 3 the colour of the organ is not mentioned, and in one it was streaked white. It may, therefore, be inferred that in cases of jaundice complicating remittent fever, the proximate cause is usually not defective action of the hepatic cells, but rather some obstacle to the passage of the bile from the liver. The occurrence of jaundice in cases of remittent fever in which there had been free use of calomel and purgatives, is a fact which has long been familiar to me, and I deduce from these two statements, and the two previously made, viz. — that gastro-duodenitis is frequently present, and that jaundice is generally not a complication of the early stage of fever — that full doses of calomel and the free use of purgatives form no part of the treatment of remittent fever complicated with jaundice. On the contrary, they are likely to cause an aggravation of the symptoms, and to accelerate the period of prostration.

As a subsidiary means benefit is sometimes derived from the use of saline diuretics, at the same time with the remedies already advised. They seem to expedite the elimination of the biliary pigment from the blood.

Remittent Fever with Hepatitis.—As already stated, the complication of remittent fever with hepatitis, either in Europeans or natives, is, according to my observation, a rare occurrence. The only question of treatment which arises is the expediency or not of inducing mercurial influence. On this point of practice it may be assumed that the doctrines advanced on the treatment by this means of a complicating meningitis, are equally applicable to a complicating hepatitis.

The management of hepatic and splenic enlargement, co-existing with or subsequent to intermittent fever, has been fully explained. The same principles apply to these enlargements when co-existing with or consequent on remittent fever.

Remittent Fever with Dysentery.—The general rule which I have endeavoured to establish in respect to the treatment of all the complications of remittent fever, should be also observed in this particular one. While we treat the fever with quinine during the remissions, we must fulfil, in so far as it may be practicable, the indications which I shall have to explain elsewhere, as appropriate in the treatment of dysentery.

Section V.—*Treatment further considered in Remarks on Blood-letting, Mercury, Cold Affusion and Wet Sheet Packing, Purgatives, Emetics, Blisters, Opiates, Quinine, Diet, and Change of Air.*

General Blood-letting. — It has been explained that general blood-letting is an expedient and useful measure — sometimes a very necessary one — in reducing the high vascular excitement of the early exacerbations of remittent fever in sthenic and lately arrived Europeans, as well as in lesser degrees of excitement, when in this state of constitution and stage of fever there co-exist considerable determinations of blood to important vital organs. The extent to which blood-letting should be carried in suitable cases is a point on which the physician must exercise his discretion — keeping in view the ultimate advantage of effecting the indication aimed at with as little loss of blood as practicable, and recollecting that the judicious removal of sources of irritation, the adoption of free ventilation, the well-timed use of emetics, cold affusion, tepid sponging, and antimonials, are all measures of considerable influence in lowering febrile excitement, which it is of essential consequence to employ with assiduity in order to lessen the necessity of large evacuations. In the treatment of remittent fever in Europeans some time resident in India, and in all classes of the native community, general blood-letting is, with few exceptions, an unnecessary and often injurious proceeding.

Throughout these observations it has been my object to inculcate the following principles: — 1. That in the great majority of instances the danger in remittent fever consists in prostration of the vital actions of the heart and nervous system. 2. That not only exhaustion, but also the protraction of the disease, is favoured by needless and undue evacuations. 3. That evacuant means used in the exacerbation have no power in shortening the duration of the attack.

The opportunity has at different times been afforded me of witnessing the treatment of the exacerbations of remittent fever by repeated venesection, and its injurious tendency was very apparent. It is true that the vascular excitement of an exacerbation may be lessened, and the symptoms depending on that excitement may be for the time alleviated by blood-letting; but the paroxysm nevertheless recurs, and after repeated depletion the febrile disturbance becomes more severe and continuous, with not unfrequently an aggravation of all the local complications. This latter fact was known to Pringle, who says: "But repeated bleedings, unless upon evident marks of a fixed inflammation, were so far from producing the desired effect, that they were apt to render the fever more obstinate."* Lind writes much to the same purpose: "This fever (remitting), unless brought to a speedy remis-

* "Observations on the Diseases of the Army." London, 1765, p. 208.

sion, is attended with considerable danger; and if large quantities of blood be repeatedly taken from patients labouring under it, by mistaking their disease for a true inflammatory fever, its obstinacy and fatality are greatly increased."* . Dr. Stokes remarks: "From what I have seen I am disposed to conclude that bleeding in the cold stage, when it does alter the type of intermittent fever, has a tendency to convert tertian into quotidian and quotidian into remittent or continued fever. I never saw any example of the converse, or in which quotidian was converted into tertian."† Mr. Twining observes: "A remarkable fact may be here noticed, namely, that the employment of blood-letting in the cold stage of intermittent fever is occasionally, though rarely, followed by continued fever."‡

The practice of blood-letting in the cold stage of intermittent fever, first recommended nearly thirty years ago by Dr. Mackintosh of Edinburgh, was warmly advocated by Mr. Twining in his clinical illustrations of the diseases of Bengal. Though this mode of treatment is not, so far as I am aware, at present followed in any part of India, I may not, on an important point of practice, pass unnoticed the opinion of one of our best authorities on Indian disease. It is not my intention to enter into any examination of the principles on which this practice is grounded, or on the evidence on which its efficacy is supposed to rest. The perusal of Mr. Twining's remarks, in connection with what I have myself written on the treatment of intermittent fever, will at once show the reasons of my dissent from the course which he recommends.

The question was ably inquired into by Dr. Stokes of Dublin in 1829; and the evidence on both sides has since been fairly stated by Mr. Martin §, and a conclusion unfavourable to the practice has been drawn by him.

Dr. Stokes thus states the results of his observations:—

"From the examination of these cases I apprehend that an impression will be received certainly against the indiscriminate or even frequent use of bleeding in the cold stages of ague. It may be remarked that, in the great majority, quinine had to be administered before the disease was eradicated; that many of them had an extremely slow and dangerous convalescence; that in several instances the disease, so far from being relieved, appeared exasperated by the practice; that local inflammatory

---

* "Essay on Diseases incidental to Europeans in Hot Climates." By James Lind, Physician to the Hospital at Haslar. 3rd Edition, London, 1777, p. 310.

† "Edinburgh Medical and Surgical Journal," vol. xxxi. p. 13.

‡ "Clinical Illustrations of Diseases of Bengal." 2nd Edition, vol. ii. p. 233.

§ "On the Influence of Tropical Climates, &c." By James Johnson and James Ranald Martin. 1841. P. 159.

affections occurred several times after the operation; and lastly, that the bleeding appears to have a tendency to convert intermittent into continued fever. In one case, that of Casey, death from pneumonia and softening of the brain occurred. In none of my cases did any bad effects from sinking of the powers of life follow the practice immediately. But I am informed that in the practice of a highly respectable individual, there occurred two cases in which the patients did not recover from the collapse produced by bleeding in the cold stage. Those facts should make us very careful how we interfere with nature by means of the lancet, when we have so certain, and, as far as I have seen, so infallible a remedy as the sulphate of quinine." *

Calomel and other Mercurials.—The circumstances under which calomel may be used with advantage in the treatment of remittent fever, with the view of increasing the excretions from the liver and intestinal canal, have been already explained.

The practice, at one time too common, of exhibiting calomel in doses of four or five grains three or four times in the course of the day, without any very definite object, and continuing it for a succession of days, cannot be too strongly condemned. Not only is it unnecessary, but, for the following reasons, often positively injurious. 1. In watching the progress of cases thus treated, it is not difficult to detect a train of symptoms more fairly attributable to the treatment than to the disease, because it is in cases thus treated that it has been chiefly observed. The symptoms alluded to are uneasy feelings, sometimes amounting to pain, with a sense of oppression or sinking at the epigastrium, and occasional griping of the abdomen, for which leeches are not unfrequently applied, and purgatives unnecessarily given. 2. The frequent repetition of the calomel keeps up a furred state of the tongue, with nausea and irritability of stomach, aggravates the febrile excitement, and produces an irritable state of the bowels, indicated by frequent watery discharges. 3. The convalescence of cases thus treated is always tedious, and frequently complicated with diarrhœa and clay-coloured dejections.

The question of the efficacy of the constitutional effect of mercury in stopping the febrile excitement of remittent fever, and the expediency of, at all hazards, endeavouring to produce it, has been at different times much debated. To induce mercurial influence with this view was, when I entered on practice in India and for many years afterwards, an article of therapeutic faith, and possibly this grave error may not yet be altogether dispelled. I shall first state the conclusions to which I have myself arrived on this question of practice, and the reasons upon which they are grounded; then notice the opinions of some other writers; and finally examine the

* "Edinburgh Medical and Surgical Journal," vol. xxxi. p. 17.

origin of the practice and the nature of the experience which gave rise to it, and exercised so much influence upon the minds of others.

Cases have occurred under my own observation in which fever persisted notwithstanding well-developed mercurial influence.

An officer in Guzerat was attacked with remittent fever on the 16th of June; he was salivated on the 18th, but the febrile state recurred and continued. The salivation ceased. The fever became adynamic with sense of great exhaustion. There was again a free exhibition of calomel, and an inefficient use of quinine; finally delirium and death on the 23rd.

Dr. Stovell, in his reports* of the European General Hospital, details two cases of remittent fever, continuing, becoming adynamic and proving fatal with co-existence of mercurial salivation: and in his statistical notice of this hospital for ten years, from 1846 to 1856, he thus concludes his matured review of this question:—

"I need not waste time by giving more proofs of the correctness of my statement. It was the observation in earlier days of cases and facts such as these that assisted in shaking my faith in the soundness of the mercurialising doctrines of Drs. Annesley and Johnson, whose works were in those days unfortunately the chief authorities for Indian practice. Greatly should I deplore a retrograding return to these mercurialising views; and I shall therefore, I trust, be excused for venturing to caution the inexperienced against the injudicious use of mercury, in any shape or form, either in remittent fever, or in any disease whatever."†

Mr. Walbran, surgeon of the 4th Light Dragoons, thus writes‡ of the fevers at Kaira in 1824:—

"To affect the system with mercury, with the object of restoring the balance of the sanguiferous system, was always kept in view as a primary object. When ptyalism was induced, the patient generally recovered. There have been, however, instances in which the ptyalism had been free for some days, the evacuations had assumed a healthy colour, and every trace of fever had gone off, yet, notwithstanding the greatest care, the ptyalism was checked, the patient immediately became anxious and restless, pulse quick and full, skin burning hot, restlessness and delirium supervened, and death followed in a few hours. This suppression of ptyalism taking place in the course of a few hours is not of very frequent occurrence in other fevers, and I can only account for it in the cases above alluded to by supposing that the inflammation of the villous coat of the stomach and intestines was incompatible with life, and the cessation of ptyalism was the forerunner of that state of the system previous to death."

If the diaries of fatal cases of remittent fever, treated on the mercurial plan, be carefully studied, it will be found that the

---

* "Transactions, Medical and Physical Society of Bombay." No. ix. p. 54, and No. x. p. 88.

† *Ib.* New Series. No. iii. p. 17.

‡ MSS. Reports.

prominent facts are a free use of calomel, persistence of febrile disturbance, and the non-induction of mercurial influence.

If, on the other hand, the diaries of recovered cases, treated on the same system, be considered, then a free use of calomel with coincidence of ptyalism and cessation of febrile disturbance will be frequently observed. This coincidence, however, is sometimes only temporary, and followed by recurrence of fever and cessation of ptyalism.

The difficulty of affecting the system with mercury during the presence of high febrile excitement is acknowledged by all; but when ptyalism and cessation of fever concur, the advocate of mercurial treatment looks upon the former as the cause, the latter the effect; and when there is coincidence of febrile recurrence and cessation of ptyalism, then the latter is regarded as the cause, and the former the effect. Such reasoning, however, is surely erroneous. It is not an unusual circumstance, in remittent fevers treated in their early stage with calomel, to observe, after the recurrence of the fever has been prevented by quinine, slight mercurial action on the second or third day; though not more than a few grains of calomel or blue pill, in combination with quinine, had been given on these days. Under these circumstances the relation of events is so evident that the question of antecedence and sequence is no longer open for argument; and surely in other instances in which the only difference is that there has been no agency employed of acknowledged power to prevent the return of fever, we ought to recollect the natural tendency of the disease to remit, and after a time to cease; and avoid the illogical position of attempting to account for the same coincident phenomena by inverting the order of causation.

For these reasons, then, an endeavour to induce mercurial action in remittent fever appears to me erroneous in theory and of no value in practice. But the question may not thus easily be disposed of. Not only is the practice unsound in theory and of no value, but it is contrary to all rational theory, and very injurious. If it be true that prostration of vital actions and a deteriorated state of the blood are very unfavourable conditions in remittent fever, and that mercury deteriorates the blood and favours prostration—on what principle of reasoning can it be maintained that mercurial influence induced by the physician can have any other than an injurious effect in remittent fever? I have, on several occasions, pointed out the tendency of malarious fever to produce a cachectic state of the system, and have endeavoured to inculcate the importance of guarding against the increase of this unfavourable diathesis by medical treatment. To all who, within the last twenty years, have had the opportunity of extensively observing disease in India, in the various classes of the European community—asthenia, dyspepsia, injured teeth, pains of sides and loins, palpitation, habitually foul tongue, constipated bowels, pale alvine evacuations, depressed spirits, and a sense of sinking at the epigastrium—all clearly traceable to the abuse of mercury—must be familiar facts.

Such then are the reasons, drawn from my own sphere of observation, which have led me to the conclusion, that the induction of mercurial influence in the treatment of malarious fever has been a great and grievous error in therapeutics. I now inquire whether other observers have held similar opinions.

Dr. Leonard Gillespie, in his observations on the diseases which prevailed in a naval squadron on the Leeward Islands Station, between November 1794, and April 1796, at a time when salivation by large doses of calomel was the system of treatment of disease in full force in the West Indies, ably discusses the practice, and unequivocally condemns it.

Dr. Robert Jackson, in the year 1817, concludes his review of the mercurial treatment of fever in the following words*:—

"Upon the whole, I venture to maintain, that if the results of what is termed mercurial treatment in fever, and even in dysentery, particularly in British military hospitals, where it has been most extensively employed, be candidly reviewed, the high, or rather the extravagant, opinion which has been, and which is even now, entertained of the salutary powers of that remedy, is not well supported. The advocates of mercurial treatment generally assert that no one dies from fever after salivation is fully established. The assertion is not altogether correct; but even if it were, and if it appear, on a reference to hospital case books, that there is one in three of the more concentrated forms of endemic fever in which calomel, given alone or in combination with opium, to the amount of a thousand grains or more, produces no increase of the salivary secretion, consequently does not produce the effect which controls the fatal tendency of the disease; and further, if it appear, through the same channel of information, that the same disease, when left to its own course or opposed by ordinary means of treatment, does not destroy life in more than one case in three, the most prepossessed in favour of the remedy will not maintain that we gain anything by the experiment; and it is evident that, if we gain nothing certain, we lose time and chances of gain from other means. But though the effect of mercury, even where it does produce an increased discharge of the salivary secretion, is not uniformly decisive of the cure of fever; and though the action of the remedy, without artificial preparation, by bleeding or other means not implied in the plan of mercurial treatment, be extremely uncertain, the practice still holds its ground, and it probably will maintain it for many years to come. It hangs on a specious delusion, viz. the expectation of

* "Sketch of the History and Cure of Febrile Diseases," &c. By Robert Jackson, M.D., 1817, p. 243.

an effect considered as in some measure specific of cure. I abstain from further remark on the subject, only adding, that if the case be viewed without prepossession, and if the hospital returns of the person* who first adopted the practice at Grenada in the year 1793, and of those who have pursued a similar practice in the different military hospitals in the West Indies since that time, be admitted as documents of effect, the arguments for the continuance of it do not appear to be strong."

Dr. Copland observes:—

"Mercury†, pushed so far as to affect the mouth, or to produce *salivation*, has been considered both a prophylactic‡ and a cure for fever. I have tried to affect the system in the most malignant forms of fever in warm climates without succeeding; and where I have succeeded there was every reason to believe that recovery would have taken place nevertheless."

Mr. Martin, in the last edition of Dr. Johnson's work on tropical diseases, after long and varied experience in India, says, "I have also seldom had occasion to urge mercury to the degree of salivation, during the whole period of my service in India."

Dr. Geddes, in his "Clinical illustrations of the diseases of India," writing of eighty-seven cases of fever in the 1st Madras European regiment, treated with mercury, concludes his remarks with the following words§:—

"The number of those altogether in whom the disease was stopped before the affection of the mouth by mercury, amounted to 48; and of those in whom this circumstance took place after such an event to 28. From these facts, there is reason to doubt whether the mouth becoming affected is not rather a consequence of the cessation of the fever than the latter a result of the system having come under the influence of mercury; but in some chronic cases, where the contrary appeared to occur, an increase of frequency of the pulse, and of feverish irritation in the remissions, has been observed to take place in a gradual manner as the mercurial action

---

* Dr. Colin Chisholm is referred to by Dr. Jackson.

† "Medical Dictionary," vol. i. p. 928.

‡ But the induction of mercurial influence has been looked upon as not only curative of malarious fever, but as also preventive of the action of malaria, and has been recommended as a prophylactic measure. It can hardly be necessary to observe, that the relation between debility as a predisposing, and malaria as an exciting, cause is well understood. It is irrational to suppose that debility caused by mercury can differ in this respect from that induced in any other way. On this question Dr. Copland remarks, "That mercury possesses no prophylactic influence against fevers has been satisfactorily shown by several able writers, and proved by my own experience. A person whose mouth was affected for the cure of syphilis was seized with malignant remittent fever in Africa, in 1817, and came under my care soon after the attack. He died a few days afterwards; the most active treatment having failed in developing vascular reaction and in supporting the vital powers. A nearly similar case is mentioned by Dr. Graves in his excellent lectures."—*Dictionary*, vol. i. p. 929.

Hunter, in his "Observations on the Diseases of the Army in Jamaica" (p. 287), writing of syphilis, says: "It is worth remarking that mercury had no effect upon the constitution to render it less susceptible of fevers; for persons under a course of that medicine were seized with the remittent fever, which, however, did not appear to be aggravated by the presence of the mercury in the body."

§ Page 189.

showed itself; and this was considered to act by breaking in upon the habitual progress of the disease, which accordingly ceased to recur. In many instances, however, after a short interval of freedom from its attacks, these have returned before the affection of the mouth had entirely left the patient; and otherwise, it will be seen from the Table now alluded to, that 37 of those who had been under the influence of mercury in the earlier months of the season had been seized with relapses before its expiration. From these circumstances—combined with a consideration of the occasional affection of the bowels, often amounting to a dysenteric state, produced by the calomel; and of what has been mentioned in speaking of the prognosis regarding the lengthened sickness of the patient, in consequence of his sore mouth—the reader will readily form an opinion of the relative value of mercury and quinine in putting a stop to that tendency to febrile exacerbation which constitutes the main feature of the remittent and intermittent fevers of the East."

The history of the mercurial treatment of fever in India may now be briefly noticed. In the last quarter of the eighteenth century, hepatic affections were treated in India by mercurial influence, and Clark thought highly of a combination of calomel and opium in allaying irritation of the bowels, and promoting their secretions in malarious fevers; but I am not aware that mercury had been much given in fevers to the degree of producing salivation, before it was used with this view, in Grenada in 1793, by Dr. Colin Chisholm.*

The general introduction of this system of treatment into India must be traced to Dr. James Johnson's work on Tropical Diseases, first published in 1813.†

At this period there were, as authorities on the treatment of remittent fever, Pringle, Cleghorn, and Jackson, who advocated the use of blood-letting and other evacuants, with bark during the

* Page 110.

† Wade, whose work was published in 1791, is mentioned as one of the earliest writers on Indian disease who recommended the mercurial treatment of fever, by Dr. H. H. Goodeve, in his very interesting "Sketch of the Progress of European Medicine in the East," published in April, 1837, in the "Quarterly Journal of the Medical and Physical Society of Calcutta." This sketch fairly represents the opinions of Bontius, Clark, Lind, and others; but from the too great prominence given to the phraseology of the time, it is evident that there was not a full appreciation of the merits of these eminent men. Indeed, it could not be otherwise, for at the time when Dr. Goodeve wrote, medical opinion in regard to the treatment of tropical disease was in a very vacillating state. I feel assured, however, that I do not go beyond my knowledge of the present opinions and sentiments of the able author of this sketch—with whom for a long series of years I have enjoyed the privilege and advantage of a free interchange of opinion on this and kindred subjects—when I say that were he now to review the progress of European medicine in the East, the sketch would, in some respects, evince a different spirit. No one more early than Dr. Goodeve became satisfied of the evils of an excessive depletory and mercurial treatment, and of the advantages of quinine, in malarious fevers. No one, whether in medical practice or in the diffusion of medical education in India, has been more liberal in his judgment of others, or has co-operated with them in a freer and a franker spirit.

remissions. Clark and Lind, on the other hand, deriving their experience from observation in Bengal, in 1762 and 1773, of an adynamic type of the disease in seamen of scorbutic taint, enjoined extreme caution in blood-letting, and recommended a moderate use of purgatives, opiates, stimulants, and bark. Moreover, in Cullen's "First Lines of the Practice of Physic," there was open to the medical inquirer a philosophic statement of the principles which should regulate the treatment of the different forms and modifications of febrile disease. At this epoch Dr. James Johnson, at an early period of his professional life, arrived in the Hooghly in the month of September, after a short run of little more than three months from England, in charge of a crew untainted, we may presume, with scurvy. He adopted, as he believed, Clark and Lind, as his practical guides, to the neglect, it would appear, of all other authority and in forgetfulness of the circumstances under which these excellent physicians had observed the disease, and to which their system of treatment exclusively applied.

Dr. Johnson * makes the following quotation from Dr. Clark: "As soon as the intestinal tubes have been thoroughly cleansed, the cure must *entirely* depend upon giving the Peruvian bark in as large doses as the patient's stomach will bear, without paying *any regard to the remissions or exacerbations of the fever.*" He then continues: "Such are the plain and easy instructions which Dr. Clark and Lind have left for our guides in this fearful endemic. They certainly are not apparently difficult to follow; and Heaven knows, I endeavoured, most religiously, to fulfil every iota of their injunctions; but with what success a single case will show."

It is true that Clark recommends the use of bark in the exacerbations, but it would have been just to that physician had Dr. Johnson extended his quotation to the sentence which immediately follows that which he has cited, viz. — "If the remissions be distinct, the bark, indeed, will have a more speedy effect in subduing the fever; but even if it become continual, by a regular and steady perseverance in the medicine, it will be effectually prevented from growing dangerous or malignant." †

It is evident from this sentence, as well as from a perusal of the

* "On the Influence of Tropical Climates." By James Johnson. London, 1841, p. 107. The italics are Dr. Johnson's.

† "Observations on the Diseases which prevail in long Voyages to hot Countries." By John Clark, M.D. Second Edition, 1792, p. 184, vol. i.

cases recorded by Clark, that his practice was to give bark chiefly in the remission; but to use it also in the exacerbation, in those cases which from the remittent had passed into the continued type.

Lind is represented by Dr. Johnson as holding the same opinion as Dr. Clark relative to the use of bark in the exacerbation. Such, however, does not appear to have been the case. Dr. Lind of Windsor, the author, referred to, of a "Treatise on the Putrid and Remitting Marsh Fever of Bengal," not only did not give bark in the exacerbations, but not even in the first remission. His words are: "For my part, I have always given the bark during the second remission, as all my care during the first was to cleanse the primæ viæ. But it is to no purpose to give the bark till the necessary purgations are over." *

I shall now quote that case in which Dr. Johnson believed that he was religiously endeavouring to fulfil every iota of the injunctions of Clark and Lind, and the ill success of which led him to abandon the therapeutic principles of a long line of able and observing men, and to promulgate a very different system of practice:—

"A young man of good constitution, in the prime of life and health, had been assisting, with several others, to navigate an Indiaman through the Hooghly. The day after he returned he was seized with the usual symptoms of this fever. I did not see him till the cold stage was past; but the reaction was violent—the headache intense, skin burning hot, great oppression about the præcordia, with quick hard pulse, thirst, and nausea. An emetic was prescribed, and towards the close of its operation discharged a quantity of ill-conditioned bile, both upwards and downwards: soon after which a perspiration broke out, the febrile symptoms subsided, and a remission, almost amounting to an intermission, followed. I now with an air of confidence began to 'throw in' the bark, quite sanguine in my expectations of soon checking this formidable disease. But, alas! my triumph was of short duration; for in a few hours the fever returned with increased violence, and attended with such obstinate vomiting, that, although I tried to push on the bark through the paroxysm by the aid of opium, effervescing draughts, &c., it was all fruitless; for every dose was rejected the moment it was swallowed, and I was forced to abandon the only means by which I had hoped to curb the fury of the disease. The other methods which I tried need not be enumerated; they were temporising shifts, calculated, in medical language, 'to obviate occasional symptoms.'

"The truth is, I knew not what to do; for the sudden and unexpected failure of that medicine on which I was taught to depend, completely embarrassed me, and before I could make up my mind to any feasible plan of treatment, my patient died on the third day of his illness, perfectly yellow, vomiting to the last a dark fluid resembling vitiated bile, and exhibiting an awful spectacle of the effects which a Bengal fever is capable of producing in so short a period on a European in the vigour of manhood." †

* Page 65.

† Page 107 of Edition of 1841.

The body was examined after death, and Dr. Johnson found —

"The liver so gorged, as it were, with blood that it actually fell to pieces on handling it. Indeed, it appeared as if the greater number of the vessels had been broken down, and almost the whole of the interior structure converted into a mass of extravasation. The gall-bladder contained a small quantity of bile, in colour and consistence resembling tar, and the ductus communis choledochus was so thickened in its coats and contracted in its diameter that a probe could scarcely be passed into it. Marks of incipient inflammation were visible in some parts of the small intestines, and the internal surface of the stomach exhibited similar appearances. The thorax was not examined, on account of the time taken up in getting at the brain. Marks of turgescence, in the venous system of vessels particularly, were there quite evident, and more than the usual quantity of lymph was found in the ventricles, but no appearance of actual inflammation."

The narration of this case is followed by remarks on the unsuitable character of the treatment, on the uncertainty of medicine, and the evils of being led by authority.

It is far from my desire to review in a critical spirit the practice of one who, after a life of active usefulness, has passed away. Still it is impossible to avoid observing, that a dispassionate consideration of this case — upon which so much of the treatment of fever in India for a quarter of a century has rested — and of the therapeutic principles of the best authorities in medicine of that day, must lead to the conclusion that these principles were not rightly appreciated or correctly applied by Dr. Johnson. To say nothing of Pringle, Clegborn, Cullen, and Jackson, I cannot suppose that either Clark or Lind would have treated a case, even of the adynamic type, with which they were familiar, in the manner which has just been detailed. Be that as it may, it is difficult to believe that either of these observant and able men would have treated remittent fever in a sthenic European after the fashion which has been attributed to them.

After this first failure, Dr. Johnson treated his subsequent cases by free blood-letting and alvine evacuations. But there were men of the crew who, from various circumstances, did not bear depletion so well as others. This led to treatment by induction of mercurial influence, by repeated doses — from five to ten grains — of calomel "as the *sine quâ non* in the medical treatment of this fever as well as many other fevers in the East." *

Dr. Johnson's treatment of remittent fever consisted, then, in free bloodletting and alvine evacuations, opium combined with calomel † in large doses when the stomach was irritable, the

* "On the Influence of Tropical Climates," p. 110.

† The combination of calomel and opium — five grains of the former and one of the latter — was highly thought of by Dr. Clark when the stomach was irritable, and as

induction of mercurial influence, with subsidiary measures, as leeches and cold applications to the head—and neglect of the use of bark.

It appears, then, that on the authority of a single case—the first seen by a young naval medical officer in the Hooghly—the principles in respect to the use of bark in remittent fever, laid down from observations made in various countries and circumstances by Pringle, Cleghorn, the two Linds, Clark, Cullen and Jackson, were ignored for a quarter of a century by the medical profession in India; and, it may be added, in tropical countries generally.

As to the treatment recommended by Dr. Johnson, we are left in ignorance of the amount of experience on which it was based. There is no statement of the length of his stay in the Hooghly, of the number of cases treated, or of the proportion of recoveries. But of this we may be certain, that the experience of a few months, in the crew of a single ship, could not be authority sufficient for that subversion of medical doctrine and practice which unfortunately resulted from it.

But, while we deplore this defection from sound principles, and the evils to which it gave rise, we must not be unjust to its author.

Dr. Johnson did not appreciate the circumstances under which remittent fever was observed by Clark and Lind. Nor have his followers in this respect been just to him.

Dr. Johnson says *, "I now carried the evacuating plan with a high hand, and with much better success than I expected. Fortunately for my patients, a great majority of them were fresh from Europe, and high in previous health and strength; these recovered wonderfully after bleeding and evacuations, though not always." Again †: "The fear of debility and putrescency still paralyses the arms of medical men in hot climates, notwithstanding the clearest evidence in favour of general and local bleeding, particularly where the subject is lately from Europe, and not broken down by the climate."

Yet—notwithstanding these clear indications that a system of treatment based at best on very limited experience, could only be successfully followed in fresh Europeans high in previous health

favouring the subsequent action of mild purgatives. It would have been right on the part of Dr. Johnson, while condemning Dr. Clark, to have acknowledged the source from which he probably derived the calomel and opium part of his own system.

* Page 109.

† Page 110.

and strength, and not broken down by climate — the followers of Dr. Johnson have applied the treatment to the long resident as well as to the lately arrived, and to asthenic natives as well as to sthenic Europeans.

But it is necessary to explain why I have now entered into these details on a mode of practice at present generally disapproved of, and one which its talented author had himself virtually abandoned before the close of his long and useful career — as we learn from the following observations written in 1841 :—

"It is necessary to observe, also, that the fevers, even of the same place, are not of the same type in all years; and consequently they require modifications of treatment. The above was the nature of the fever on the banks of the Ganges thirty-five years ago, and the general mode of treatment described was found most beneficial. I have no doubt, however, that fevers in such places will often be effectually combated by early depletion, especially purging, and then, when a remission takes place, by administering bark, particularly the quinine, so as to prevent the return of the paroxysms. Particular organs are to be guarded by local blood-letting and blistering, while the glandular secretions of the chylopoietic viscera are to be kept in order by appropriate doses of calomel or the quicksilver pill."*

My reasons for having enlarged on this subject are—

1. The importance of the lesson which it teaches. The caution which it enjoins against accepting new systems of treatment without a careful examination of the evidence and the principles on which they rest. The practice of medicine will never be free from errors of this kind, unless all who exercise it give their minds to patient observation and the study of principles, and are fully impressed with the responsibility which it involves.

2. In the second number of the "Indian Annals of Medicine," † there is a paper on "Tropical Fever and Dysentery" by Mr. Hare. He speaks with much truth of the opinions of several of the older physicians, and also treats of those historical details with which we have just been engaged.

But in Mr. Hare's communication are the following remarks, from which, after the opinions expressed in various parts of this work, I need hardly say that I altogether dissent :—

"There cannot be a doubt, that if not calomel, yet certainly salivation, *is* an antidote to malarious fever. The instant a patient's mouth is sore the fever leaves him; the mercury produces not the slightest effect till then, but from that moment the disease vanishes as if charmed; the change is from death to life, from extremity of suffering to calm and comfort." ‡

* Page 113.

† April, 1854.

‡ "The Annals of Medicine," No. 2, pp. 468, 469.

Again :—

"Numerous instances, too, of the safety which salivation gives from the effects of the malarious poison may be found in Dr. Johnson's book, viz. patients salivated for syphilis sleeping with impunity in places which were fatal to every one of their companions; and also many cases on record of officers in India passing in a state of salivation by dâk unharmed through the most deadly jungles."

It is this revival at the present day of doctrines from whose evil influence the practice of medicine has too slowly emerged, that has induced me to deviate from the course which I pursued in 1843, when writing on this disease.* Then I assumed that the necessity of discussing the question of the treatment of remittent fever by mercurial salivation had passed away.

The *supposed sedative influence of large doses of calomel* on the mucous membrane of the stomach, first assumed by Sir James Annesley, and then adopted by many writers on materia medica and on tropical disease, may now be shortly noticed.

Annesley's opinion was founded on the results of some experiments on dogs. In the year 1841 Mr. Murray, at the time surgeon of the convalescent station on the Mahubuleshwur Hills, and well known to his professional brethren in India as a zealous and successful cultivator of medical science, published in the fourth number of the "Transactions of the Medical and Physical Society of Bombay" a paper entitled "Experiments illustrative of the physiological effects of calomel on the gastro-intestinal mucous membrane of dogs," which proved that Annesley's conclusion was erroneous — and that large doses of calomel increased the vascularity and secretions of the gastric as well as of the intestinal mucous membrane.

But the question is now one of comparatively little importance, for the latest investigations seem to show that only a very small portion of the insoluble preparations of mercury — blue-pill and calomel — are dissolved by the gastric and enteric secretions and absorbed. Dr. Headland thus alludes to the subject † :—

"Some have, without sufficient reason, assumed calomel to be a sedative when given in large doses. To act in this way, very large doses have been recommended, and given in fever and malignant cholera. Calomel is naturally an insoluble substance; and in these cases the function of absorption is at the very lowest ebb; so that it is probable that the large doses are often left unabsorbed, and pass out of the bowels very much as they entered, producing scarcely any more effect than so much chalk mixture."—Page 391.

---

* "Transactions, Medical and Physical Society of Bombay," No. 6, p. 199.

† "An Essay on the Action of Medicines." By F. W. Headland, M.D. &c. Third Edition, 1859.

Again:—

"Their action does not in reality depend much on the dose given. This may be often increased with little effect. Until the amount of solvent matter in the stomach or bowels is increased, the amount of mercury taken into the system will be much the same. In fevers and cholera, when the dissolving power is little, and the function of absorption at a low ebb, calomel may often be poured in with no effect at all. As the patient recovers, a dangerous salivation may occur; and in some idiosyncrasies, some peculiarly susceptible states of the absorbent surfaces, one to two grains of calomel in the stomach, or one drachm of mercurial ointment rubbed into the skin may be followed by violent mercurialism, or produce necrosis of the jaw and death."—Page 381.

Cold Affusion—in cases and stages of the paroxysm in which the skin is dry and steadily above the natural temperature, and the pulse of good volume — is of great use, by lessening vascular excitement, and, when the head is the organ affected, alleviating the headache, and either doing away with the necessity of applying leeches, or reducing considerably the number required. But it is contra-indicated in fever, as in other diseases, when there is complication of pectoral affection, and also probably when gastro-enteric symptoms are present.

When cold affusion is doubtful, or when the suitable stage has passed, tepid sponging may be had recourse to with very good effect whenever the skin is above the natural temperature. And in all cases of remittent fever extending to two or three paroxysms, in which the vascular excitement during the stage of exacerbation is considerable, or in which the head is affected, the scalp should be shaved, and cold assiduously applied.

Wet-Sheet Packing. — Within the last few years the treatment of remittent fever and other acute forms of disease by this method has at different times been brought under my notice in India; and it has seemed to me that injury to medical practice is not unlikely to result from the routine and injudicious use of the wet-sheet.

I have tried it in a few cases, and have watched its application by others in a greater number, with the following results:—

1. In the conditions which justify cold affusion, it is possible enough that the wet sheet, renewed every ten minutes, or quarter of an hour, for two or three times, may be a convenient and effective manner of reducing the temperature of the body; but on this point I do not speak from experience. Should there be tendency to hepatic or splenic congestion, then the wet sheet used in the manner above stated is likely to do harm by increasing the congestion: this statement is made from personal observation.

2. The treatment of the height of the exacerbation, by wet-

sheet packing after the manner of the hydropathic system, has been to my knowledge adopted in some cases. Without denying that the moisture of the surface of the body may somewhat modify the action, there can be little doubt that this mode of treating fever is a retrograde movement towards that sweating system which, nearly two centuries ago, the genius of Sydenham banished from the practice of medicine. But even if it can be shown that wet-sheet packing is useful in lessening the exacerbation of remittent fever, surely it is well understood that this is not a leading indication in the cure of the disease; and that means which merely aim at this can never occupy other than a subsidiary position.

3. If wet-sheet packing be used towards the close of an exacerbation, when the circumstances have been such as to render undue collapse at this period an event not improbable, then there can be no doubt that the increased diaphoresis caused by the wet sheet will increase exhaustion, and may produce it when it otherwise would not have occurred. I have never witnessed this effect from the wet sheet in remittent fever; but I have observed it in the treatment of tetanus — a disease in which a tendency to death by failure of the action of the heart is also well marked. In the case alluded to, death was undoubtedly hastened by this proceeding.

4. A routine system of wet-sheet packing, by directing the chief curative means to the reduction of febrile heat, must tend to withdraw attention from the sedulous use of those methods by which local inflammation or other disease may be detected. It is opposed to careful and accurate diagnosis. Then in regard to the diaphoretic action of the wet sheet in the treatment of disease, there can be no question of the advantage of making the skin perform its share of increased elimination when this becomes an indication of cure; but can there be a greater error in practice than that of acting on the skin alone, and neglecting the other important excretory organs?

These are not theoretic objections. I have witnessed the diagnosis of local inflammation overlooked, and the symptomatic fever treated by wet sheets to the neglect of the inflammation — under circumstances in which I felt convinced that treatment conducted on generally received principles, and by ordinary means, would have led to a different course and termination of the disease.

On the Use of Purgatives. — Of the necessity in remittent fever of the moderate use of purgatives, more or less active according to the circumstances of particular cases, no question can arise; but the bad effect of keeping up a constant state of irritation of the intestinal lining is equally certain.

After the first two or three days, if the secretions dependent directly or indirectly on the portal system have been freely solicited, further purging is unnecessary. It will be sufficient that the bowels are moved once gently in the course of twenty-four hours. The effect of the opposite and too common practice is to irritate the mucous membrane, to hurry on and very much aggravate the adynamic symptoms in protracted cases; and, in recoveries, to leave during the convalescence a deranged condition of the bowels, with a decided proclivity to attacks of dysentery, more especially in the cold season.

Whether purgatives should be given during the exacerbation or the remission of remittent fever, is an important point to determine. In the Medico-Topographical Report of the Presidency division of the army, published by the Medical Board of Madras, a very decided opinion on this point is expressed by the surgeon of the Presidency General Hospital. He is opposed to the use of purgatives in the exacerbation, because they do not act readily, and they tend to perpetuate the exacerbation and interfere with the access of the remission. There is much practical truth in this remark, but it is hardly sufficiently precise and discriminating.

There can be no doubt that a state of febrile disturbance is adverse to the action of all remedies, purgatives included. It is also true that the too free use of purgatives favours the continuance of the exacerbation and interferes with the remission, partly from undue evacuation, and partly from irritation of the intestinal mucous lining. This influence is most likely to be exercised in asthenic constitutions.

In the fevers of sthenic individuals, however, evacuation by purgatives is adopted with the view of moderating the excitement of the exacerbation; and if this be one of the indications for their use, it is evident that it can only be carried into effect during the exacerbation itself. But in following out the other indications for which purgatives are given, as removing constipation, correcting deranged secretions, or eliminating morbid matter from the blood, the remission is the suitable period for their exhibition. They should be administered in moderate doses early in the remission; and probably there is no better method than by combination with the first doses of quinine in the manner already recommended.

The imperfect action of purgatives in the exacerbation of fever is partly due to defective secretion and partly to impaired irritability of the intestinal muscular fibre. This latter condition is sometimes made evident by the retention of enemata when used in the exacerbation: this circumstance is known to me from my own observation; and Gillespie, in his remarks on the diseases of the Leeward Islands station, notes the retention of enemata during the exacerbation, and their action during the remission.*

The practice of Cleghorn, as explained in his observations on the epidemical diseases in Minorca, was to give purgatives in the morning with the first remission. He attaches importance to their use at this stage, but does not allude to their exhibition in the exacerbation.

Balfour recommends purgatives at the commencement of the remission, or, when this is not well marked, at the periods when the remissions usually occur. He says: "I have learnt by experience that all laxative and purgative medicines, as well as injections, are very uncertain in their operation, and generally disappoint so long as any degree of fever is present." †

Emetics. — The occasional utility of emetics in the early stage of fever, and the circumstances for which they are suitable, have been already explained.

The treatment of fevers by a solution of tartar emetic and Epsom salts in frequently-repeated doses, to the causing of free vomiting and purging, is unsuited to febrile disease as occurring in Bombay, and as a routine system of practice must always be hazardous. Even in the quotidian and ephemeral fevers of more phlogistic type, in the Deccan, in well-conditioned Europeans, I have witnessed an alarming state of collapse brought on by this mode of treatment. It is not disputed that many cases of fever, thus managed, recover well; but they must be selected with care, for in every epidemic of tropical fever there occur many cases for which this kind of treatment is not only unsuited, but also very dangerous.

Blisters applied with the intention of controlling local capillary derangement when the stage appropriate for topical blood-letting has passed have already been adverted to; and I would only here repeat what has already been previously stated, that when blisters are used in remittent fever the stage of remission is the suitable time.

On the Use of Opiates. — In my remarks on the treatment of

* Page 73.

† "Collection of Treatises on the Effects of Sol-lunar Influence in Fevers." By Francis Balfour, M.D., late President Medical Board, Bengal. First Edition, 1816.

ordinary remittent fever the circumstances in which an opiate often acts with advantage, and the precautions which should be kept in view, have been explained. At the period when this practice was followed by me in the European General Hospital, I was not aware that Lind * had given opium still more freely and with less precaution in the hot stage of intermittent fever. His belief was, that, when administered early in the attack, it shortened the duration of the hot stage, and favoured the access of the third stage and of the intermission. He did not give opium when delirium was present, but considered that headache was no contra-indication to its use.

Whether the favourable opinion entertained by this high authority on tropical fevers, of the beneficial effects of this free use of opium, be just or not, I am unable to judge from experience. As already explained, I have always, before exhibiting opiates in the hot stage of fever, had recourse to certain precautionary measures for reducing general and cerebral vascular action : these I still think must be very expedient. But, whatever view be taken of Lind's opinions, there are certainly other conditions of fever, in some respects analogous, in which a full dose of opium cannot be given without much hazard. I allude to its use after a lengthened period of restlessness, in which the skin is not steadily warm or rather is coldish, and in which the pulse is frequent and feeble. This state occurs either in cases which have been for some time protracted, or towards the end of a paroxysm. These symptoms indicate that the nervous influence on the organs of circulation is failing, and the sedative action of a *full* opiate, under these circumstances, is apt † to increase the state of collapse, to mask the degree in which it exists, and to hurry on coma and death. Such cases should be treated by the assiduous use of stimulants.

Again, when in the remittent fevers of the intemperate, there exist delirium and tremors with slight febrile heat and a pulse frequent and compressible, there is — in consequence of the resemblance of these symptoms to those of delirium tremens, and of the erroneous views entertained on the treatment of this latter disease — often a great temptation to give a full opiate to *overcome* the delirium and to cause sleep. This is, assuredly, in general, a most hazardous and not unfrequently a fatal proceeding, as is illustrated by cases 23, 24, 25. It is very probable that in the treatment of

* "Lind's Essay on Diseases incidental to Europeans in Hot Climates," 1777, p. 343.

† Case No. 9 is an illustration.

such cases the exhibition of quarter-grain doses of tartar-emetic, with five minims of tincture of opium, on the principles advocated by Dr. Graves, in the management of some forms of delirium in European continued fever, may prove appropriate and useful.

The use of opium in remittent fever demands our careful study, for the cases which have been now specially alluded to are not the only instances of error which I have myself witnessed; and others have been noted by me in the perusal of the diaries of cases which had not come under my own observation. These circumstances have fixed my attention on this question of practice, and after much reflection it has seemed to me that the following are the principles which should be kept in view in giving full opiates in remittent fever.

1. Opium can be used with safety only in the restlessness of the early stage of remittent fever, when there are not symptoms of marked determination to the brain, and when the pulse is of good volume, and soft, and not much above 100.

2. When remittent fever has persisted for six or seven days, each recurring exacerbation is attended with increasing frequency and decreasing strength of the pulse. This depression of the heart's action is most observable towards the close of the paroxysm, and is not unfrequently attended with general restlessness, and then the temptation to give an opiate is often great, in the hope that sleep and its consequent advantages may be secured; but, under these circumstances, the proceeding is always dangerous. A pulse that ranges towards 120, or one not so frequent, but feeble and compressible; or still more, a pulse that has the frequency of 120, and is, at the same time, feeble and compressible, are conditions which may be held to contra-indicate the use of a full opiate — even though they should not be associated with headache, wandering, delirium, or tendency to drowsiness. Nor is it difficult to understand why this should be. These conditions of the pulse indicate that the tendency to death is by syncope — a tendency sure to be most marked towards the close of the paroxysm, and to increase with each returning exacerbation of fever. In this depressed state of the heart's action, the functions of the brain also become impaired, and, under the influence of a full opiate, are not unlikely to be suspended; in other words, the opium is apt to induce coma, and its sedative influence on the brain, acting through the nervous system, still further depresses the action of the heart; and thus, under these circumstances, an opiate, injudiciously given, favours death both in the way of syncope and coma.

3. As yet no derangement of the brain itself has been assumed. But in a great proportion of cases of remittent fever, of six or seven days' duration, the earlier exacerbations are marked by flushing and headache, the later ones by slight wandering or tendency to drowsiness. This condition of the cerebral functions, *whatever the state of the pulse may be*, contra-indicates the use of opium; for in such cases the tendency to death is by coma. If the opiate be given at the close of the earlier paroxysms, it may only increase the restlessness; but if it be given at the close of the later paroxysms, when wandering or tendency to drowsiness is present, it will most surely expedite the supervention of coma, and ought to be most scrupulously abstained from.

4. But in those cases of remittent fever in which the wandering delirium, or drowsiness of the later paroxysms shows a tendency to death by coma, there is also, most generally speaking, a frequent and failing pulse. Whenever an exacerbation of remittent fever which has been attended with wandering delirium, or a tendency to drowsiness, terminates with a quick and feeble pulse, it may be inferred with tolerable certainty that death by coma is not far distant, is only to be warded off by the most judicious management, and is most certain to be hurried on if we commit the grievous error of attempting to lessen the delirium and restlessness by the exhibition of opium. To conclude, then, whenever in remittent fever the pulse is towards 120, feeble and compressible, and whenever there is wandering delirium, or slight drowsiness, the exhibition of a full opiate is a measure of danger, more particularly towards the close of a febrile exacerbation. In other words, whenever in remittent fever the tendency to death by asthenia or by coma is well marked *, a full opiate will expedite the fatal result.

On the Use of Quinine.—The manner in which quinine has been used by me in the treatment of intermittent and remittent fever has already been fully detailed.

On investigation it is evident that the principles inculcated differ little from those of the older writers, chiefly the Linds †, Cleghorn, and Balfour, in respect to bark.

* I need hardly observe that, in these remarks, I refer exclusively to opiates given with the intention of, and in doses calculated to produce the soporific action of the drug. Whether opiates given in small doses, with a view to their stimulant effects, may or may not be admissible in some of the states of fever adverted to by me, is a question altogether apart from my present subject, and one in regard to which I am unable to express any opinion from experience.

† I may here state that there are two Dr. James Linds; one of Haslar Hospital,

Cleghorn remarks:—

"Inflammations of the abdominal viscera are likewise natural effects of tertian fevers. For we find that they often come on little by little, and increase with every paroxysm till at last they end in a gangrene. Whereas the cortex, by bringing the fever to a speedy conclusion, impedes the further progress of the inflammation, so that it afterwards goes off gradually of its own accord; as I have had occasion to observe in a multitude of instances, where acute fixed pains, tension, and other symptoms made the nature of the disease too plain to be doubted."

Again:—

"Upon the whole I am convinced that the unhappy metastases, which some have observed to follow the use of the bark, are exceeding rare, and ought rather to be ascribed to other causes than to this medicine. And I will venture to affirm that more bad consequences ensue from giving it too late than too soon. Prostration of the strength, sudden death, or the most obstinate chronic diseases, if the sick recover, being the usual effects of delay. Whereas the worst that commonly happens from the too early use of it is that it does not at once restrain the paroxysms, like a charm without any sensible evacuation as it frequently does when given after the fever has arrived naturally to its height, and begins to decline of its own accord." *

Balfour's principles, in respect to the use of bark, are, on the whole, practical and sound. He advocates evacuants in the first exacerbation, and then gives bark in powder freely, increasing the retaining power of the stomach by opium. He prefers the intermission and remission, but does not scruple to use it under some circumstances in the exacerbation. His words are: "This becomes absolutely necessary when you happen to be called too late, for after the third or fourth day the fits are protracted so long as to run into one another; and when this is the case, whoever waits for complete remission will find himself wofully disappointed." † He recognises cases, however, in which reaction is high, remissions short, evacuations more required, and bark less. He insists upon bark being of as great importance in remittents as in intermittents. "All the arguments," he observes, "I have been advancing in favour of an early exhibition of the bark in intermittents are equally applicable in the case of remittents, whether attended or not with symptoms of obstruction. And as these disorders are more rapid in their progress, and more dangerous, so is the necessity of this practice in proportion more urgent." ‡ After stating that a complicating hepatitis, or other inflammation in intermittent and remittent fever, is to be met by venesection, other evacuants and blisters, he adds: "If it be not likely to stop

who writes on scurvy and diseases incidental to Europeans in hot climates; the other, Dr. James Lind, of Windsor, who writes on putrid and remitting marsh fever of Bengal.

* "Observations on the Epidemical Diseases in Minorca, from 1744 to 1749." By George Cleghorn, pp. 223 and 225.

† Page 34.

‡ Page 39.

by prosecuting this plan, the bark is to be given without hesitation, for in all the partial determinations I have met with, I have ever found the fever do much more harm in one fit than all the bark that is necessary to stop its return."

The following are the rules laid down by Cullen:—*

"1. That the bark may be employed with safety at any period of intermittent fevers, providing that, at the same time, there be neither a phlogistic diathesis prevailing in the system, nor any considerable or fixed congestion present in the abdominal viscera.

"2. The proper time for exhibiting the bark in intermittent fevers, is during the time of intermission; and where intermissions are to be expected, it is to be abstained from in the time of paroxysms.

"3. In remittents, though no entire apyrexia occurs, the bark may be given during the remissions; and it should be given, even though the remissions be considerable, if, from the known nature of the epidemic, intermissions or considerable remissions are not to be so soon expected, and that great danger is apprehended from repeated exacerbations.

"4. In the case of genuine intermittents, while a due quantity of bark is to be employed, the exhibition of it ought to be brought as near to the time of accession as the condition of the patient's stomach will allow.

"5. In general, in all cases of intermittents, it is not sufficient that the recurrence of paroxysms be stopped for once by the use of the bark; a relapse is commonly to be expected, and should be prevented by the exhibition of the bark, repeated at proper intervals."

When we recollect the difficulties with which the older physicians had to contend in the exhibition of the crude bark, we cannot sufficiently admire the ingenuity with which they endeavoured to overcome them, and the constancy with which they adhered to those sound principles of therapeutics which the means at their command enabled them so inadequately to apply. The great advantage which the modern physician enjoys, is simply this, that he is able by means of quinine to carry out those same principles more easily, completely, and safely.

Dr. Geddes was, at an early period (1828), instrumental in establishing the use of quinine in India. In his later work published in 1846†, there are valuable practical suggestions on the use of quinine in fever, which well deserve attentive consideration. They are too long for insertion here, but I cannot deny myself the satisfaction of quoting that part of Dr. Geddes' remarks which relates to the exhibition of quinine in complicated cases.

"The exhibition of quinine," he writes‡, "can go on along with that of any remedy for attendant symptoms; and, inasmuch as the latter may depend upon or be aggravated by the febrile accession, this medicine must be considered as an auxiliary to any

* Thomson's Edition, vol. i. p. 673.

† "Clinical Illustrations of the Diseases of India." By William Geddes, M.D., p. 175.

‡ *Ibid.* p. 176.

remedial means, even of a supposed discordant nature, which may be employed for the relief of such symptoms. Thus quinine has been combined with the treatment suitable to inflammatory, dysenteric, and other affections; and by preventing the increased febrile action of the paroxysmal disease, it has tended, in a material degree, to the diminution and ultimate removal of all the accompanying morbid phenomena."

Dr. Haspel *, in his treatise on the diseases of Algeria, inculcates the same principles on the use of quinine in complicated cases of remittent fever.

In the year 1851 the treatment of Bengal remittent fever with scruple doses of quinine repeated several times during the height of the exacerbation, was advocated by Mr. Hare of the Bengal Medical Service. The subject attracted considerable attention at the time, and was much discussed. The tendency of the system is to favour superficial clinical observation, as is evident in the following extract from Mr. Hare's Report:—†

"I thus treated 421 cases in all of Bengal fever, and during the experiment some remarkable facts were observed. My orders to my apothecary in both wards were to give scruple doses of quinine to every patient with symptoms of fever, from the very first moment of admission, and they often thus got forty grains of quinine before I saw them. During part of the year, viz., March, April, and May, small-pox and measles raged like an epidemic in Calcutta. Numbers of these patients in their early stages, before the appearance of any eruption, were sent to my ward as fever cases, and were treated as the rest with large doses of quinine, sometimes for thirty-six hours before I could detect their disease. Almost all these cases terminated fatally. Latterly, however, I was able to avoid these errors, by watching the effect of the first dose of quinine. For in cases not malarious it invariably caused great uneasiness, without any benefit to the general symptoms. Moreover, deafness and singing in the ears were very quickly induced; whereas in malarious fever, with the same ardent symptoms, the quantity of quinine taken without producing any cinchonism was often extraordinary, and so far from uneasiness, it seemed always to give relief, and the febrile symptoms yielded rapidly under its use."

We may, with Balfour, admit, that when the exacerbations so run into each another that the remissions are hardly observed, quinine may be given with care at the periods which, in the ordinary course of the disease, are those of remission.

The question of the free use of quinine in the exacerbations of remittent fever is so important, that no apology is necessary for submitting the reflections which its consideration has suggested to me.

1. There is no evidence that quinine has the power of diminishing existing febrile excitement in the manner of evacuants and cold. The disturbed action of the heart and nervous system, described by Briquet ‡ as resulting from large doses of quinine,

* "Maladies de l'Algérie," vol. ii. pp. 176, 184.

† "The Indian Annals of Medical Science," No. 2, p. 474.

‡ "Medical Times and Gazette," May and June, 1855; "Indian Annals of Medical Science," vol. iii. p. 281.

resembles that from hydrocyanic acid; and it cannot be safe in therapeutics to produce such disturbance of these important organs.

2. When the action of a remedy is distinct in its nature, and opposed to that of a morbific cause, it is a therapeutic law that such remedy will be more effective before the action of the morbific influence is in full force. For example: an anodyne, in anticipation of pain, an anti-spasmodic in anticipation of a paroxysm of asthma, a soporific in anticipation of a season of restlessness, are more certainly effective than when postponed till these several derangements are in full force: in the latter case they often fail. Anti-periodics are so called because their peculiar action is unquestionably of this character. They are comparatively powerless if not given to anticipate derangement, as appears in intermittent fever and neuralgia: why should it be otherwise in remittent fever?

3. Admitting that quinine in the exacerbation may be beneficial rather than otherwise, still we know that the greater the febrile disturbance, the less likely the action of remedies which require to be previously absorbed and assimilated. The exacerbation must therefore be the period least suited for ensuring their action, and if not then injurious they are at best in a great measure useless, because necessarily inert.

4. That quinine has no power of directly reducing febrile excitement is clear from its inutility in continued fever, symptomatic fever, and the eruptive fevers: why should it be otherwise in the exacerbation of remittent fever?

5. Febrile disturbance in zymotic continued fevers may be increased by injudicious and moderated by judicious management; increased by stimulants, heat, imperfect ventilation, and moderated by evacuants, cool and pure air, sponging, affusion, and the wet sheet. It is of as much, if not more, importance to attend to this indication in remittent fever, not only on account of the reaction and the immediate danger to important organs, but also because it favours an early and more complete remission—that is, brings about the opportunity of giving with good effect—quinine—the agent most potent in the cure of the disease.

6. By administering quinine in the exacerbation, we give it at a time least appropriate for its peculiar action, and when its action, if any, is as likely to be injurious as useful. Moreover, attention thus misdirected tends to induce neglect of those means for reducing febrile excitement,—applicable to all types of fever,—

and which are additionally useful in remittents, because they favour the access of a distinct remission.

7. Under wavering principles the appropriate treatment of the exacerbation is liable to be neglected. The difficulty seems to be in keeping clearly before the mind, that the principles for the exacerbation are distinct from those for the remission; that both are important, and require to be modified in particular cases, but should never be confounded and transposed.

8. We cannot, with certainty, distinguish remittent fever, first seen during the exacerbation, from continued fever, or the initiatory stage of an eruptive fever, or that type compounded of remittent and common continued fever—for all of which large doses of quinine are unquestionably unsuitable.

9. I know, from clinical experience, that there are febrile states in which quinine is injurious, and others in which large doses do harm, and small ones good. All that we practically know of the action of anti-periodics is, that when given, at seasons of subsidence of deranged action, in diseases in which there are remissions and exacerbations, they are efficacious; that the dose varies, that it ought to be sufficient to prevent the recurrence of the derangement, but not to cause its own abnormal actions. If we use these agents at other periods of disease, and with other views, we are misapplying remedies, and acting with needless empiricism.

10. The indications of treatment in remittent fever are three, and each has its own appropriate means. 1. To control the excitement and complications of the exacerbation. 2. To act in the remission so as to prevent a recurrence of the exacerbation. 3. To ward off exhaustion by the timely use of stimulants and nourishment.*

I would, in conclusion, remark, that my opinions respecting quinine are the result of clinical observation, and were formed irrespective of those of other observers. This statement (and a similar one might be made relative to my opinions on the mercurial treatment of fever) is advanced simply that the authority of my own investigations may be added to that of others who,

* *Warburg's fever drops* have at times acquired a reputation in parts of India. In 1844, when attached to the European General Hospital, eleven bottles were tried by me. In one or two of the cases there was a decided sudorific action from the medicine, and the febrile paroxysm seemed to be shortened, and did not recur for several days; but in none was a cure effected. In other cases there was no sudorific action from the medicine, and the fever was in no respect benefited by its use. In one case the fever was checked for a time, but marked subacute inflammation of the stomach was excited. From these trials I drew the conclusion that Warburg's drops were an addition of very little value to the means which we already possess of con-

through the same process, have arrived at similar and independent conclusions.

On the prophylactic use of Quinine.—The prevention of intermittent and remittent fever in malarious districts by the daily use of a small quantity of quinine is an important consideration, but the evidence in its favour is as yet neither extensive nor conclusive.

There is no want of instances which are supposed to prove this prophylactic power, but they are generally deficient in some of the conditions essential in experiments of this nature. For example: detachments of the 18th Royal Irish, the 92nd Highlanders, the 3rd Dragoon Guards, with the 4th troop Bombay Horse Artillery and native details, were engaged on field service in the latter half of November and beginning of December, 1858, in the jungly tracts along the southern base of the Sautpoora Hills, in localities usually considered to be malarious at that season of the year. The men of the 92nd took two grains of quinine twice daily from the 27th November to 6th December, and the immunity from fever which they enjoyed was attributed by the medical officer to this measure. On inquiring into the state of health of the other detachments, I found that they had been equally free of fever, though they had not used quinine as a prophylactic. The comparison of the 92nd and Horse Artillery troop was instructive: the men of the 92nd had been conveyed to the scene of service by bullock train, but the troop had reached it by forced and fatiguing marches. The men of the latter were consequently more predisposed, yet they did not suffer from fever. The immunity of the 92nd therefore did not depend on the small quantity of quinine consumed daily, but, with that of the other troops engaged, on the circumstance that the malarious season had passed. Further careful investigation is, in my opinion, necessary before the prophylactic value of quinine can be received as an established fact.

Diet.—In order to control the undue vascular action of the exacerbation, the regimen must in all respects be antiphlogistic.

trolling the fevers of India; and that, in some cases, their use is not unattended with risk of injury.

In 1851 I was asked to see an English merchant in Bombay, who in the month of July, from residence in a swampy locality, became affected with remittent fever complicated with diarrhœa. He was moved to a better situation. The state of the bowels interfered, it was said, with the use of quinine. I saw this gentleman on the eleventh day of the fever, the third after it had become continued, and one after a bottle of Warburg's drops had been given. It caused profuse sweating, which continued at the time of my visit; the adynamic symptoms were well marked. He died twenty-four hours afterwards. Here the profuse diaphoresis from the medicine must have increased the exhaustion.

It has, however, been stated, that in remittent fever we must be on the outlook for prostration, and prepared to prevent it by the adequate use of farinacea, milk, and animal broths during the remission. The usual error in practice on this point — a very serious one — is to postpone the use of nutritious food till prostration is urgently present. The judicious physician, however, foresees its advent, appreciates its earliest signs, and strives to prevent it by the timely and skilful use of nourishment and stimulants. The adjustment of the food and of stimulants to the state of the constitution and type and stage of the fever is a very important part of the management, and one on which, in bad cases, success very often mainly depends.

Change of Air.—To place a fever patient in the most advantageous circumstances at our command as respects house and apartment, ought to be an invariable rule. If the situation be decidedly malarious, and that in which the fever has been acquired, then the removal of the patient to a more suitable adjoining locality, where medical treatment and care are also available, is a very necessary measure. But this necessity does not frequently occur in India, for hospital patients, by their removal to hospital, experience the benefit of change from the locality in which the attack has been excited; and officers do not frequently suffer from fever caused by malaria generated in the neighbourhood of their residences, but from exposure on the occasion of a hunting, shooting, or pic-nic expedition. When remittent fever persists, uncontrolled by remedies, change of air often holds out the prospect of benefit, particularly when residence on the sea-coast admits of change to sea, provided the patient can enjoy at the same time the advantages of careful nursing and medical treatment. The necessity for a measure of this kind will be frequent or rare, according to the knowledge and skill evinced in the medical treatment. The contingency often occurred in former years, when remittent fever was treated with mercury, without bark or quinine; and the change was so generally carried into effect, without sufficient provision for the essential medical management of the patient, or reference to fatigue and exposure, that much suffering and increased mortality resulted from it.

That this evil has really existed, is very evident from the following facts:—

A medical officer, on the 10th October, 1829, was taken ill with fever at Jumbooseer, in Guzerat. The attack was treated with depletion and mercurials, and was characterised by tendency to exhaustion. He went to Tankariabunder, and embarked there for Bombay on the 19th; suffered in the boat from nightly exacerbations, and sense of exhaustion in the day. He reached Bombay on the morning of the 23rd with a thready pulse, and died at 9 P.M.

A military officer was taken ill with remittent fever at Rajcote on the 18th October, 1834; treated with mercurials and purgatives; and sent on the 22nd to the coast and Bombay, supplied with fever pills and purgatives. He died on the road on the 26th.

An officer at Ahmudnuggur, in Guzerat, after ailing for two or three days, became affected with remittent fever on the 13th August, 1835. There were noon and midnight exacerbations and morning remissions. He was bled, used calomel and purgatives, and was sent to Hursole on the 18th. He reached it exhausted on the 19th, and died on the 20th. He was on his way to the sea-coast.

A military officer, in the month of October, 1839, was ill for a week with fever at Ahmedabad. He was sent to Cambay; was exhausted; there was wandering delirium, with oppression of breathing. Leeches were applied to the head, a blister to the epigastrium, and several free doses of calomel were given. He was then embarked for Bombay, and died at sea the night of his departure from Cambay.

The wife of the subject of the last case, also ill with remittent fever, left Cambay at the same time in another boat. I went on board to receive this lady on her arrival at Bombay, and found her suffering from adynamic fever. I attended her for two or three days, when she died. It was this case that first fixed my attention on the evils of this routine and injudicious system.

An officer ill with remittent fever at Tatta, in Scinde, in December, 1840, was sent to Kurrachee, and was seen there three days afterwards in a state of febrile excitement with delirium and fulness of both hypochondria. He was bled, and purgatives were given, also a draught with half a drachm of solution of muriate of morphia. He became comatose, and died twelve hours after his arrival. The head was not examined. The liver and spleen were enlarged, congested, and friable.

An officer of intemperate habits, and often injudiciously exposing himself to the sun, suffered from two or three attacks of fever at Tatta in December, 1840; these were followed by dysentery. He proceeded to Kurrachee, and arrived there in an adynamic state, and died the following day. The liver was much enlarged, and there was softening of the gastro-intestinal mucous lining.

A gentleman had fever at Poona on the 21st of November, and was first seen on the 23rd. The morning remission and noon exacerbation were marked on the 24th, 25th, 26th, 27th, 28th, and 29th. He was treated with leeching, mercurials, purgatives; and general blood-letting on the 28th: no quinine. He was sent from Poona on the morning of the 29th, and was seen at Bombay on the evening of the 30th. There was exacerbation with stupor and asthenia. On the morning of the 1st, a remission; at noon, an exacerbation with increasing stupor. He died comatose at 10 A.M. of the 2nd.

These cases will suffice*; they show unmistakeably the injurious effects of the excitement and fatigue of travelling, and the neglect of medical treatment. It is not difficult to understand how this system of mismanagement obtained currency. It is very evident that depletory measures and mercury are quite unequal to the cure of remittent fever. In this difficulty medical men and the public clung to the hope of benefit from change of air, and have been slow to interpret rightly the casualties which have resulted from it.

When treating of splenic cachexia, I pointed out the necessity of change of air with the view of improving the state of the constitution. When health has been injured by remittent fever, and convalescence is in progress, then change of air becomes, on the same grounds, a very useful and important measure.

* To satisfy myself on the question of change of air in remittent fever was a principal object with me in examining the cases of sick officers. From the ninety fatal cases of which I have notes, I have selected the eight just quoted. On the other hand, of 1,388 successful cases of officers recommended for change of air on different accounts, I do not find that I have noted a single instance of benefit from the measure adopted under those circumstances of fever to which these remarks have been directed.

Note.—The principles of treatment of remittent fever have been considered at somewhat greater length, and with more precision than in the first edition of this work. The discussion on the mercurial treatment has been reproduced with a greater conviction of its importance and necessity, because the nature of my duties on my return to India has afforded me the opportunity of becoming acquainted on a more extended scale with the present state of medical practice in that country, and I have been often astonished at the want of sound principles on the use of mercury, and of fixed principles of any kind on the general treatment of fever.

CHAP VI.

ON CERTAIN OBSCURE PHENOMENA, PROBABLY RELATED TO MALARIA.

INTERMITTENT and remittent fever are attributed to malaria as a cause, and the presence of these diseases may be received as evidence that this agency is active.

The observations made on the symptoms of the cold stage of intermittent fever, and on the diagnosis between remittent and symptomatic fever, have evinced my belief that the influence of malaria may be indicated by phenomena less marked, but still partaking somewhat of the character of those of intermittent and remittent fever. This subject may be pursued still further, and with much advantage by the practitioner in malarious countries. Careful observation in tropical climates will satisfy the inquirer that there is a tendency in all forms of disease to put on more or less of a periodic character in the malarious months of the year. This feature is more likely to be observed in the natives of India, and in long resident Europeans, than in the recently arrived. It is practically important; for when observed, it may be viewed as suggesting caution in the use of antiphlogistic means, and indicating the expediency of quinine.

After a period of residence in tropical countries, occurring sooner in some localities and constitutions than in others, an influence becomes operative on the system, produced perhaps by general climatic conditions, but more probably by malaria. There are many phenomena which may be taken as indicating the presence of this influence, — as restless nights, pain of limbs, frequent yawning, depression of spirits, giddiness, booming sounds in the ears, a sense of faintness or chilliness with vomiting, defective secretion of the liver leading to pale alvine discharges without jaundice; defective irritability of muscular fibre giving rise to palpitation, a feeble, sometimes intermitting pulse, constipation and dyspeptic symptoms. In these phenomena, if watched, a marked periodic tendency may often be observed. They are more apt to occur at times of considerable atmospheric changes, and very frequently about full or new moon.* All these symptoms are distinctly controlled by the use of quinine. The occurrence of night paroxysms of malarious fever is a familiar fact. The phenomena of the lesser influence of malaria may occur at the same diurnal period. In this way restless nights may often be explained: at all events, five or six grains of quinine, given at bed-time under these circumstances, cause sleep more certainly than opium.

The correct interpretation of these symptoms of deranged health leads to the use of quinine, and, to great caution in local blood-lettings, purgatives, and mercury; but the measure which they most clearly indicate, is change to a suitable temperate climate free from malaria. This is a most necessary step; for in the state of constitution of which these phenomena are the evidence, there is unquestionably a general tendency to fatty or other degeneration of tissue, which can only be prevented by forethought on our part, in recommending a suitable change of climate. To wait for the occurrence of structural change as the signal for removal from India, is a great practical error, and pathology has been studied to little purpose if its lessons have not taught us when to expect structural lesions, and how best to prevent them.

* The question of lunar influence on disease in India has been much discussed at different times. In the 2nd and 6th numbers of the "Transactions of the Medical and Physical Society of Bombay," the reader will find the latest consideration of this subject with which I am acquainted. The first paper, by Mr. Murray, details what the author conceived to be illustrations of lunar agency in chronic disease. The second is by Dr. Peet, and embraces an inquiry into the evidence on which the opinion rests.

On this question I shall merely observe: 1. To find on the same day several of the asthenic inmates of his wards affected with febrile disease, though all had been free of it for many days previously, is a fact familiar to the hospital physician in India. The days on which this is observed are often coincident with new or full moon.

2. To find those who have suffered from malarious fever experiencing recurrences at the periods of new and full moon, is a fact familiar both to patients and to medical men in India.

3. When this coincidence of febrile disease and these lunar phases are noted, there will generally be found to be present an appreciable atmospheric change of temperature, of moisture, of direction of the winds, &c. It is this atmospheric vicissitude, I apprehend, which is the determining cause of the febrile disturbance. Dr. Balfour, the great advocate of sol-lunar influence, admits this coincidence of atmospheric changes. His words are: "But I can declare in general that in India the meridional periods, both diurnal and nocturnal, were distinguished by remarkable changes or paroxysms in the state of the weather; and that these paroxysms were most remarkable at the lunar periods."

CHAP. VII.

ON ADYNAMIC REMITTENT FEVER OF SUSPECTED INFECTIOUS CHARACTER.

THAT malarious fevers are liable, under circumstances favourable to the spread of infection, to become infectious, is an old opinion. Fordyce held this view, and Clark and Lind believed that Bengal remittent was at times invested with this character.

We shall do well to bear this old doctrine in recollection, because, though with our present greater attention to cleanliness and ventilation, remittent fever is not infectious, it does not follow that it may not become so from overcrowding and neglect. From 1815 to 1820 a febrile disease* of very adynamic type prevailed in Kattywar, Kutch, and parts of Guzerat. A similar affection appeared at Pali in Marwar in July, 1836; was more or less present there, and extended to the towns in the adjacent districts up to the middle of 1838. Again, we have notices of a like disease in 1849 in Gurhwal, in Kumaon, and, more lately still (1853), in Rohilcund.

The fever was remittent in character, with great tendency to become continued, and the adynamic phenomena were well marked. It was attended, in the great majority of instances, with glandular swellings of the groins, axillæ, and neck; and, in the cold season, there was in some of the fatal cases dyspnœa, with cough and bloody expectoration. In none were carbuncles and petechiæ or purple patches present.

The number of cases seen by Dr. Forbes† at Pali, from January

* The terms Pali disease and Mahamurree have been given to this fever. It is much to be desired that the too common practice of giving local or native names to diseases in India be altogether abandoned, as tending to lead to careless diagnosis and vague pathology; I allude to such terms as Scinde, Guzerat, Mysore, Bengal, Deccan, Jungle, Pucka fever, Liver, Spleen, Beri-beri, Hill diarrhœa, and many others.

† "Transactions, Medical and Physical Society of Bombay," No. 2, p. 14.

29th to February 3rd, 1848, amounted to forty-eight. He thus describes the symptoms:—*

"Of these many had reached from the tenth to the twentieth day of the disease, with large buboes, no particular degree of fever, parched skin, tenderness of epigastrium, tongue white and moist, eyes dull and watery, bowels generally very slow, but sometimes loose, and the greater part with more or less cough; some few complained of little else than the pain of the buboes, with great weakness and loss of appetite. All, without exception, had buboes, but I met with no instance of carbuncle or vibices.

"In the mildest form the buboes make their appearance with little constitutional disturbance, attended only by languor, debility, and a general feeling of indisposition; they go on slowly to suppuration, and health is very gradually restored.

"In the most common variety the invasion is sudden, not being preceded by any feelings of disorder or uneasiness sufficient to engage the notice of the patient, generally takes place in the evening, and is rarely attended with rigors. The occurrence of the febrile symptoms, and the pain and swelling of the glands, appear to be in most cases simultaneous; in many the buboes showed themselves before the fever, while in none were they developed at a later period than the second day of the disease. The symptoms most generally present are great prostration of strength, giddiness, headache confined to the forehead, excessive thirst, dry burning skin, tongue moist and white, pulse from 110 to 130, small and weak, slight vomiting and tenderness of epigastrium, bowels confined, urine scanty and high coloured, great indifference as to recovery, and disinclination to speak or answer questions. The fever is of the remittent type, with marked tertian exacerbations, often attended with low delirium, but the crises are very imperfect. If uncomplicated with any thoracic or abdominal affection, and if the patient survives the fifth day, it commonly abates in violence after the seventh or eighth, so that in the third week little else remains but extreme debility, and sympathetic evening flushes from the buboes, which by this time have advanced to suppuration. In most of these cases, however, more or less cough is present through the height of the disease; it is generally dry, but sometimes accompanied by white frothy expectoration.

"In the more violent and malignant forms the attack sets in suddenly, with severe headache, staggering, and giddiness, quickly followed by delirium. The morning remission is scarcely perceptible, except by the abatement of the delirium. No glandular swellings appear, or they remain small, hard, and exquisitely painful; vomiting of bilious matter, and latterly of dark coffee-coloured fluid, comes on; the bowels are either constipated or the stools black and fetid, the teeth are covered with sordes, and the patient tosses and moans in bed. A dry cough now supervenes, attended with severe pain in the region of the heart, and laboured respiration; partial insensibility passes into profound coma with trismus, and death takes place early in the morning of the fourth day, or, in cases where the symptoms are less violent, on the morning of the sixth.

"The most fatal modification of the disease, from which no recovery has been known, sets in without any febrile excitement whatever, if we except a very slight acceleration of the pulse. The most prominent symptoms from the commencement are slight cough, and expectoration of blood; the cough appears to an observer more like a voluntary act to relieve oppression or constriction about the chest than to be caused by pain or irritation. The body is covered with frequent clammy sweats; the countenance exceedingly anxious and wild; thirst urgent, tongue clean, bowels slow; the urine increased in quantity and loaded with blood, which also oozes from

* This enterprising officer subsequently lost his life in Central Asia, while travelling on his return from Europe to India.

the gums. The expectoration of blood becomes more copious. To the anxiety and oppression of the chest is added pain in the cardiac region, the pulse becomes quick and thready, the action of the heart tumultuous, faintness and complete exhaustion come on; and a fatal syncope puts an end to the sufferings of the patient, generally within forty hours from the attack, the intellectual faculties remaining perfect till nearly the last moment.

"It is, however, by no means rare to see the different forms mixed or merging in each other. The attack may be at first mild and apparently without much danger, the buboes well developed and the fever slight; when from the third to the fifth day, and sometimes so late as the seventh, the occurrence either of delirium, coma, bloody expectoration, diarrhœa, retention of urine, or recession of the bubo, point out an unfavourable change, and the fatal termination soon follows, as in the more aggravated forms."

Dr. Forbes alludes to the treatment, and points out the inapplicability of all depressant remedies.

This fever has been observed at all periods of the year, and has prevailed chiefly amongst the poor, in filthy, badly-ventilated houses and villages, and has been preceded by seasons of famine. The mortality has been very great. Dr. Forbes thinks four-fifths of those attacked died. The circumstances just stated sufficiently explain the occurrence of adynamic fever; but they have been viewed chiefly with reference to the question of the contagious character of the fever, and its identity, or not, with the plague of Egypt and the Levant. Hence speculations arose relative to the manner of its introduction into India in the course of commerce from the Red Sea or Persian Gulf; and quarantine measures were on occasions strictly enforced.

It would be unprofitable, and foreign to the objects of this work, to enter into discussion on a subject of which I have no personal knowledge; but my impression is in favour of the opinion that it was a fever of endemic origin, of very adynamic type from the state of constitution of the attacked, assuming infectious properties from filth, crowding and imperfect ventilation, and having features in common with the plague of Egypt,—as is more or less the case in every fever in which adynamic symptoms and deteriorated blood are well marked.*

* The first known reports of this disease are by Messrs. McAdam, Whyte, and Gilder, in the 1st Number of the "Transactions of the Medical and Physical Society of Bombay."

The disease, as appearing at Pali and the adjoining districts, has been described by Messrs. McLean, Irvine, Keir, and Russel, of the Bengal Medical Service; and the results of their observations have been brought forward in an able memoir, by Dr. James Ranken, at the time Secretary to the Medical Board of Bengal. It was also reported on by Mr. Cramond and Dr. Forbes, of the Bombay Medical Service. The latter gentleman published a very interesting report of his observations in the 2nd Number of the "Transactions of the Bombay Society," already referred to in the text.

The accounts of the disease in Kumaon and Rohilcund are given by Drs. Pearson,

The description of jail or hospital fever by Pringle, in the seventh chapter of the third part of his work on the diseases of the army, has considerable resemblance to that of the fever observed at Pali. There were the same kind of adynamic phenomena, with suppuration of the axillary and parotid glands, with, in addition, the frequent presence of petechial spots. The causes were supposed to be crowding, filth, and effluvia from decomposing animal and vegetable matters. In some cases it was attributed to the effluvia from putrefying marshes; and in these the type was more remitting. The fever was regarded as infectious, but in no great degree, unless there had been continued exposure to the foul air.

In a Report on the Medical Topography and Diseases of Aden*, by Mr. Ruttonjee Hormuzjee, it is stated that intermittent fever is not so common there as in India; but the station is not exempt from the occasional visitation of febrile disease of severe type. During two of the years embraced in the report, 270 cases of remittent fever of adynamic type were treated, and of these 77 proved fatal. It prevailed with greatest severity from February to April, 1856, during which time there were 188 admissions and 60 deaths. The outbreak occurred among the native labourers engaged in the public works, and was attributed to undue crowding in a hot and badly-ventilated valley, in close, badly-constructed huts, in the proximity of sources of foul effluvia from decomposing animal excreta and other matters, coupled with poor living, and especially an inadequate supply of fresh water. The fever was characterised by evening exacerbations and morning remissions. The complications were various: cerebral disturbance in some indicated by delirium, drowsiness, and coma, attended with adynamic phenomena, as subsultus tendinum and dry tongue. Pneumonia, bronchitis, dysen-

Francis, Renny, and Stiven, of the Bengal Service, and are noticed in the 2nd and 3rd Numbers of the "Indian Annals of Medical Science."

The subject is also ably discussed by Dr. Mackinnon, in his treatise on the "Prevailing Diseases of Bengal and the North-west Provinces," published in the same journal.

In the 4th Number of the "Indian Annals of Medical Science," received since these remarks were written, I find a report, by Dr. Farquhar and Mr. Wallick, of an adynamic remittent fever which prevailed in the valley of Peshawur in 1852 and 1853, and was believed to be contagious. The worst cases were complicated with jaundice, and a relapsing tendency would seem to have been well marked in the disease.

It is important to note that this form of fever would seem to be confined to extra-tropical India, or to districts—Cutch, Kattywar—not much to the south of the tropic.

* Grant College Medical Society, Retrospective Address for the year 1857, by the author.

tery, diarrhœa, and jaundice were the complicating conditions in other cases. In the general immunity from intermittent fever at Aden, there is evidence that the true ague-malaria is not abundantly generated there, and this view is further supported by the physical characters of the locality—the absence of vegetation and moisture. It is therefore reasonable to conclude that this fever of bad type was due, in great part, to the defective sanitary conditions which existed, and was probably allied to the fever described in this chapter as having occurred at Pali, and other localities in the northern parts of India. The question of infection is not noticed by Mr. Hormuzjee in his report.

CHAP. VIII.

ON TYPHOID FEVER.

In the first edition of this work I stated that typhoid fever was unknown in India. Shortly after my return to Bombay a case of fever came under my observation towards the end of November, 1856, which led me to doubt the correctness of this opinion. The subject was a European female, and the attack commenced the day after her arrival from England by the overland route. The symptoms were febrile heat without distinct remissions, much prostration, febrile expression of countenance, tremulous hands, dry lips, the tongue dry and brownish in the centre, and some degree of tympanites. The bowels were very readily acted on by small doses of laxatives, and on one or two occasions blood was intermixed with the feculent discharges. Quinine was given without effect, and then omitted after two or three days, when the treatment consisted of small opiates, and attention to suitable nourishment. The fever persisted for twenty-one days, after which there was slow amendment, but the patient was not able to leave the house till the thirty-fifth day from the commencement of the illness.

This seemed to me to be a mild case of typhoid fever, and not long after its occurrence the reports* of Dr. Ewart and Mr. Scriven on typhoid fever came under my notice, and, more recently, the doubts which I still entertained were removed by a clinical lecture† by Dr. Edward Goodeve, in which seven cases of undoubted typhoid fever are detailed. As the object of this work is to record my personal experience, a detailed description of typhoid fever would be misplaced, as it could only be drawn from sources equally open to my readers.

The investigation which has thus been commenced is of much practical importance, in consequence of the principles of treatment

* "Indian Annals of Medical Science," vol. iv. pp. 65, 511.

† *Ibid.* No. xi. p. 141.

of typhoid fever differing so materially from those of malarious fevers; and it will require to be prosecuted with much care, in order that the tendency so common in medical research to exaggerate the importance of new subjects of inquiry, to the neglect of established truths, may be sufficiently controlled. With this view I would venture to suggest:—

1. That the locality, season and supposed causes be always stated, for it is not improbable that typhoid fever will be chiefly found in extra-tropical India, or in inter-tropical provinces, in the near proximity of the tropics and in the winter rather than the autumnal malarious season.

2. That it be recollected that disease of Peyer's glands, either in the stage of turgescence or ulceration, is not a morbid state peculiar to typhoid fever. It occurs in cholera, in protracted diarrhœa, in acute muco-enteritis, as an occasional complication of remittent fever, and a frequent one of phthisis pulmonalis.

3. From the last statement it follows, that we are not justified in asserting the existence of typhoid fever from the mere character of the post-mortem appearances. These require to be interpreted by the symptoms which have been present during life, in order that they may be correctly understood.

4. The observation made by Dr. Jenner, and confirmed by Dr. Watson, that they never saw jaundice in typhus or typhoid fever, is important to remember.

5. That the so-called typhoid (adynamic) symptoms are not peculiar to one form of fever, but may occur in all, is well known, and should not be forgotten.

CHAP. IX.

ON COMMON CONTINUED FEVER—FEBRICULA—AND ARDENT CONTINUED FEVER.

SECTION I.—*General Remarks.*

IN India and other tropical countries, in addition to intermittent and remittent fevers, there occur forms of idiopathic fever produced by ordinary exciting causes,—as vicissitudes of temperature, great heat, violent exercise, excitement of mind, excesses in eating, intemperate habits, and imperfect excretion. The fevers thus excited differ in degree rather than character. To the milder form, the terms ephemeral fever, common continued fever and febricula, have been almost indiscriminately applied. To the severer form, the designation ardent fever has been given.

They are most common in those parts of India which do not experience much of the influence of the monsoon rains, and whose hot season is not tempered by regular breezes from the sea. They are more met with in the central parts of the table land of the Deccan and Mysore, the Ceded districts, the coast of Coromandel, Scinde, and the Punjaub, than in Bengal or Bombay, and the western coast line south of Surat. They chiefly occur in March, April, and May; but also prevail in June and July in localities where the temperature is elevated, and the conditions of malaria are absent.

SECTION II.—*Common Continued Fever—Febricula.*

The mildest variety—*ephemeral*—may proceed from any of the ordinary exciting causes which have been mentioned, and though most common in unseasoned Europeans, may occur in Natives as well as in Europeans who have been some time resident in India. It consists of febrile symptoms without local complication, commencing with chills, followed by reaction, and this by perspiration, and thus is removed in from twenty-four to thirty-six hours. But the febrile reaction may continue for periods of four or five days; and then the term *common continued fever* is more correctly applied. It would be convenient, however, to substitute for these two designations, the single name, *febricula.* For the treatment of ephemeral and common continued fever, such means as an emetic, purgatives, tepid sponging, diaphoretics, and antiphlogistic regimen are employed. In plethoric individuals, when there is much headache and flushing of the face, a moderate general blood-letting, or leeches to the temples, may be an expedient measure, but they are not often necessary. These are not serious affections, and do not differ from the *febricula* of the colder climates; but the degree of reaction has always relation to the state of constitution, whether sthenic or not.

This form of fever occurred under my observation in the troops at Poona, in 1858 and 1859. In March, April, and May, the 17th Lancers, the 3rd Dragoon Guards, the 18th Royal Irish, and the D Troop, Horse Artillery—all recently arrived—suffered from febricula, marked by headache, flushed face, coated tongue, and pains of loins and limbs, subsiding and disappearing in from two to four days under moderate treatment. The 3rd Dragoon Guards were affected in greatest degree, consequent, as was supposed, on an imperfect head-dress, late morning parades, and suspected excesses in drinking. In the D Troop there was in some cases an eruption of roseola, or erythema, about the loins and thighs, which came and disappeared with the fever. The recruits of the Native Regiments at Poona were also sickly from febricula during the rains—June, July, August—of this year, consequent, in all probability, on too much drill and insufficient protection from cold and wet, owing to the badness of their huts.

A comparison of the state of health, as respects febricula, of the 31st Regiment and the German Legion, at Poona, from December 1858, to April 1859, is interesting, because both regiments arrived from the Cape of Good Hope about the same time, and the difference was doubtless due to the different sanitary conditions of the two bodies of men.

The 31st was composed of seasoned, well-equipped, and disciplined soldiers, and not, as was the case with many regiments sent to India to meet the late exigency, in great part of young recruits. They also occupied the best barracks at the station.

The German Legion consisted of badly-selected volunteers, who had been ill-cared for at the Cape, and a considerable number of whom left the colony tainted with scurvy and syphilis, and reached India in that condition. They were ill-equipped, occupied the worst barracks at Poona, were, perhaps, too much exposed at drill, but were not intemperate. The Indian ration was much more than they had been accustomed to. The scorbutic taint rapidly disappeared, and the men gained in flesh and strength. In fact, the Indian ration, and the Deccan cold season, so raised the constitution of these men, that it was, at the commencement of the hot months, similar to that of troops freshly arrived at that season. They were therefore more predisposed than the men of the 31st, who had not, in the cold months, undergone a change of this kind.

The general symptoms in the German Legion were considerable febrile excitement, flushing, headache, coated tongue, occasional vomiting, and sometimes cramps of the legs: with recovery in from three to four days. In a small proportion a remittent tendency was noticed. The treatment consisted of an ipecacuanha emetic,—which generally acted also on the bowels—acid drinks, and antiphlogistic regimen. There was no fatal case; seldom a readmission.

ADMISSIONS FROM FEVER IN THE 31ST REGIMENT AND THE GERMAN LEGION, AT POONA, FROM DECEMBER, 1858, TO APRIL, 1859.

	31st Regiment. Strength ranged from 864 to 1116.	German Legion. Strength, 1027.
December	3	8
January	14	65
February	24	127
March	37	283
April	25	65
	103	548

During the hot season, a squadron of the 6th Inniskilling Dragoons (late arrival) suffered from severe febricula at Sattara, consequent chiefly on insufficient protection in temporary barracks. The 22nd Native Infantry were sickly at Ahmednuggur from febricula at the same time; of a strength of 886, there were 214 cases of fever, chiefly febricula, admitted in April.

SECTION III.—*Ardent Continued Fever.*

Ardent continued fever is almost confined to tropical countries, and is a very serious disease. The exciting causes are elevated temperature, exposure to the sun, excessive exercise, mental excitement, excesses in eating, intemperance, defective excretion. There may be several of these causes combined. But in order to produce the disease in its most aggravated form elevated temperature is a necessary condition; and another is, that there should be present that kind of predisposition peculiar to the robust European lately arrived in a warm climate. This form of fever, then, is almost confined to the hot and dry months of the year in arid localities, and to regiments or recruits recently arrived from Europe.

Symptoms.—The attack is generally sudden, often without much chilliness. The face becomes flushed, and there is giddiness with much headache, and intolerance of light and of sound. The heat of skin is great, and the pulse frequent, full and firm. There is pain of limbs and of loins. The respiration is anxious. There is a sense of oppression at the epigastrium, with nausea and frequently vomiting of bilious matters. The bowels are sometimes confined; but, at others, vitiated bilious discharges take place. The tongue is white, often with florid edges. The urine is scanty and high coloured. If the excitement continues unabated, the headache increases, and is often accompanied with delirium. If symptoms such as these persist for from forty-eight to sixty hours, then the febrile phenomena may subside, the skin may become cold, and there will be risk of death from exhaustion and sudden collapse; or in cases in which the cerebral disturbance is great, death may take place at even an earlier period in the way of coma; or when symptoms of gastritis are very prominent, exhaustion may hasten the fatal result; or jaundice may appear and increase the danger.

The continuance for two or three days of excessive vascular action, such as that now described, must necessarily be followed by a corresponding depression; and in this we have the explanation of the collapse and exhaustion which become developed as the febrile excitement subsides. Again, the excessive action, with the addition of retained excretions, must vitiate the blood; and in some cases there is evidence of this condition in the dark grumous matters vomited and evacuated from the bowels. When these phenomena are present, exhaustion and collapse become very prominent, and are no doubt in a great measure attributable to the influence of the deteriorated blood.

The diagnosis between this form of fever, and inflammatory remittent has been already considered (p. 57), and the remarks then made should now be referred to.

Pathology.—In the excessive vascular action of this form of fever there is risk to important organs, as in the stage of exacerbation of the severer remittents. There is also danger from prostration, after a time, in consequence of continuance of high febrile excitement.

But between the pathology of ardent and remittent fever there is believed to be this great difference. In the former there is no materies in the blood, as in the latter, exercising a sedative influence on vital actions, and requiring time for its elimination. Therefore, we may hope that by subduing the vascular excitement at the outset of ardent fever we are adopting the most efficient means for shortening the duration of the disease.

Treatment.—There is much more scope in the treatment of ardent fever for the use of free and repeated general and local blood-letting, cold affusion, tartar emetic when tolerated, and mercurial and other purgatives. It must, however, be borne in mind, that these means are only effective when used promptly in the early periods of the fever, and that, if they be delayed till the third or fourth day,—when in the course of the disease the phenomena of prostration may be looked for,—their effect must be to hurry on the fatal result. They must be adopted also in recollection of the difficulties which sometimes beset the diagnosis of this from the remittent form of fever, and of the greater caution required in their use in the latter disease.

The symptoms of ardent fever, and the success of prompt and active treatment, are well illustrated in Dr. Arnott's Medical History of the Bombay Fusileers in the Punjaub.* The fever prevailed chiefly in the months of June, July and August at Peshawur, when the men were in tents under a temperature ranging from 70° to 114°, described by the author as intense, with hot blasts and thick suffocating clouds of dust, and as fearfully oppressive day and night, and completely breaking and disturbing rest. In these months 884 admissions from fever took place, and not a single death.

Dr. Arnott thus describes the character of the fever and the nature of the treatment which he followed:—

"The character of the epidemic fever which prevailed in July and August may be inferred, when I mention that out of the 798 cases admitted in these two months, not a man died. The symptoms on admission, it is true, were often very urgent, and demanded the most prompt and decided measures for their relief. There was pungent

* "Transactions of the Medical and Physical Society of Bombay," 1st Series. 10th Number, p. 34.

heat of skin; great thirst; parched, red, and dry tongue; quick, full, and strong pulse; racking pains in different parts of the body and acute headache, with flushed countenance; throbbing of the temples, restlessness, nausea, and vomiting of bilious matter, &c.; which symptoms, no doubt, were in many instances aggravated by the indifferent shelter the men had from the inclemency of the weather in that hot valley. The autumnal fever, which afterwards appeared, was almost equally mild, as we lost only three men from fever in October, November, and December.*

"To describe the plan of treatment of a disease having such marked symptoms seems almost superfluous. Evacuants fully and freely employed, with copious and repeated venesection, cupping and leeches (in fact, I never at any former time had occasion to prescribe bleeding, either to the same extent or so frequently), aided by tartar emetic, till all local determination and the chief urgent symptoms were removed, and afterwards quinine, were the means had recourse to."

It is not to be supposed that all the cases in the Fusileers were of the ardent variety, and presented the symptoms and required the treatment described by Dr. Arnott; doubtless, the greater number were febricula, and yielded to moderate measures. But as there was a proportion of ardent cases, and no deaths, the statement shows that the active treatment followed in these was appropriate.

* In these three months the range of the thermometer was from 42° to 91°.

CHAP. X.

ON THE FEBRILE AFFECTIONS OF CHILDREN IN INDIA.—FEBRICULA. INTERMITTENT AND REMITTENT FEVER.

THE fevers of children in India are best understood by keeping in view the principles which have been stated in respect to adults.

During the period of infancy—from birth to the end of the second year—attacks of febricula occur from errors in diet or the irritation of teething, just as in the colder climates, and they require the application of the same general principles of treatment. It is also necessary in the management of the febrile affections of early life, in India as elsewhere, to be careful in our diagnosis, and not to mistake the fever symptomatic of an internal inflammation for simple febricula. This caution is very necessary in regard to native children in the cold season in Bombay, for I have seen several cases in which pneumonia had been overlooked.

Intermittent or remittent fevers are, according to my experience, not common in the period of infancy; they doubtless occur, and probably much more frequently, in very malarious districts, than I have myself witnessed. The most striking instance that I have seen was early in November 1837. On the Bhore Ghaut, midway between Campooly and Khandalla, on the route from Bombay to Poona, there is a small house situated on the margin of a ravine for the accommodation of the gatherer of the tax levied on carts and bullocks passing over the mountain. At the time adverted to it was occupied by an old European pensioner and his wife; they had both suffered from intermittent fever. In the woman the indications of malarious fever were well marked in her sallow countenance and emaciated frame, and at the time I saw her she was suffering from tertian fever. She had an infant six weeks old, whom she was nursing, and it also experienced regular febrile paroxysms commencing with a well-marked cold stage. I saw the child in the cold stage of one of the attacks.

During the period of childhood, from the third to the tenth year and upwards, febricula is met with as in colder climates, proceeding from the same ordinary causes, and exhibiting that feature of remittence characteristic more or less of all the febrile affections of early life. These should be treated on the same principles as in other countries.

But in India, during childhood, just as in the adult, malarious fevers are by far the most frequent idiopathic forms. I have before me the diaries of many cases of intermittent and remittent fever treated by me in the Byculla Schools, while I held medical charge of that institution. They resemble the same affections in the adult, and require the same means of treatment modified to difference of age and peculiarities of constitution. Quinine may be used with the same freedom as in the adult, and it constitutes as essential a part of the treatment. There has been hesitation on this point in the minds of many; but I can state, on the authority of my own experience, and that of friends in whose judgment I place confidence, that two or three-grain doses may be given with safety, in necessary cases, in a child of three years of age. A European child of about seven years of age, ill for several days with intermittent fever, uninfluenced by a grain and a half dose of quinine, was brought to me. The recurrences were at once prevented by five or six-grain doses.

From the results of recent research, it may be concluded that occasional attacks of typhoid fever may also be looked for in children in India.

CHAP. XI.

STATISTICS OF FEVER IN THE EUROPEAN GENERAL HOSPITAL, THE JAMSETJEE JEJEEBHOY HOSPITAL, AND BYCULLA SCHOOLS, AT BOMBAY.

SECTION I.—*European General Hospital.—Total Fevers.*

TABLES V., VI., VII. represent the total* admissions of fever (4,037) into the European General Hospital at Bombay for the fifteen years from 1838 to 1853, arranged in quinquennial periods. Table V. is for a period during which I was assistant surgeon in the hospital, and includes cases from which a part of the clinical observations recorded in these pages has been drawn. For Tables VI. and VII. I am indebted to Dr. Stovell, when surgeon of the hospital.

When we compare the proportion of fever admissions in these three quinquennial periods, we find a remarkable difference between the first and the last. In the former (1838 to 1843) the fevers to the total admissions were 24·2 per cent. In the latter (1849 to 1853) only 13·5. In the middle period (1844 to 1848) they were 20·6.

In the three tables the greater proportion of admissions in the six months, from June to November, is well shown—it is 24·1; whereas that from December to May is 14. And if we omit the last quinquennial period—that in which fever admissions were comparatively few—we find that the proportion differs still more widely. That from June to November the fevers are 28·8 per cent. of the total admissions. From December to May they are 15. The month of October, however, is that of greatest prevalence—they amount to 37·5 per cent.

When we regard the mortality from fever in this hospital, we find it to be very uniform for these three periods. In the first table it is 3·5 per cent. of the admissions; in the second 3·3;

* They are chiefly intermittent and remittent. The proportion of ephemeral fevers is very small; it is only given for the first quinquennial period, in which they amounted to 8·7 per cent. of the total fever admissions.

in the third 3·1.* From 1838 to 1848 the proportion of fever mortality to total hospital deaths is 12·1; but from 1849 to 1853 it is only 6·7.

TABLE V.—*Admissions and Deaths, with Per-centage, from Fever of all kinds, in the European General Hospital at Bombay, for the Six Years from July* 1838 *to July* 1843.

	July 1838 to July 1843.		Monthly Average of the Six Years.		
	Admissions.	Deaths.	Deaths on Admissions.	Admissions on total Admissions.	Deaths on total Deaths.
January . .	105	5	4.7	19·1	11·5
February . .	55	2	3·6	13·3	6·2
March . . .	74	3	4·	14·5	9·
April . . .	88	5	5·6	15·1	12·1
May . . .	154	3	1·9	17·9	3·7
June . . .	219	6	2·7	28·4	11·7
July . . .	219	7	3·1	30·5	18·9
August . . .	179	8	4·4	29·3	22·8
September . .	141	8	5·6	25·8	15·3
October . .	318	6	1·8	44·	22·2
November . .	193	5	2·5	28.1	10·6
December . .	94	8	8·5	15·3	12·1
Total . .	1839	66	3·5	24·2	12·1

TABLE VI.—*Admissions and Deaths, with Per-centage, from Fever of all kinds, in the European General Hospital at Bombay, for the Five Years from* 1844 *to* 1848.

	1844 to 1848.		Monthly Average.		
	Admissions.	Deaths.	Deaths on Admissions.	Admissions on total Admissions.	Deaths on total Deaths.
January . .	105	6	5·7	17·0	13·0
February . .	85	4	4·7	16·5	11·5
March . . .	59	1	1·7	12·2	3·3
April . . .	67	2	3·0	13·1	6·5
May . . .	99	4	4·0	16·9	13·3
June . . .	172	5	2·9	24·1	15·2
July . . .	196	4	2·0	28·8	11·1
August . .	154	4	2·6	28·1	26·6
September . .	100	2	2·0	21·8	9·1
October . .	188	8	4·2	31·1	21·0
November . .	136	5	3·7	24·3	16·4
December . .	58	2	3·4	11·1	5·0
Total . .	1419	47	3·3	20·6	12·1

* Dr. Stovell's report ("Statistics of European General Hospitals for Ten Years," "Transactions of Medical and Physical Society, Bombay," New Series, No. 3) extends to March 1856; and shows a decreasing mortality from fever, that for the five years from 1851 to 1856, being 0·789.

TABLE VII.—*Admissions and Deaths, with Per-centage, from Fever of all kinds, in the European General Hospital at Bombay, for the Five Years from* 1849 *to* 1853.

	1849 to 1853.		Monthly Average.		
	Admissions.	Deaths.	Deaths on Admissions.	Admissions on total Admissions.	Deaths on total Deaths
January	48	4	8·3	10·6	10·3
February	38	3	7·8	10·3	16·6
March	43	0	—	9·8	—
April	45	3	6·6	8·7	12·0
May	91	0	—	17·5	—
June	78	1	1·3	13·6	3·4
July	87	4	4·6	16·4	12·1
August	62	3	4·8	12·0	7·8
September	49	0	—	13·8	—
October	52	0	—	13·2	—
November	93	5	5·3	17·8	16·6
December	93	1	1·1	15·3	2·5
Total	779	24	3·1	13·5	6·7

SECTION II.—*European General Hospital.—Intermittent Fever.*

Tables VIII., IX., X. give the admissions from intermittent fever, from 1838 to 1853, also arranged in three quinquennial periods. They show that the proportion of this type to the total admissions from fever has been 73·6 per cent.

We found from Tables V., VI., VII. that the proportion of fever admissions from June to November was nearly double that of from December to May; but the present Tables show that the excess of the first half year is not due to admissions of the intermittent type, for the proportions of intermittents to total fevers is from June to November 72·3, and from December to May 75·1.

The deaths are 1·1 per cent. of the admissions. It has been stated (p. 24) that we have no data which correctly show the mortality from simple intermittent fever. Much of the mortality stated in these tables (and I may add in hospital returns generally) is, I am satisfied not accurately recorded as directly proceeding from intermittent fever. It occurs from inflammations arising in malaria-tainted constitutions, and should be entered under the head of the inflammation, whatever it may be.

Table XI. shows the ephemeral fevers from 1838 to 1843.

TABLE VIII.—*Admissions and Deaths, with Per-centage, from Intermittent Fever, in the European General Hospital at Bombay, for the Five Years from July* 1838 *to July* 1843.

	July 1838 to July 1843.		Monthly Average.		
	Admissions.	Deaths.	Deaths on Admissions.	Admissions on total Fever Admissions.	Deaths on total Fever Deaths.
January . .	77	1	1·3	73·3	20·0
February . .	43	1	2·3	78·2	50·0
March . . .	59	2	3·4	79·7	66·0
April . . .	60	2	3·4	68·2	40·0
May . . .	109	1	0·9	64·3	33·3
June . . .	169	1	0·6	77·2	16·7
July . . .	136	1	0·8	62·1	14·3
August . . .	113	0	—	63·1	—
September . .	92	2	2·2	65·2	25·0
October . .	262	3	1·15	82·4	50·0
November . .	151	0	—	78·2	—
December . .	73	4	5·5	77·7	50·0
Total . .	1344	18	1·3	72·0	27·3

TABLE IX.—*Admissions and Deaths, with Per-centage, from Intermittent Fever, in the European General Hospital at Bombay, for the Five Years from* 1844 *to* 1848.

	1844 to 1848.		Monthly Average.		
	Admissions.	Deaths.	Deaths on Admissions.	Admissions on total Fever Admissions.	Deaths on total Fever Deaths.
January . .	87	1	1·1	82·9	16·6
February . .	69	1	1·4	81·2	25·0
March . . .	51	0	—	86·5	—
April . . .	57	0	—	85·1	—
May . . .	88	0	—	88·8	—
June . . .	144	1	0·7	83·7	20·0
July . . .	163	3	1·8	83·2	75·0
August . . .	116	0	—	74·0	—
September . .	81	0	—	81·0	—
October . .	167	4	2·4	88·8	50·0
November . .	114	2	1·7	83·8	40·0
December . .	44	0	—	76·0	—
Total . .	1181	12	1·02	83·2	25·0

TABLE X.—*Admissions and Deaths, with Per-centage, from Intermittent Fever, in the European General Hospital at Bombay, for the Five Years from* 1849 *to* 1853.

	1849 to 1853.		Monthly Average.		
	Admissions.	Deaths.	Deaths on Admissions.	Admissions on total Fever Admissions.	Deaths on total Fever Deaths.
January	32	2	6·3	66·6	50·0
February	25	0	—	65·8	—
March	32	0	—	74·4	—
April	30	1	3·3	66·6	33·3
May	60	0	—	65·9	—
June	46	0	—	58·9	—
July	53	1	1·9	60·9	25·0
August	37	1	2·7	59·7	33·3
September	30	0	—	61·2	—
October	32	0	—	61·5	—
November	67	0	—	72·0	—
December	67	0	—	72·0	—
Total	511	5	0·98	65·6	20·8

TABLE XI.—*Admissions and Deaths, with Per-centage, from Ephemeral Fever, in the European General Hospital at Bombay, for the Five Years from July* 1838 *to June* 1843.

	July 1838 to June 1843.		Monthly Average.		
	Admissions.	Deaths.	Deaths on Admissions.	Admissions on total Fever Admissions.	Deaths on total Fever Deaths.
January	13	0	0	12·4	0
February	5	0	0	8·9	0
March	8	0	0	10·8	0
April	9	0	0	10·2	0
May	21	0	0	13·6	0
June	23	0	0	10·5	0
July	8	0	0	3·7	0
August	17	0	0	9·5	0
September	15	0	0	10·5	0
October	23	0	0	7·2	0
November	9	0	0	4·6	0
December	8	0	0	8·5	0
Total	159	0	0	8·7	0

SECTION III.—*Jamsetjee Jejeebhoy Hospital.—Total Fevers.*

Table XII. gives the total admissions of fever into this hospital from 1848 to 1853, a period of six years; they amount to 2,473.* Compared with the European General Hospital, it shows a smaller proportion of fevers to total admissions; it is 9·8, that in the European General Hospital for the same years is 13·5 per cent. In the half year from June to November the excess is also less; the proportion is 10·8 per cent. of the total hospital admissions, while in the half year from December to May it is 8·6. But in comparing this proportion with the average of the European General Hospital we must bear in mind that for the years included in this Table (XII.) the difference between the two half years was in the European General Hospital much below that of the ten preceding years. It was from June to November 14·4; from December to May 12.

The mortality from fever in this Hospital has been 12·4 per cent.; that in the European General Hospital was 3·3.

In this difference we have an illustration of the kind of errors to which statistical statements must inevitably lead when applied to etiology and therapeutics, unless used by those who are familiar with all the circumstances of the individuals to whom the figures relate.

A statistical inquirer, from a comparison of the mortality in the European General Hospital for Europeans, and the Jamsetjee Jejeebhoy Hospital for Natives, as shown in Tables V., VI., VII. and XII., might infer that fever is a more fatal disease in Natives than in Europeans, and that the treatment of the disease was not so well understood in the one hospital as in the other.

But I, who have had a lengthened clinical experience in both hospitals, know that these inferences would be altogether erroneous. The high mortality in the Jamsetjee Jejeebhoy Hospital is simply due to the very destitute state of a large proportion of its inmates, and the very advanced stages of disease at which they seek for admission.

* The clinical cases, so frequently adverted to, were selections from this number.

TABLE XII.—*Admissions and Deaths, with Per-centage, from Remittent and Intermittent Fever*, in the Jamsetjee Jejeebhoy Hospital at Bombay, for the Six Years from* 1848 *to* 1853.

	1848 to 1853.		Monthly Average.		
	Admissions.	Deaths.	Deaths on Admissions.	Admissions on total Admissions.	Deaths on total Deaths.
January	183	40	21·8	8·7	8·9
February	146	30	20·6	7·2	9·4
March	139	23	16·5	6·5	5·9
April	168	16	9·5	7·9	4·6
May	218	20	9·1	9·9	6·9
June	194	20	10·3	9·3	6·5
July	210	19	9·04	10·4	6·2
August	214	18	8·4	10·8	5·5
September	202	26	12·3	9·8	8·3
October	274	27	9·9	12·8	7·9
November	251	26	10·3	11·6	7·8
December	274	43	15·7	11·8	10·8
Total	2,473	308	12·4	9·8	7·5

SECTION IV.—*Jamsetjee Jejeebhoy Hospital.—Intermittent Fever.*

The proportion of admissions of this type to the total fevers is 69·1; that for the half year from June to November being 72·5; that from December to May 63·9. The mortality is 0·9.

In the proportion of intermittents in the two half-yearly periods, we have the converse of what is stated in respect to the European General Hospital: in it the greater proportion is in the half year including the cold months of the year. In the Jamsetjee Jejeebhoy Hospital it is in the half year which includes the malarious months.

This discrepancy is to be explained by the fact, that, in the European General Hospital, a considerable proportion of the admissions from intermittent fever are of individuals who have arrived from other malarious countries, and who, reaching Bombay in the cold season, have the disease re-excited, not by the malaria of Bombay as an exciting cause, but by cold or other atmospheric states acting on a tainted system. This is not the case in the Jamsetjee Jejeebhoy Hospital to nearly the same extent.

* This Table might have been entitled "Fevers of all Kinds," for the admissions under the head "Ephemeral" have been very few.

TABLE XIII.—*Admissions and Deaths, with Per-centage, from Intermittent Fever, in the Jamsetjee Jejeebhoy Hospital at Bombay, for the Six Years from* 1848 *to* 1853.

	1848 to 1853.		Monthly Average.		
	Admissions.	Deaths.	Deaths on Admissions.	Admissions on total Fever Admissions.	Deaths on total Fever Deaths.
January . .	107	6	5·6	58·5	15·0
February . .	89	3	3·4	60·6	10·0
March . . .	79	0	—	56·8	—
April . . .	111	0	—	66·1	—
May . . .	148	2	1·4	67·8	10·0
June . . .	152	0	—	78·3	—
July . . .	169	3	1·8	80·4	15·8
August . . .	140	1	0·7	65·4	5·5
September . .	141	0	—	69·8	—
October . .	185	1	0·5	67·5	3·7
November . .	186	0	—	74·1	—
December . .	202	1	0·49	73·7	2·3
Total . .	1709	7	0·9	69·1	5·5

SECTION V.—*European General Hospital.—Remittent Fever.*

Tables XIV., XV., XVI. show that the proportion of this type, to the total fevers, is 16·6 * per cent.

When we compare the proportion in the half-years, from June to November, and December to May, we find that it was 19·8 per cent. in the former, and 13·6 in the latter.

The mortality from this type is, for the 15 years †, 15·1 per cent. on the admissions, and 76·1 per cent. of the total deaths from fever.

In regarding the mortality from remittent fever in this hospital, it must be borne in mind that, from the variety in the inmates, and the not unfrequent advanced periods of admission, it is necessarily higher than that of European regimental hospitals.

* That 16·6 of this type, with the proportion of Intermittents, does not complete the total admissions, is to be explained by the abstraction of 8·7 for Ephemerals in the first quinquennial period.

† Dr. Stovell's decennial Report shows a remarkable decrease in the mortality, from 1853 to 1856. For the five years from 1846 to 1851, the ratio keeps up to that in the text—it is 15·423; but for the five years from 1851 to 1856, it falls to 4·838 per cent.

TABLE XIV.—*Admissions and Deaths, with Per-centage, from Remittent Fever, in the European General Hospital at Bombay, for the Five Years from July* 1838 *to June* 1843.

	July 1838 to June 1843.		Monthly Average for the Five Years.		
	Admissions.	Deaths.	Deaths on Admissions.	Admissions on total Fever Admissions.	Deaths on total Fever Deaths.
January	15	4	26·6	14·1	80·0
February	7	1	14·2	12·7	50·0
March	7	1	14·2	9·4	33·3
April	19	3	15·7	21·5	60·0
May	24	2	8·3	15·5	66·6
June	27	5	18·5	12·3	83·3
July	75	6	8·0	34·7	85·7
August	49	8	16·3	27·3	100 0
September	34	6	17·6	24·1	75·0
October	33	3	9·0	10·3	50·0
November	33	5	15·1	17·0	100·0
December	13	4	30·0	13·7	50·0
Total	336	48	14·2	17·6	72·7

TABLE XV.—*Admissions and Deaths, with Per-centage, from Remittent Fever, in the European General Hospital at Bombay, for the Five Years from* 1844 *to* 1848.

	1844 to 1848.		Monthly Average.		
	Admissions.	Deaths.	Deaths on Admissions.	Admissions on total Fever Admissions.	Deaths on total Fever Deaths.
January	16	5	31·3	15·2	83·3
February	10	2	20·0	11·7	50·0
March	5	1	20·0	8·5	100·0
April	10	1	10·0	14·9	50·0
May	11	4	36·4	11·1	100·0
June	25	4	16·0	14·5	80·0
July	25	3	12·0	12·7	75·0
August	36	4	11·1	23·4	100·0
September	16	2	12·5	16·0	100·0
October	21	5	23·8	11·2	62·5
November	20	3	15·0	14·7	60·0
December	11	2	18·2	18·9	100·0
Total	206	36	17·4	14·5	76·6

TABLE XVI.—*Admissions and Deaths, with Per-centage, from Remittent Fever, in the European General Hospital at Bombay, for the Five Years from* 1849 *to* 1853.

	1849 to 1853.		Monthly Average.		
	Admissions.	Deaths.	Deaths on Admissions.	Admissions on total Fever Admissions.	Deaths on total Fever Deaths.
January . .	8	2	25·0	16·7	50·0
February . .	7	3	42·8	18·4	100·0
March . . .	2	0	—	4·6	—
April . . .	4	2	50·0	8·9	66·6
May . . .	13	0	—	14·2	—
June . . .	16	1	6·2	20·5	100·0
July . . .	21	3	14·3	24·1	75·0
August . . .	15	2	13·3	25·8	66·6
September . ,	8	0	—	16·4	—
October . .	16	0	—	30·8	—
November . .	13	5	38·4	13·9	100·0
December . .	15	1	6·6	16·1	100·0
Total . .	138	19	13·7	17·7	79·2

SECTION VI.—*Jamsetjee Jejeebhoy Hospital.—Remittent Fever.*

The proportion of remittents to intermittents is 32·1 per cent.: double that of the European General Hospital. If the inference be drawn from this statement that the remittent is more frequent in Natives, compared with the intermittent type, than in Europeans, it would be a correct deduction from the tables; but it would be an application of the figures to a question which they are not calculated to solve. The fact is, that natives do not readily resort to a civil hospital for mild attacks of fever; therefore the proportion of the severer type is greater than in a European hospital, partly civil and partly military in its character.

In the half year from June to November the proportion of this type is 29; in the half year from December to May it is 36 per cent. We have found that, from June to November the proportion of remittents was greater, but that of intermittents was less, in the European General Hospital; whereas in the Jamsetjee Jejeebhoy Hospital the proportion of remittents was less, that of intermittents was greater. On the other hand, in the half year from December to May intermittents were proportionally greater, and remittents less, in the European General Hospital; but in the Jamsetjee Jejeebhoy Hospital the proportion of remittents exceeded that of the intermittents, and fell short of that of the other half year.

It may be suggested, in explanation of the greater proportional prevalence of remittent fever in the native inmates of the Jamsetjee Jejeebhoy Hospital, in the half year including the cold months, than in that including the malarious months — that many of them are instances of malarious fever, assuming the remittent character in consequence of inflammatory complication—pneumonia or other—induced by cold, to the influence of which, as an exciting cause, the badly fed and clothed classes of the native community are very susceptible.

The greater proportion of fever deaths in natives in Bombay, in the half year from December to May, also appears in Mr. Leith's Mortuary Returns; it is—for the five years from February 1848 to January 1853 — 54·44 of the total mortality; whereas the proportion for the half year from June to November is 45·55. This fact is also to be explained in the same manner, with the addition that, as a large number of the returns are made from non-professional sources, it is probable that part of the mortality recorded as due to fevers has been caused by inflammations with symptomatic fever. This is Mr. Leith's opinion.

I have already explained the probable cause of the proportional excess of intermittents in the European General Hospital in the non-malarious half of the year. We have found, however, that the remittent type is in greatest proportion in the malarious six months —for then we have a more fixed community, and more of the influence of the malaria of the island as an exciting cause.

TABLE XVII.—*Admission and Deaths, with Per-centage, from Remittent Fever, in the Jamsetjee Jejeebhoy Hospital at Bombay, for the Six Years from* 1848 *to* 1853.

	1848 to 1853.		Monthly Average.		
	Admissions.	Deaths.	Deaths on Admissions.	Admissions on total Fever Admissions.	Deaths on total Fever Deaths.
January	76	34	44·7	41·5	85·0
February	57	27	47·3	39·04	90·0
March	60	23	38·3	43·1	100·0
April	57	16	28·1	33·9	100·0
May	70	18	25·7	32·1	90·0
June	42	20	47·6	21·6	100·0
July	51	16	31·4	24·3	84·2
August	74	17	22·9	34·6	94·4
September	71	26	36·6	35·1	100·0
October	89	26	29·2	32·5	93·3
November	65	26	40·0	25·9	100·0
December	72	42	58·3	26·3	97·7
Total	784	291	37·1	32·1	94·5

SECTION VII. — *Byculla Schools. — Intermittent and Remittent Fever.*

The averages are not given in the following table, because the "strength" of the children and the total admissions are not known. The strength has ranged from about 235 to 355.

It will be observed that there are no deaths from intermittent fever, and that the ratio of mortality from remittent fever is 2·8 per cent. of admissions.

TABLE XVIII.—*Admissions and Deaths, from Intermitent and Remittent Fever, in the Byculla Schools, for the Seventeen Years from* 1837 *to* 1853.

	Intermittent Fever.		Remittent Fever.	
	Admissions.	Deaths.	Admissions.	Deaths.
January	160	0	16	1
February	149	0	21	1
March	153	0	17	0
April	172	0	11	0
May	184	0	9	0
June	214	0	20	1
July	284	0	47	2
August	260	0	19	1
September	250	0	20	0
October	226	0	9	0
November	197	0	12	0
December	117	0	12	0
Total	2,366	0	213	6

CHAP. XII.

ON ERUPTIVE FEVERS.

SECTION I. — *Prevalence in the Native Army.*

THE following statement exhibits the comparative prevalence of the different kinds of eruptive fever in the native army of the Madras and Bombay Presidencies for the five years from 1851–52 to 1855-56: —

	MADRAS.		BOMBAY.	
	Admissions.	Deaths.	Admissions.	Deaths.
Variola	495	22	310	21
Varicella	1,229	1	612	—
Rubeola	114	1	113	—
Scarlatina	1	—	—	—
Total . . .	1,839	24	1,035	21

The proportion of small-pox in the Bombay Presidency is probably understated, in consequence of cases being returned "varicella," which are in reality modified small-pox. At all events, I observed in the hospitals at Poona, in the early part of 1858, when small pox prevailed, several cases in which this error of diagnosis had been committed.

SECTION II.—*Small-pox, as observed in Bombay.—Prevalence.— Prevention by Vaccination.*

During five years of my service in the European General Hospital, from July 1838 to July 1843, 32 cases of small-pox were admitted. Of these 25 took place in the months of January, February, March, and April; 4 in the month of November, that of 1839; and 3 — one in each month — in May, June, and July; and in the months of August, September, October, and December, there was not, during these five years, a single admission from small-pox. There were 5 deaths, which gives a mortality of 15·6 per cent.

During the ten succeeding years — from 1844 to 1853 — there were 49 admissions of small-pox into the European General Hospital, and of these 44 were in the five months from January to May. The deaths were 12, being a mortality rate of 25·6 per cent.

In the course of the seventeen years from 1837 to 1853, 23 children of the Byculla Schools suffered from small-pox, and 3 of them died, a mortality of 13 per cent; but the disease did not prevail in each year of this period, 1838, 1841, 1843 to 1848 inclusive; 1852 and 1853 were exempt.

The subjoined tabular statement shows the admissions from small-pox into the Jamsetjee Jejeebhoy Hospital for the six years from 1848 to 1853: —

	Total.		Monthly Average.		
	Admissions.	Deaths.	Deaths on Admissions.	Admissions on total Admissions.	Deaths on total Deaths.
January	32	9	28·1	1·5	2·0
February	59	18	30·5	3·1	5·6
March	74	29	38·8	3·4	7·5
April	52	28	53·8	2·4	8·1
May	17	11	64·6	0·7	3·8
June	6	1	16·6	0·2	0·3
July	10	3	30·0	0·5	0·9
August	2	3	15·0	0·1	0·8
September	1	—	—	0·05	—
October	—	—	—	—	—
November	1	1	100.0	0·05	0·3
December	7	1	14.3	0·3	0·3
Total	261	104	39·8	1·03	2·5

Though daily visiting the small-pox ward during the prevalence of the disease in these six years and the three preceding ones, it was in the months of December 1845, January, February, and March 1846, that I took immediate charge of the small-pox patients, and made the following notes on the disease, as it occurs in the hospital frequenting classes of the native community of Bombay.

The number of admissions, and deaths from small-pox, during these four months, are shown in this tabular statement: —

Years.	Months.	Remained.	Admitted.	Total.	Discharged.	Died.	Remaining.
1845	December	—	5	5	2	—	3
1846	January	3	10	13	4	5	4
"	February	4	8	12	2	6	4
"	March	4	26	30	7	12	11
	Total . . .	—	49	—	15	23	—

It exhibits a mortality of 46 per cent. The fatal cases were, with very few exceptions, markedly confluent, and death took place on the 3rd, 4th, 6th, 7th, 8th, 9th, 10th, and 11th days of the eruption.

The cases which proved fatal before the seventh day of the eruption, were generally instances in which the eruptive fever had been characterised by very urgent symptoms, as delirium, much anxiety, vomiting, pain of loins, badly-developed pulse, and had extended beyond the usual period, having in two instances continued till the fifth day. These symptoms were succeeded by a badly-developed eruption. In these cases the urgent symptoms abated somewhat on the first appearance of the eruption, but they in general recurred on the second and succeeding days, and proved fatal about the fourth and fifth, with delirium, sinking pulse, and coma. Such form of fatal result is to be accounted for, in a majority of cases, by the circumstance of the febrile state being more or less congestive and adynamic in type. There are, however, cases occasionally to be observed which prove fatal under very much the same train of symptoms, and at the same stage, in consequence of congestion taking place in important organs, — as the lungs, — during the eruptive fever, and, by its presence, preventing the free development of the eruption. I have seen more than one case fatal on the third or fourth day of a badly-developed eruption, with complication of pneumonia marked by hurried breathing and rusty sputa, dating back to the period of the eruptive fever.

The cases fatal after the seventh day of the eruption (and they constitute the greater number) were generally those in which the eruption had been copious and very confluent, and in which there had been present hoarseness, with more or less dyspnœa and cough. These signs of laryngeal and tracheal irritation increased towards the eighth day, and proved fatal then, or in the early stage of the secondary fever. The eleventh was the latest day of fatal termination.

In none of the fatal cases were the symptoms usually termed malignant observed, as petechiæ, the pustules filling with dark-coloured serum, hæmaturia or other hæmorrhage. In a few of the successful cases, glandular swellings, and the formation of small abscesses, were troublesome during convalescence. In none of them did injured vision take place.

The admissions from small-pox were, with four exceptions, confined to Mussulmans and Portuguese: many of the former were sailors, and probably strangers in Bombay; several of the latter had recently arrived from Goa. Of the affected with small-pox 7 were females, the rest males. The ages of 48 of the number were —

5 years and under	4
15 " "	3
15 " to 20	6
20 " to 30 inclusive	29
30 " to 40	4
40 " to oldest, 55	2
Total	48

It is probable that almost all the admissions were of parties unprotected by vaccination or previous small-pox, but on this point it is often impossible to obtain trustworthy information from the inmates of our hospitals; for they are admitted, not unfrequently, at stages of the disease when incapable of giving a connected history of themselves, and are often unattended by friends able to supply the deficiency.

Of the admissions which form the subject of these notes, there was only one in which vaccination was undoubted and the marks on the arms distinct. In this case the disease was very modified, and confined to a few vesicles on the face, — and this, though (as is usually observed) the initiatory fever had been very well marked.

Several interesting cases of the modifying influence of vaccination came under my notice at Poona in 1858, especially one in the hospital of the Bombay Artillery, and another in that of the 18th Royal Irish. In both the initiatory fever ran high, and the eruption came out copiously, with confluence on the face, and up to its fifth day there was every indication of a dangerous attack, when the distinct vesicles acuminated, and became turbid. On the sixth day desiccation was in progress on the face, and before the acme of the natural disease — the eighth day — had arrived, convalescence was well advanced.

As already stated, I have reason to think that modified small-pox, in its mildest form, is liable to be mistaken for chicken-pox. In chicken-pox there is little initiatory fever. The pellucid vesicles are without central depression; they come out in successive crops, seldom appear on the face, and their contents become turbid before desiccation begins. In modified small-pox the initiatory fever is always well marked, often severe. The eruption first appears on the face, then on the trunk and extremities, and is often very scanty. The vesicles are depressed in the centre at first, but they acuminate on the fifth day, their contents become turbid, and on the sixth day they dry into small dark-coloured crusts. In consequence of the eruption on the face preceding that on the other parts of the body,—the character and development by successive crops is in a measure simulated. But the liability to err in the diagnosis turns on this point, that the period of depression of the vesicles is of short duration, probably not more than twenty-four hours, and is therefore very apt to be overlooked. When there has been marked initiatory fever, acuminated vesicles, with turbid contents, on the face, on the fourth or fifth day of the eruption, with desiccation on the fifth or sixth, and at the same time (fifth or sixth day) acuminated vesicles on the trunk and extremities, there should be no hesitation in regarding the case as modified small-pox — not varicella.

Treatment. — In the mild distinct small-pox with a moderate eruption we may look for recovery; and, with the exception of mitigating the febrile disturbance by diaphoretics, aperients, if necessary, and attention to purity of air and cleanliness, further medical interference is unnecessary.

In the confluent form we have another illustration of the speedy prostration of vital actions from the sedative influence of the morbific cause, often aggravated by complicating derangement of important organs.

All that can be attempted under these circumstances is to endeavour, by stimulants, nourishment, and opiates, to sustain the system till the natural course and processes of poison elimination have been gone through. It need hardly be added that attention to purity of air and cleanliness are most important parts of these arrangements.

Finally, in respect to the initiatory fever the treatment should always be very guarded, and conducted in recollection that the dangers of prostration are likely soon to arise.

Prevalence and Prevention of Small-pox. — The best means of prevention of this still very prevalent and fatal disease continue to engage the attention of the Indian Government. In the report of the Small-pox Commissioners apppointed by the Government of Bengal in 1850; in Mr. Bedford's Statistical Notes on Small-pox, Vaccination, and Inoculation in India*, and in Dr. Mackinnon's paper on the Epidemics of the Bengal and North-West Presidencies†, we have the latest and fullest consideration of this subject in relation to Bengal and the North-Western Provinces.

In the following remarks, however, I shall confine myself in a great measure to the island of Bombay; for I believe that in the published mortuary registers of Bombay, prepared since the year 1848 with so much care and ability by Mr. Leith, we have data far more trustworthy than are to be obtained of any other part of India.

From these we learn that during the five years from 1st February 1848, to 31st January 1853, 4,038 deaths took place from small-pox in Bombay, and of these 3,203 occurred in children under seven years of age. The proportion of deaths from this disease to the total deaths was, for the five years, 5·83 per cent., the highest being 7·80, in the year 1848, and the lowest 2·70, in 1849.

The observation made by me in 1846 ‡ — founded on hospital records, and on Dr. Stewart's report of the small-pox epidemics in Calcutta of 1833, 1838, 1843 — that small-pox prevailed more in some months of the year than in others, is amply confirmed by Mr. Leith's registers, for in these we find that the deaths from small-pox bear, in the different quarters of the year, the following proportions to the total deaths: —

1st	Quarter from	1st February	to 30th April	11·15	per cent.
2nd	"	1st May	to 31st July	6·24	"
3rd	"	1st August	to 31st October	1·19	"
4th	"	1st November	to 31st January	1·36	"

The tables enable us to enter into still further details, and to allot the proportion of deaths from small-pox to the different months of the year. Thus — still taking the average of the five years — the proportion in different months is —

January	4·18
February	11·17
March	20·34
April	24·24

* "Indian Annals of Medical Science," No. 2, 1853.

† *Ibid.* No. 3, 1854.

‡ "Transactions, Medical and Physical Society of Bombay," No. 8, p. 28.

May	17·47
June	11·36
July	4·51
August	2·20
September	1·21
October	·51
November	·90
December	1·84
Total	99·93

The tabular statement of small-pox in the Jamsetjee Jejeebhoy Hospital (p. 183) illustrates this feature of small-pox, viz. that it prevails most in Bombay in the first half of the year, and more in March and April than in other months. The same general law is also true of Calcutta.* A similar characteristic, but much less marked, may probably be observed of small-pox epidemics in Europe. Sydenham distinctly states that the season about the vernal equinox is that most favourable to epidemic small-pox; and the same fact may be traced more or less through Huxham's "Observations on Air and Epidemics." In the Second Annual Report by the Registrar-General of births, deaths, and marriages in England, there is an account of an epidemic small-pox in England in the years 1838, 1839, in which this law may be traced, but not so clearly as in the Bombay and Calcutta records. For example, from 1st January to 1st July of 1838, there were 8,631 deaths from small-pox; from 1st July to 1st January 7,536 deaths, being a decrease of 1,095 in the last half year. From January to July 1839, there were 5,487 deaths; but from July to January 1840, there were 3,263, being a decrease in the summer and autumn of 2,224.†

* Report of the Small-pox Commissioners, Calcutta, 1850, table A. page 9; also the following abstract, taken from p. 24 of the same Report.

TABLE showing the Total Monthly Mortality by Small-pox during Eighteen successive Years, from 1st May 1832, to 1st May 1850, inclusive:—

November	120	March	3,689	July	551
December	512	April	2,846	August	189
January	1,316	May	1,419	September	181
February	2,372	June	761	October	134

† This observation, written in 1846 and published (Transactions, Medical and Physical Society of Bombay, No. 8, p. 29) in 1847, does not altogether accord with the statement made by Mr. Bedford at page 192 of the able and interesting paper already referred to; nor with that of the Small-pox Commissioners of Calcutta at page 24 of their Report. I have not at present the opportunity nor the time to mak another and more extensive reference to the Report of the Registrar General.

In 1846 (Transactions, Bombay, Medical Society, No. 8, p. 29), adverting to these facts, which seem to show that the prevalence of small-pox in particular seasons, so

The question of the degree to which the prevalence of small-pox may be attributed to the practice of inoculation, has been discussed in the Bengal reports; but as respects the island of Bombay it need not be entertained. The practice of inoculation is not, it is believed, followed by any of the classes of the native community of Bombay; but a greater mortality from small-pox in some years than in others is very observable in Mr. Leith's reports: for example,—

In 1848.	1849.	1850.	1851.	1852.
7·80	2·70	7·635	3·57	7·45

We gather, then, from Mr. Leith's registers, that the mortality from small-pox in the island of Bombay is very nearly 60 in 1000.

Small-pox inoculation is not practised in the island, but it is so to some extent in the adjoining Concans; therefore, though the native population of Bombay is not in general protected by inoculation, still, from its fluctuating character, a proportion of it probably is so.

I am unable to state precisely the number of annual vaccinations in Bombay, but the proportion which it bears to the total native population is very small indeed. The mortality from small-pox in

remarkable in India, may also be traced in European countries, I remarked, "Though, then, this law of epidemic small-pox is not peculiar but only more marked in tropical countries, it is only, as far as I am aware, in this country, that a similar law has been observed in a remarkable way to influence the propagation of the vaccine disease.

"Now that there is not any longer doubt in regard to the identity of small-pox and cow-pox, the difficulty of propagating the latter in some parts of India during the hot months may be considered as in accordance with the epidemic law, and as additional evidence of the identity of the two diseases. The difficulty which has attended the propagation of the vaccine disease in some months, in some of the Bengal provinces, has been the subject of much discussion, and too much weight has in all probability been attached to it, as an *impediment* in the way of the diffusion of the protective influence of vaccination in India. While the law of preference of certain seasons has been so much dwelt on with reference to the cow-pox, it has been too much lost sight of in regard to the small-pox. For what is the practical inference? It is this: if, in the seasons in which there is difficulty, if not impracticability, in propagating the vaccine disease in its perfect form, there is also very seldom prevalence of epidemic small-pox—does it not follow that this obstacle to the diffusion of the vaccine is a matter of no great regret, and speaking generally, the absence of vaccination in these seasons no great evil, because there is no great demand for the exercise of its protective influence? While, on the contrary, if the seasons, to which epidemic small-pox is almost exclusively confined, are those, or immediately succeed those, in which there is no difficulty in keeping up the vaccine disease,—then, does it not follow that vaccination, assiduously and carefully practised in those seasons, will afford to the people almost the full measure of its protection?"

Mr. Bedford, at page 194 of his "Notes," shows, that in the Upper Provinces of India, successful vaccinations in July amount only to 10 per cent. and in October to 7 per cent.

Bombay represents that of a very partially protected community. But when we direct our attention to the European residents of Bombay, whose number, according to the census of 1850*, was 5,088, we find that, during the five years from 1848 to 1852 inclusive, 1,177 deaths are registered, and of these 12 were from small-pox. This is a fraction more than 10 deaths in 1000; double that of the average of European countries in which vaccination is *compulsory*, but not half that of England and Wales, and not more than one-fifth of that of the native population of Bombay. There can be no doubt that the instances, if any, must be few of inoculated Europeans in Bombay, and that therefore the smaller proportion of mortality from small pox in them can only be attributed to the protective power of vaccination.

The results deducible from my notes of the fatal cases of European officers do not seem so favourable to vaccination. Of 311 deaths 7 were from small-pox, which is at about the rate of 22 in 1000. The fatal cases† occurred in the years 1834, 1848, 1849, 1850, 1851.

Though the attention of the Indian Government was called to the subject of vaccination very shortly after Jenner's discovery, and notwithstanding the exertions which have been made, it is to be feared that as yet little influence has been exercised on the health of the civil population of India by the systems of vaccination which have been adopted. The tabular returns, from the impossibility, owing to the prejudices or fears of the people, of verifying the success of the operation in a large proportion of cases, and from the ignorance, dishonesty, and unskilfulness of much of the native agency employed, are unworthy of being received as evidence for or against a question so important as the prophylactic power of vaccination.

Nor can it be said that vaccination in the Native army and followers has been attended with that degree of success which might fairly have been anticipated from the more effective agency of military system. It was, I believe, never enforced in the Bengal Native army; but the rule both in Madras and Bombay has been to vaccinate all unprotected recruits.

The prevalence of small-pox at several of the military stations

* I have not alluded to this census (which make the total population of the island 566,119), relative to the native population, because it is considered untrustworthy. But in respect to Europeans there is no reason for questioning its accuracy.

† One at each of the following stations: Seroor, Nassick, Poona, Mooltan, Mahubuleshwur. Of two the station is not mentioned in my notes.

in the Poona division of the Bombay army, in the early part of 1858, led to the system of vaccination and its results being submitted to close scrutiny. The returns of all kinds were communicated to me, as Superintending Surgeon of the division, by Major-General Michel, who at that time commanded; and the report which was prepared by me from these documents was afterwards published by the Commander-in-chief in the general orders of the army.

From this report the following extracts are taken :—

"1. The tables exhibit a total of 7,189 natives; that is, 58·2 per cent. of the strength who have at some time or other suffered from small-pox. As the returns do not separate those who have been inoculated for small-pox from those who have had the natural disease*, it is impossible to estimate correctly the mortality represented by this number of attacks. If these had been all instances of natural small-pox, and if the average rate of mortality in European countries, viz. 1 in 4, obtains also in India, then 7,189 attacks represents about 1,797 deaths. If, however, the impression entertained by some, though as yet unsubstantiated by statistical data, that small-pox is a less fatal disease in India be correct, and 1 in 7 be assumed as the rate of mortality, then the number of attacks in question will have been attended by about 1,027 deaths in the communities of which the individuals were members.

"2. The same tables show the numbers vaccinated to be 4,299—that is, 34·8 per cent. of the strength; and the numbers unprotected to be 855—that is, 7 per cent. of the strength. Of the unprotected, 539 are children under 10 years of age, which gives a per-centage 20·3 of unprotected children.

"3. This proportion of small-pox and unprotection, viz. 65·2 per cent., and of vaccinated 34·8, exists in a native army in which "every recruit is to be vaccinated, if requisite, on enlistment," and in respect to which medical officers are told "that it is particularly imperative on those serving in the army to fulfil this duty (vaccination) in their respective regiments or other charges, as well as among the women, children, and camp followers belonging to the same."

"4. Of adult male sepoys and followers the following are the general per-centages:

	Small-pox.	Vaccinated.	Unprotected.
Sepoys . . .	61·8	34·5	3·5
Followers . . .	68·8	27·1	3·4

"If these be alone regarded, then it may be inferred that the per-centage of small-pox shows the proportion existing at the period of enlistment, and merely indicates the degree in which vaccination is neglected in the communities of which the individuals in question were originally members. But when the difference exhibited in the several regiments is considered, then the following range becomes apparent:—

	Small-pox.	Vaccinated.	Unprotected.
Sepoys . . .	23· to 86·3	7·1 to 72·9	0· to 13·6
Followers . . .	13·8 to 100·	0· to 86.2	0· to 20·

* On this question it may be stated that inoculation is not practised in the upper provinces of India, is so in a very limited degree in the Deccan, but in greater degree in the Concan.

"It may be advanced, in explanation of this difference in the proportion of small-pox, that inoculation is probably more practised in the communities from which some regiments are chiefly recruited than in those from which others are; and to account for the greater proportion of vaccination in some, it may be that it is practised in these more indiscriminately than in others—that is, without regard to the fact of previous small-pox; and that such operations, though unsuccessful, have been erroneously recorded as vaccinations. Still, making every allowance for these explanations in abatement of the difference in the number of adult males vaccinated in different regiments, it is impossible to avoid the conclusion that vaccination, as respects this class, is more carefully conducted in some regiments than in others.

"5. Of the wives of sepoys and followers the general per-centages are—

	Small Pox.	Vaccinated.	Unprotected.
Sepoys' Wives	69·7	29·3	0·9
Followers' ditto	73·7	21·3	5·7

"The range is as follows:—

	Small Pox.	Vaccinated.	Unprotected.
Sepoys' Wives	40·4 to 97·3	2·7 to 55·	0· to 4·4
Followers' ditto	16·6 to 100·	0· to 85·3	0· to 17·5

"The several remarks made in the preceding paragraph on the different proportions of small-pox and vaccinated among the males in different regiments, are, to some extent, also applicable to females. But this further observation may be hazarded—that the differences in the number vaccinated show that scruples and prejudices are more readily overcome in some regiments than in others.

"6. Of the children of sepoys and followers the general per-centages are—

	Small Pox.	Vaccinated.	Unprotected.
Sepoys' Children	27·	57·3	15·5
Followers' ditto	40·6	34·3	25·1

"The following is the range:—

	Small Pox.	Vaccinated.	Unprotected.
Sepoys' Children	17·9 to 54·3	22·5 to 77·7	0· to 50·
Followers' ditto	4· to 100·	4·4 to 96·	0· to 71·2

"The difficulty in determining the number of adults, male and female, affected with small-pox before coming under regimental observation, renders the returns of these classes an imperfect test of the degree of observance or neglect of vaccination. But in respect to children, this uncertainty does not exist; for it may be fairly assumed that a large proportion of them have been born and reared in the regimental lines, and that $27 + 40·6 = 67·6 \div 2 = 38·8$ per cent. small-pox, and $15·5 + 25·1 = 40·6 \div 2 = 20·3$ per cent. unprotected prove a very defective state of vaccination in the community in which they exist.

"7. The number returned 'vaccinated' is shown in the 2nd paragraph to be 4,299; that is, 34·8 per cent. of the strength. But even this small proportion of 'vaccinated' is in excess of the nominally 'vaccinated' under ordinary circumstances, and very considerably in excess of the truly protected by vaccination. (*a.*) On the prevalence of small-pox at Poona being reported, the acting superintending surgeon called the attention of the medical officers in charge of native troops in the division to the subject of vaccination by circular, dated 10th March, and required not only a return of the numbers vaccinated monthly, but also of those who remained unprotected. From the 1st March to the 30th June 1,138 vaccinations were returned from native regiments, which is 26·4 per cent. of the total vaccinated shown in the 2nd paragraph. It is therefore a just conclusion that the proportion of vaccinated shown on the 30th June had been raised above the usual standard by a temporary impulse. (*b.*) The native regimental vaccinations for the official year 1857-58 (from 1st April 1857, to 31st March 1858) amounted to 1,627, viz.:—Men, regiments, 460; men, followers, 2; woman, 1; children, sepoys, 713; children, followers, 451: total, 1,627. Of these the proportion returned as failed or doubtful is:—Men, regiments, 273; men, followers, 2 or 59·3 per cent. this class; children, sepoys, 202; children, followers, 126 or 28·1 per cent. this class. The total of vaccinations in 1857-58, not affording the certainty of protection, was 602, or 37 per cent. of the whole number vaccinated. It may be reasonably assumed, that of the total vaccinations given in the 2nd paragraph, 37 per cent. were failures or doubtful; and that, in consequence, the proportion of real protection from vaccination is not 34·8 per cent. of the strength, but only 22·1.

"8. It is of importance to determine the cause of the large proportion of unsuccessful vaccinations in the native army. They may be stated as follows:—1st. The want of general and systematic vaccination leaves the medical officer too often dependent on lymph, preserved on glasses,—often sent from a distance, and perhaps carelessly taken and transmitted. 2nd. Vaccination is too much left to hospital assistants, who, from want of practice, are unskilled in the operation, and, from defective knowledge, are not well acquainted with the conditions of its success. 3rd. A portion of the failures in adults is due to protection by previous small-pox.

"9. Another table shows the number of European soldiers, with their wives and children, who have had small-pox, been vaccinated, or are unprotected. The percentage to strength is as follows:—

	Small Pox.	Vaccinated.	Unprotected.
Soldiers	13·5	83·5	3·4
Ditto Wives	11·6	86·2	0·5
Ditto Children	2·8	93·0	4·1

"The contrast between the proportions of vaccinated here shown and that in natives, in paragraphs 4, 5, 6, is striking. Still the proportion of those who have had small-pox illustrates the well-known fact, that in the classes in Great Britain and Ireland, from which recruits for the army are drawn, vaccination is also imperfectly conducted.

"10. The information communicated in these returns, relative to the proportion of protected and unprotected in cantonment military bazaars, is quite inadequate for the object in view. The facts recorded amount to this: that the estimated population is, in

Poona Bazaar	35,000
Kirkee	5,000
Ahmednuggur	6,405
Malligaum	3,949
Sattara	2,142
Dapoolie	3,615
Total	56,111

"The number protected in the Poona, Kirkee, and Malligaum bazaars is unknown. In the other, the residents are supposed to be all protected, with the following exceptions:—

Ahmednuggur	236
Sattara	11
Dapoolie	111

"If the ratio of the successfully vaccinated in the native army, under the more favourable circumstances of smaller numbers, greater control, and professional agency, is only 22 per cent. of the strength, it may be fairly assumed that the ratio of annual vaccinations in large military bazaars as that of Poona, does not, under ordinary circumstances, exceed that of the general civil population of the Bombay Presidency, which, estimating the population at 15,578,992*, and the successful vaccinations at 202,535†, is 1·3‡ per cent.

"Though the quarterly returns, from which the several statements in this memorandum have been deduced, cannot be regarded as statistical data, on which full reliance may be placed, yet they safely justify the following conclusions. 1st. Vaccination is very insufficiently carried on in the general communities from which the recruits of the native army are drawn. 2nd. Vaccination is unequally practised in native regiments, and though this may in part be explained, as respects adults, by circumstances antecedent to enlistment, yet the great degree of difference, and the facts relative to small-pox and to vaccination in children, prove that this important sanitary measure, inadequate in all regiments, receives much greater attention in some than in others.

"12. The representations which led to the issue of the Division Order would seem to be amply confirmed by the analysis of these returns, and it is not to be doubted that the imperfect practice of vaccination, thus made apparent, calls for active and sustained efforts on the part of the military and medical officers connected with the native army and with military bazaars. This subject, though of great importance to the interests of the native military population, also involves the welfare, in some degree, of a large body of European troops brought into constant association with the Sepoys of the native army and the residents in the military bazaars. Though it is true that Europeans in India enjoy, for the most part, the advantage of protection from small-pox through a well-organised system of vaccination, still occasional instances occur when, from some cause or other, this protection has ceased, and lives, of the highest value to the State, may thus fall a sacrifice to that extensive diffusion of small-pox which the neglect of vaccination permits to exist." §

SECTION III. — *On Measles in Bombay and the Deccan.*

My clinical knowledge of measles has been chiefly obtained in the sick wards of the Central Schools at Byculla.‖ This institution is for the maintenance and education of children of the European soldiers of the Bombay Presidency. The children are partly of unmixed European extraction, and partly Indo-Britons. During

* "Thornton's Gazetteer."

† "Report on Vaccination, Bombay Presidency, for 1854-55," p. 53.

‡ In Agra and Delhi, 0·054 per cent. In Bengal, where inoculation is practised, the annual vaccinations are 0·98 per thousand.—*Indian Annals Medical Science*, vol. i. (*Bedford.*)

§ This memorandum was written shortly after the lamented death of Sir William Peel, by confluent small-pox, at Cawnpore, in April 1858.

‖ In the Island of Bombay.

the last twenty years, their numbers, both sexes included, have ranged from 235 to 355, and their ages from 3 to 16.

There are two buildings, one for boys, the other for girls; both situated in the same grounds, with an interval of about 100 yards. About eight years ago, a separate hospital was added to the institution; for before this period, the sick wards were in the school buildings.

Measles prevailed in the schools in October 1832*; but no record has been preserved of this visitation. The next occurrence of the disease was in December 1838; it commenced on the 21st of that month, and continued till the 2nd of April 1839. At this time I held medical charge of the institution. The schools, with the exception of a single case in January 1840, remained free of measles till December 1846, when it commenced on the 21st of the month and ceased on the 10th March 1847. It reappeared on the 13th March 1852, and prevailed till the 22nd of May. It was again absent till the 10th March 1857, when it returned and continued till the 14th of April. No further notice will be taken of the visitation of 1832; and in the subsequent remarks, I shall designate the remaining four the first, second, third, and fourth epidemics.

The disease commenced in the girls' school in the three first, and in the boys' in the last epidemic, and in the second and third the importation of the infection was traced to a fresh arrival. The period that elapsed between the commencement of the disease in the one school and its appearance in the other was in the first epidemic twenty-six days, in the second twenty-seven, in the third twenty-four, and in the fourth eleven. During the first and second epidemics there was no separate hospital building. During the first epidemic the healthy children were removed to a building at some distance†, and the school-rooms were converted into sick wards. This course was adopted because, in the months of February and March 1837, 74 cases of mumps occurred in the girls' school, but not a single case in the boys' school; and in the months of March and April 1838, 29 cases of varicella occurred in the boys' school, but not a single case in the girls' school. I had therefore, on the outbreak of measles in the girls' school, some expectation

* Measles was very prevalent at Calcutta and the vicinity in March, April, and May 1832, as stated by Mr. Corbyn. — *Transactions, Medical and Physical Society of Calcutta*, vol. vi. p. 477.

† The imperfect accommodation for the sick was also a reason for the adoption of this measure.

that it would not extend to the boys' school, and in consequence did not recommend in the first instance any measures of prevention in addition to those already afforded by the school buildings.

But the removal of the healthy children, after the disease had shown itself also in the boys' school, had no effect in checking the further spread of the epidemic.

There have been, in the course of twenty-two years, four visitations of measles in these schools, with intervals of five and eight years. The first and second commenced on the 21st December, and the third and fourth on the 13th and 10th of March, and none of them continued later than the 22nd of May. Epidemic measles then, in Bombay, shows a preference for the same months as small-pox and (as has just been shown) mumps and varicella are similarly characterised.

The following is a note of the admissions and deaths in the four epidemics:—

	Admissions.	Deaths.	Mortality per cent.
1838-39	100	5	5·
1846-47	144	5	3·4
1852	107	,,*	5·4
1857	117	10	8·5

These four epidemics have been described in the Transactions of the Medical and Physical Society of Bombay. The first † by myself, the second ‡ by Dr. Coles, and the third and fourth § by Mr. Carter.

But my information relative to measles is not confined to this single institution or to the island of Bombay. In 1857 it prevailed among the general native population in Bombay. Mr. Moreshwur Junardhun, in a report addressed to the Grant College Medical Society mentions that between January and May of that year he treated 83 cases, of which 15 died — a mortality of 18 per cent. In March and April of the same year the disease visited the infant branch of the Byculla Schools, located at Poona; 31 children were affected and 7 died, — a mortality of 22·5 per cent.

The children of the 1st battalion of Artillery at Ahmednuggur suffered from measles in May, June, and July of 1857, with this result:—

	Admitted.	Died.
Indo-Britons	12	4
Europeans	52	14
	64	18

This high mortality — 28 per cent. — may in part be accounted

* The number is not distinctly stated in the Report.

† 2nd No. ‡ 9th No. § 1st No. and 4th No. New Series.

for by the children having come off a long and fatiguing journey from Nusseerabad, and their accommodation at Ahmednuggur being overcrowded.

Again, as regards the general population of the island of Bombay, it appears from Mr. Leith's Register that during the five years from 1st February 1848, to 31st January 1852, 323 deaths from measles are recorded; and of these 212 occurred in children under seven years of age. In the following classification of these deaths, made with reference to the months of their occurrence, the preference shown by the disease for the first six months of the year is again well illustrated:—

Month	Deaths	Month	Deaths
January	32	July	15
February	48	August	4
March	47	September	1
April	63	October	7
May	57	November	4
June	41	December	4
	288		35

Among the children of the better classes of Europeans at Bombay, I do not recollect an instance of its epidemic prevalence. But sporadic cases have been met with from time to time. I remember, however, only two as coming under my personal observation. They occurred in the month of June 1853.

In the fatal cases of European officers, from 1829 to 1848, I find only one case of measles. It occurred at Belgaum in February 1832, in an officer of the staff. The initiatory febrile symptoms were congestive in character; they continued from the 9th to the 13th, when the eruption came out on the 14th. This officer imprudently sat up, exposed to cold, and attended to some of the duties of his office. On the evening of that day he complained of sore throat, which had increased on the following day with addition of oppression of the chest and delirium; symptoms of collapse came on, and he died on the 15th.

It is unnecessary for me to describe the symptoms and treatment of a disease so well known to medical observers in all countries; but there is one circumstance in the character of the symptoms, as it has been observed in the Byculla schools, which it is of importance to note. In the accounts of measles as occurring in European countries, paleness of the eruption is stated to be of unfavourable import. This doubtless is true of the more sthenic children of these countries, and equally so of well-conditioned European children in India. But in all Indian epidemics we may expect frequently to meet with the disease in children more or less anæmic; and in them the eruption will be found occasionally to present a faintness of tint, which in a sthenic child might excite apprehension, but which in the asthenic is quite compatible with a mild and favourable course.

In respect to treatment, I would only observe that it is of much importance in the feeble children of India to be very careful not to debilitate, but to watch for a failing pulse and other symptoms of asthenia, and then to give chicken broth or beef tea freely, and wine if necessary; to omit all depressant medicines, and use squills and carbonate of ammonia with camphor mixture. I am satisfied that several lives were saved in the first epidemic from observance of this principle, and if errors were committed in the general management they were on the side of too much depression.

Measles in the Byculla schools has been usually followed by troublesome catarrhal ophthalmia.

The fatal cases which I had an opportunity of examining were those of the first epidemic. They were five in number. In all there was pneumonia, which in four had passed on to hepatization, with, in one, gangrenous excavations. In two the pneumonia was general, in two lobular, and in one vesicular. In all there had been muco-enteritis, which in two had led to granular exudation on the mucous lining of the lower part of the ileum and of the colon; in one to turgescence and ulceration of Peyer's agminated glands; in one to redness of the mucous membrane of the lower part of the ileum and turgescence of Peyer's glands; and in one merely to vascularity of the end of the ileum.

When we compare the history of measles in India with that of the disease in colder climates, we find the mortality to be much higher in the former. The rates of mortality stand thus:—

European countries *			3·	per cent.
Byculla Schools, Bombay, —	1st	Epidemic	5·	
„	2nd	„	3·4	„
„	3rd	„	5·4	„
„	4th	„	8·5	„
Moreshwur Junardhun's cases			18·	„
Infant Schools, Poona			22·5	„
1st Battalion, Artillery, Nuggur			28·	„
Bengal and N.W. Provinces †			8.	„

Nor is it difficult to understand how this should be. The prone-

* "Lectures on Diseases of Infancy and Childhood," by Dr. West. 4th edition, p. 712.

† Dr. Mackinnon, in his remarks on the Epidemics of Bengal and the North-western Provinces, states the mortality from measles in the children of European soldiers to be eight per cent.—*Indian Annals of Medicine*, No. 3, p. 171.

ness of the asthenic constitution in India to become affected with pneumonia has been already alluded to, and will be more fully illustrated in a subsequent part of this work. It has been also shown that January, February, March are months in which measles is apt to prevail. Though the absolute temperature of these months in India is high compared with that of European countries, yet the daily range is great relatively to other seasons of the year; and the more or less prevalence of north-easterly winds in these months also increases the heat-abstracting property of the atmosphere. When these facts are considered with the additional one, that the heat-generating power of the animal system has relation to temperature of season and climate, we can be at no loss in understanding how the predisposed become affected with pneumonia in India and how cold is an exciting cause.

There is probably moreover greater danger in measles from gastro-intestinal inflammation in India than in the same disease in more temperate climates. And as an additional cause of high mortality, the greater obscurity of pneumonia in asthenic states, and the less control over its course, are deserving of notice.

SECTION IV. — *Scarlatina.* — *Erysipelas.* — *Varicella.* — *Hooping Cough.* — *Cynanche Parotidea.*

Scarlatina. — We have not any satisfactory account * of the occurrence in India of the scarlatina simplex, anginosa, and maligna of European countries.

A fever, remittent in character and attended with scarlet eruption, has prevailed epidemically on several occasions, since 1824 to 1853, in Bengal and the North-western Provinces. In some instances the mucous membrane of the mouth and fauces has been inflamed; but in others this feature has not been observed. In the earlier epidemics rheumatic pain of the joints was frequently noticed; but this has not been the case in the later visitations of the disease.

I am not acquainted with the occurrence of a similar epidemic in any part of the Bombay Presidency.† I have however met with an occasional case of remittent fever in natives attended with an eruption resembling roseola. The same kind of eruption has also

* The single case entered in the Madras return at the commencement of this chapter cannot be received. The fact of a single case of an infectious disease returned of an unprotected community, is of itself proof of inaccurate diagnosis.

† Dr. Peet reports that it has prevailed at Bombay and Poona in 1850. "Transactions, Medical and Physical Society," New Series, No. 5, p. 211.

been observed by me in a few instances in the secondary fever of cholera, and I have already stated that it was present in some of the cases of febricula in the D troop, Royal Artillery, at Poona in the hot season of 1858.

The Bengal epidemics have been described by Drs. Mellis, Twining, Cavell, Mouat, and H. H. Goodeve *; also by Dr. Edward Goodeve†, and by Dr. Mackinnon.‡ None of these authors have considered the disease described by them as identical with European scarlatina. It is, however, similar to the Dengue of America and the West Indies.

Erysipelas.—The remark made by Dr. Mackinnon, that "idiopathic erysipelas, as it appears on the face and lower extremities unconnected with wounds, is a rare affection in India," § is fully confirmed by observation in Bombay. I have met with very few cases either in Europeans or in natives.

But traumatic erysipelas is of more common occurrence, and at times evinces almost an epidemic tendency. It was common in the Jamsetjee Jejeebhoy Hospital in November and December 1851, after wounds of the scalp and lower extremities, but was easily subdued. It did not in all cases originate in the hospital, but in some was present on the admission of the patient; thus showing that it was not, at least in all cases, due to the air of the hospital. On one or two occasions I have also noticed the liability to erysipelas after the application of blisters so well marked as to render it expedient to discontinue, for the time, the use of this remedy.

Varicella.—In my observations on measles, allusion has already been made to the occurrence of twenty-nine cases of varicella in the boys' school at Byculla in March and April 1838, but notes of this epidemic have not been preserved by me. Since then, however, cases of this disease have come under my observation, and I am satisfied that the term varicella has not been applied by me to an affection varioloid in character. The diagnosis of the two diseases has been already explained in the remarks on small-pox.

Mr. Carter states that, in the year 1849, a varioloid form of varicella affected twenty-four boys in the school, but only one girl, in

* "Transactions, Medical and Physical Society, Calcutta," vols. i. ii. ix.

† "Indian Annals of Medical Science, No. 2."

‡ "Treatise on Public Health. Indian Annals of Medical Science," No. 3.

§ "Indian Annals of Medicine," No. 3, p. 177. It may be well to bear in mind immunity from scarlatina and erysipelas in India, in reference to the question raised by some pathologists of relation between these affections.

the months of March, April, and May. I am unable to say whether this epidemic differed from that of 1838, or whether the term varioloid used by Mr. Carter merely indicates a difference of opinion on the part of the observers.

Hooping-Cough.—In Dr. Coles' Report on Measles in the Byculla schools, allusion is made to the presence of three cases of hooping-cough at the same time. I do not find any account of the epidemic prevalence of this disease in these schools; but my impression is that it has occurred, from time to time, during the last twenty years.

Cynanche Parotidea attacked the girls' school in February and March 1837. Seventy-four girls were affected, not a single boy. Mr. Carter reports that it broke out among the boys in October and November 1851. Seventy-five boys were affected, but only two girls.

CHAP. XIII.

ON EPIDEMIC CHOLERA.

SECTION I. — *Remarks on the Seasons of Prevalence and on the Causes of Cholera.*

THE leading statistical facts of cholera amongst European and native troops in India are *:—

PRESIDENCY	EUROPEANS.			NATIVES.		
	Per-centage of Admissions to strength.	Per-centage of Deaths to strength.	Per-centage of Deaths to Admissions.	Per-centage of Admissions to strength.	Per-centage of Deaths to strength.	Per-centage of Deaths to Admissions.
Bengal	2·87	0·97	33·70	0·53	0·16	30·54
Bombay	2·64	0·86	32·53	0·96	0·32	33·06
Madras	1·98	0·69	34·83	1·35	0·58	42·91

In the European General Hospital 234 cases of cholera, and in the Jamsetjee Jejeebhoy Hospital 1259, were treated during my periods of service in these institutions. I have also had the opportunity of investigating this disease in other parts of the presidency as well as among the better classes of the community, both European and Native, in the island of Bombay.†

The following remarks on cholera combine the results of my own experience, and of a careful consideration of much that has been written on the subject, both by Indian and European writers.

My connexion with hospitals in Bombay extends from June

* "Vital Statistics of the European and Native Armies in India," by Joseph Ewart, M.D., pp. 147, 160.

† It may be stated here, that during my service in India, from August 1856 to September 1859, subsequent to the publication of the first edition of this work, I have again had extensive opportunities of observing cholera, both in the Jamsetjee Jejeebhoy Hospital, and the Hospitals of the 61st Regiment and the German Legion, at Poona. Notwithstanding, the text is left very much as originally written, for this further experience has in no respect modified my opinions.

1838 to May 1854; and from these sources I learn, that in the years 1841, 1847, and 1848, there was very little cholera in the island. It, however, prevailed extensively in the years 1842, 1846, 1849, 1850, 1851, 1853, and 1854. But the partial character of the visitations of cholera is shown by the returns from the Byculla schools, in which 1840, 1844, and 1845 were the years of greatest prevalence, and 1848, 1850, 1852, and 1853 were those of exemption.

The greater prevalence of cholera in some years than in others in Bombay is also apparent in Mr. Leith's Mortuary Register. There we learn that the proportion which the deaths from cholera bore to the total deaths in the island in different years, was as follows: —

1848 . . .	·63 per cent.	1851 . . .	27·75 per cent.
1849 . . .	17·40	1852 . . .	8·40
1850 . . .	27·850		

The greater prevalence of cholera in the warmer months of the year in European countries, has been supposed to depend on elevated temperature favouring an impure state of the atmosphere by increasing decomposition.* But as the heat of an Indian climate must always be sufficient to cause atmospheric impurity in this manner, it may be inferred, if the view stated in respect to European countries be correct, that cholera in India will not show a preference for particular seasons. The admissions into the European General Hospital at Bombay, from 1838 to 1853, are, for the half year from April to September, 234, and for that from October to March, 114: those into the Hospital of the Byculla schools, from 1837 to 1853, are, for the first period, 68, and for the second 21. Cholera prevailed extensively in many places in the southern Mahratta country and Deccan from April to June 1859; and the Artillery, the 61st Regiment, and the German Legion at Poona suffered considerably from the 24th May to the 7th June.

This statement seems to countenance the relation of the disease to the hot and rainy months of the year; but then this inference is corrected by a reference to the Jamsetjee Jejeebhoy Hospital, in which (from 1848 to 1853) 417 admissions took place in the first half year, and 637 in the second. Mr. Leith's Mortuary Returns, from 1848 to 1852, also give the greatest number of cholera deaths in the half year which includes the cold season, viz. 7,112 for the half year, from October to March, and 5,110 from April to September.

* "Report on the Cause and Mode of Diffusion of Epidemic Cholera." By Wm. Baly, M.D. 1854.

But it may be supposed from these statements, considered in connexion with remarks in Mr. Webb's report on the medical statistics of European troops in the Bombay presidency *, that cholera affects Europeans in greatest degree in the hot and rainy months, but Natives in the cold season. This conclusion is, however, corrected by tabular statements before me, relative to the disease in Calcutta. The first † refers to the general population of the city, from 1832 to 1838, and shows, for the half year from April to September, 9,560 deaths, and for that from October to March, 8,555. The second ‡ relates to the European General Hospital at Calcutta from 1842 to 1853, and gives from April to September 358 admissions, and from October to March 383.

I conclude, then, that though partial data may suggest that cholera has also in India its seasons of preference, the conclusion is not as yet sustained by general and extensive inquiry.

The *cause* of cholera — that is, the nature of the poison — is as yet undetermined. If we regard the various opinions which have been put forth on this subject, the want of precision and completeness in many of the statements and the hypothetical character of much of the reasoning on which the opinions rest, it is impossible to avoid the conclusion, that at the present time the records of medical science are inadequate for the solution of this question.

In the course of three epidemics of cholera in Bombay (from 1849 to 1854), 158 inmates of the Jamsetjee Jejeebhoy Hospital, while under treatment for other diseases, have been attacked with cholera, and 73 of them died. At the time of these events, a record was kept, showing the date of the attack, the bed of the patient, the date of admission into hospital, and the disease for which he was under treatment.§ I entertained the hope that these facts might throw some light on the etiology of cholera; but their careful consideration has brought me to this conclusion, — that though a considerable part of them are trustworthy, so far as they go, yet they are defective in so many particulars, necessary to justify positive inferences, in an inquiry so difficult and important, that their detailed statement is not here submitted. This course

* "Transactions, Medical and Physical Society of Bombay," New Series, No. 1, p. 104.

† Mr. Martin, "Influence of Tropical Climates," &c. p. 346. Edition of 1854.

‡ "Notes on Cholera," by John Macpherson, M.D. "Indian Annals of Medical Science, "No. 1, p. 111.

§ This unsatisfactory state of matters continues. During my absence from India, and also subsequent to my return: viz. from July 1854 to April 1857, there were 84 seizures from cholera in Hospital, with 79 deaths, and yet the explanation is no further advanced.

is adopted, because I am satisfied that nothing so surely impedes the progress of medical science as the irrelevant use made by some inquirers of the observations and statements of others.

The occurrence, however, of so many attacks of cholera in one institution have seemed to point to the following general inferences: —

1. Cholera prevailed in the divisions of the town adjacent to the hospital, so that the cause may be assumed to have been operative on the residents of both.

2. A considerable proportion of the seizures was of individuals only a few days resident in the hospital, and who may therefore have been infected before admission.

3. A considerable proportion was simultaneous with an increase of the disease in the island generally, and therefore justified the inference that a general cause was in operation.

4. They occurred more or less in all the fourteen wards of the hospital, but in considerably greater number in those in which from position, nature of disease, or number of inmates, atmospheric impurity was most likely, at times, to be present.

5. The greater number of attacks was in cachectic or debilitated individuals: the influence of predisposition was very apparent.

6. The cholera sick in the hospital, whether admissions or seizures, were treated in the verandahs of certain wards, and were so arranged as to be widely apart from each other. The ward which adjoined the verandah in which cholera patients were most constantly present, was that in which, in one epidemic, the fewest cholera seizures took place; and in which, in another epidemic, the seizures were fewer than in several other wards.

These statements seem to indicate a relation between the cause of cholera and an atmospheric state, external to, as well as in, the hospital; also a relation to impure conditions of the atmosphere and states of individual predisposition.

The portable or contagious property of the cholera poison is not supported by these statements; and it is chiefly with reference to this question that facts more complete, precise, and detailed than these, or than any as yet observed and recorded, are required.*

* In the "Lancet" of the 4th and 11th December 1858, circumstances relative to the arrival of two coolie ships at Mauritius are narrated by Dr. Ayres, the superintendent of quarantine at Mauritius, which appear to him convincing proof of the conveyance of cholera, its communicability, and the value of strict quarantine. The narrative is very interesting, but the conclusions appear to me in part questionable. The following is a summary of the leading facts. The quarantine station at Mauritius is on two small islands, Gabriol and Flat Islands, separated from each other by a

My present impression on this point is, that if any of the spread of cholera be due to human intercourse, the degree is very limited; but my practice with reference to it has always been to pay great attention to scrupulous cleanliness and ventilation around cholera patients, and to place them widely apart from each other; for setting aside the suspicion of communicability, nothing is so likely,

coral reef. Flat Island is about one mile in diameter, and it had been inhabited for many months by about 150 persons, Europeans and coolie workmen, and servants of the quarantine establishment. On the 16th October 1857 a coolie ship arrived from Madras, after twenty-six days' voyage; thirty-six cases of cholera, with eighteen deaths, the last five days before arrival, had occurred. Shortly afterwards, another coolie ship, in which there had been cases of cholera during the voyage, arrived from Calcutta. The coolies of both ships numbered between six and seven hundred. Those of the Madras ship were landed on 16th October, and accommodated in Flat Island; and those of the Calcutta ship on the 26th, and placed in huts on Gabriol Island. There had been no trace of cholera in Mauritius or the adjacent islands for upwards of a year. The Madras coolies were in a much better physical condition than those from Calcutta.

The following cases of cholera, or choleraic diarrhœa, occurred in Flat and Gabriol Islands:—

Date.	Madras Coolies.	Calcutta Coolies.	Quarantine Servants.
October 26	1		
„ 27	..	2	
„ 29	..	..	2
„ 30	1	1	
„ 31	..	4	
November 1	1	1	
„ 2	..	4	
„ 3	..	4	
„ 4	1	1	
„ 19	..	1	
„ 20	..	..	1

Consequent on the greater number of cases in Gabriol island, the Calcutta coolies were removed to Flat Island on the 5th November, and the disease entirely disappeared after the 20th.

From these facts, Dr. Ayres concludes:—1. That cholera was conveyed from India to Mauritius. 2. That the quarantine servants were infected. 3. That the disease would have been introduced into Mauritius, which it was not, had rigid quarantine not been enforced.

I would rather substitute for these conclusions the following suggestions:—1. That the probably tainted with cholera poison, on departure from India, were with the others, placed, from crowding and other defective sanitary conditions on board ship, in circumstances favourable for the development of the disease. 2. That, congregated together in huts on two small islands, the unfavourable conditions of the ship were continued after arrival; the disease was therefore kept up, and extended to others, who had also become exposed to the same adverse local sanitary state. 3. That had the coolies on arrival, instead of being collected together, been distributed, well housed, clothed, washed, and fed, the probabilities are that cholera would not have reappeared amongst them, and would not have affected others.

as exhalation from the discharges and bodies of the sick, to produce that impure state of the atmosphere, which is undoubtedly an efficient condition in favouring the spread of the disease.

There were circumstances connected with the outbreak of cholera at Aden, in October 1858, and in part of the troops at Poona, in May 1859, which bear evidence on questions involved in the etiology of cholera, and which it may be useful briefly to state.

In the summer of 1858 *, cholera prevailed to a great degree along the Arabian coast, at Jedda, Loheia, Hodeida, Mocha, and Musawa. Native vessels from these ports were in constant communication with Aden; and in a ship with pilgrims from Mecca it was said that two deaths from cholera occurred as they approached Aden, but none were reported after the vessel came to anchor; but the date of arrival is not stated in the report. Aden had been exempt from cholera, with the exception of an occasional spasmodic case, from the period of its occupation in 1839 to the 29th of September 1858, when the first case occurred among the labourers on the public works. The temperature ranged from 80 to 98, and dew fell in the early morning. Between the 29th September and the 13th October, when it ceased, 136 individuals, partly labourers, partly Sepoys and others, were seized, and 85 deaths occurred, a mortality of 62·5. The mortality among the Sepoys was less than amongst the labourers: it was 52·6 in the former and 65·6 in the latter; and the difference was attributed to the Sepoys being in better condition, and nearer to their hospitals. The disease became more amenable to treatment after the 8th October.

Of the number attacked, 108 resided in the Koosaff Valley, in one side of which there was an open privy ground near to the huts, and a source of foul emanations.

After ceasing at Aden, the disease appeared at Lahadge, a short distance inland, and also at Berbera, on the opposite Somauli coast. Both these places were in free communication with Aden, but the date on which cholera appeared in them is not stated in the report.

Mr. Hormuzjee was of opinion that the outbreak was caused by the poison imported from affected places acting on people generally predisposed by debility, and favoured by a privy atmosphere and elevated temperature; but the evidence of importation is incomplete.

In May 1859, cholera, though prevailing in different places of

* Report by Mr. Ruttonjee Hormuzjee. "Transactions, Medical and Physical Society, Bombay;" New Series, No. 5.

the Deccan, was, in the military cantonment of Poona, confined to the Artillery, the 61st Regiment, and the German Legion. These troops occupied a consecutive line of barracks, in a direction from east to west. The buildings, with the exception of one block, were the oldest and worst constructed at the station, and had long before been condemned. They were, moreover, overcrowded, but the exigency of the times had continued to render their occupation an unavoidable measure. The 61st Regiment, after distinguished services before Delhi and Lucknow, were marched to Bombay for embarkation to Europe, but an unlooked-for contingency led to their temporary detention, and with this view they were sent to Poona, where they arrived in May, disappointed and depressed. The condition of the Germans, on arrival from the Cape, and their subsequent sickness in March and April, from febricula, have already been described (p. 163).

The regiments exempt from cholera were the 31st Infantry, and the 6th and 14th Dragoons, situated at considerable distances from the others, in more open positions, and in better barracks.

The 31st and 6th Dragoons had been healthy throughout the cold and hot seasons, and though the 14th Dragoons had, as the 61st, been marched to Bombay for embarkation, and also temporarily detained, the circumstances were very different. The 14th returned from service to their families and to a favourite station, which had for many years of their Indian service been their home. The 61st had served exclusively in the Bengal Presidency, and found themselves in a new place and among strangers.

Before concluding my remarks on the causes of cholera, I would observe, that the occurrence of the disease after exposure to cold or wet, has been occasionally noticed; and it may be presumed that the relation which subsists between these ordinary exciting causes of disease and the special cause of cholera, is the same as that which obtains between them and malaria in respect to occasional attacks of intermittent fever. They are determinining causes.

Section II.— *Symptoms considered in reference to their degrees of severity. — Diagnosis from Bilious Cholera, Irritant Poisoning, and Collapse of Remittent Fever.*

It is assumed that the student of clinical medicine is already familiar with the leading features of epidemic cholera — that the disease frequently comes on in the night, often without previous warning, but, at other times, preceded by diarrhœa of longer or shorter duration — that the characteristic symptoms are the rice-water-like alvine discharges, the vomiting of watery fluid, spasms of the extremities or muscles of the abdomen, restlessness and anxiety, skin cold, damp and clammy, sunken eyes and shrunken features, a quickly failing, and finally imperceptible pulse, much thirst, suspended secretions, a whispering voice, intelligence languid but not deranged.

There is considerable range in the degree and rapidity of the collapse; and neglect of this fact has led to much inaccurate statement on the value of different remedial means.

The characteristic alvine discharges are the pathognomonic symptom of cholera. They may be present in varying amount, associated with more or less — sometimes hardly appreciable — muscular spasm, and with different degrees of collapse. The following classification is convenient for practical purposes.

1. Cases in which, after three or four hours of the characteristic vomiting and purging, with some amount of spasm, the countenance becomes somewhat collapsed; but the tempe rature of the skin remains still good, and the pulse of tolerable strength. There is generally a varying proportion of this class of cases met with in epidemic visitations in European regiments in India; and if they are judiciously treated, a very considerable number may be expected to recover. This mildest form of the disease occurs very seldom in natives, or in the classes of Europeans who resort to general hospitals in India.

2. Cases in which, after six or seven hours of more or less characteristic purging, vomiting, and spasm, the countenance becomes sunken, the skin cold and damp; but the pulse, though small and feeble, is still distinct, and the respiration without hurry or oppression. This degree of the disease is met with both in natives and Europeans. It may be considered the mildest form in natives as well as in Europeans in general hospitals. It does not seem to be merely the first degree aggravated by longer duration; for it will be found that the greater collapse has been present from the very outset, and little under the control of medical treatment. Still, a considerable proportion of this form of the disease recovers, probably more than one half.

3. Cases in which, after from one to six hours of characteristic vomiting and purging, with discharges often inconsiderable in quantity, the skin becomes cold and clammy, the countenance sunken, the voice almost gone, the restlessness great, the pulse imperceptible, and the respiration begins to be hurried and anxious. This

degree of the disease occurs both in Europeans and natives, and recoveries, though occasional, are few in number. The very speedy collapse, unattended by the usual evacuations mentioned by some writers, has not come under my observation; but I should think it a very possible occurrence, for the scanty watery secretion may take place into, and be retained in, the intestinal canal.

The two last degrees of the disease are by far the most common, at the present time, in India, and have been so during the whole period of my service in that country. The first degree would seem to have been met with more frequently in the epidemics between 1818 and 1824, as suggested by Mr. Martin, and many of the cases detailed by Sir James Annesley confirm this opinion.

I have not thought it necessary to notice particularly a train of symptoms described as occurring in sthenic Europeans in India, and consisting of urgent cramps, a warm skin, a flushed countenance, and a pulse full and firm. This must be a rare form of disease, for I can bring to my recollection only one instance, and that was in the year 1830, in a soldier of her Majesty's 40th Regiment, at Vingorla; yet it has been erroneously classed with epidemic cholera, and its successful treatment by general blood-letting was one of the circumstances which led to the adoption of that remedy in the very different form of disease now under consideration.

In following the course of the three degrees under which the symptoms of epidemic cholera have here been classed, we find that in the first, recoveries are numerous, derangements pass away, and the several functions are gradually restored to their normal state; and that when cases prove fatal this result is brought about by increasing collapse, or by consecutive fever with or without the complication of secondary inflammations. I do not, however, enlarge on these milder instances of the disease, because my clinical experience has been chiefly of the severer forms.

In a large proportion of the second and third degrees, the pulseless collapse, which has taken place in periods longer or shorter, persists, though the serous discharges from the bowels may have ceased, and the cramps have abated; the respiration becomes hurried, and death follows in from four to thirty-six hours, dating from the commencement of the symptoms. When, however, a fatal result has not occurred in the stage of collapse, then the disease may pursue one of the following courses: —

1. There is gradual and slow improvement of the pulse; the

skin loses its dampness, and its heat slowly returns; the alvine discharges become less frequent and watery, assume first a turbid and milky appearance, then become coloured, and gradually restored to their normal state; and the secretion of urine, which had been suspended during the stage of collapse, is slowly established. It is when the collapse has not been of long duration — not exceeding seven or eight hours — that we may hope for this favourable course of the disease. It is, on the other hand, when the collapse has endured eighteen hours or upwards (though recoveries may still take place in the manner just described), that we may apprehend one or other of the remaining more unfavourable terminations.

2. The restoration of function, and final recovery, may be retarded by gastro-enteric irritation, or inflammation, characterised by a florid tongue with central yellow fur, uneasiness at the epigastrium, vomiting of ingesta, yellow watery, or greenish gelatinous dejections, associated with a dry skin, and often some degree of febrile heat and frequency of pulse.

3. Whilst the pulse and the heat of the skin have been gradually restored, the alvine and renal excretions may continue suppressed, the conjunctivæ become gradually injected, and the manner sluggish; then distinct drowsiness may come on and pass into coma. In these cases the stupor is occasionally preceded by low delirium; and a preternatural slowness of the pulse is sometimes the first symptom to direct attention to the cerebral functions. This train of symptoms, if not passing beyond the state of drowsiness, is sometimes recovered from.

4. The stage of collapse may be immediately succeeded by febrile reaction, adynamic in character, sometimes complicated with gastro-enteritis, cerebral or pulmonic symptoms, or suppressed alvine and renal excretion.

5. In asthenic individuals there may be restoration of function, and yet death from secondary exhaustion, without any very evident local complication.

Though the favourable import of restored urine and coloured alvine discharges in the course of cholera is not to be doubted, yet, I am certain, that needless alarm is often experienced from their absence, as well as too much hope sometimes entertained from their reappearance.

So long as the skin continues cold and the pulse imperceptible or very feeble, it is not in accordance with sound physiology to look for restoration of the biliary or urinary secretions. Again:

if the collapse has not exceeded eight or ten hours, the non-appearance of the excretions during the succeeding twelve or eighteen hours of the *gradual* return of the circulation and of animal heat need not occasion apprehension.

But if the collapse has endured for eighteen hours and more, then, as already explained, with the return of the circulation and of animal heat, all secondary dangers — those arising from defective excretion included — are increased. The more completely and speedily the circulation becomes restored after this long collapse, the greater is the risk incurred by the continued suppression of urine.

These statements, derived from clinical observation, are in strict accordance with physiology. While the processes in which the capillary circulation is concerned are suspended during the stage of collapse, metamorphoses of tissue and the formation of products of excretion are necessarily in abeyance; but the longer the collapse has endured and the more completely it has been removed, the more surely and quickly will effete products be formed and the necessity for their elimination created.

Though we may admit that there is a probable relation between uræmia and cerebral disturbance, and perhaps other local derangements, yet we shall be disappointed if we always expect to find head symptoms removed on the return of the urinary secretion.

Again, in attributing the cessation of drowsiness to the restoration of the renal secretion, care is necessary in order that the stupor occasionally present in the stage of collapse may not be mistaken for that which is secondary, which occurs after reaction, and which alone can be related to uræmia.

There is still another clinical remark to be made with reference to the urine. The early observers of cholera confounded suppression with retention of urine, and used the catheter; but there is now an occasional risk of retention being mistaken for a continuance of suppression and the use of the catheter being neglected.

It has been already mentioned that as the profuse watery alvine discharges cease, they become less thin, and assume a milky appearance; there is, in fact, less of water and more of epithelial debris. This change, in favourable cases, is a state intermediate between the clear watery and the coloured discharges, and may continue for twelve hours and more after reaction has taken place. Nor are we to assume from the continuance of these scanty milk-like discharges that the case is progressing unfavourably. They were present in the intestinal canal as the residue of the transudations of the stage of collapse, antecedent to the commencement of reaction, and must necessarily be evacuated before more normal excretions can reappear. Moreover, if during the period of transudation much of the intestinal epithelium has been thrown off, it is reasonable to suppose that its restoration will be amongst the earliest actions of returning health, and one desirable to accomplish before biliary secretions are brought into relation with the lining membrane. Then, just as in respect to the urine, clinical observation and physiology lead to the practical conclusion that for twelve or eighteen hours after the commencement of reaction, more particularly when the collapse has been of short duration, we need not attach any importance to the alvine discharges not becoming of normal colour.

In occasional instances dejections during the collapse are of pinkish tint; they may be so, and not profuse, from the commencement, or they may present this appearance at a later period when they have ceased to be very watery. Discharges of this kind, caused, no doubt, by partial transudation of the colouring matter of the blood, have been observed by me only in natives. They are of most unfavourable import, for I have never met with an instance of recovery.

Dr. Macpherson* cites two interesting cases of hæmatemesis in the course of cholera, which occurred to him in the General Hospital at Calcutta; and it is not improbable, though I am not aware that the observation has been made, that the pink-coloured discharges are of more frequent occurrence in Bengal than in Bombay, because hæmorrhage from the bowels is more common in that province.

The remark, in the report on cholera by the Madras Medical Board, that hiccup is not the unfavourable prognostic in this disease which it is in many others, accords with what I have myself noticed. It occurs generally in cases in which the collapse has been long, and the reaction slowly established, is coincident with the latter state, and though often, is not necessarily, associated with gastric irritation.

The *diagnosis* of epidemic cholera is well marked when the disease is fully formed. The cramps and the prostration co-existing with the peculiar discharges, are sufficiently characteristic to distinguish it from bilious cholera, with its bile-tinged discharges, coated tongue, transient prostration, and occasional cramps. If a

* "Notes on Cholera. Indian Annals of Medical Science," vol. i. p. 120.

conclusion may be drawn from my own field of inquiry, I would say that bilious cholera is a rare form of disease in Indian hospitals, particularly in those for native sick. On referring to the returns of the European General Hospital at Bombay, I find, that of 20,147 admissions in fifteen years, only 74 were from bilious cholera, and 52 of those were during the six years of my service in that hospital. The deaths recorded under this head were 3, occurring from 1845 to 1847; and as during this period the admissions amounted only to 4, we have a mortality from bilious cholera of 75 per cent.—a result so contrary to all experience, leads to the conclusion that these were cases of epidemic cholera, and the record therefore further shows that an error in diagnosis is a possible contingency. Then in respect to the Jamsetjee Jejeebhoy Hospital, it appears that out of 25,190 admissions in six years, there were only 2 of bilious cholera.

These facts justify the statement that bilious cholera is not a common disease in India in numerous classes of the community.

It is not denied that in sthenic Europeans in India bilious vomiting, a flushed countenance, a coated tongue, and more or less derangement of the bowels after debauch, are sufficiently common; but this form of disease, even if correctly designated bilious cholera, cannot possibly be mistaken for epidemic cholera.

But another and very important question of diagnosis may present itself in India.

In one * of the reports of the Bengal charitable dispensaries, it is stated that advantage is sometimes taken of the prevalence of cholera for the perpetration of acts of criminal poisoning, in consequence of the lessened chance of detection which exists under such circumstances of the public health. This remark is just; for my own observation in Bombay enables me to say, that criminal poisoning, chiefly by arsenic, is, unfortunately, not rare, and that the great collapse which speedily comes on after a large quantity of this poison has been taken, sufficiently resembles that of cholera as to render the mistake in cholera seasons, when suspicion has not been aroused, by no means improbable. If we have the opportunity of examining the vomited and dejected matters during life, there should be no difficulty in determining the question. The florid tongue and tender epigastrium of gastritis, will also assist in the diagnosis; but if in fatal cases doubt still remains, a *post mortem* examination will at once remove it.

* I regret my inability at the present time to refer particularly to the Report and its author.

At a time when cholera prevailed, two children, a brother and sister, were brought to the European General Hospital ill with vomiting and purging. They died shortly afterwards, and there had not been any opportunity, subsequent to their admission into hospital, of observing the character of the evacuations. There were circumstances connected with the commencement of the illness of these children which raised the suspicion that something deleterious had been exhibited. An inquest was held. The parents were unwilling that the *post mortem* examination should be more minute than was sufficient to remove the doubt. The stomach and the end of the ileum were opened, and in both cases the mucous coat of the former was pale, that of the latter was studded with prominent Peyer's glands. On these appearances, coupled with the circumstance that cholera was prevalent, I grounded the opinion that death had been caused by cholera, and not by an irritant poison.

When treating of remittent fever it was explained that the paroxysm sometimes terminates with unlooked-for prostration, thready pulse, cold skin, and death by syncope. I have known such an event viewed as an attack of cholera coming on in the course of fever; but we must be on our guard against an error of this kind. Cholera may doubtless occur in the course of fever, and lead to a fatal issue; but there can be no difficulty in distinguishing such cases from prostration at the close of a febrile paroxysm. The diagnosis will turn upon the relation of the prostration to alvine discharges, to the period of the paroxysm, and to the general course of the disease.

SECTION III. — *The general rate of mortality. — Its relation to age, period of epidemic, and duration before admission considered. — General pathology shortly noticed. — Morbid anatomy described.*

The following statement, with that at p. 202, illustrates the well-known mortality occasioned by this disease: —

	Proportion of Mortality from Cholera to total Mortality.
In European troops, Bombay Presidency	10· per cent.
European officers, ditto	7·7 "
In Population, Bombay, for four years	20·35 "
European General Hospital, Bombay	14·5 "
Jamsetjee Jejeebhoy Hospital	13·9 "

In regard to the rate of mortality there is a good deal of discrepancy in published statements. But this is easily understood, when we recollect that the severity of the disease varies in different epidemics, and at different periods of the same epidemic, and in different classes of individuals.

As an approximate statement, we may estimate the mortality in India at from 30 to 45 per cent. in regimental hospitals, 50 to 55 in European general hospitals, and 60 to 65 in general hospitals for the civil native population of large towns, as the Jamsetjee Jejeebhoy Hospital in Bombay.*

The only investigations which I have made on the variation of the ratio from age †, the period of the epidemic, and duration of attack, refer to 159 individuals admitted into the Jamsetjee Jejeebhoy Hospital from the 17th August to the 31st December, 1849; of these, 94 died, and 5 remained under treatment on the 1st of January. The results are shown in the following tables: —

A.

Ages noted.	Numbers.	Rate of Mortality.
Under 10 years	13	69 per cent.
Between 10 and 20	19	63 "
" 20 and 40	112	58 "
Above 50	10	50 "

These numbers are too limited to be of much value on the question of age. The high mortality shown in the tables in very early life probably accords with the results of the epidemic cholera in England in 1849.‡ But in that epidemic the lowest mortality was from five to fifteen years of age: this does not appear to be a feature of cholera in India, judging from the above table and one in Dr. Macpherson's notes.§ The low mortality above the age of fifty, in my statement, is opposed to the results obtained by Dr. Gull and Dr. Macpherson, and illustrates the errors into which we may be led by partial statistics.

* This is a considerably higher rate than appears in the appended return of this hospital for six years, and I so state it because the mortality has been higher in other years and patients occasionally are removed in a precarious state by their friends, but entered discharged in the returns, and rated as recoveries.

† The rate of mortality in the Byculla Schools may also be considered—it has been 48·2.

‡ "Report on the Morbid Anatomy, Pathology, and Treatment of Epidemic Cholera." By William W. Gull, M.D. &c. p. 147.

§ "Annals of Indian Medical Science." No. 1, p. 113.

The varying ratio at different periods of the epidemic is clearly exhibited in the following table: —

B.

Dates of Admission.	Rate of Mortality.
17th August to 3rd September	84·6 per cent.
4th September to 17th September	72·0 ,,
18th September to 1st October.	75·0 ,,
2nd October to 15th October	47·0 ,,
16th October to 29th October	28·0 ,,
30th October to 12th November	50·0 ,,
13th November to 26th November	50·0 ,,
27th November to 10th December	55·5 ,,
11th December to 31st December	43·3 ,,

With the view of endeavouring to determine to what extent the mortality was influenced by admission into hospital at early or advanced periods of the attack, I made the following note in respect to 157 cases: —

C.

Duration of Disease on Admission.	Numbers.	Rate of Mortality.
Under 5 hours	38	63·3
,, 5 to 12 hours	49	61·3
,, 12 to 24 hours	48	45·9
Above 24 hours	22	59·0

That the highest mortality should be in those admitted at the earliest period of the disease, and the lowest in those in whom it had been present for upwards of twelve hours, may seem an unexpected result; but it is easily explained by those who are acquainted with the habits of the individuals represented by these figures, — with their unwillingness to resort for hospital relief in the early stages of illness. The conclusion to be drawn from the statement is, that the admissions under five hours were cases of great severity, enforcing an early application for relief, hence the high mortality. On the other hand, those between twelve and twenty-four hours were milder, and had not yet entered on the risks of reaction. In the admissions above twenty-four hours there is again a rise in the mortality, depending, no doubt, on the fact that a proportion of these cases had been neglected, and that the secondary dangers had been incurred before admission.

To determine the proportion of deaths in the stage of collapse, and in that of reaction, is a question of interest, for it probably differs in India and in European countries; I have no data bearing on this point. Dr. Gull * estimates the proportion of death from consecutive fever in England at one-tenth. Though the opinion generally entertained, that the proportion of deaths in the stage of collapse in India preponderates over that of the same stage in England, is probably correct; yet it is an error to suppose that the practitioner in India is not perfectly familiar with all the secondary phenomena and dangers of cholera.

Pathology. — In considering the pathology of cholera, the first circumstance on which to fix the attention is, that the general and capillary circulation of the blood, and all their dependent actions, are more or less arrested. That this arrest is favoured, but not mainly caused, by the copious watery discharges, is shown by the facts that not unfrequently the collapse is great, and the discharge is small; and that occasionally the prostration is moderate, and the discharges copious and long continued.

Whether the morbific cause acts first on the blood or on the ganglionic nervous system, is a question which physiological and pathological science are, in their present state, unequal to determine, and the discussion of which does not come within the scope of a clinical treatise.

I proceed to notice the morbid anatomy of the disease. Of 17 fatal cases now before me, 15 occurred in the stage of collapse, and 2 with secondary complication — one of the head, the other of the lungs and pericardium. These cases show that the morbid appearances which chiefly attract attention after death, in the collapsed stage of cholera, are the following: —

Head. — The vessels of the membranes are congested with dark-coloured blood, and the substance of the brain, when incised, shows numerous bloody points. There is generally increased effusion of serum in the cavity of the cranium, but this state is not necessarily an evidence of drowsiness or other head symptoms having been present during life.

Chest. — The lungs are usually well collapsed; the anterior surface is pale, with sometimes an inflated, or emphysematous state of their edges. There is, for the most part, a reddened colour at their posterior aspect, with moderate congestion. The heart is sometimes flaccid, at others not so. The left ventricle is almost invariably empty; but the right one is more or less filled with blood, dark-coloured, generally quite fluid, sometimes with co-existing fibrinous coagula.

* Report, p. 142.

Abdomen.—Very commonly there is a blush of redness on the visceral peritoneum. The stomach is frequently distended, and its mucous surface, commonly pale, sometimes presents dotted or marbled red patches. The small intestines usually contain some amount of watery or milk-like contents similar to the cholera discharges; and their mucous surface is, for the most part, pale, with the villi very distinct. The isolated and agminated glands of Peyer are very generally prominent; this has been chiefly observed at the lower part of the ileum, where the surface is often studded with pale solitary glands, enlarged to about the size of a mustard seed. The large intestines are often contracted, and the mucous membrane of the colon is pale, and the solitary glands prominent: the mucous follicles, with their dark depressed centres, are frequently distinctly seen. The mesenteric glands are usually enlarged, but pale in colour. There is commonly little to notice in the appearance of the liver; sometimes, when incised, it bleeds more freely than usual. A distended state of the gall-bladder was observed in only one of the cases, and from this it may be inferred that there has not been usually anything in the state ofthis viscus to arrest my attention. In my cases little notice is taken of the condition of the spleen, from which it may be concluded that it was not enlarged; the free evacuations must tend to cause this organ to shrink, and, indeed, I have had evidence of this in the great decrease of a much enlarged spleen in an individual who became affected with cholera. The kidneys are sometimes healthy in external apppearance, sometimes they are congested. In one case, that of an individual (with abdominal pleuritic effusion, with commencing Bright's disease and old tubercular peritonitis), attacked with cholera, the collapse was incomplete, and the disease protracted for four days—evidently in consequence of the dropsical effusions, which gradually disappeared, supplying to the blood the water which was being lost by the discharges. In this case absorption took place because the pulse continued distinct till shortly before death.

In cases of cholera fatal in the secondary stage, the morbid appearances found after death are the results of inflammation of the structures which have been chiefly affected during life.

Such is a summary of the morbid appearances in the collapsed stage of cholera, drawn from my own observation, and I am not aware that any important addition can be made to it from the writings of the latest observers, with exception of a minuter description of the condition of the kidneys.* I allude to the epithelial debris found in the uriniferous tubes and pelvis of the kidney as explanatory of the albuminous state of the urine † on its re-appearance after reaction.

The chemistry of the alvine discharges and of the blood in cholera has also been investigated; but as yet the inquiry has done little more than confirm and give precision to inferences already fairly deducible from clinical observation and morbid anatomy.

According to Dr. Parkes ‡, there are in 1000 parts of cholera evacuations: water, 987·95; organic matter and insoluble salts (earthy phosphates), 3·9; soluble salts (chlorides, phosphates, and sulphates of soda and potash), 8·1. The same careful inquirer has particularly noted the small amount of organic extractives in the discharges of cholera, and he believes that this circumstance indicates the suspension during the collapsed stage of cholera of the proper excreting functions of the intestinal mucous membrane. I need hardly remark that this belief is quite in accordance with clinical inferences relative to the general state of the vital actions of the system in this stage of the disease.

The density of the blood is necessarily much increased in consequence of the transudation from the capillaries and discharge from the bowels of so much of its watery constituent. The degree of increase of density will have relation to the duration of the attack, the amount of transudation, and the absence of replacement of water. It need hardly be observed, that the loss of the water of the blood does not merely affect the constitution of the liquor sanguinis, but must also, in accordance with the laws of endosmosis and exosmosis, influence that of the contents of the blood corpuscles. The proportion of the inorganic salts of the blood would seem to be increased in the early stages of the disease in consequence of the greater proportional transudation of the water. But in the more advanced periods the salts gradually sink below their normal ratio.§

Dr. Garrod ‖ thus states the conclusion which may be drawn from his experiments on urea in the blood in cholera: "That urea usually exists in increased quantities in cholera blood,

* Dr. Gull's Report, p. 32.

† Of this condition of the urine I am unable to say much from my own observation; in the few cases in which the urine was tested it was found albuminous.

‡ "Report on the Morbid Anatomy and Pathology of Cholera," pp. 25 and 26, by Dr. Gull.

§ Dr. Gull's Report, p. 45.

‖ Dr. Gull's Report, p. 53.

but that the amount differs considerably in the different stages of the disease; being but small in quantity in the intense stage of collapse, increasing during re-action, and in excess when consecutive febrile symptoms occur."

This statement — that urea is present in the blood in small quantity in the intense stage of collapse, increased with reaction, and is in excess when consecutive febrile symptoms occur — quite accords with the general tenour of the remarks, based on clinical observation alone, which I have already made relative to the importance attributable to the absence of the urinary secretion in cholera (pp. 211, 212).

SECTION IV. — *Treatment in the different degrees and stages of the disease.*

My remarks on the treatment of cholera will be restricted to a statement of the conclusions to which I have been led by reflection, and the clinical observation of cases not only immediately under my own care, but also of those treated by others in the same or different hospitals. I place the more confidence in the opinions thus formed, — many years ago in part elsewhere expressed, — because they rest on principles very similar to those entertained by the latest and best writers * on this disease.

Extensive clinical experience of epidemic cholera leads the unbiassed mind to this conclusion. That there are degrees and stages of cholera, as of other zymotic diseases, beyond the direct resources of medical art, and that in the management of these the physician best consults the interests of humanity and the character of his profession, when he abstains from rash and restless empiricism, and is satisfied with placing the patient in the circumstances most favourable for the revival of vital actions, under the influence of their ordinary stimuli. That, on the other hand, there are degrees and stages of the disease which are frequently readily controlled by medicine, and that these demand careful study and attention. Guided by these principles, I proceed to the consideration of the treatment of cholera.

The prevalence of diarrhœa in seasons of epidemic cholera, obtains in India as well as in European countries; but this event is more common in the latter than in the former. The relation, however, which these two affections bear to each other is the same

* Chapter on Treatment in Dr. Parkes' "Researches into the Pathology and Treatment of Cholera;" also Dr. Gull's "Report on the Treatment of Cholera."

in both countries. The diarrhœa, if neglected, is very apt to pass into cholera; and, on the other hand, is amenable to ordinary treatment in a large proportion of cases. We may state these facts in other words by saying that cholera is not unfrequently preceded by a premonitory, and often readily curable, diarrhœa. The practical rule of carefully regarding and treating all cases of diarrhœa, and of being very cautious in the use of purgatives, antimonials, or other intestinal irritants, in the general treatment of disease, in cholera seasons, is very familiar to the experienced practitioner in India; and there can be no doubt that its observance has led to much saving of life. It has for many years been the judicious practice of the authorities in Bombay, in seasons when cholera is epidemic, to station qualified individuals, with suitable remedies, in the different divisions of the native town; and to encourage those affected with diarrhœa to apply for relief.

The medicines which have been used for this premonitory diarrhœa are numerous; but in natives or Europeans who have been long resident in India, a simple opiate is the best means we can adopt. One or two grains of solid opium, or twenty to forty minims of the tincture with peppermint water, and two or three drachms of brandy, may be given. If the diarrhœa has been early noticed, and if at the same time diet and the temperature of the surface of the body have been carefully attended to, a single dose of opium will very generally suffice. Should, however, it prove otherwise, then after a suitable interval a smaller dose may be repeated.

In sthenic Europeans in India, in whom this premonitory diarrhœa frequently co-exists with a coated tongue, it is advisable to combine the opium with calomel, in the proportion of two grains of the former to ten of the latter. This course is followed, not so much on account of any direct expected benefit from the calomel, as on the supposition that it modifies or prevents the astringing effect of the opium on the biliary excretion.

In cases in which the diarrhœa has been neglected, and allowed to continue for some time unchecked, in which the discharges are becoming very watery, and the pulse and countenance beginning to change, then attention to such adjuvants as confinement to bed in the recumbent posture, and warmth by suitable clothing to the surface of the body, must at once be enforced; while at the same time the opiate remedies are given and repeated, combined with a larger proportion of alcoholic or ammoniated stimulant.

Should such means, however, used under these circumstances, fail in speedily checking the diarrhœa, and should the true cholera discharges not as yet have been established, then we are no longer to trust to opium alone, for it will prove inefficacious in small doses, and injurious in large ones frequently repeated. Recourse must be had to astringent remedies given more or less frequently, either alone or combined with small doses of opium. Acetate of lead, diluted sulphuric acid, preparations of kino or catechu, gallic acid, with many others, may be named. The first * is the astringent of which my experience has been the greatest, but I have no great bias in its favour, and would prefer any of the others, if, as is very probable, they should prove of equal efficacy.

But should the symptoms still continue, and the diarrhœa pass into cholera, and collapse be more or less established, then the principles for the treatment of this stage of cholera, presently to be explained, ought to be applied.

After these few remarks on the treatment of, and the importance of attending to, the diarrhœa prevalent at cholera seasons, I next consider the management of the disease after it has become fairly developed. And here it is necessary, in the first instance, to state certain principles which seem to me to be true, and to rest on clinical observation.

* I have always used the formula recommended by Dr. Graves, from whose writings I adopted this system of treatment, viz.: "A scruple of acetate of lead combined with a grain of opium, and six grains of powdered liquorice made into a mass with mucilage, divided into twelve pills."

In the year 1839, I published in the second number of the "Transactions of the Medical and Physical Society of Bombay" cases of cholera treated with acetate of lead, after the manner recommended by Dr. Graves. They seemed to me favourable. Further experience led me, in the seventh number of the Transactions of the Society, in 1845, to write in a more qualified manner. Again, after my experience in the Jamsetjee Jejeebhoy Hospital, I expressed myself in the tenth number of the Transactions, p. 323, in 1850, to the following effect:—

"In the "Transactions of the Medical and Physical Society" I have expressed my opinion on the efficacy of the acetate of lead, if given while the pulse is of tolerable strength, also of its inapplicability to those extreme cases of the disease in which great collapse follows trifling discharges; and I would now add, as the result of my experience in this epidemic, that the acetate of lead has proved altogether powerless in restraining the serous discharges occurring after collapse has fully set in. Whether an attempt to restrain these discharges after fully formed collapse has taken place is an indication to be kept in view, is probably an open question in the pathology of the disease, which need not be discussed here. The acetate of lead, however, has been inefficacious for the purpose, and I should be indisposed again to have recourse to it under the same circumstances of the disease; the more so, as it is possible enough that the drug lying inert in the alimentary canal during the period of collapse may have an injurious influence by its rapid absorption on the occurrence of reaction." My present opinion, then, is not corroborative of the estimate entertained by Dr. Graves of the value of this medicine in cholera, and the above statement will show that it has not been hastily formed, but is the result of upwards of fifteen years' attention to the question.

1. In the collapsed stage of cholera, the capillary circulation, and the processes in which it is concerned, are in a great measure suspended; hence there cannot be absorption or action of medicinal agents.

2. In cases in which the collapse is recovered from, the return of the general and capillary circulation, and consequent vital processes, is gradual and slow, and more likely to be disturbed than aided by medicines; while, at the same time, the gastro-intestinal mucous membrane is very predisposed, from defective epithelium, to take on inflammatory action.

3. Medicinal agents given in the stage of collapse and not at that time absorbed, are liable to accumulate in the intestinal canal, to become absorbed as reaction is re-established, and then to interfere with the restoration of secretion and other functions; or they may, by their mere presence, act as irritants on the predisposed mucous surface, and excite gastro-enteritis.

In the first and milder degree, described at page 209, — in which, though the cholera discharges are present, the pulse is still of moderate strength, — it is not improbable that absorption still may be carried on at the intestinal surface, and that therefore there may be indication for the use of medicines. It is right to act cautiously on this probability; but, with every allowance for it, my belief still is, that when cholera discharges are fairly established, they are, whatever the state of the circulation may be, very little under the control of astringent or other remedies.

In my further remarks on treatment, it is assumed that the reader bears in mind not only the statement of principles which has just been made, but also the degrees of the disease as already explained in connection with the symptoms.

When cases of cholera come under treatment with the pulse distinct, then the remedies recommended for the treatment of the preliminary diarrhœa may be used. We must be careful, however, not to give more than one or two * full doses of opium; for this will be test sufficient of its efficacy, and more will be likely to prove injurious. If the collapse increases and the pulse becomes indistinct, or if, after four or six hours of the use of astringents, the discharges persist unchecked, the discontinuance of these remedies, even though the pulse is still distinct, will be advisable, for under both circumstances a fair trial of them will have been made. The want of success justifies the inference that the state of the system

* I assume, of course, that opiates have not been previously given at earlier stages.

has not been compatible with the action of the medicines, and that their further use may lead to the subsequent risks attendant on their accumulation.

A considerable proportion of the cases of the first degree of the disease, — those in which, after three or four hours of characteristic vomiting and purging, the temperature of the skin remains still good and the pulse of tolerable strength, — will do well under this treatment without any material augmentation of the collapse. It was in this form of the disease — common in the early epidemics in India, but rare in later years — that general blood-letting and repeated doses of calomel and opium acquired a therapeutic fame, which subsequent and more general experience has not confirmed. The truth is simply this, — that when the degree of the disease is such as to stop short of any considerable amount of collapse, then attention to the recumbent posture, to warmth of the surface of the body by suitable coverings, and the exhibition of a full opiate with or without calomel, according to the state of the tongue, are means sufficient for the cure. That more than this is in general not only unnecessary, but likely to be injurious rather than beneficial.

But, as already stated, a large proportion of the cases in Indian epidemics are of those degrees in which collapse, complete or great, comes on more or less quickly. In these the skin is cold and damp, the pulse thready or imperceptible, and the features shrunken. When these symptoms are present — it matters not whether they have come on quickly or slowly, or whether treatment has been previously followed or neglected, or whether the discharges continue or have ceased — the period for the exhibition of opiates or alteratives or astringents has passed; the condition of the system is incompatible with their action. This state of the disease is best managed by directing attention to those ordinary stimuli necessary to the maintenance of vital actions in health, and to their restoration when depressed. The patient should be placed in a well-ventilated room; the surface of the body should be wiped from time to time, lightly covered with two or three blankets, over which warm bricks, or other similar means of imparting external heat, may be applied. Water should be given frequently in small quantities, according to the desire of the patient, if he is alert; or it should be offered to him if he is sluggish and apathetic. It has been my practice, in addition to these means, to give a drachm of aromatic spirit of ammonia every hour or second hour, and a little wine with thin sago every third hour; for it is well to assume the possibility of some degree of absorption, and to regard it to this extent. A recumbent posture should also be strictly observed. The cramps and restlessness, if distressing, may be palliated by gentle rubbing and shampooing.

The proportion of recoveries from the stage of complete or great collapse is considerable, certainly not less than 40 per cent.: but I believe that if the attention of the practitioner were more generally confined to assiduously enforcing the simple indications just explained, and not distracted with the vain hope of benefit from rash empirical experiments, the mortality in this stage would be still further reduced. Of the cases in India, which recover from the collapse, the larger proportion is restored to health by a gradual return of the functions to their normal condition; but the remainder is more or less exposed to the risks of secondary fever or inflammation, and a portion of them die. Though my impression, — that by treating the stage of collapse in the manner just recommended, an increase in the number of recoveries from that state is probable, — may admit of doubt, still I am very confident that, by abstaining from the use of opiates, astringents, alteratives, and excessive stimulants, we materially lessen the proportion of subsequent secondary risks, and, consequently, diminish the absolute mortality of the disease.

Let us now follow the treatment when collapse is passing away and reaction is taking place, noticing, first, those cases in which there is gradual restoration of function without febrile excitement or secondary inflammation. When writing on the treatment of cholera in the European General Hospital in 1845, I made the following observations *: —

"The most satisfactory recoveries which I have witnessed from states of extreme and almost hopeless collapse—the purging having in great measure ceased—have been under the use of camphor and blue pill, in doses of three grains of the former and two of the latter, given every second or third hour, with effervescing draughts, light nourishment, and occasional stimulants.

"In successful cases, when the collapse is passing off, and the indication of cure is to restore the secretory functions which have been paralysed, I am clearly of opinion that this, in most cases, can be most satisfactorily effected by combinations of camphor, or quinine, and blue pill; perhaps calomel in small doses, with or without a small addition of opium, according to circumstances, and accompanied with the occasional exhibition of effervescing draughts, or small doses of castor oil. This course seems to me safer than to attempt the same indication by calomel in large doses and purgatives; it being probably more in accordance with the operations of nature. For it seems a fair assumption that functions after having been completely checked, will be more likely to recover their natural course by degrees; and that, consequently, the indication seems rather gently to guide, than attempt by strong measures to propel."

* "Transactions of Medical and Physical Society of Bombay," No. 7, p. 192.

In the fifteen years which have elapsed since these remarks were written, my opportunities of treating cholera, and of witnessing the treatment by others, have been extensive; but my principles have undergone very little change. On considering the diaries of recovered cases now before me, I observe that not unfrequently twenty-four hours, after return of pulse and warmth of the surface, have elapsed before the urine has been restored, or the alvine discharges become coloured: such facts prove that these processes are restored to their normal condition slowly and gradually, and that, if active alteratives and eliminants are used, harm rather than good is likely to result. Again, some cases show that calomel may, under these circumstances, be given in considerable doses, and yet not exercise any perceptible effect on the biliary secretion; while, at the same time, its irritant action on the gastro-intestinal surface may be suspected: from these events we may draw the inference, that for some time after the commencement of reaction the secretory processes are not readily susceptible of influence from alteratives or eliminants, and that, therefore, when these remedies are used, the hazard of gastro-enteric irritation without the counter-balancing advantage of more quickly restored secretions, is incurred. It follows, then, that, in my remarks of 1845, an importance was accorded to the combination of blue pill with camphor and quinine to which it was in all probability not entitled. My present opinion is, that the recoveries would have taken place equally well under the use of occasional effervescing draughts and diluents, light nourishment and occasional stimulants; and that, by the needless use of mercurials and purgatives, restoration is delayed, and gastro-enteric irritation is apt to be excited. In individuals asthenic before the attack, it will sometimes be of advantage to give small doses of quinine every third or fourth hour; and it will be very necessary in such cases to pay much attention to frequent and appropriate nourishment, for asthenic individuals recovered from collapse are liable to sink unexpectedly from subsequent exhaustion. Occasionally, after reaction has been established, the alvine discharges continue so frequent as to indicate the expediency of restraining them by small opiates or astringents; but I believe that this seldom occurs, unless secondary enteric irritation is present, and is chiefly observed when irritant remedies have formed a part of the previous treatment.

Next we have to notice the treatment of cases recovered from collapse, but in which the restoration to health has been delayed, and risk to life occasioned, by secondary fever or inflammation.

The secondary febrile and inflammatory states are more or less adynamic. In India the febrile state is seldom simple, but generally accompanied with gastro-enteric, cerebral, pulmonic, or other inflammation; but when it does occur in its uncomplicated form, it must be treated on the general principles applicable to adynamic fever, however arising.

When the injected conjunctivæ, delirium, or drowsiness, and slow pulse, indicate cerebral disturbance, and threatening secondary meningitis; or the florid tongue, the tender epigastrium, the vomiting, the diarrhœa, indicate gastro-enteritis, then general principles of treatment, by leeches and blisters according to the state of constitution, must be adopted, and cases before me show that success may attend the use of these means.

But an important practical question remains to be considered. It is the tendency of current pathological theory to relate these secondary inflammations, more particularly the cerebral, to the retention of excretions in the blood, and to point to elimination by the usual channels, as an indication in their treatment. Clinical observation is sufficiently in accordance with this theory to justify our acceptance of the therapeutic principle; but it requires to be carried into effect with much caution.

Whenever the collapse has been of such duration as to render it probable that secondary dangers may arise, then, with the returning pulse and warmth of the surface, we may commence the use of a saline diuretic, and give it every third or fourth hour: the acetate or nitrate of potass in combination with spiritus ætheris nitrici, answers very well, and, at the same time, simple diluents should be given. Should cerebral complication threaten, and there be no symptoms of gastro-enteric irritation present, then recourse may be had to one or two ten-grain doses of calomel, followed, if necessary, by two or three drachms each of castor and turpentine oil. These means, however, must be very cautiously used, because, as already shown, under this state of the secretions calomel is slow to take effect on them, but quick to excite gastro-enteric inflammation. When, however, the threatening of cerebral complication co-exists with gastro-enteric irritation, we must abstain from the use of mercurial or other purgatives, for the excitement of gastro-enteritis will more certainly aggravate the head symptoms and endanger life than the eliminatory action of the mercury effect good.

On the whole, there is more scope for the use of mercurial and other purgatives in cerebral complication after cholera in sthenic individuals, than in those debilitated before the attack, because in asthenic constitutions cerebral complication with gastro-enteritis is more common than the simple form, and when this coincidence occurs, the remedial means are restricted to local depletion, counter-irritation, diuretics, and diluents.

Still, however, another practical question may be asked: May we not endeavour to control the secondary inflammations of cholera, more especially the cerebral, by constitutional mercurial action? My opinion is distinctly opposed to this proceeding, both because the adynamic state of the system generally contra-indicates it, and the risk of gastro-enteric irritation, from the internal use of mercury, more than counterbalances any advantage likely to arise from its theoretic adoption.

Before concluding the treatment of cholera, it is desirable that I should state the estimate entertained by me of remedies which at times have been much used, but which, as yet, have not been alluded to in these remarks.

General Blood-letting, at one time so much used in India in the treatment of cholera, is now nearly abandoned. In the few instances in which I have myself adopted it, no good effect was apparent, and the recoveries which took place under its use in the early epidemics, were probably generally of the mild form of the disease now seldom seen, and for the cure of which rest and an opiate usually suffice.

My estimate of opium, *calomel*, *astringents*, and *stimulants*, may be gathered from the observations which have already been made on the general treatment of the disease.

The *Hot bath*, with the view of restoring the heat of the body and thus lessening the collapse, has been had recourse to. On this means of treatment Dr. Parkes * thus expresses his opinion: "The depressing effects of the warm bath were sometimes marked and unmistakeable. I have seen a man walk firmly to the bath, with a pulse of tolerable volume, and a cool but not cold surface, and in five or ten minutes have seen the same man carried from the bath with a pulse almost imperceptible, and a cold and clammy skin. I cannot find in my notes a single case in which the warm bath appeared beneficial." In the second number of the "Transactions of the Bombay Medical and Physical Society," in 1839, I thus stated the result of my own observation on the effect of the

* "Treatise on Cholera," p. 209.

hot bath in cholera patients. "I used the hot bath in this case, and watched the effect, that I might have an opportunity of satisfying myself on this point of practice. The bath was plainly injurious." *

Further, it may be asserted that a reference to the works of authors on Indian cholera will show a very general condemnation of the hot bath in the stage of collapse. This important fact would seem to have been disregarded in the treatment of cholera in London in the epidemic of 1854, for I find † in the metropolitan hospitals it was used in nearly 37 per cent. of the cases treated.

Emetics have been given in the collapse of cholera in expectation that the act of vomiting might favour reaction. In the cholera epidemic of 1849, in Bombay, a Cholera Infirmary was temporarily established by Dr. Mosgrove, for the treatment of the disease chiefly by the plentiful imbibition of cold water and the application of external heat. When this institution passed under the care of the late Dr. Larkworthy, I visited, through his kind permission, the patients almost daily, and sometimes twice a day, for the period of a month. One of the objects in giving large draughts of water was, that the act of vomiting, and its assumed stimulant action on the pulse, might be from time to time induced. As I had never exhibited emetics in my own practice, I gladly availed myself of the opportunity of testing the accuracy of the principle on which they have been recommended; and the result of my observation was, that in a large majority of cases in which collapse was fairly present, the draughts of water and the vomiting were not followed by any sensible effect on the pulse. I witnessed many cases of ultimate recovery, in which the state of pulseless collapse continued from six to twenty-four hours after the commencement of the exhibition of the cold water; and it may be further remarked, that in some instances the frequent imbibition of water in large quantity seemed to keep up an irritable state of the stomach, which it was afterwards troublesome to subdue. ‡

Hot Saline Enemata were used by me in the European General

* "Transactions of Medical and Physical Society of Bombay," No. 2, p. 240.

† "Report on the Results of the Different Methods of Treatment pursued in Epidemic Cholera, addressed to the President of the General Board of Health." By the Treatment Committee of the Medical Council.

‡ At p. 321, No. 10, "Transactions, Medical and Physical Society of Bombay," there will be found a letter on the treatment followed in the Cholera Infirmary, addressed by me to the Superintending Surgeon.

Hospital, but without any effect in lessening the state of collapse.

Rubefacient Liniments, Turpentine, and *Sinapisms* have been generally applied in the stage of collapse, but I have no faith in their utility; and there is a disadvantage in the disagreeable odours which arise from some of them, and in their probable interference with the functions of the skin.

Of *Saline Injections into the Veins* I have no experience; but it may be taken for granted that the experiments which have been already recorded are conclusive against them.

The *Inhalation of Vapours* seems to be a therapeutic means to which some still incline with hope. I have not had any opportunity of witnessing this mode of treatment, nor am I of those who see in it the prospect of good. If it be that the pulmonary is obstructed as well as the general capillary circulation, then the pulmonary channel of absorption into the blood is as much closed as the intestinal one: and when it begins to be re-established, can there be a doubt that pure atmospheric air will more surely minister to the restoration of depressed vital actions than medicated vapours?

Galvanism has been applied with the view of exciting the action of the heart and the respiratory function in the stage of collapse, but without any results calculated to inspire hope. The coil machine has also, to my knowledge, been used after reaction with the view of re-exciting the secretory function of the kidney. In this therapeutic theory I have no belief. The statements which have been made to me of urine having been passed shortly after the transmission of the electric current in the course of the kidneys and ureters are not called in question; but it may be suggested that the action has been on the muscular fibre of the bladder, into which the urine for hours previously had been slowly trickling, and not on the secretory structure of the kidney.

Cold Affusion and Wet Sheet. — Of these I cannot speak from personal knowledge; but I quote * Dr. Gull's summary: —

"On the continent, in the former and in the last epidemic, cold affusion was highly spoken of as a means of producing reaction. The patient was placed in a warm hip bath, and cold water poured or thrown over the head, back, and chest. This was done quickly, and the patient then placed between warm blankets. If the first application was followed by any improvement, the operation was repeated every three or four hours. The results appear to have been on the whole more satisfactory than from the hot bath.

"The 'wet-sheet envelope' was more commonly used in this country. The effects

* Report, p. 206.

varied according to the state of the patient; in the milder cases it favoured reaction, but when the disease was severe it was useless or injurious. The sweating caused by it added to the exhaustion, and had no influence in arresting the intestinal discharges. In none of the cases, which were many, in which we saw it tried, did it produce any good effect."

Results such as these are surely sufficient to induce medical men henceforth to abstain from a restless and too often injurious empiricism in the management of this disease.

RECAPITULATION.

My practical conclusions may be shortly re-stated under the following heads: —

1. In cholera epidemics there is a proportion of cases ushered in by premonitory diarrhœa, which if early treated by simple means are frequently curable, and the cholera attack is prevented. In some instances, however, the diarrhœa is not checked by treatment, and cholera becomes developed.

2. Cases of cholera occur — common in the early Indian epidemics, but rare in the later ones — in which the state of collapse is moderate in degree. In these the tendency is to recovery, not to death; but restoration is materially favoured by judicious moderate medical treatment.

3. When collapse is considerable, then we have a condition somewhat analogous to the cold stage of ague, or the initiatory fever of small-pox, — a state which cannot be checked, but which must run on a certain course, varying in intensity and duration in different instances — in which all that we can pretend to attempt, is to place the patient in circumstances as favourable as possible for enabling the system to outlive this stage of the disease while we at the same time carefully abstain from the use of means which may be injurious, not only then, but in subsequent stages of the attack.

5. When reaction from collapse is taking place, the restoration of the various functions is a slow process requiring careful watching, mild assistance, and avoidance of officious interference. This expectant course is more certainly correct when the stage of collapse has not exceeded eight hours; but when it has been longer, the probability of secondary danger is increased; and when this arises it must be met, or when it threatens it may be modified, by cautious judicious medical treatment, directed with the fact constantly before us, that in this state of the disease gastro-enteritis is readily excited.

5. The secondary dangers of cholera are to be treated, on general principles, with that care and caution which it is always necessary to observe in all forms of disease present in states of constitution which tend to be adynamic.

6. In a disease amenable in its milder degrees to ordinary medical treatment — and in its severer ones, though beyond the influence of medicines, still often recovered from — the value of remedies cannot be tested by statistical data as hitherto recorded. Therapeutic principles drawn from this source are very likely to be erroneous.

7. It is to be feared that cholera — as some other zymotic diseases in their severer forms, for example, plague, yellow fever, small-pox — will, in its severer forms, always prove little under the control of medical treatment; and that therefore in it, as in these others, the chief hope of lessening the mortality rests on our being able to understand its causes, and to prevent their action. To these important objects the attention of the medical profession should be earnestly given.

SECTION V. — *Statistical Tables relative to Epidemic Cholera in the European General Hospital, the Jamsetjee Jejeebhoy Hospital and the Byculla Schools at Bombay.*

TABLE XIX. — *Admissions and Deaths, with Per-centage, from Epidemic Cholera in the European General Hospital at Bombay, for the Six years from* 1838 *to* 1843.

	1838 to 1843.		Monthly Average.		
	Admissions.	Deaths.	Deaths on Admissions.	Admissions on total Admissions.	Deaths on total Deaths.
January	1	1	100·0	0·18	2·3
February	—	—	—	—	—
March	13	4	30·8	2·5	12·1
April	11	9	81·8	1·8	21·9
May	56	28	50·0	6·5	35·0
June	23	13	56·5	2·9	25·5
July	19	9	47·4	2·6	24·3
August	11	5	45·5	1·8	14·3
September	14	5	35·7	2·5	9·6
October	10	6	60·0	1·3	22·2
November	14	8	57·1	2·04	17·02
December	31	18	58·06	5·05	27·3
Total	203	106	52.2	2·7	19·5

TABLE XX.—*Admissions and Deaths, with Per-centage, from Epidemic Cholera, in the European General Hospital at Bombay, for the Five years from* 1844 *to* 1848.

	1844 to 1848.		Monthly Average.		
	Admissions.	Deaths.	Deaths on Admissions.	Admissions on total Admissions.	Deaths on total, Deaths.
January . .	4	4	100·0	0·6	8·7
February . .	6	3	50·9	1·1	8·6
March. . .	5	4	80·0	1·03	13·3
April . . .	3	4	133·3	0·5	12·8
May . . .	11	8	72·5	1·9	26·6
June . . .	29	12	41·4	4·6	36·7
July . . .	7	5	71·4	1·03	13·9
August . .	1	—	—	0·18	—
September . .	1	—	—	2·2	—
October . .	—	—	—	—	—
November . .	—	—	—	—	—
December . .	—	—	—	—	—
Total . .	67	40	59·6	0·98	10·3

TABLE XXI.—*Admissions and Deaths, with Per-centage, from Epidemic Cholera, in the European General Hospital at Bombay, for the Five years, from* 1849 *to* 1853.

	1849 to 1853.		Monthly Average.		
	Admissions.	Deaths.	Deaths on Admissions.	Admissions on total Admissions.	Deaths on total Deaths.
January . .	7	6	85·7	1·5	15·4
February . .	2	1	50·0	0·5	5·5
March . . .	4	2	50·6	0·9	5·9
April . . .	3	2	60·6	0·5	8·3
May . . .	5	3	60·0	0·9	12·5
June . . .	9	7	77·7	1·5	24·1
July . . .	5	5	100·0	0·9	15·1
August . .	16	9	56·2	3·2	23·7
September . .	10	7	70·0	2·8	28·0
October . .	1	—	—	0·25	—
November . .	7	3	42·8	1·3	10·0
December . .	9	5	55·5	1·5	12·5
Total . .	78	50	64·1	1·3	13·9

TABLE XXII.—*Admissions and Deaths, with Per-centage, from Epidemic Cholera, in the Jamsetjee Jejeebhoy Hospital at Bombay, for the Six years, from* 1848 *to* 1853.

	1848 to 1853.		Monthly Average.		
	Admissions.	Deaths.	Deaths on Admissions.	Admissions on total Admissions.	Deaths on total Deaths.
January	158	95	60·2	7·5	21·1
February	69	36	52·2	3·7	11·3
March	141	71	50·3	6·6	18·4
April	138	73	52·9	6·5	21·3
May	84	41	48·8	3·8	14·3
June	50	30	60·0	2·4	9·8
July	37	20	54·1	1·8	6·5
August	41	27	65·9	2·05	8·2
September	66	43	65·1	3·3	13·8
October	65	31	47·7	3·04	9·1
November	94	45	47·8	4·3	13·6
December	110	62	56·3	4·7	15·6
Total	1053	574	54·5	4·1	13·9

TABLE XXIII.—*Admissions and Deaths, with Per-centage, from Epidemic Cholera in the Byculla Schools, at Bombay, for the Seventeen years from* 1837 *to* 1853.

	1837 to 1853.		Monthly Average.		
	Admissions.	Deaths.	Deaths per cent. of Admissions.		
January	2	1	50·0		
February	3	1	33·3		
March	14	6	42·8		
April	6	4	66·6		
May	15	5	33·3		
June	31	17	54·8		
July	14	8	57·1		
August	—	—	—		
September	2	1	50·0		
October	—	—	—		
November	1	—	—		
December	1	—	—		
Total	89	43	48·2		

CHAP. XIV.

ON DYSENTERY.

SECTION I.—*The Importance of Dysentery in India—Order in which the subject will be treated.*

THE following facts relative to the sickness and mortality, from dysentery and diarrhœa, amongst European and Native troops in India, are extracted from Dr. Ewart's very instructive work:—*

	EUROPEANS.			NATIVES.		
	Per-centage of Admissions to strength.	Per-centage of Deaths to strength.	Per-centage of Deaths to Admissions.	Per-centage of Admissions to strength.	Per-centage of Deaths to strength.	Per-centage of Deaths to Admissions.
Bengal . . .	30·41	2·02	6·65	6·18	·173	2·80
Bombay . .	27·13	1·71	6·30	6·57	·196	2·98
Madras . . .	23·43	1·24	5·30	3·08	·190	6·17

During the six years of my service in the European General Hospital, 736 cases of dysentery were treated; and during nine of the years of my charge of the Jamsetjee Jejeebhoy Hospital, 1642 cases were admitted. To these latter may be added† 1470 cases of diarrhœa treated during the same period; making an aggregate of 3112 affections of the bowels.

This disease also came under my observation in its severest form in the hospital of Her Majesty's 40th Regiment at Belgaum, in 1830; also in Her Majesty's 4th Light Dragoons at Kirkee, in 1832, as well as more or less in all the other fields of practice in which I have been engaged in India.

* "Vital Statistics of the European and Native Armies in India," pp. 86, 121.

† My reason for classing diarrhœa with dysentery will appear in the sequel of this chapter.

The importance of this disease is at once shown by the facts just quoted from Dr. Ewart's work, as well as by those exhibited in the following tabular statement:

	Per-centage of Deaths from Dysentery and Diarrhœa on treated.	Per-centage of Deaths from Dysentery and Diarrhœa on aggregate Mortality.
European General Hospital, Bombay (Dysentery)	18·3	24·1
* Do. Officers, Bombay Presidency . .	. .	5·7
Jamsetjee Jejeebhoy Hospital	38·9	21·8
† General Population of Bombay . . .	. .	13·50

The ratio of deaths to treated varies according to the class of the sick, and the stage of the disease when submitted to treatment: it is therefore less in regimental than in general hospitals. It is very high in the Jamsetjee Jejeebhoy Hospital, because, as has been explained in respect to other forms of disease, the admissions often take place in hopeless states and stages of disease. The rate of mortality from these affections would seem to be greater in native than in European troops, more particularly those of the Madras Presidency; but the reason is not apparent.

My remarks on dysentery will be arranged in the following order: 1st. Pathology; 2nd. Causes; 3rd. Symptoms; 4th. Treatment.

Section II. — *Pathology.* — *Detailed Statement of the Morbid Anatomy.*

Dysentery is inflammation of varying extent and degree, of more or less of the constituent parts of the mucous membrane, — sometimes also of the other tissues, — of the large intestine.‡

* My own Notes.

† Mr. Leith's Deaths in Bombay.

‡ When we consider the structural analogy of cutaneous and mucous tissue, it is reasonable to anticipate more or less resemblance in their pathological phenomena, which future research may establish.

Inflammation of the skin exists in various forms. (*a.*) General redness with or without desquamation of the cuticle — the orders *exanthemata* and *papulæ.* (*b.*) The cutis may become thickened in patches of greater or less extent, with an excoriated surface, and excessive development and shedding of epidermal scales—the order *squamæ.* (*c.*) The upper layer of the cutis, inflamed at points more or less numerous, more or less aggregated together, may lead to serous or puriform effusion, confined by the superimposed epidermis, in collections of various size, and termi-

In describing the morbid anatomy of the disease, I shall, though occasionally referring to the writings of others, chiefly follow my own observations.

The subject may be appropriately arranged under the following heads: —

I. The morbid appearances presented by the mucous membrane of the large intestine.

II. The complication of inflammation, or its results, of the mucous membrane of the large intestine, with peritonitis, general or partial.

III. Tumefaction in the region of the cœcum, or sigmoid flexure of the colon.

IV. Displacements of the colon.

V. Complication of ulceration of the mucous lining of the large intestine, with abscess in the liver.

VI. Complication of dysentery with morbid lesions of the stomach or small intestine.

VII. The co-existence of enlargement of the mesenteric glands.

I.—The morbid appearances of the Mucous Membrane of the large Intestine may be classed under the following heads: — 1. Changes of colour and texture of the membrane; 2. Exudation on the free surface and into the interstices of the membrane; 3. Implication of the ordinary mucous follicles, or of the solitary glands; 4. Different forms of ulceration of the mucous membrane; 5. The

nating in desiccation, incrustation, and desquamation—the orders *vesiculæ*, *bullæ*, and *pustulæ*. (*d.*) Inflammation of the skin may extend to the subcutaneous tissue, and end in serous or puriform effusion, or gangrene and sloughing—*erysipelas*, *carbuncle*, *furunculus*. Consequent on these various forms of inflammation, there may be solution of continuity—destruction—of portions of the skin, more or less extensive, by processes of ulceration or sloughing.

The several orders of cutaneous inflammations have been further subdivided into genera and species. The opportunity of observing inflammation of the skin from its earliest appearance to its close has enabled us to determine these facts of its pathology. Similar processes may fairly be assumed to occur in some degree in the mucous membrane of the large intestine; but, for very evident reasons, they are, and must always be, insusceptible of proof, except in a very limited degree.

If the skin during life were removed from the cognizance of our senses, and all that we know of its inflammations were derived from symptoms caused by deranged function or constitutional sympathy, desquamated products, and post mortem appearances, we should be, in respect to the pathology of the skin, in a position analogous to that in which we now stand in respect to the pathology of the mucous membrane of the large intestine. In this hypothetical state of ignorance of cutaneous inflammation, our positive knowledge would probably be fully expressed by a single term — as *dermitis*—just as our present positive knowledge of inflammation of the mucous membrane of the large intestine is expressed by the single term—*dysentery*.

cicatrisation of ulcers; 6. The separation of parts of the mucous coat in patches, shreds, or tubular portions.

1. *Changes of Colour and Texture of the Membrane.* — A bright red and turgid state of the mucous membrane must be the earliest change produced by acute inflammation; but death takes place so seldom in this stage that the appearance is very rarely observed. Occasionally in cases of disease which have proved fatal with the symptoms of chronic dysentery, the only morbid appearance found after death is dark red or grey, sometimes black (melanosis), discoloration of the mucous coat of the large intestine. This state may be attended with softening, thinning, or thickening of the tissue. Hypertrophy is more common than the other alterations of texture, and sometimes in consequence of its having taken place unequally, the surface of the membrane presents an irregular mammillated or tubercular appearance. I have not satisfied myself that there are any particular symptoms which enable us to determine during life, that these only, and not other morbid changes, have taken place. It is not improbable that they exist most generally in cases in which dysentery has alternated with other diseases — as rheumatism — and in which it is reasonable to infer that there may be something special in the character of the inflammatory action.

The following three cases are illustrative: —

46. *Under treatment nine months.—Dysentery alternating with rheumatism, probably syphilitic; terminating in general cachexia with febrile symptoms.* — Charles ———, aged twenty-eight, after ten days' illness with dysentery, was admitted into the General Hospital on the 3rd November, 1841. The symptoms were for some time urgent, and considerable abdominal tenderness was complained of. He remained under treatment with alternation of dysentery, swelling and pain of joints, with thickening in the course of the tibiæ and increasing cachexia, and died on the 1st August, 1842.

Inspection fourteen hours after death made and reported by Mr. J. Peet. — Body emaciated, crude tubercles interspersed through the substance of both lungs. Rather more fluid than usual in the pericardium; heart healthy. *Abdomen.*—The stomach and duodenum contained a quantity of dark chocolate-looking fluid, and the mucous membrane of both presented distinct patches of injected vessels; these were most distinctly seen near the pyloric extremity of the stomach. The mucous membrane of cœcum of a dark, nearly approaching to a black, colour, but without thickening or ulceration. The transverse portion of the colon upon its inner surface was in a state of excessive congestion, but there were no distinct ulcers, although in some parts the mucous membrane was soft and pulpy; the mucous surface of sigmoid flexure healthy. Coats of the ileum at its termination in the colon thickened, in other respects, as well as the jejunum, healthy. Other viscera presented no abnormal appearance.—*Head* not examined.

47. *Chronic dysentery, discoloration with thickening of parts of the mucous membrane of the large intestines.* — Antone de Cost, of African extraction, but brought up at Goa, of twenty years of age, and following the occupation of cook on board a ship. For about two months before his admission, on the 28th June, 1849, he had been

affected with bowel complaint. He was much emaciated, and the pulse was very feeble. The tongue was moist and florid. He was purged from six to ten times in the twenty-four hours. The discharges were of slimy feculence, sometimes pale, at others of various tints of gray. He improved somewhat from the 2nd to the 10th July, then the purging increased, the discharges being more copious and watery. He died on the 21st.

Inspection. — *Chest.*—The lower part of the second lobe of the left lung was in a state of red hepatisation, the upper lobe was somewhat œdematous. The right lung adhered by old adhesions to the costal pleura, but was crepitating in its structure. *Abdomen.*—The liver was undiseased; the small intestine was somewhat attenuated. About three feet of the lower end of the ileum were laid open, but no morbid changes of the mucous membrane were observed. The mucous lining of the cœcum, colon, and rectum was in many places discoloured, of dark red, of brownish and of greyish tints, and in parts seemed somewhat thickened; in the sigmoid flexure and at the upper part of the rectum there were well-marked cicatrices of former ulcers. *Kidneys.*— In the central part of both there was commencement of yellow degeneration.

48. *Melanosis of the colon.— No ulceration.—Tubercles in the liver.*—Private F. L., aged forty-five, of the Bombay European Regiment. Had frequently been a patient in hospital, with symptoms of dyspepsia. He was admitted for the last time at Bombay on the 13th April, 1829. He then complained principally of flatulence and debility. Seldom had pain of abdomen, but when present it was generally removed by carminatives and remedies of that description. He gradually became emaciated, without the symptoms becoming more distinct. Finally diarrhœa came on, and the dejections were of dark colour. He sunk slowly, and died October 29th, 1829.

Inspection.—The transverse colon was much distended, except at the middle portion, where it was a good deal contracted. The peritoneal surface was of dark colour. The coats of the large intestine throughout its whole course were much thickened and indurated. The mucous membrane was of dark colour, in some places almost black, and presented a very irregular surface, which was caused by numerous small globular bodies, each about the size of a pea, apparently situated in the sub-mucous tissue. There were not any traces of ulceration throughout the whole course of the large intestine. The stomach was small, and owing to the distension of the colon, was forced upwards; but its coats were free from disease. The small intestine was healthy. The liver was of light colour externally, with tubercles the size of cherry stones in the substance of the left lobe. With the exception of old costal adhesions the thoracic viscera were healthy.

2. *Exudation on the Free Surface and into the Tissue of the Membrane.* — The uniform effusion of lymph for some extent over the surface of the mucous coat, in such manner as to lead to its separation in shreds or tubular portions, as obtains in the croupous forms of inflammation of the mucous membrane of the air passages, has been noticed by several writers on this disease. The occasional occurrence of this exudation in tropical dysentery may probably be admitted, but the following is the only instance of this morbid state which has come under my own observation, and it was not a case of dysentery: —

49. *Membranous mucous exudation on the inner surface of the large intestine.*—Private William Todd, aged 29, admitted into the hospital of the Bombay European Regiment, October 28th, 1829, ill with fever. There was much headache, with full and frequent pulse. He became drowsy, the skin assumed a yellow tint; he sunk and died November 1st. On the 29th he shrunk on the abdomen being pressed; but there was no

purging except from the use of medicine. About one hundred grains of calomel were given during the three days preceding death.

Inspection. — Vascularity of the membranes of the brain and effusion of patches of lymph. The greater part of the mucous surface of the large intestine was covered with a dark red effusion, in some places loosely attached to the membrane, and having the appearance of red currant jelly; in other places the effusion was firmer in consistence, and could be peeled from the mucous tunic in an almost membranous form. In the cœcum the effusion was evidently of longer standing from its firmer consistence, and from its being connected with the subjacent mucous tissue, through the medium of what appeared to be small capillary vessels. The mucous membrane underneath the effusion was vascular.

A yellow or greyish granular exudation — sometimes small, like grains of sand, at others larger and thicker — not unfrequently occurs on the mucous surface of some part of the colon or rectum, as well as of the ileum in cases of disease which have proved fatal with symptoms of chronic dysentery. It presents itself in patches more or less extensive, frequently coursing round the intestine in transverse bands, and preferring the elevated part of the rugæ of the membrane. The granules are generally found adherent to the surface of the membrane, which is commonly of a red tint more or less dark. The mucous membrane and the sub-mucous tissue are also usually thickened, sometimes to a considerable degree, and when cut, the edges of the incision present a fleshy appearance.

The granular exudation and the thickening are, however, distinctly preceded by a state of simply increased redness; whence it follows that the appearance adverted to under the first head — discoloration — may be merely the earlier stage of that now under consideration.

This granular deposit, which probably consists partly of modified epithelial debris, and partly of amorphous lymph exudation, is noticed by Rokitansky, Baly*, and other pathologists.

It has been observed by me most commonly in dysentery in persons whose constitutions have been in some degree cachectic, and an analogy between it and the squamous order of cutaneous inflammation may be suggested. The two cases which follow are instances of this appearance: — †

50. *Chronic dysentery in an opium eater.—The mucous coat of the colon covered with a firm granular layer.— The lungs tubercular.— Cartilaginous contraction of the pyloric orifice of the stomach.*—Wm. C., aged about thirty-five, of dissipated habits, an acknowledged opium eater, of spare habit, with narrow chest, came to Bombay as the surgeon of a ship from Australia, and was under treatment in the General Hospital for delirium tremens. He was discharged cured, and remained out of hospital for about

* Gulstonian Lectures, Medical Gazette.

† Also 34, 36, 42, 95, 98, 99.

a fortnight or three weeks, when he was again admitted on the 10th of July, 1840, with dysentery, which had attacked him four or five days previously. It became chronic, and he gradually sunk and died on the 3rd September. The treatment consisted of free opiates with bismuth, quinine and blue pill, wine and brandy.

Inspection seven hours after death.—Body much emaciated. *Head.*—There was a veil of serum below the arachnoid membrane on the convex surface of the brain. *Chest.*—The lungs partially collapsed, adhered here and there to the costal pleuræ. A considerable part of the upper lobe of the left lung was condensed from tubercular infiltration, and at its apex there was a cavity the size of an almond. In the lower lobe of the left lung there were many scattered miliary tubercles. There were numerous miliary tubercles in the right lung, but nowhere condensation of any considerable portion of the pulmonary tissue. *Abdomen.*—The intestines were collapsed. The liver was of dark red colour. The mesenteric glands were not enlarged. Four feet of the end of the ileum and the large intestine were laid open. The contents of the end of the ileum were mucous and tenacious. The lining membrane was of dark red colour without alteration of texture. The mucous coat of the cæcum was dark red, the surface slightly roughened, as if sprinkled with sand, but the texture was natural. The inner surface of the colon was of dark red colour throughout, and granular. But in the rectum the granular exudation was greatest, and most firmly adherent to the mucous coat, which was somewhat thickened, and when cut, had a fleshy appearance. There was one ulcer in the colon. The mucous coat of the stomach was of dark brown colour towards the cardiac end. The pylorus was much contracted from a cartilaginous ring in the sub-mucous tissue. The mucous coat of the duodenum was dark red in colour, but healthy in texture. The kidneys were healthy.

51. *Diarrhœa tedious.— Granular yellow exudation on the mucous surface of the large intestine with thickening of the tunic.*—James Grady, aged twenty-three, private in Her Majesty's 15th Hussars, admitted on the 12th October, 1839, with febrile symptoms. Diarrhœa followed and continued troublesome. The dejections were generally of pale yellow colour and thin. There was frequently irritability of stomach, with fulness and tenseness of the abdomen, and florid tongue. Under these symptoms he became much emaciated and sallow, and died on the 13th January.

Inspection.—Abdomen.—The chief disease was a yellow warty granular layer on the mucous coat of the large intestine, closely adherent to, and attended with thickening, and a thickened state of the mucous, and subjacent tunics. Where this granular exudation was still thin and only formed here and there, the mucous coat had not become thickened; thus proving that the granular state preceded the thickening of the tissue.

3. *Implication of the Mucous Follicles and of the Solitary Glands of the Colon.*—In the normal state of the lining membrane of the colon, the mucous follicles are hardly apparent to the naked eye, but on the occurrence of increased secretion consequent on active or passive congestion, they become more or less prominent, and their orifices — dark coloured, slightly depressed points — are very distinct. This condition of these follicles is very generally observed in the examination of fatal cases of cholera; also occasionally after death from remittent fever (26); and it is very probable that it always occurs in cases of transient diarrhœa, as well as during and immediately after the action of an active cathartic: it merely indicates an excess of the ordinary secretion of the mucous crypts.

The enlargement of the follicles in these several circumstances has as yet been unaccompanied by inflammatory action; but there is reason to believe that inflammation very readily takes place, and that its early stage is marked by general redness of the mucous membrane, or merely by a circle of vascularity around the orifice of the follicle, associated in some cases with thickening of the tissue, in others with ulceration. These conditions of the ordinary follicles of the colon, though not frequently noticed in fatal cases of dysentery, are very important with reference to that disease, because they are the early stages of morbid changes, which, in their advanced states, are often observed.

The solitary glands of the colon are also often implicated in this disease. In cholera, they, as well as the ordinary follicles of the colon, and Peyer's solitary and agminated glands of the ileum become distinct, pale in colour, about the size of a mustard seed, and are scattered here and there over the inner surface of the bowel. Under continued irritation, these glandular structures are liable, consequent on an increase of their secretion, to become larger and more elevated, sometimes attaining the size of a split pea. On the occurrence of inflammation of the mucous membrane, that part of it which is placed over the swollen solitary glands must, consequent on the pressure from within, readily give way, partly by an ulcerative process, partly by simple rupture. So frequently are these glands engaged in dysentery, that some observers, as Dr. Parkes, are of opinion that the disease always originates in them; but it seems to me that the utmost that can be said is, that they share with the other constituent tissues of the bowel in the morbid action. There has been much obscurity in the descriptions of the morbid appearances presented by the glandular structures of the large intestine, partly in consequence of the ordinary follicles and the solitary glands being confounded, and partly from the terms used by some observers. It may be useful to explain this statement more fully. Rokitansky uses the term mucous follicles, and it is not always clear, whether in his descriptions he speaks of the ordinary crypts or of the solitary glands. Pringle*, in describing the morbid appearances in dysentery, mentions certain protuberances of light colour, roundish, the twelfth of an inch in elevation, closely set, and resembling the small-pox at the height of the disease. Dr. Murray, of the Bengal Service, many years ago† drew attention to appearances similar to those

* "Diseases of the Army," p. 245.

† "Transactions, Medical and Physical Society of Calcutta," 7th volume.

attributed by me to enlarged follicles; but he uses the term vesicles, and loses sight of the fact that they were probably more related to the cholera of which his patients died, than to the dysenteric symptoms under which they had previously suffered: he hence conceived—on erroneous grounds, as seems to me—an analogy between dysentery and small-pox. Whether it is the follicular development, or the enlargement of solitary glands, which Dr. Bleeker describes under the term "Lenticular exudation*," I am unable to determine.

Rokitansky also alludes to vesicles formed by the epithelium raised by clear serum, and this in connection with the granular deposit of which I have already treated. Rokitansky implies that both appearances are different stages of the same process; that, after the discharge of the serum the epithelium subsides in the form of branny scales. It does not, however, clearly appear whether this statement refers to what has been actually observed, or to a hypothetical explanation of the commencement of morbid changes witnessed only in their after stages. The elevation of the epithelium in the form of vesicles by small collections of clear serum, has never been seen by me; and yet I have had the opportunity of frequently observing the different stages of the process connected with this granular exudation: 1, as reddened mucous membrane without thickening or exudation; 2, some slight degree of thickening and sandy-looking deposit; 3, increased thickening of the membrane and increased exudation—morbid processes more related, it seems to me, to the order Squamæ than Vesiculæ.

The term pustular appearance has been used by Mr. Twining in reference to the early stages of dysentery; but he does not explain to what altered anatomical condition of the membrane it is applied: small puriform collections in the sub-mucous tissue, not elevations of the mere epithelium, are probably referred to. Though inflammation of the mucous membrane of the large intestine, analogous to vesiculæ and pustulæ of the skin, is a reasonable hypothesis,

* "Indian Annals of Medical Science," No. 1, p. 4. I have read Dr. Bleeker's very able paper with much interest and care, but I cannot satisfy myself that I rightly understand his description of the morbid appearances of dysentery. When I compare it with my own observations I find a sufficient resemblance to give me the impression that we have both looked upon the same objects; but I cannot avoid the suspicion that Mr. Bleeker has marred the distinctness of his pictures by a too exclusive generalisation and by the unappreciated influence of a preconceived theory. This remark I make with great diffidence, being very sensible that the error may be with myself and not with the acute Batavian pathologist, whose co-operation I, equally with the able editors of the "Indian Annals of Medical Science," have hailed with much and sincere pleasure.

yet, in determining its probability, we must not forget the physical difference of the epithelium in the two situations.*

4. *Different Forms of Ulcer of the Mucous Membrane.*—The term ulcer is here used to express destruction, more or less extensive, of the mucous membrane, irrespective of whether it has been caused by a true process of ulceration, or by one of more rapid fusion of tissue, or by a process of gangrene and sloughing.

Ulcers of the mucous membrane of the large intestine may be conveniently classed under the heads *transverse*, and *circular*, as elementary types. These two forms, however, though often distinct, are not unfrequently combined; and in their advanced stages they may coalesce, and thus form extensive irregular surfaces of ulceration. The *transverse* form,—either in separate bands, or in several bands coalescing and occupying a greater or less extent of the inner surface of the large intestine,—is generally found after acute attacks of dysentery, and is most commonly associated with more or less thickening of the walls of the intestine. The appearance of the ulcer varies according to its stage, and the state of the contiguous tissues. Its bed may be occupied by a greyish slough; or the slough having been thrown off, the muscular coat may be exposed, and the edges of the ulcer may be irregular and thickened, or thinner and more rounded, with commencing cicatrisation. On the mucous membrane surrounding the ulcer granular exudation is sometimes observed.

In regard to the manner of formation of these transverse ulcers, it may in the first place be remarked, that one of the early effects of inflammation of the mucous lining of the large intestine is to stimulate the muscular coat to increased contraction; and, in consequence, to dispose part of the free mucous surface to arrange itself in transverse folds, as well as in rugæ in other directions. This fact has, I am satisfied, not been sufficiently taken into account in the explanation of the irregularity of surface frequently presented by the mucous membrane in its morbid conditions.†

* Since this passage was written the translation of the Rudiments of Pathological Histology, by Carl. Wedl, M.D. by the Sydenham Society, has come into my hands, and I observe at page 213 the following observation:—

"When the delicacy of the epithelial layer of the mucous membranes in general, except in the *mouth*, *œsophagus*, *vagina*, and *palpebræ*, is considered, it is easy to comprehend that exudations poured out from the corium cannot produce any vesicular elevation of the epithelium. The single layer of epithelial cells is easily detached by the exudation collected beneath it; and the elements newly formed from the exudation, are seen upon the exposed surface of the mucous membrane, and often become the subject of observation when eliminated from the living organism."

† I called attention to this in a paper published in the 7th volume of the "Transactions of the Medical and Physical Society of Calcutta," in 1835.

It has been stated that the granular exudation is frequently found on the summit of the transverse folds of the membrane. This is true of the ileum as well as of the large intestine. Why inflammatory action should show this preference for these situations I do not pretend to explain; but the fact is undoubted.

Let it be further remembered that, in the advanced stages of the granular exudation, there is always considerable thickening of the mucous membrane and sub-mucous tissue; and that the transverse ulcers are most commonly associated with thickening of the intestinal coats.

These facts justify the inference that transverse ulcers, co-existing with thickening, are merely the last stage of that morbid process which, commencing with redness, terminates, in its chronic form, in thickening and granular exudation; but which, under acuter inflammatory action, either original or superadded, passes on to gangrene and sloughing, and the formation of the kind of ulcer of which I now treat, as well as of others of different forms, also associated with thickening of tissue.

Under this view, then, it is assumed that when the morbid process — which going on slowly, gives rise to the symptoms of chronic dysentery, and does not pass beyond a state of thickening of the mucous membrane with granular exudation on the free surface — runs a more rapid course, it gives rise to the symptoms of acute dysentery, and ends in gangrene and sloughing. This view also explains how it is that we not unfrequently meet with cases of dysentery in which, after two or three days of apparently a simple diarrhœa, acute symptoms rapidly evolve themselves. In such we may suppose that the first stage — that of redness — of the process has gone on mildly, but that, from some cause or other, exacerbation has arisen, and that then the morbid action has rapidly gone through its full course.

But there is still further evidence of this relation between transverse ulcers and granular exudation in the fact, that cases of dysentery are not unfrequently met with in which we find sloughy ulceration of the mucous membrane, and granular exudation on the free surface immediately adjoining.

The following thirteen cases illustrate this last statement:—

52. *Dysentery with adynamic febrile symptoms.—Granular exudation on the mucous coat at the end of the ileum.—Sloughy ulceration of the large intestine.*—John Thompson, aged thirteen, of the Garrison Band, a delicate boy, frequently in hospital with intermittent fever, was admitted on the 27th November, 1840, stating that he had suffered from bowel complaint for two or three days. The tongue was without fur, the abdomen supple, dejections yellowish, thin, and the iliac regions tender. He was freely leeched and treated with ipecacuanha, gentian, and blue pill without purgatives.

On the 29th pyrexial symptoms came on. The dejections thin and partly feculent. Abdomen tender. He was again leeched and the ipecacuanha and blue pill treatment continued. The purging became more urgent, the pulse rose to 120, the skin became dry and the tongue brownish. He lost flesh and continued to pass light yellow dejections sometimes with streaks of blood. Enemata, opiates, a blister, &c. were used. He died on the 10th December.

Inspection twelve hours after death. —Body considerably emaciated. *Head.*—The membranes of the brain rather vascular and there were more bloody points than usual on incising the brain. There was an ounce of serum at the base of the skull. *Chest.* —The lungs collapsed and were healthy. Heart healthy. *Abdomen.*—Liver healthy. The omentum was matted over the transverse colon and the cœcum, and adhered to folds of the small intestine. The descending colon adhered to the lateral parietes, and the sigmoid flexure, by tender bands, to the walls of the pelvis. The mesenteric glands were enlarged, and reddened. The small intestine contained much thin yellow adhesive feculence. For three feet of the end of the ileum a layer of granular lymph adhered closely to the mucous coat, in transverse bands, following the summit of the valvulæ conniventes. There was little of the mucous coat of the large intestines left except in the form of sloughy transverse patches; the muscular coat was distinct and denuded. The stomach was healthy.

53. *Granular exudation on mucous surface of ileum and colon, with irregular ulceration of the latter.—No disease of the liver.—Displacement of the colon.*— Henry Green, aged thirty-six, private 4th Light Dragoons, ten years resident in India, suffered from fever twice at Kaira, but never from hepatitis, was admitted into the hospital at Kirkee, on the 21st April, 1832, with diarrhœa, was discharged on April the 25th. Re-admitted on June 1st, with mild dysentery, and was discharged on the 26th. Re-admitted on the 15th July, affected with frequent purging. The evacuations contained blood and mucus and were passed with griping and straining. There was constant pain around the umbilicus increased by pressure. The disease progressed, and by the 21st the discharges were reddish brown, watery, with clots of blood and shreddy matter. The pulse was frequent and small, the countenance collapsed, and hiccup present. He died on the 30th July.

Inspection five hours after death.— The omentum was vascular, and adhered firmly to the surface of the transverse colon, to the left side of the pelvis, and to the sigmoid flexure of the colon. The large intestine throughout was thickened. The upper portion of the ascending colon adhered to the under surface of the liver. The commencement of the transverse portion doubled down towards the umbilicus, thence ascended obliquely upwards towards the left side, passed to the left of the great arch of the stomach to which it was closely united, reached the diaphragm, and thence, after an acute duplicature, descended closely adherent to the left side of the abdominal parietes. The mucous coat of the ileum for about three inches from its termination was of dark red colour, and covered with granular lymph. The inner coat of the large intestine was irregular, and in many places fungus-like from granular lymph. There were many large transverse ulcers, some covered with thick pus, and others with black sloughs in the centre. Surrounding the ulcers, and in most part of the inner coat not occupied by ulceration, there was tenacious red transparent mucus effused; and here and there on its surface there was granular lymph. The stomach was displaced to accommodate itself to the displacement of the transverse colon; its inner surface was not examined. Liver healthy. Gall-bladder not distended. Lungs healthy. Heart healthy. There were one or two small points of deposit at the commencement of the aorta.

54. *Dysentery alternating with febrile accessions.—Bands of granular deposit at the end of the ileum.—Sloughy ulceration of the colon.*—Goolab Poorie, a Hindoo beggar, of twenty-seven years of age, was admitted into hospital on the 17th June, 1851. He had suffered for about two months from quotidian fever, which commenced with chills in

the evening. For fifteen days he had been affected with diarrhœa. From the time of admission to the 1st July, frequent thin feculent evacuations were passed with griping and straining. The tongue was florid and glazed, and there was occasional vomiting. The pulse was feeble, but febrile accessions were absent. He was treated with astringents, opium, diluted hydrocyanic acid, opiate enemata, and small blisters. From the 1st to the 16th July, the bowels were composed, the vomiting ceased, the tongue lost its florid appearance, but the febrile accessions recurred and were tertian in type. He was now treated with hydrocyanic acid and quinine in small doses. From the 14th to his death on the 20th July, dysenteric symptoms recurred and the discharges contained blood-tinged mucus, and the febrile accessions ceased.

Inspection five hours after death.—The body generally was much emaciated, but there was a thick layer of fat in the parietes of the abdomen as well as in the omentum. The peritoneal covering of the small intestine was in some places slightly vascular, and some of the convolutions adhered to each other by tender lymph. A part of the great omentum (that covering the ascending and the transverse colon) was fleshy looking and of rose-red colour. *Intestines.*—The mucous lining at the end of the ileum presented red transverse streaks, the surface of which was studded with granular deposit. The ascending and the transverse colon were much thickened throughout, and presented internally almost a continuous surface of ulceration covered with greyish sloughs. In the mucous membrane of the descending colon and of the sigmoid flexure the ulcers were not so continuous. They were circular in character, each about the size of quarter of a rupee. The liver was of natural size and texture, but of pale yellow colour, both externally and internally. The mucous membrane of the stomach was pale-looking and soft, chiefly towards the cardiac end. Both the kidneys were healthy but ex-sanguine. *Chest.*—The lungs collapsed, were of spongy texture and free from adhesion. The heart was of natural size, and its surface covered with fat, chiefly towards the margin of the right ventricle.

55. *Dysentery.—Sloughy ulceration of large intestine.— Granular deposit in transverse bands in the ileum.—Peritonitis and matting of the omentum.—An opium eater.*—Dhyam, a Mussulman water-carrier, of forty years of age, emaciated and addicted to the habitual use of opium, a native of Delhi, and not long resident in Bombay, was admitted into hospital on the 10th December, 1848. He had been ill with bowel complaint and febrile symptoms for twenty days. On admission, the abdomen was soft and collapsed, but uneasy on pressure at the umbilical region. During his stay in hospital the alvine discharges were frequent, consisted of slimy mucus tinged with blood, and were passed with griping, tenesmus, and occasional prolapsus. Febrile heat was frequently observed, and the pulse was feeble; the tongue was moist and without fur. He died on the 24th December. He was treated first with ipecacuanha and full opiates; then acetate of lead or sulphate of copper or trisnitrate of bismuth were substituted for the ipecacuanha. A small blister was applied to the pained part of the abdomen.

Inspection six hours after death.—Chest.—Lungs extremely collapsed, crepitating and healthy. Pericardium and heart healthy. *Abdomen.*—The liver was healthy. The great omentum, red, and thickened, was matted over the transverse colon, and adhered by friable lymph to folds of intestine (small and great) and to parts of the abdominal parietes. The convolutions of the intestines adhered by flakes of lymph to one another, to the viscera of the pelvis, and the parietes of the abdomen; and there was a blush of redness over them. The cœcum, the ascending colon, and the right half of the transverse colon were internally in a state of sloughy ulceration, and all the coats were tender, of greyish colour, and pultaceous consistence, and tore readily on separating the adhesions; the contents of the gut were thin and of greyish colour. The sigmoid flexure of the colon was in a similar sloughy condition. The rest of the colon was somewhat thickened with the mucous lining softened, but without any distinct ulceration. The ileum was laid open for about three feet of its length;

there was general redness of the mucous coat ranged in transverse streaks, corresponding to the valvulæ conniventes; and at the lower part of the intestine, the reddened surface was covered with a layer of firm, granular lymph, and the mucous coat underneath was thickened. This effusion of granular lymph lessened as the cœcum was receded from, and ceased two and a half feet from the cœcum, but the redness in transverse streaks without the granular deposit extended somewhat higher. The kidneys appeared tolerably healthy. Head not examined.

56. *Probable scorbutic taint.—Dark, irregular, ragged, internal surface of the colon, with thickening.—Granular deposit on mucous membrane of ileum, with thickening.*—Dhondoo Essew, a Maratha labourer, twenty-one years of age, recently returned from Aden, where he had been employed for two years, was admitted into hospital on the 16th October, 1848, after ten days' illness from diarrhœa and febrile symptoms. He was reduced in strength. He died on the 8th of November. The symptoms observed were frequent alvine discharges, scanty, passed with griping, and consisting of adhesive pasty or slimy feculence of palish colour, and frequently streaked with blood. There was no fulness or induration of abdomen, and seldom uneasiness on pressure. The tongue was sometimes coated in the centre, but was not florid. There was frequently an evening febrile exacerbation noted. The skin was always dry; the pulse feeble, sometimes irritable, and it ranged from 80 to 94. There was no sponginess of the gums, yet residence at Aden is well known to engender a scorbutic taint. The urine showed no traces of albumen. He was treated first with acetate of lead and opium, then with quinine and full opiates, and a small blister was applied to the abdomen. Diet, milk, sago, port wine.

Inspection thirteen hours after death.—The body much emaciated. *Chest.*—The lungs collapsed freely. *Abdomen.*—The intestines collapsed. No peritoneal adhesions. The large intestine was rather contracted, and very much thickened. The inner surface presented a dark green, very irregular and ragged surface, and the dark tint extended into the interstices of the tissues, and gave the cut edges of the thickened walls an almost black colour, in places. The inner surface of the ileum, for about two feet above the ileo-colic valve, was diseased; the mucous membrane red, thickened, and covered with a layer, more or less thick, of granular, closely adherent lymph. The kidneys were healthy. The liver was healthy.

57. *Thickening and sloughy ulceration of large intestine, with here and there a small encysted abscess in the thickened tissue.— Granular deposit on inner surface of ileum.— Peritonitis.— Old pericarditis and heart disease.*— Corporal C. W., aged thirty-one, of Her Majesty's 40th Regiment, after four days' illness, was admitted into the hospital at Belgaum, on the 8th July, 1830. There was tenderness of abdomen, and frequent purging, attended with tenesmus. The skin was hot and dry. The tenderness of abdomen, never entirely removed, was much aggravated on the 14th. The purging continued frequent, and he died July 16th. No ptyalism induced.

Inspection.—The peritoneal covering of all the intestines and of the convex surface of the liver was vascular and covered with flakes of effused lymph. The caput cœcum had formed firm adhesions, and in endeavouring to separate it from the iliac fossa, its coats readily gave way. The disease of the mucous membrane commenced at the termination of the ileum, where there where several vascular patches covered with a slight effusion of granular lymph, but unattended with ulceration. In the cœcum and ascending colon the whole mucous coat was ulcerated and broken down, and the subjacent coats were much thickened, with here and there a small encysted secretion of pus in their tissue. In the transverse and descending colon the ulcers were large, but circumscribed, of an olive green colour in their centre, surrounded by a blush of redness, and uniformly attended with thickening of the other tunics. The parenchyma of the liver was of lighter colour than natural. The gall-bladder contained little bile. *Chest.*—The pericardium adhered firmly to the whole surface of the heart, from which it could not be separated without the knife. The heart was natural in size, but of darker colour. The mitral valve was thickened and cartilaginous; the aortic valves were in a similar state, and instead of being applied to the sides of the vessel projected into its cavity, leaving dilated pouches behind them.

58. *Dysentery.—Sloughy ulceration in transverse bands, and the follicles of the colon in different stages of disease.—Insensibility for an hour before death.—Two ounces of serum at the base of the skull.*—Edward Clark, aged twenty-four, a seaman of slight frame and dark complexion, was under treatment in the General Hospital from May 26th to 31st, 1839, ill with rheumatism, chiefly marked by rigidity of the muscles of the back of the neck, and of the masseter muscles. He was discharged well, and joined the Indian Navy. On the 6th June he was re-admitted into the hospital, ill with dysentery. It was the fifth day of the disease. There was considerable fulness and pain of the abdomen, with tenesmus and pain at the anus. The countenance was anxious, the pulse frequent, and feeble, the tongue white, but not coated, and the evacuations were yellow, slimy, and streaked with blood. Five dozen leeches were applied to the abdomen, a warm bath used at bed-time, and pills of calomel seven grains, ipecacuanha and opium, each one grain and a half, were given, and followed on the succeeding morning by four drachms of castor oil. During the night he was several times disturbed; the evacuations were watery, and tinged red. On the morning of the 17th, the abdomen continued full, and was somewhat tense and tender at the umbilicus. There was also considerable pain at the anus; the countenance was anxious; the pulse 116, of moderate strength, and the tongue pretty clean. Five dozen leeches were again applied to the abdomen, and fomentations directed to be used every second hour, and an anodyne enema to be exhibited at noon. The evacuations continued frequent, watery, and tinged with blood. The tenderness and fulness of the abdomen persisted, the skin was above natural temperature, the pulse 120, and irritable.. At the evening visit the fomentations were continued, and calomel six grains, with opium and ipecacuanha two grains, given at bed-time. The purging continued during the night, and on the morning of the 18th the skin was dampish, pulse 92, and feeble. There was less fulness of the abdomen, and less straining. A large blister was applied to the abdomen, and the anodyne enema was repeated, and three ounces of port wine ordered. At the evening visit the blister was found to have acted well; the purging, however, persisted, and the evacuations consisted of bloody serum with flocculi of blood. Pulse frequent and small, skin hot, much thirst, but the tongue not furred. There had also been frequent vomiting. Calomel and opium each two grains and ipecacuanha one grain, in the form of a pill, were ordered every four hours. The purging was unchecked, and he died at 7 P.M., having become comatose half an hour before death.

Inspection twelve hours after death. — The abdomen was moderately distended. *Head.*—There was about two ounces of serum in the cavity, chiefly at the base of the skull. *Chest.*—The lungs were emphysematous and not collasped; but the thoracic viscera were otherwise healthy.—*Abdomen.* The omentum adhered to the cœcum, and to the colon; and many of the mesenteric glands were enlarged. At the hepatic flexure of the colon, an ulcer was patched by the opposing side of the angle. The whole of the inner surface of the large intestine was more or less diseased. There were sloughly ulcerations and elevated transverse ridges coated with a layer of granular lymph. The mucous follicles were also in different stages of disease; in some the orifice was merely apparent, in others it was enlarged by ulceration, and ranged from a mustard seed to the size of a sixpence. The mucous coat of the stomach was mammillated. The liver was pale in texture, and in the left lobe there was a small abscess, the size of a walnut. The kidneys were healthy.

59. *Dysentery neglected for thirteen days, attended with abscess in the liver.—Sloughy ulceration of the mucous coat of the colon, with fringe of granular exudation.* —Charles Mitchell, aged twenty-four, of stout habit, four years resident in India. After thirteen days' illness, was admitted into the General Hospital on the 14th December, ill with dysentery. There was a good deal of uneasiness of the abdomen, and much tenesmus, and the dejections contained much blood mixed with mucus or serum. He died on the 3rd January.

Inspection.—Abdomen.—In the right lobe of the liver there was an abscess the size of an orange, and in the left lobe there was one the size of a walnut. The large intestine was thickened, and there were large patches of sloughy ulceration of the mucous surface fringed with a layer of granular lymph. This layer of lymph was plainly secreted by the inflamed surrounding mucous coat, and not by the surface of the ulcer.

60. — *Acute dysentery.— The large intestine ulcerated in transverse ridges.— The mucous follicles enlarged.— Considerable effusion of serum in the head without symptoms.*— John Billing, aged twenty-three, a stout muscular man, a seaman of Her Majesty's ship *Volage* was admitted into the European General Hospital, on the 28th December, 1838. On the 22nd he had been affected with slight diarrhœa, from which it was stated he had recovered. He was allowed to go on shore on leave, and returned to the ship complaining of inability to void his urine, and of pain and tenderness of the hypogastrium. A catheter was introduced, and the bladder was found empty. Subsequently, after the exhibition of diuretics, the urine was voided naturally. On the morning of the 28th there was griping and purging, pain and tenderness of the abdomen on pressure, a small and rapid pulse, cold perspiration, and a dark brown fur on the tongue. He was bled to twenty ounces, a blister was applied to the abdomen, some castor oil exhibited, and he was sent to the European General Hospital. On admission, at 5 P.M., the pulse was very feeble, the skin was cold, the respiration was somewhat hurried, the tongue had a thin brown coat in its centre, and the chief complaint was of debility, faintness, and frequent ineffectual calls to stool. The blister on the abdomen had risen well. An ounce of camphor mixture, with a drachm of aromatic spirit of ammonia and five grains of the sesquicarbonate of ammonia, was given on admission, and ten grains of calomel and two of opium at bed-time. The respiration became more hurried, the pulse thready, the skin cold and damp. Mulled wine was given every hour. He died at 2 A.M. of the 29th.

Inspection eleven hours after death.—Head.—The vessels of the pia mater were moderately congested. On the convex surface of the brain between the pia mater and the arachnoid membrane, there was considerable effusion of serum, and the latter membrane was somewhat thickened and opaque. There were about six drachms of serum in each lateral ventricle, and about two ounces at the base of the skull. *Chest.*—The lungs with exception of emphysema of the upper lobes were healthy. *Abdomen.*—The omentum adhered by fleshy points to the cœcum, the iliac fossa, and different parts of the ascending and descending colon. The sigmoid flexure of the colon was doubled down, and adhered to the fundus of the bladder, and to the rectum. The inner surface of the cœcum and colon was much ulcerated, under the form of closely set transverse elevated indurated ridges, with an ulcerated suface fringed by a layer of granular gritty yellow lymph, or red gelatinous mucus. In many places, when the layer of lymph was removed, the ulcer was found in process of cicatrisation. Many of the mucous follicles in the colon were enlarged, and some were ulcerated. Throughout the greater part of the large intestine, the sub-mucous tissue was thickened. The liver was healthy, and the gall-bladder full of bile. The small intestine was healthy. The mucous membrane of the stomach was somewhat softened, with marbled dark redness at its cardiac end, and in some places it was mammillated and thickened. The spleen, the kidneys, and bladder, were healthy.

61. *Acute dysentery.— The ulceration in transverse ridges.—Considerable effusion of serum in the head, without symptoms.* — John Gale, aged fifty-two, a tall man of sallow complexion, who had served for forty-two years in India, had generally enjoyed good health, but had led an intemperate life. After six days' illness, he was admitted into the European General Hospital on the 12th December, affected with frequent purging and pain of the abdomen. He described the evacuations to have been of various appearance, and frequently to have contained much blood. On the

night before admission he had been constantly purged, and much blood had been dejected. There was acute tenderness in the course of the colon and over the cœcum. Pulse 120, feeble. Skin of natural temperature; tongue furred. He was ordered four grains of acetate of lead with two grains of opium, at bed-time, and to be repeated the following morning; port wine was also given in small quantities. During the night there was much purging, the evacuations being red and watery, and on the morning of the 13th the pulse was almost imperceptible. The purging continued, the sinking increased, and he died at midnight.

Inspection eight hours after death.—Head.—The vessels of the pia mater were turgid. There was considerable effusion of serum between the arachnoid tunic and the pia mater on the convex surface of the brain, and there was also considerable effusion at the base of the skull. *Chest.*—The lungs were of dark colour and emphysematous, but otherwise healthy. The heart was healthy. *Abdomen.*—The liver was of natural size, externally of pale colour, with an irregular surface. When incised the texture was found to be indurated, was of a pale buff colour, and mottled. The mucous lining of the middle of the great arch of the stomach was mammillated; at the cardiac end it was thin, and in places almost removed. The end of the ileum was natural. The colon from beginning to end presented internally an irregular surface of sloughy ulceration, chiefly ranged in dark red fungous, closely set transverse ridges, some of which were half an inch thick, and fleshy when cut across. The free surface of these ridges presented either a foul ulceration or a granular gritty surface from effused lymph. The small intestine was contracted. In the right kidney there was a serous cyst of the size of a walnut, and the parenchyma of the organ was congested. The spleen was healthy.

62. *Dysentery in an advanced state obscured by secondary peritonitis.— Granular deposit on the mucous surface of the large intestine.*—Shawah, a Hindoo washerman, of thirty years of age, was admitted into the Jamsetjee Jejeebhoy Hospital on the 25th December, 1851. He was emaciated, had been ill for a month, and could not give a connected history of his illness. He complained chiefly of uneasiness of abdomen, which was somewhat full and resisting. The bowels were open sometimes two or three times in the day, and the evacuations were thin and feculent; at other times they were not opened. The pulse was feeble. The case was looked upon as one of subacute peritonitis, and was treated with leeches, opium, ipecacuanha, and castor and turpentine oils in small doses. He died on 1st January.

Inspection.—The small intestine was full of air, and its convolutions were adherent to each other by bands of friable lymph. The transverse colon was displaced downwards at its central part. The omentum was matted over it, and was also closely adherent to the larger curvature of the stomach. There was a pouch-like dilatation of the upper part of the ascending colon. The coats of the large intestine were generally thickened; the mucous coat was pulpy, and generally softened, and studded over with large patches of ulceration and granular deposit. The other viscera were healthy, with the exception of slight encroachment on the tubular part of the kidney.

63. *Several attacks.— Colon thickened.— Sloughy ulceration, with granular deposit on other parts of the mucous surface of the colon.— Slight peritonitis.*—Private J. A., aged thirty-five, of Her Majesty's 40th Regiment, was admitted into hospital at Belgaum, on the 8th July, 1830, ill with dysentery. The attack was acute, but he was discharged well on the 31st July. Re-admitted 10th August with tender abdomen, and other dysenteric symptoms. Ptyalism not induced. He was discharged on the 18th September, after having been in hospital a long time convalescent. Re-admitted September 23rd with tender abdomen and frequent purging. He complained for the first time of pain of the right hypochondrium. Was subjected to the usual treatment. No ptyalism. Died on the 1st October.

Inspection.—There was much fat in the omentum and about the mesentery. The omentum adhered slightly to the intestines. The small intestine had a blush of redness on its peritoneal surface. The caput cœcum was drawn upwards from its usual situation in the iliac fossa. The colon was thickened, covered with fat, and firmly adherent to the fundus of the gall-bladder, which latter organ adhered also to the pyloric portion of the duodenum. The transverse arch was closely connected to the stomach. The sigmoid flexure formed several folds in the hypogastrium, and the sides of the folds adhered to each other. The mucous membrane of the large intestine was discoloured and ulcerated, and when floated in water exhibited a flocculent surface. Where less diseased there was a granular white effusion on the vascular mucous surface. The liver was rather enlarged, and of lighter colour than natural; no adhesion. The viscera of the chest were healthy.

64. *Dysentery admitted in the last stage.—Peritonitic inflammation.—Sloughy ulceration of the mucous coat of the colon.* — Robert Hunter, aged thirty-eight, a seaman of Her Majesty's ship *Endymion*, was admitted into the European General Hospital on the 21st August, 1841. He stated that he had suffered from dysenteric symptoms for five weeks, but had not reported himself sick till ten days previously. On admission the countenance was sallow, reduced, and anxious. The skin dry, and above the natural temperature. The pulse 116, feeble and easily compressed. The abdomen was rather full and tender on pressure at the right iliac region. The tongue was florid at the tip, dryish in the centre, and without fur. He had been frequently purged during the previous night, but the straining, formerly great, had considerably decreased. Thirty-six leeches were applied to the right iliac region, a warm bath was used, and the ipecacuanha pills with opium given. During the night, there were frequent dejections of ochreous red colour, with intermixed sloughy shreds. On the morning of the 22nd pulse 88 feeble. The other symptoms as on the previous day. Two grains of opium, with an equal quantity of blue pill and ipecacuanha, were given every four hours. On the 23rd, the frequent purging continued, the dejections being of claret-red colour, attended with hiccup and sinking pulse. Acetate of lead and opium were given every four hours, two grains of each. The purging continued unchecked, and on the 24th, the opium was combined with sulphate of copper, instead of the acetate of lead, without benefit. He died on the morning of the 25th.

Inspection six hours after death.—The omentum, vascular and fleshy, extended over the intestines, adhered to the cœcum and to the abdominal parietes. There was dark vascularity, with exudation of lymph and tender adhesions of the peritoneal surface of the small intestine. The cœcum, ascending and transverse colon were thickened and tender, tearing readily and showing an inner surface of irregular ulceration, covered with dark-coloured adhesive secretion. Liver healthy. Thoracic viscera healthy.

Transverse ulceration may also exist with thickening of the coats of the intestine, but without granular exudation. It may occur also, though rarely, without thickening, and then the morbid process is of a different nature — it is one of serous and lymph exudation and suppuration in the sub-mucous tissue of the transverse fold, followed by gangrene and sloughing of the mucous layer. But this lesion will be more fully considered in connection with the second form of ulcer — the *circular*.

Circular ulcers are generally found in dysentery of long duration, in which the symptoms have never at any time been very acute.

According to Drs. Parkes and Baly they originate in the solitary glands. The latter author has described well the process of sloughing by which the gland is thrown off and the circular ulcer is formed. That some circular ulcers of the large intestine are formed in this manner is not to be disputed. They, however, constitute, probably, but a small proportion of the circular ulcers which are met with in that situation; for many of them have seemed to me to originate in the ordinary follicles. It has been already explained that when these structures are irritated to increased secretion they become turgid and their orifices distinct; then a vascular ring surrounds them and exudation of serum and lymph in small quantity takes place into the mucous membrane of the follicle and the areolar tissue around it, soon to be followed by destruction of these tissues, through a process of fusion or sloughing.

Circular ulcers may probably also be formed by the same process as transverse ones, viz. by thickening of and granular exudation on circular patches of the membrane followed by grangrene and sloughing. But this mode is suggested rather hypothetically than stated as an observed fact.

Circular and other forms of ulcer may originate in circumscribed sub-mucous suppuration, of greater or less extent, followed by sloughing of the superimposed mucous layer; or, to express it otherwise, exudation of circumscribed portions of lymph takes place into the sub-mucous tissue, degenerates into pus, and is succeeded by gangrene and sloughing of the mucous coat which covers it. This manner of ulceration in dysentery has been described by Haspel*; and if I comprehend Dr. Bleeker† rightly, it is the explanation of destruction of tissue in dysentery, which he exclusively adopts. That ulcers are thus formed does not admit of doubt. The process is analogous to that by which some kinds of cutaneous ulcer are caused, viz. by small circumscribed sub-cutaneous abscesses with sloughing or ulceration of the superimposed cutis. But in the writings of Haspel and Bleeker it does not distinctly appear whether these observers have met with the small sub-mucous abscesses frequently or only very occasionally. If the latter,—which would be in accordance with my own experience,—then their opinion that intestinal ulcers are *frequently* formed in this way is in great measure hypothetical. If, however, on the other hand, they have frequently observed this morbid process in the *stage* of sub-mucous abscess, then the inference is, either that this process is rare in India compared with Algeria and

* "Maladies de l'Algérie," tome ii. p. 71.

† "Indian Annals of Medical Science," No. 1.

Batavia, or that death in these latter countries takes place more frequently at an earlier period of the disease.

I have met with only one instance of sub-mucous abscess in my own researches; for this state is not to be confounded with that of intestinal thickening from lymph deposit with subsequent destruction, partly by sloughing, partly by suppuration.*

The following is my only case of sub-mucous abscess:—

65. *Patches of sub-mucous puriform infiltration in colon.*—A Hindoo, with febrile symptoms, abnormal dulness of the lower part of right chest, with crepitus, was considered to be affected with pneumonia, and was treated in part with tartar emetic. He died, and a large abscess was found in the upper and central part of the right lobe of the liver, approaching the diaphragm; its walls were ragged and shreddy. On the inner surface of the cœcum, ascending and transverse colon, there were sloughy elevated dark grey patches, of the size of a rupee, not separating, but pulpy, and chiefly remarkable for the distinct puriform infiltration into the sub-mucous tissue beneath. The kidneys were in a state of granular degeneration. Diarrhœa had not been present as a prominent symptom.

Circular ulcers of the mucous membrane in cachectic individuals may be caused in still another manner—by gangrenous patches consequent on sub-mucous œdema, just as in similar states of constitution cutaneous ulcers may be formed by a like process.

The following is an illustrative case:—

66. *Sloughy patches of mucous membrane of colon, with sub-mucous œdema.*—Ram Dial, treated in the clinical ward, in February 1852, for emphysema, dropsy, and dysentery. The surface of the mucous membrane of the large intestine was elevated from sub-mucous œdema. The elevated patches were grey, circular, and gangrenous in the centre, and ranged in size from a rupee to a quarter of a rupee. In none had separation of the slough taken place.

There is then, it seems to me, still considerable uncertainty, in regard to the precise mode of formation of ulcers in dysentery, more particularly of those which are circular in form.

Pathologists in India will do well to direct their attention to this subject, and to pursue it with minuteness and care. The questions to be determined are,—the relative proportion of these ulcers which originate: 1, in the solitary glands; 2, in the ordinary mucous follicles; 3, in patches of mucous membrane thickened by exudation process; 4, in sub-mucous abscess; and perhaps, we may add, in vesicular and pustular processes of the superficial parts of the membrane. The circumstance of surrounding thickening of the mucous membrane, or sub-mucous tissue, or of both, should also be carefully noted. My expectation is that it will be found that circular ulcers are associated with surrounding thickening, chiefly when they are formed in the third manner.

I now quote four cases illustrative of circular ulceration:—

* Cases 57 and 75.

67. *Numerous small circular ulcerations of the colon.*—Kuneem Khajee, a Mussulman pilgrim, of twenty years of age, on his way from Lahore to Bombay, with the view of proceeding to Mecca, was exposed to vicissitudes of weather, and three months before admission into hospital, on the 28th September, 1862, became affected with bowel complaint. When he came under observation, he was a good deal emaciated. The face was puffed, the feet were œdematous, and the abdomen full, with indistinct sense of fluctuation and uneasiness in the course of the transverse colon. The bowels were opened eight or ten times in the twenty-four hours, and the evacuations, passed with griping and straining, were thin, slimy, and sometimes streaked with blood. The urine not scanty, had generally a specific gravity of 1020, and showed no traces of albumen. He died on the 4th October.

Inspection five hours after death.—The body was much emaciated. *Chest.*—There were about six ounces of serous fluid in the sac of the left pleura. Both lungs were pale, crepitating, and without adhesion. The sac of the pericardium contained about four ounces of serous fluid. The heart was of natural size, and the valves healthy; but there was more than usual quantity of adipose tissue, both over the base and apex of the organ. *Abdomen.*—The sac of the peritoneum contained about ten ounces of clear serum. The liver was smaller than natural, and the external surface and substance were of pale yellow colour. The gall-bladder and the gall-ducts were quite pervious. Stomach and small intestines collapsed, their peritoneal surface was pale. The large intestine was not collapsed; its coats were thickened apparently from œdema; the mucous membrane was mottled red and white, and numerous small circular ulcers — some about the size of a pin's head, and others that of a split-pea — were seen scattered throughout the whole inner surface. They were most numerous about the sigmoid flexure of the colon, and many of them presented an appearance of cicatrisation. The mucous membrane of the ileum was healthy, except close to the ileo-colic valve, where several circular ulcers were also observed. The kidneys were healthy.

68. *Chronic dysentery in a person of broken constitution. Numerous circular ulcers in the large intestine, many of them cicatrising. Serous effusion in the head without symptoms.*—Henry Heming, aged forty-seven, an Indo-Briton, broken in constitution, feeble in mind, and subject to dysentery for many months, was admitted into hospital on the 2nd November, 1840. Both legs were œdematous, and the surface of the right one was of dark red colour. The diarrhœa continued notwithstanding the different remedies used, which were chiefly bismuth, sulphate of copper, and quinine in combination with opium. The dejections were generally pale in colour and thin. He died on the 14th November.

Inspection thirteen hours after death.—Head.—There was a thin veil of serum between the arachnoid and pia mater on the convex surface of the brain, and about an ounce at the base of the skull. *Chest.*—The lungs were fully collapsed. The right auricle of the heart was distended with blood. *Abdomen.*—The liver, not enlarged, was mottled red and white, and blood flowed from it when incised. The sigmoid flexure of the colon was much dilated, and filled the space between the pelvis and umbilicus, and overlaid the cœcum. The end of the ileum and the large intestine were laid open. The mucous coat of the end of the ileum was of natural appearance, and contained light yellow formed feculence. The coats of the colon were not thickened, except, in places, the mucous coat itself. The inner surface throughout was very closely studded with circular ulcers ranging from a silver penny to a small split pea in size. In some places the ulcers ran together, and formed irregular longitudinal vertical bands. For the most part the edges of the ulcers were rounded and cicatrised, and the bed of the ulcers presented a dark grey cicatrised surface somewhat fleshy when incised. The surface generally had very much the appearance of deep small-pox pits, shortly after desquamation. The mucous coat between the ulcers presented generally a dark reddish tint, but was not softened. The ulcers were most crowded in that part of the sigmoid flexure which was dilated. The mucous coat of the stomach, the kidneys, spleen, and mesenteric glands were healthy.

69. *Dark grey discoloration, with some degree of thickening of mucous membrane of colon, with numerous circular ulcers.*—Luximan, a Hindoo beggar, of twenty-five years of age, after eighteen days' illness, was admitted into hospital on the 30th November, 1850. He was frequently purged; the evacuations consisted partly of thin feculence, blood, and mucus, and were passed with much griping and tenesmus. The abdomen was full, and tender on pressure, chiefly at the iliac regions. He suffered from febrile disturbance also. The symptoms continued with occasional alleviation, but at times hiccup was present with a gradually failing pulse, till 23rd December, when he died. Leeches were used at the commencement, followed by small blisters. Quinine and opium and then acetate of lead were given, and towards the end opium alone. Milk, sago, wine, and chicken-broth as diet.

Inspection eleven hours after death.—*Chest.*—The lungs did not collapse readily, and adhered closely to the costal pleura. The upper lobe of the right lung was crepitating, the middle and inferior lobes were œdematous, as was also the inferior lobe of the left lung. The heart was healthy. *Abdomen.*—The cavity contained about three pints of clear serum. The mucous membrane of the large intestine was of dark grey colour, was somewhat thickened, and did not move freely on the subjacent tissue. There were many round superficial ulcers, several of which were in process of cicatrisation. The ulceration, in its most active state, was in the cœcum and ascending colon. The glands at the end of the ileum were more developed than natural. The mucous membrane of the small intestine was healthy. The mesenteric glands were somewhat enlarged, but free from tubercular deposit. The liver somewhat congested. Kidneys normal.

70. *Circular and transverse ulcers of the large intestine.—Matting of the omentum over the colon, with displacement.—Liver healthy.—Distention of the urinary bladder.*—Antonio Ignatio, of twenty-two years of age, and of spare habit, a native of Lisbon, a sailor by occupation, and once the subject of yellow fever at Rio de Janeiro, was admitted into hospital on the 25th July, 1851. He suffered from tertian fever for eighteen days, and some degree of enlargement of the spleen was noted. Dysenteric symptoms had been present for five days before admission, and there was pain of the abdomen on pressure at the umbilicus. While under treatment, the alvine discharges —from six to twelve in the twenty-four hours—are described as thin and feculent, passed with tenesmus, and occasionally with prolapsus. The tongue was coated, and latterly florid at the top. The febrile accessions occasionally recurred. He died on the 10th August. He was treated with opium and ipecacuanha, anodyne enemata, and the application of a small blister to the pained part of the abdomen.

Inspection ten hours after death.—*Chest.*—Both lungs collapsed freely. They were soft and crepitating, but pale, and adhered firmly to the walls of the chest. The pericardium contained about two ounces of clear serum. The valves and structure of the heart were natural. *Abdomen.*—The liver was of normal size; its structure healthy. The spleen was somewhat enlarged. A small portion of the omentum matted over the cœcum, dragged the transverse colon downwards, to the right side. The cœcum adhered to the anterior parietes of the abdomen by tolerably firm bands. The whole of the colon was distended by flatus. The mucous membrane of the large intestine throughout presented numerous ulcers of various sizes. The smallest was the size of a split pea, others—the largest—that of a dollar. Some were circular, others oval or transverse, and others were rendered very large and irregular, by the coalescence of several smaller ones. The base of all these ulcers was formed by the muscular coat. The mucous coat presented here and there a blush of redness chiefly around the margins of the ulcers. The sub-mucous coat of the cœcum was swollen by serous infiltration. The kidneys were slightly enlarged, but their structure was healthy. The bladder was much distended by urine, and reached above the pelvis.* The ureters were also distended up to the kidneys. The mucous membrane of the anterior wall of the stomach presented a blush of redness.

5. *The separation of Parts of the Mucous Coat in Shreds and Tubular Portions.*—The description of the processes by which destruction and sloughing of the intestinal mucous membrane are effected in dysentery is not yet completed. The mucous membrane of the large intestine is liable to be affected with a form of inflammation, acute and generally extensive, which, from the course it follows, and the appearances it presents after death, may reasonably be regarded as analogous in character to erysipelatous inflammation of the skin. It is commonly, but not exclusively, met with in Europeans who have not been long resident in India, and whose constitutions have been deteriorated by debauch and climatic influences. The mucous membrane is discoloured and swollen from exudation of serum and badly plastic lymph, which, also diffusively infiltrated into the sub-mucous tissue, quickly degenerates into sero-pus, and leads to gangrene of this tissue as well as of the mucous membrane itself. Hence the separation of patches and shreds of sloughy mucous tissue—often seen in the dejections during life, and found after death in various states and stages of separation. Cases 71 to 76 illustrate this condition of the intestinal structures.

71. *Dysentery.—Death in early stage by cholera.—Gangrenous patches of mucous membrane of large intestine, but no separation.*—A soldier of the German Legion at Poona, under treatment for affection of the bowels with bloody discharges, mistaken for hæmorrhoids, was seized on the 4th June, 1859, with cholera, at the time prevailing, and died.

Inspection.—The mucous membrane of the colon and rectum was somewhat œdematous; there were numerous large, grey-black, tumid, chiefly transverse, patches; none had separated, but some were very easily lacerable and gave out sero-pus, others were firmer. The intervening mucous membrane was pale, with enlarged solitary glands and follicles.

72. *Dysentery.—Sloughs of the mucous coat passed before death.—Much displacement of the colon to the left side. Abscess in the Liver.*—Joseph Slayman, aged thirty-two, a seaman, was admitted into hospital on the 20th August, 1840. He had been ill with dysentery for fourteen days. On admission the abdomen was tender, the skin and tongue were dry, and the pulse moderately full. On the 22nd there was tenderness of the left iliac region, with perceptible hardness. Throughout his illness there was a good deal of tenesmus. The abdomen was moderately full, and there was more or less dysuria. Dejections watery, brown, and with dysenteric fœtor. On the 4th, 5th, and 6th September, considerable patches of sloughed mucous coat were passed. There were no peritonitic symptoms during the last days. He died on the 10th September. *Treatment.*—He was once bled at the arm, was leeched several times on the abdo-

---

* The distention of the bladder would seem not to have been detected before death. This is an oversight which ought never to occur in the treatment of dysentery, as attention to the state of this viscus should be a rule of practice.

men, and around the anus. The abdomen was blistered. At first two or three doses of calomel with opium and ipecacuanha were given, then ipecacuanha, gentian, and blue pill, without purgatives; afterwards free opiates frequently repeated in combination with blue pill and ipecacuanha, or quinine and bismuth, according to the state of the pulse and skin. For two or three days acetate of lead and opium were freely used with partial alleviation of the symptoms. Light nourishment and wine.

Inspection eight hours after death. Body emaciated.—*Chest.*—Old adhesions of the right pleura; no emphysema. Viscera healthy. *Abdomen.*—The omentum adhered to the left lateral parietes, and had so dragged the colon from its natural situation that the cœcum was lodged in the pelvis and adhered to the bladder. The right iliac fossa and all the right side of the abdominal region were occupied by the small intestine. The ascending and transverse portions of the colon passed vertically in the mesial line, extended under the stomach, and formed various turns before passing into the descending colon; these duplicatures adhered to each other, and the intestine was laccrated in many places, in separating them. The mucous coat of the end of the ileum was healthy. In the cœcum there were hanging loose dark sloughed patches of the mucous tunic. Lower down the mucous coat had separated and been thrown off, and a pearly glistening surface was left, with here and there bands and isolated patches of the mucous coat tolerably healthy, and standing out in relief. The liver was enlarged, and extended into the left hypochondrium. It was mottled red and white; and in the right lobe towards the diaphragm there was an abscess about the size of a large orange, and about half an inch from the surface. The pyloric end of the mucous coat of the stomach was mammillated. The kidneys were healthy.

73. *Acute Dysentery.—Extensive sloughy ulceration of the inner surface of the large intestine.—Dark red grumous discharges.*—Charles Thompson, aged forty-two, a sailor of intemperate habits, who had been five years in the Indian Navy, and who had made frequent voyages to China during the twelve previous years, was admitted into the European General Hospital on the 17th July, 1838, after he had been ill with dysentery for five days. On admission the symptoms were not urgent. The skin, pulse, and tongue were natural. There was no distention or pain of the abdomen, or straining, when he was purged. The discharges varied in frequency; they were generally tinged deeply with bile, and contained mucus. As the disease advanced, the purging became more urgent, and tenesmus more complained of. The dejections were more mucous and scanty; latterly they became dark red and serous, and contained clots of blood. The pulse became frequent and feeble, and the skin damp. He died on the 11th August. It would be tedious to detail the varied and ineffective treatment that was pursued.

Inspection five hours after death.—Body not very emaciated. *Abdomen.*—The omentum extended over all the intestines, and in the hypogastrium and iliac regions adhered to the walls of the pelvis by fleshy vascular fringes. The intestines generally were of dark grey colour, and more distended than natural. The cœcum adhered by tender dark-coloured layers of lymph to the lateral parietes, and in these places the coats of the bowel were black, and tore readily. The tunics of the ascending and transverse portions of the colon were also tender, and the latter part of the gut passed the left side of the stomach, was applied to the diaphragm, and united by adhesions to the spleen. The descending colon adhered to the left lateral parietes, and, on attempting to separate it, the coats readily gave way, and dark grumous blood escaped. The sigmoid flexure of the colon, before turning to reach the top of the sacrum, had dipped more into the pelvis than is natural; it adhered to the peritoneal lining of the pelvis, and its coats also tore readily. The same lacerable condition characterised the tissues of the rectum; so much so that it was only separable in fragments. The whole of the large intestine was filled with dark grumous blood. The inner surface of the last two feet of the ileum was dark and red, vascular and softened. The coats of the cœcum were much thickened, and the lining membrane completely disorganised, was replaced by large dark purple sloughy shreds. In the transverse colon the ulcers were more defined, and where there was no ulceration, there the mucous coat was dark red, and softened. The condition of part of the internal surface of the descending colon, the sigmoid flexure and rectum, was similar to that of the cœcum. The lining membrane along the small curvature of the stomach presented marbled, red, extravasated patches, and was softer than natural. The liver was healthy. The kidneys were paler than natural. The thoracic viscera were healthy.

74. *Dysentery.—General peritonitis before the fatal termination.—Serous effusion in the head; no head symptoms.—The mucous coat of the colon in process of separation from the other tunics.*—William Anderson, aged twenty-one, stout, seaman of the ship *Lord Auckland*, after ailing more or less with dysentery for a fortnight, but much aggravated during the last two or three days before admission into the General Hospital on the 25th July, 1840, when the abdomen was full, tender, and resisting; pulse frequent and slightly sharp, but compressible. He was once bled from the arm, and leeches in considerable numbers were applied to the abdomen, so long as any tenderness remained. He was also blistered twice. Calomel in free doses with opium and ipecacuanha was given at the commencement at bed-time, followed during the day with pills of ipecacuanha blue pill and extract of gentian. The dejections were, for the most part, of light yellow colour streaked with blood, and generally passed without much tenesmus. The disease not yielding, mercury was exhibited, partly by the mouth, partly by inunction, with the view of affecting the system. On the 17th August he was under the influence of mercury, and an abscess formed at the right angle of the lower jaw. The purging, however, continued. Free opiates, in combination with bismuth, sulphate of copper, or acetate of lead, were given, and opiate enemata were used. On the 29th August the abdomen became tender, continued so, and became full and somewhat tense. The sinking increased rapidly, the purging continued, and he died on the 1st September.

Inspection five hours after death.—Head.—The vessels of the membranes were deficient in blood, and the substance of the brain was pale. Between the arachnoid membrane and pia mater, at the posterior part of the hemisphere, there was a thin veil of serum, and there was also about an ounce at the base of the skull. *Chest.*—The viscera were healthy. *Abdomen.*—The omentum thickened was spread over the intestines and adhered to them, and to parts of the abdominal parietes by a red-coloured fringe. The convolutions of the intestines, great and small, adhered to each other by flakes of lymph, and, on separating these, sero-purulent effusion oozed from among them. The end of the ileum and the large intestine were laid open. The mucous coat of the end of the ileum was healthy, and its contents were feculent and partly formed. The mucous coat of the large intestine was of dark grey colour and pulpy aspect, and throughout almost the entire extent of the bowel large patches were detached from the muscular coat. Between the mucous and muscular coats there was a yellow lymph-like lacerable layer. The stomach was healthy. The kidneys were healthy. Blood flowed from the liver where it was incised, and the substance of the viscus was in part mottled buff.

75. *Sloughy state of mucous membrane of the colon.—Sub-mucous puriform infiltration forming little cavities.—General peritonitis.—Matting of omentum.—Retention of urine.*—Mahdoo Suggujee, a Hindoo labourer, aged fifty years of age, and of feeble constitution, was admitted into hospital on the 2nd July, 1848. There was retention of urine, the abdomen was painful, and the pain was increased by pressure. He had also frequent calls to stool, and the discharges consisted of blood-tinged serum; he had been ill four days; he died on the 11th July. During the time he was under treatment the alvine discharges were frequent, consisted of blood-tinged mucus or serum, mixed with more or less feculence. The abdomen was full, doughy, or tense, with some degree of hardness in the right iliac region; was tender on pressure, and a

sense of burning was at times complained of. The catheter had frequently to be used. From the 4th the countenance was anxious, and dysenteric fœtor was observed. The tongue was more or less coated, the pulse was never above 92, at first well developed, latterly becoming small. Leeches were several times applied. The treatment was commenced with grains ten of calomel and two of opium, followed by castor oil; then ipecacuanha and blue pill were given at intervals, latterly combined with quinine. Turpentine stupes were applied to the abdomen.

Inspection twelve hours after death.—The abdomen distended, the body emaciated. *Abdomen.*—The small intestine was much distended from the duodenum downwards, and adhered to the abdominal parietes, and the convolutions to each other by flakes of lymph. The chief adhesions were to the pelvic walls and pelvic viscera, and over the descending colon. In the pelvis and in the lumbar regions there was a good deal of pus effused. The peritoneal surface under the flakes of lymph had a dotted red appearance. The large intestine was contracted. The omentum was matted over the transverse colon. The inner surface of the large intestine, throughout its entire extent, was of a grey black colour, pulpy, thickened, softened from disorganisation; and here and there apparently in the sub-mucous tissue were little cavities with ragged sides, containing grey fœtid, sero-puriform fluid.

76. *Mucous membrane of colon sloughy and separating in shreds.—General peritonitis and matting of the omentum.*—Enam Khan, a Mussulman water-carrier, of twenty-five years of age, was admitted into hospital on the 6th August, 1850. He was reduced in flesh. The abdomen was tense and generally tender on pressure, but more particularly so in the right iliac, epigastric, and left iliac regions. There was no dulness or induration. The skin was above the natural temperature. The pulse was frequent and somewhat irritable. The tongue was coated with a thin dark brown fur, and was florid at the tip and edges, but moist. The lungs and heart showed no signs of disease. He stated that he had been ill for a month with relaxed bowels, that at first the evacuations were thin and feculent, but after a few days consisted chiefly of scanty discharges of blood and mucus, passed with griping and straining; that for fifteen days there had been febrile symptoms, with tender abdomen. At the time of admission he was purged from fifteen to twenty times daily, and the urine was scanty and high coloured. On the 7th the scanty bloody mucus discharges continued, the pulse became more irritable, and there was hiccup. On the 8th the abdomen was more tense, full, and tympanitic, and he died at noon of that day. He was treated with quinine, opium, and ipecacuanha.

Inspection twenty-one hours after death.—Chest.—There were firm adhesions between the greater part of the pleural surfaces of both lungs. The substance of the lungs was soft and crepitating. The heart was healthy. Abdomen tense and tympanitic. On opening the cavity of the peritoneum, some gas escaped. The great omentum was contracted, and matted over the colon, and was also attached by tender lymph to the adjoining convolutions of the small intestine. The small intestines were somewhat distended, and at points of their contact with one another there were continuous stripes of redness, about one-third of an inch broad. There was also slight effusion of lymph between the uppermost convolutions of the small intestine and the transverse colon and stomach. There were five or six ounces of sero-puriform effusion in the pelvic cavity. The mucous membrane, throughout the whole extent of the large intestine, was in a sloughy state. It was detached from the subjacent tunic, and in some places hung in loose shreds. There was some mottled redness of the mucous membrane near the pyloric extremity of the stomach, but this tissue was otherwise healthy. *Head.*—The vessels of the membranes of the brain were a good deal congested. The substance of the brain was apparently healthy.

There is one form in which these sloughs of mucous membrane

are separated, which has given rise to some discussion among pathologists, and which therefore calls for more particular notice, viz.: the separation of tubular portions of several inches in extent. Of this lesion eight cases have come under my observation:— 1. In a soldier of the 15th Hussars in the European General Hospital in 1839. The slough, of about one foot in length, was perfectly tubular, and evidently consisted of the mucous coat of part of the intestine. Recovery took place. 2. Four in the Jamsetjee Jejeebhoy Hospital, with one death, and the result in the other three not known. 3. A gentleman, at Poona, in August 1859. The slough was tubular, nine inches in length, and death took place by hæmorrhage eighteen hours after its separation. 4. One in the practice of Mr. Sebastian Carvalho, the wife of a European pensioner, fatal; one with Mr. Bhawoo Dhajee, a Parsee female, pregnant four months. She miscarried, but ultimately recovered.

Dr. Stovell * thus records his experience:—

"In four cases there was separation and expulsion per anum of some portion of the mucous lining of the large intestines. In each of these cases the portion was about six inches in length, and in one of them it retained its tubular form. It occurred in the case of a seaman belonging to the ship *Euterpe*. He died two days afterwards. In a second case, the patient, a sergeant in the Ordnance Department, lived three months after the separated portion came away. The third case recovered. The fourth case was more remarkable. It occurred in a boatswain of the Indian Navy. The separated portion was twenty inches in length, the greater part retaining its tubular form. The membrane was passed on the 29th January, 1852; yet he lived till June 28th—five months. This was the largest portion of membrane which was ever passed in my care."

Of the twelve cases observed by Dr. Stovell and myself, there have been three recoveries, six deaths, and of three the result was unknown. In two of the fatal cases the result was postponed for three and five months after the separation of the slough. In only one hæmorrhage was present, and caused death.

The nature of the sloughs has been considered at great length by Haspel.† He adopts the view that they consist of mucous tissue, and quotes confirmatory cases strengthened by microscopic observation. Annesley was acquainted with this morbid process, but Twining would seem not to have been familiar with it; indeed, he almost doubts its occurrence.

Intus-susception,—strangulation, sloughing, and discharge—of part of the end of the ileum, consequent, probably, on previous destruction of the ileo-colic valve, may be confounded with the morbid lesion which has just been described. I have never seen an instance of it. Twining, in the course of eight years, met with

* "Transactions, Medical and Physical Society, Bombay." New Series, No. 3, p. 29.
† "Maladies de l'Algérie," tome ii. p. 78.

five cases; and in two of them recovery took place. Dr. Stovell* reports an interesting case of intus-susception in its early stage.

6. *The cicatrisation of ulcers.*—The cicatrisation of intestinal ulcers has been mentioned, by several late writers, as a process with which Indian pathologists are not well acquainted, but I cannot bring to my recollection the time when it was not as familiar to me as any other fact of the morbid anatomy of dysentery. It is distinctly noticed by me in papers published in 1832 †, 1833 ‡, and 1845.§

The stage of the disease when this healthy action may be expected to commence, and its duration, are points which it is impossible to foretell in any given case, because they are dependent more or less on coincident circumstances — as the state of constitution, the degree in which the process of repair has been promoted by judicious management, or counteracted by too active interference. It doubtless may be assumed that the less the constitution has been impaired, the more kindly cicatrisation will progress after it has commenced. Moreover, it is evident from some of the cases to which reference will presently be made — and it is a satisfactory fact, — that the repair of intestinal ulcers may go on under very adverse circumstances, such as the co-existence of abscess in the liver. The process of cicatrisation has been minutely and well described by Drs. Parkes and Baly. It consists of exudation and organisation of lymph with contraction of the edges of the ulcer. The appearances which it presents are illustrated by the following cases, 77 to 79. Also in 80, 81.

77. *Dysentery attended by general peritonitis.—The ulcers in different stages of progress, some cicatrised, one perforating, but patched up.*—John Murphy, aged eight, was admitted into the sick ward of the Byculla Schools on the 25th September, 1837, ill with dysentery. After ten days he had recovered, the gums having become affected from the moderate use of hydrargyrum c. creta. Shortly afterwards, however, the dysenteric symptoms recurred, but were slight. On the 17th November they had increased, and were attended with tenderness to the left of the umbilicus. The gums were still affected with mercury. From this time to the period of his death, on the 28th November, the symptoms were more or less urgent. There were frequent calls to stool, attended by tenesmus, and scanty discharges of blood-tinged mucus or serum. There was more or less tenderness of the abdomen, though never very acute; it was sometimes of the right iliac region, at others of the left, and unattended at any time with much distention. The skin was often hot and dry. The pulse ranged from 120 to 130, and was occasionally sharp and irritable. The tongue was generally clean and moist, but towards the end of his illness it became florid at the edges and tip. The

* "Transactions, Medical and Physical Society of Bombay." No. 10, p. 312, First Series.
† "Edinburgh Medical and Surgical Journal," April, 1832.
‡ "Transactions, Medical and Physical Society of Calcutta," vol. vii.
§ "Transactions, Medical and Physical Society of Bombay." No. 7.

treatment consisted of leeching and blistering, opiate enemata, opium combined with ipecacuanha, and with acetate of lead, &c.

Inspection six hours after death.—Abdomen.—There were three or four ounces of sero-purulent fluid in the cavity. The omentum was vascular, spread over the small intestines, and adherent to them. The peritoneal surface of the anterior parietes, that of the ileum, the sigmoid flexure of the colon, and the rectum, was dotted red, and the convolutions of the ileum adhered to each other by flakes of lymph. The sigmoid flexure of the colon and the rectum adhered in a similar manner to their opposing serous surfaces. The cœcum was thickened, and perforated by a small ulceration, which had been patched up by one of the convolutions of the ileum. On the inner surface of the cœcum there were large sloughy ulcerations, with much thickening of the subjacent coat, except where the perforating ulcer existed; and its bed was a portion of sloughy-looking lymph, lying immediately upon the peritoneal coat. The perforation existed at one corner of the ulcer. On the inner surface of the transverse colon there were puckered dark grey cicatrices, and also others, round, depressed, the size of a sixpence. Cicatrisation had commenced at the edges and the centre, but the mucous layer had not been replaced in these situations. About two inches above the sphincter of the anus there was thickening of the mucous coat; and for about an inch in breadth, and throughout the whole circumference of the gut, a portion of that tunic had been removed, and the muscular coat was exposed, and presented a shreddy surface. There was no ulceration of the ileum. The other abdominal and the thoracic viscera were healthy.

78. *Chronic dysentery.—Enlarged mesenteric glands.—Mucous coat of the colon firm and thickened. The cicatrices of ulcers.*—Abraham Johnson, aged twenty-eight, a seaman of the ship *Triumph*, suffered from chronic dysentery from July 12th to January 22nd, when he died, much emaciated.

Inspection.—Abdomen.—Many of the mesenteric glands were as large as an almond without the shell. The intestines were generally contracted. At the end of the ileum there was vascularity in transverse streaks, but the tunics were sound. The colon was in many places contracted; the mucous surface was in parts white, in others dark grey, and slightly roughened; it was firm, and adhered closely to the sub-mucous tissue. There were the cicatrices of several ulcers in the upper part of the colon.

79. *Pleuritis cured, succeeded by hydrocele radically cured; followed by rheumatism, succeeded by dysentery, cachexia, and recurrence of dysentery.—Colon ulcerated.*—Phillip Steer, aged twenty-five, a marine on board Her Majesty's ship *Endymion*. On the 25th June, 1841, suffered from an attack of pleuritis, for which he was bled largely. On the 22nd July he was admitted into the European General Hospital with swelling of the left testicle and hydrocele of the same side of ten days' standing. On the 2nd August the hydrocele was tapped and port wine injection was used. On the 23rd August the testicle was nearly well, and the fluid had not re-accumulated; but swelling, pain, and heat of the left knee (to which he had formerly been subject) came on and continued at times very acute, and with much febrile excitement; treated with leeching, colchicum, and mercurials. After a few days' steady improvement, on the 21st September dysenteric symptoms came on, and the knee-joint improved more rapidly; and he was discharged, free of complaint, though weak, on the 11th October. On board the *Hastings* he became affected with dysentery on the 25th October, and continued under treatment there till the 30th, when he was sent again to the General Hospital. He was reduced in flesh and strength, pulse 120 and very feeble. The tongue aphthous at the edges and coated in the centre; the abdomen collapsed, but without tenderness. There had been no return of the pain or swelling of the knee-joint. Sago and port wine were ordered, and an anodyne enema at bed-time. During the night he was purged frequently, the dejections being feculent and lumpy, and passed without griping or straining. Subnitrate of bismuth, four grains, opium one grain,

were ordered every four hours. On the morning of the 31st the purging continued; drowsiness came on with a febrile evening accession. The quantity of opium in each dose of the pills was reduced to half a grain, but the drowsiness increased to coma, and he died at 8 P.M. of the 31st.

Inspection twelve hours after death.—The body was much emaciated. The left knee in every respect similar to the right. The left testicle much wasted; no effusion into the tunica vaginalis of that side. *Chest.*—There were firm adhesions of the right lung to the costal pleura. The serous covering of the heart presented a general pearly appearance, with here and there opaque spots very slightly thickened; no enlargement of the heart. *Abdomen.*—The liver was pale and bound to the side by partial peritonitic adhesions. The intestines generally pale and washy-looking; and there were a few ounces of serous effusion in the cavity of the abdomen. The colon presented on its inner surface numerous puckered ulcerations, many of them in process of cicatrisation.

In cases of frequently recurring attacks of dysentery, appearances are sometimes observed which are best explained on the supposition that under the fatal recurrence the cicatrices of former ulcers have lost their vitality, and assumed the appearance of dark-coloured thin pellicles, some attached, some separating, and some detached, and exhibiting underneath a dark red or black, moist, infiltrated surface, with a layer of pale condensed areolar tissue interposed between it and the muscular tissue.

II. THE COMPLICATION OF INFLAMMATION, OR ITS RESULTS, OF THE MUCOUS MEMBRANE OF THE LARGE INTESTINE, WITH PERITONITIC INFLAMMATION, GENERAL OR PARTIAL. — Under this head are included, 1st, those cases of general peritonitis terminating in vascularity of the membrane, deposit of flakes of lymph on its suface, or sero-purulent effusion, traceable, perhaps, in some cases, though certainly only in a small proportion, to rupture of an ulcer and consequent escape of part of the contents of the intestine into the sac of the peritoneum. It is remarkable how very generally perforation of the intestinal wall, from sloughy or other ulceration, is patched by adhesions, and effusion in this manner prevented.*

2nd. Those very frequent instances of partial peritonitis which cause adhesions of the omentum over the transverse colon or the cœcum, to the margin of the liver or to different parts of the peritoneal lining of the abdominal walls,—the most common being over the transverse colon and in the neighbourhood of the cœcum.†

The first complication, when not dependent on effusion into the peritoneal sac, will be found generally to occur in persons who have suffered for some time from dysentery, have been previously in indifferent health, or who, not having had the advantage of appropriate treatment at its commencement, have experienced an exacer-

* Cases 58, 72, 73, 77, 80, 81, 82, 87, 96, 135, 178, 179.
† Do. 52, 54, 55, 60, 72, 96.

bation of inflammatory action terminating in gangrene of the mucous membrane. The second complication most frequently takes place in acute attacks, and is generally associated with thickening of the walls of the intestine, and sloughy ulceration of the mucous coat in transverse bands. Sometimes, as a result of omental adhesion, a tight band passing over the cœcum, and adherent to the iliac fossa, is found calculated by its pressure to obstruct the passage through the gut.

The following cases from 80 to 86 illustrate these observations; as do also 52, 54, 55, 60, 72.

80. *Sloughy ulceration of colon.—General peritonitis and matting of the omentum.*—Shaik Abdoolla, a Mussulman sailor of twenty-two years of age, using spirituous liquors moderately, but not opium, was, after four months' illness with bowel complaint, admitted into hospital on the 23rd August, 1850. He was much reduced. The abdomen was full and soft, and painful on pressure at the umbilicus. The tongue was moist and slightly florid. The pulse was 76, small, and easily compressed. He continued under observation till the 21st September, when he died. During that time the bowels were opened from six to ten times in the twenty-four hours. The evacuations were scanty, thin, yellowish, greyish, or greenish feculence tinged with mucus and blood, and passed with griping and straining. There was occasional evening febrile exacerbation. The countenance became pinched, the feet œdematous. The urine was of low density, but showed no traces of albumen. He was treated with opiates, astringents, and the application of small blisters, sago, milk, and wine.

Inspection seven hours after death.—Chest.—On opening the chest, both lungs were found fully collapsed. No effusion into the sacs of the pleura, nor any adhesion observed. There was some degree of emphysema of both lungs at their thin edges. The lungs were spongy in every part. Some degree of redness of the mucous membrane of the bronchial tubes was observed, but no dilatation. *Heart.*—There were opaque points of deposit on the inner surface of the aorta; also on the aortic valves, but not to the extent of injuring their pliability. *Abdomen.*—About eight or ten ounces of serum were effused into the cavity of the abdomen. There was a blush of dotted redness on the peritoneal surface of several of the convolutions of the small intestine, with effusion of flakes of lymph. The omentum, vascular and matted over the transverse colon, had a sloughy appearance at one part—that over the hepatic flexure of the colon; and under this sloughy part there was an ulcerated opening into the intestine. About the omentum, and also over part of the mesentery, there were greyish flakes of lymph deposited. *Pelvis.*—There were five or six ounces of serum in the cavity of the pelvis. Its peritoneal lining, including that covering the fundus of the bladder, was covered with thick yellowish flakes of lymph. The mucous membrane of the large intestine presented numerous ulcerations, some of them with soft and granular surfaces, in others more or less cicatrisation had taken place. The opening at the hepatic flexure of the colon was about the size of half a rupee. The kidneys were healthy. Liver of natural consistence and structure, but rather pale. The spleen was not enlarged. The brain was healthy.

81. *Sloughy ulceration of large intestine without thickening.—Commencing abscesses in liver. Peritonitis.*—Private W. H., aged thirty-eight, of Her Majesty's 40th Regiment, after two days' illness, was admitted into hospital at Belgaum, on the 14th July, 1830. There was purging, with much pain and tenderness in the course of the colon. Pulse full, frequent, and sharp. He was freely bled and leeched, and was free of pain for some days; but the purging continued, attended with tenesmus. The dejections

contained neither mucus nor blood, but were watery, light-coloured, fœtid, and filmy. On the 23rd there was again tenderness of abdomen. The symptoms continued unaltered. He died July 27th. No ptyalism induced.

Inspection.—The omentum adhered to both iliac fossæ. The peritoneal covering of all the intestines was vascular, and in some places covered with effused lymph. The ascending colon and commencement of the transverse arch adhered to the concave surface of the liver. The mucous membrane of the large intestine was ulcerated in many places. In the cœcum one ulcer had perforated the coats of the bowel, but effusion was prevented by adhesion to the abdominal parietes. Some of the ulcers had the appearance of commencing cicatrisation, and were covered with firmly adhering yellowish shreds. In no situation were the coats of the intestine thickened; on the contrary, they were generally thinner than natural. The liver, more compact and tougher than in the healthy state, was externally of olive colour, and in its substance some points of purulent effusion were observed. The gall-bladder was shrivelled and nearly empty.

82. *Sloughy ulceration and thickening of large intestine.—Matting of omentum. Dysuria.—Peritonitis of bladder.*—Private J. T., of Her Majesty's 40th Regiment, twenty-six years of age, and of slight make, was, after two days' illness, admitted into the hospital at Belgaum on the 30th May, 1830. He complained of tenesmus, and passed frequent scanty dejections, which contained blood and mucus. There was not any febrile excitement or tenderness of abdomen. He gradually improved, and was discharged free of complaint on the 14th June. He was readmitted on the 18th June with a return of his former symptoms. Still neither pain nor tenderness of abdomen. On the 22nd, however, slight tenderness of the right iliac region was present, but it was removed by the application of a few leeches. On the 26th he complained of dysuria. On the 27th the dejections were brown and watery. He gradually sank without return of pain of abdomen, and died on the 30th June. Ptyalism had not been induced.

Inspection.—There was evidence that extensive inflammation of the peritoneum had existed. The colon and rectum adhered to every organ in contact with them, the former to the under surface of the right lobe of the liver, the latter by more recent adhesions to the urinary bladder, and to the pelvic wall at the symphysis pubis. The large intestine throughout its whole course was thickened. The mucous membrane was much ulcerated, and in many places gangrenous. The omentum was drawn down like a cord of small vessels, and adhered firmly to the cœcum.

83. *Much sloughy destruction of the colon.—Peritonitis and matting of the omentum. Former attack of hepatitis.—Puckered fibrous bands in liver.*—Private B. M., aged twenty-seven, of Her Majesty's 40th Regiment, was admitted into hospital at Belgaum on the 22nd July, 1830. He had been ill in hospital with hepatitis from January 16th to January 24th. Had been well ever since, till three or four days before admission, when he became affected with purging of mucous and bloody dejections, and with tender abdomen. He died on the 6th August. No ptyalism. Tender gums.

Inspection.—The whole omentum, vascular, thick, and fleshy, embraced firmly the colon from the cœcum to the sigmoid flexure; and on attempts being made to separate it, the contents of the bowel escaped. In some places, where covered by the omentum, the natural coats of the intestine were entirely destroyed. All the intestines, great and small, were connected together in one mass, and adhered to the parietes of the abdomen. The liver was smaller than natural. Its whole surface, both convex and concave, was covered with depressed and puckered cicatrices, which, when cut into, were found to be firm and membranous. The liver adhered slightly to the diaphragm.

84. *Thickening of the colon.—Numerous deep ulcers.—Matting of the omentum. Liver with fibrous puckered bands.*—Private J. P., aged thirty-one, of leuco-phlegmatic habit, was admitted into hospital at Belgaum, on the 27th June, 1830, with ophthal-

mia, which terminated in obstinate opacity of the cornea with interstitial ulceration. While under treatment for ophthalmia, he complained for the first time of dysentery on the 9th October; but it was ascertained that he had been ill during the two days preceding. The symptoms were urgent. The dejections very frequent, mucous, and bloody, were passed with griping and tenesmus, and there was tenderness in the course of the colon. The skin was hot and dry, and the pulse frequent. He was treated in the usual way. Ptyalism was not induced. He died on the 15th October.

Inspection.—The omentum spread over the intestines adhered firmly to the cœcum, where that intestine was united by unnatural adhesions to the iliac fossa. At the points of adhesion the coats of the cœcum were black and tender. The walls of the large intestine, which were in general thickened, were at the upper portion of the ascending colon quite cartilaginous. The mucous membrane was ulcerated. The ulcers were numerous, defined, and deep. The liver was natural in size, but hard and much mottled; there were few adhesions, but the peritoneal covering of the organ was thickened and of pearly colour. Old firm adhesions attached the gall-bladder to the colon. Around the situation of the gall-bladder and elsewhere the liver had a puckered depressed appearance, as if from the adhesion of the surfaces of the cyst of an abscess. In these situations the structure of the liver was almost cartilaginous. The gall-bladder contained numerous concretions. In the chest the costal and pulmonary pleuræ were connected by old adhesions.

85. *Thickening and sloughy ulceration of large intestine.—Matting of omentum. Congestion of the liver.*—Private M. C., Her Majesty's 40th Regiment, aged twenty-eight, after suffering for thirteen days from pain in the epigastrium and right hypochondrium, on motion and pressure, was admitted into hospital at Belgaum on the 26th June, 1830. His bowels had generally been confined, but he had been purged the day before admission. The purging became more frequent. The dejections contained mucus and blood, then finally became watery and of a reddish brown colour. He sunk and died July 5th. No ptyalism induced.

Inspection.—The colon was distended, and its peritoneal covering was vascular, and had contracted adhesions. Those between the cœcum and right iliac fossa were pale and firmly organised. The omentum was very vascular, and adhered by one corner to the caput cœcum and right iliac fossa, so that the commencement of the transverse arch of the colon was drawn down towards the right iliac region, and a bend was produced in the course of that intestine. The ascending colon was more diseased than the rest of the intestine, and it adhered to the gall-bladder. The mucous membrane of the cœcum, ascending colon, and transverse arch, was not vascular, but thickened, and presented an irregular and softened surface, resembling the walls of a tubercular excavation. The liver was much enlarged, and contained much blood, but was free from adhesion or abscess. The gall-bladder was full of bile.

86. *Habitual constipation.—Colon contracted in parts and strictured by a band of the omentum.—Tubercular infiltration of the lungs.—Ulceration of the ileum and cœcum, probably from softening of tubercles.*—A lady of strumous habit and feeble conformation, aged about twenty-two, had whilst in England, for some years before her departure for India, suffered habitually from constipation, sometimes urgent, attended with fulness and pain in the right iliac region, supposed to be caused by fœcal accumulations. In January 1834, after a year's residence in Bombay, in the enjoyment of comparatively good health, this lady became the subject of a severe attack of dysentery, for which, about the end of February, she was sent to the Mahubuleshwur Hills. She was pale, weak, and very much reduced; the bowels acted irregularly, sometimes loose and irritable, the dejections being watery and containing mucus,—at other times confined for two or three days in succession, and then relieved by sudden and copious evacuation. The monsoon was passed at Poona, where her bowels were more irritable and relaxed, and where she latterly experienced frequent attacks of dyspnœa. Much

emaciated, she returned to the Mahubuleshwur Hills on the 31st October, and died on the 24th November.

Inspection seven hours after death.—The body was much emaciated and the abdomen collapsed. *Abdomen.*—The stomach was small and contracted. A band of the omentum reached from the first third of the transverse colon, passed across the cœcum, and adhered to the hollow of the os ilium. Underneath the peritoneal coat of the end of the ilium there were small miliary tubercles, and underneath that of the cœcum the tubercles were numerous, and of the size of a pea. The coats of the cœcum were much thickened, and there was adhesion to the hollow of the os ilium. At the hepatic flexure the colon was contracted, and formed a double angle; it then passed obliquely upwards to the left, became applied to the cardiac end of the stomach, and to the diaphragm; thence it doubled acutely downwards, and formed the descending colon, considerably contracted, but without thickening. The rectum and the sigmoid flexure of the colon were dilated. On the inner surface of the ileum, close to the ileocolic valve, there was a ragged ulceration the size of half a crown, with edges dark red, elevated, rounded, and centre irregular. The inner surface of the cœcum presented an irregular hard fungoid surface, the elevated parts coursing in transverse bands with an occasional intersection of longitudinal ones; their colour was dark red, grey black, in parts ink black; the colouring matter infiltrating deeply the thickened tissues. The mucous coat of the ascending colon was of dark red colour, and much softened. The mesenteric glands were enlarged, and had undergone tubercular degeneration. *Chest.*—Both lungs contained tubercular masses in a crude state, and adhered to the costal pleura at the points of tubercular deposition. Around the tubercles the substance of the lung was quite healthy, and collapsed, so that the tubercles stood in relief from the surface of the lung.

III. Tumefaction in the Region of the Cœcum or Sigmoid Flexure of the Colon. — The first is the more common, and is caused by matting of the omentum over the cœcum, with more or less thickening of the coats of the latter, or by thickening of the coats of the cœcum without adhesions of the omentum.* It may be caused also by intus-susception of the ileum. In case 88, perforation of the cœcum and effusion of its contents into the cellular tissue surrounding the gut, followed by gangrene of the abdominal walls, took place.

The opinion that the tumefaction is frequently caused by fœcal accumulation does not accord with my experience in India; and belief in the frequent occurrence of this morbid condition has, to my knowledge, led to serious errors in practice.

87. *Chronic dysentery.—A palpable tumour of the cœcum.—The lungs studded with tubercles not suspected during life.—Considerable effusion of serum in the head.*—Patrick Fox, aged forty-two, a pensioner, emaciated and of broken constitution, was admitted into the European General Hospital on the 8th March, 1839. He had served twenty-three years in India, had been pensioned two years and a half, and had, he said, generally enjoyed good health. On admission he stated that since the 10th of January he had been affected with purging; that at first the evacuations were scanty and slimy, but that latterly they had become watery; and that he had not used any remedies. The abdomen was not distended, but it was somewhat tense;

* Cases 87, 133.

and on pressure in the course of the colon there was tenderness, and over the cœcum a distinct defined hardness. The pulse was 92 and small; the skin cool; the tongue, coated yellow, was rough in the centre and florid at the edges and tip. There were in general eight or ten pale, yellow, watery, sometimes frothy, evacuations passed in the twenty-four hours, with dysenteric fœtor, but unattended by either griping or straining. At no time was there cough or other pectoral symptoms complained of. He died on the 22nd.

Inspection sixteen hours after death. Head.—About three ounces of serum in the cavity. *Chest.*—The lungs collapsed partially. There were old adhesions of the upper lobes of both sides, and a good deal of puckered irregularity of the external surface of the lung at the site of these adhesions. Both lungs and all the lobes were more or less studded with small grey tubercles, the size of a mustard-seed. At the posterior part of both lungs, these tubercles had become so numerous and aggregated that the tissue was almost impermeable. On the anterior part of the lungs they were scattered with considerable intervals. Here and there there was a small cavity, the size of a pea; and there were one or two nodules which, when cut, presented a pearly cartilaginous appearance. *Abdomen.*—The coats of the cœcum were about half an inch thick, firm and cartilaginous, with round tubercular deposition, intermixed · the inner surface ragged and ulcerated, and a perforation on the anterior aspect was patched up by the omentum. The rest of the colon was little diseased. The liver was pale, mottled, and softened. The stomach was healthy; so were the kidneys.

88. *Dysentery.—Perforation of the cœcum, with consequent formation of a circumscribed sac, with gangrene of the muscles and integuments.*— — Walker, private of Her Majesty's 6th Regiment, aged 28, after six days' illness, was admitted into hospital with dysentery, and died after a month. The bowels were generally very loose, and the dejections frequently contained clots of blood with dysenteric fœtor. The pulse was feeble and the skin damp. Latterly there was much defined fulness over the cœcum.

Inspection.—There was fulness of the right iliac region, with a dark gangrenous patch of the integuments about three inches in diameter; and underneath the muscles were found in a gangrenous state. Over the cœcum there was a circumscribed sac, about the size of an ostrich egg; the inner surface dark olive green, fœtid, and sloughy. The contents of the sac were dark olive green, watery, fœtid,—the evident contents of the cœcum which communicated with the sac by an opening of an inch and a half in diameter.

IV. Displacements of the Colon—are, 1st, of the commencement of the transverse arch. This is very frequent, and is produced by adhesion of the omentum to the cœcum or iliac fossa, causing that portion of the intestine to double down parallel to the ascending colon. 2nd. The transverse colon passing in the line of the great arch of the stomach, adherent to the left side of the diaphragm, and then doubling acutely down to form the descending colon, is a form of displacement occasionally observed, but not nearly so frequently as the one first described. I have witnessed it in four cases. 3rd. The sigmoid flexure dragged to the right, and adherent to the brim of the pelvis or to the bladder, is a displacement, also caused by adhesions, but it is not very common.

I would refer to cases 53, 60, 63, 68, 70, 72, 178, 179, as affording illustrations of various displacements of the colon.

V. Complication of Ulceration of the Mucous Lining of the Large Intestine, with Abscess in the Liver. — This is very common; but the subject will be more appropriately considered in a subsequent chapter in connection with hepatitis and hepatic abscess.

VI. Complication of Dysentery, with Morbid Lesions of the Small Intestine or of the Stomach. — When the small intestine is affected, the morbid changes will be generally found at the end of the ileum. They consist of ulcers more or less circular, originating in Peyer's glands; or in increased redness, with granular exudation, as already stated.*

In the following cases circular ulcers of the stomach were associated with similar ulcers of the colon:—

89. *Circular ulcers with sloughs in mucous membrane of colon and stomach.—No thickening.*—Mahadoo Mallee, a Hindoo flower-seller, of thirty-five years of age, of feeble constitution, in destitute circumstances, and often exposed to vicissitudes of weather, and occasionally indulging in the moderate use of spirits, was, after twelve days' illness, admitted into hospital on the 22nd June, 1850. During that time he had suffered from relaxed bowels; the evacuations at first had been thin and feculent, but latterly had shown traces of blood and mucus, and were attended with tenesmus and sometimes with prolapsus. Such continued to be their character during the time the patient was under observation. On admission, the lungs and heart were found to be healthy. There was some fulness of abdomen, but no induration. There was no febrile disturbance. The pulse was small, feeble, and easily compressed. The tongue was clean, moist, and pale. These symptoms continued with little change till the 25th, when the bowels became more relaxed; he sank rapidly, and died at 9 P. M. of that day. He was treated with quinine, in three-grain doses, combined with a grain each of ipecacuanha and blue pill, and latterly half a grain of opium, every fourth hour; and had milk, sago, and wine as diet.

Inspection seventeen hours after death.—Chest.—The lungs were collapsed and crepitating, but in parts old adhesions united the costal and pulmonary pleuræ of both sides. The heart was of healthy size and structure. *Abdomen.*—There was a small quantity of serous fluid in the peritoneal cavity. The liver was healthy in size and structure. The spleen was healthy. There were five or six patches of ulceration in the mucous membrane of the stomach; one or two of them were quite circular, with dark yellow or brownish sloughs in the centre; the others were larger, and more or less irregular, but also had central sloughs attached to them. The mucous membrane at the cardiac extremity of the stomach had a dark brown marbled appearance, but its substance was not soft. The mucous membrane of the large intestine, from the rectum to the cœcum, was studded with ulcers, with dark grey sloughy surfaces of different sizes,—the smallest being circular, and the larger irregular. There was no thickening of the coats of the intestine, and the mucous membrane was not more firmly adherent to the subjacent coat than natural. No ulceration of the mucous membrane of the end of the ileum. The kidneys were apparently healthy.

90. *Gray softening, with a few ulcers of the mucous lining of the stomach and colon.—Cicatrices of ulcers in the former.*—John Knapp, a private of the 4th Light Dragoons, aged twenty-two, who had suffered twice from dysentery in the year 1830, was, after two days' illness, admitted into the Hospital at Kirkee, on the 17th April, 1832. The evacuations were scanty, frequent, of light colour, tinged with blood, and passed with

* Cases 46, 52, 55, and 56.

griping and tenesmus. The iliac regions were tender on pressure. The tongue was coated in the centre and florid at the edges. There was occasional retching and vomiting, and frequency of pulse. He died on the 22nd. He had been bled; a blister was applied to the epigastrium; mercury with opiates was given. The mouth was sore, but there was no salivation.

Inspection.—There were not any traces of peritoneal inflammation, and no distention of the bowels. The mucous membrane at the end of the ileum was somewhat vascular, perhaps thinner, and peeled easily off with the nail. There was one ulcer in the cœcum about the size of a silver penny, not deep, and unsurrounded by thickening or vascularity. The mucous lining of the great intestine throughout, perhaps thicker than natural, of a light ash-grey colour, was here and there dotted red, and peeled off readily with the nail in shreds. The contents of the large intestine were green and feculent. The mucous membrane of the stomach, thickened and somewhat softened, presented there and here an ash-grey dotted red appearance, with the marks of one or two small cicatrising ulcers. The small intestine was not opened, with exception of the end of the ileum. The liver was healthy. The gall-bladder was full of bile. The thoracic viscera were healthy.

VII. Co-existence of Enlargement of the Mesenteric Glands with Dysentery. — An enlarged, reddened, and somewhat sero-infiltrated state of the mesenteric glands is not unusual in dysentery, depending, it may be supposed, on the increased flow of blood through the mesenteric arteries, which is probably present in this disease. These glands were enlarged in cases 52, 69, 101.

Part of the intestine chiefly affected. — On this point observers have somewhat differed in their statements. The tendency of the inflammation is to affect the entire mucous surface of the large intestine. In some cases it is general; in others present in greater degree in one portion than another, but very seldom exclusively limited to a particular part. The situation of the disease is noticed distinctly in forty-six of my fatal cases. Of these it is described as general in twenty-four; as predominant in the cœcum and ascending colon in fifteen; in the cœcum and transverse colon in three; in the cœcum and rectum in one; in the cœcum and sigmoid flexure in one; and in the transverse colon in two.

Concluding remarks. — My observations on the morbid anatomy of this important disease do not include any results of microscopic inquiry, for I have not any information from this source to communicate. A careful use of the microscope will, doubtless, give precision to descriptions of the discharges and of the exudation matter on the surface and in the interstices of the membrane, and serve to distinguish the tissues and structures affected in different forms of the disease. Still, making full allowance for this, and not estimating lightly the addition of positive facts to our knowledge, however unimportant they at first sight may appear, I must frankly avow that I do not anticipate much increase to our practical acquaintance with dysentery from this method of investigation; and I would venture to caution the young pathologist, when engaged with microscopic details, to take care that his mind does not lose the grasp of large principles of Pathology, Etiology, and Therapeutics.

SECTION III. — *Etiology of Dysentery. — Importance of distinguishing exciting and predisposing Causes. — Exciting Causes. — Cold, Food.—Predisposing Causes. — Cachectic States. — Action of Malaria discussed.*

In explaining the etiology of dysentery it is necessary carefully to distinguish between exciting and predisposing causes, for neglect of this distinction has led to much of the confusion which exists in the descriptions of this disease. I shall treat first of the exciting, then of the predisposing causes; and lastly state my reasons for dissenting from the common opinion that malaria is an exciting cause, and for believing that the important influence which it undoubtedly exercises in the causation of dysentery, is predisposing.*

Exciting causes. — The atmospheric states which unduly or suddenly depress the temperature of the surface of the body are the most common exciting cause. They consist of absolute lowness of temperature, of considerable diurnal ranges, of much atmospheric moisture, and of currents of dry or humid air. The action of these conditions is often favoured by imprudent exposure of the body deficient in resisting power in consequence of that lowered capacity of generating animal heat which is its physiological state in tropical climates.

My hospital experience shows that the proportion of admissions

* In a note on the pathology of dysentery, p. 237, reference is made to certain theoretic analogies between inflammation of the skin and that of the intestinal mucous membrane; and, in considering the causes of dysentery, these analogies are again suggested to the mind. Some inflammations of the skin — the eruptions of *measles*, *scarlatina*, *small-pox* — are caused by the reception of specific poisons into the blood. To apply a similar principle of causation to some forms of dysentery, and to suspect contagious or infectious properties, is within the limits of rational speculation. But it may be safely affirmed that such conclusions are as yet altogether without proof.

Again, it is sufficiently probable that the blood, vitiated by a specific poison, or by retained or altered excretions, may give rise to other forms of cutaneous inflammation — as *erysipelas*—or some of the *squamous*, *vesicular*, and *pustular* eruptions; and that this theory may also be reasonably applied to some forms of dysentery.

But, as it is not pretended that every inflammation of the skin is caused by the blood being vitiated in one or other of these ways, it is contrary to analogy to propose an etiological theory of this kind in respect to all forms of dysentery.

from dysentery is greatest in those months of the year in which the atmospheric state is most likely to be one or other of those which have just been mentioned; and in this category I am careful to include June and November, — months in which marked atmospheric changes occur in Bombay. In June the hot season terminates, the rains begin to fall, and damp winds to blow. In November the sultry heat of October ends, and north-easterly winds set in.

The following statement gives the proportion of admissions from dysentery per cent. of the total admissions in the European General Hospital, and the Jamsetjee Jejeebhoy Hospital at Bombay, in different seasons of the year: —

	European General Hospital.	Jamsetjee Jejeeb-Hospital.*
Cold months.—November, December, January	10·8	10·2
Wet months.—June, July, August	7·0	10·7
Transition from cold months. — February, March	6·3	6·4
Transition from rains.—September, October	5·4	8·9
Hot months.—April and May	5·1	7·2
Annual proportion	7·4	9·1

The same result is shown by the per-centage of monthly admissions, from dysentery and diarrhœa, to the total annual admissions from these diseases in the European General Hospital for the ten years from 1846 to 1856, and in the Byculla Schools for the seventeen years from 1837 to 1853. Thus: —†

	European General Hospital.		Byculla Schools.
	Dysentery.	Diarrhœa.	Dysentery and Diarrhœa.
January	12·470	8·172	5·634
February	5·827	5·836	6·933
March	6·177	8·300	8·422
April	7·266	7·652	7·769
May	7·266	6·485	8·956
June	7·342	9·597	12·633
July	10·839	12·840	16·903
August	7·459	9·987	11·565
September	5·827	5·966	5·753
October	5·447	6·255	4·922
November	9·440	8·819	5·634
December	14·685	10·116	4·863

* This column gives the proportion of dysentery and diarrhœa combined.

† The figures relative to the European General Hospital, are taken from Dr.

Unsuitable food — impure water included — may excite dysentery; but it is not a common cause.

Fæcal accumulation, and what are usually termed vitiated excretions, in the large intestine, may act as exciting causes of dysentery; but my experience on this point is not confirmatory of the doctrines of Annesley and others on the frequency and importance of these conditions: it is more in accordance with the opinion of Dr. Mackinnon, that fæcal accumulation is not a common pathological state in India.* The question is practically important, from its evident bearing on the use of calomel and purgatives, not only in the treatment of dysentery, but of disease in general.

Predisposing causes.— The exciting causes of dysentery cannot be justly appreciated unless we carefully note those predisposing states of the system which very generally determine their action. Therefore, in order to discover the causes of dysentery, it is not sufficient merely to regard the atmospheric states to which the affected have just been exposed, or the food, clothing, and houses with which they have been supplied. It is fully as necessary that we should be informed whether or not, and in what degree, they have been *previously* subjected to those various well-known influences designated predisposing causes, which are as essential to the development of the disease as the application of the exciting cause itself.

The chief predisposing conditions of dysentery may be thus briefly stated.

The European lately arrived in India, consequent on the exhausting effects of elevated temperature, or on the want of adaptation of food and habits to the altered assimilation and elimination induced by climate, has a state of constitution engendered favourable to the occurrence of dysentery, under the influence of exciting atmospheric conditions, and which is often still further favoured by imprudent exposure of the perspiring surface of the body. It is in

Stovell's report. "Transactions, Medical and Physical Society," No. 3, New Series, pp. 22—34. Those of the Byculla Schools, from my own notes, Table XXIX., p. 322. There is a striking contrast in the ratios of the General Hospital and of the Schools for December and January; but as respects the schools, the necessary data are incomplete. It is not improbable that a "strength," greatly reduced by absence in the Christmas holidays, may explain the low ratio in December and January. When we compare the column diarrhœa of the hospital with the conjoint column of the schools, the inference may be drawn that the high ratio of June, July, August, in the latter—is due to diarrhœa rather than dysentery.

* Treatise on Public Health, by Dr. Mackinnon, p. 314.

these circumstances that the erysipelatous form of dysentery is usually produced in Europeans in India.

All *cachectic states* of the system, however developed, are very predisponent of dysentery. So much so, that when they are present in considerable degree, a very slight exciting cause is sufficient; and when present in great degree, inflammation of the intestinal mucous lining is apt to arise, almost without appreciable exciting cause, — being, as it were, the closing act of the cachexia. Let me point to some illustrations of this position.

1. There is no more common cause of cachexia in India than malaria, and recurrences of malarious fever. It consequently happens that whenever persons cachectic from malaria are exposed to atmospheric states, which depress the temperature of the surface of the body, dysentery becomes prevalent and very fatal. Evidences of this etiological law, which have passed under my own observation, have been already brought forward in reference to the mortality from intermittent fever (p. 24), and it would be easy to add to their number. For example, the experience of the Himalayan Hill Sanitaria, as set forth by Mr. Grant and Mr. Green in their papers * on Hill Diarrhœa and Dysentery may be instanced.

2. Again, continued elevation of temperature, habitual residence in an atmosphere vitiated by excess of carbonic acid, or emanations from decaying vegetable or animal matter, or too much moisture, will induce cachexia; so will the habitual use of food defective in quantity or quality (scurvy), intemperance of all kinds, too much bodily fatigue, and the influence of depressing passions, as anxiety, fear, &c. A cachectic state may also arise from long-continued disease, from injudicious and too-prolonged antiphlogistic medical treatment, from mercury, and the poison of syphilis, &c.

3. The occurrence of dysentery in crowded barracks, transport ships, jails, standing camps, besieged garrisons, beaten and retreating armies, are illustrations of the importance of considering cachectic conditions in explaining the causes of dysentery. And, if the history of events of this kind be rightly investigated, the influence of cold or wet, from undue exposure, defective clothing, and houses, or of unsuitable food, or impure water, will always be evident, and prove the preventible character of both the predisposing and exciting causes.

The opinion that malaria is an exciting cause of dysentery may now be considered. I do not pretend to name all the able writers

* "Indian Annals of Medical Science," Nos. 1 and 2.

who have advocated this doctrine; but, amongst later authors, Dr. R. Williams, Dr. Baly, Haspel, Mr. Hare, and Mr. Grant may be mentioned.

The circumstances in which dysentery have occurred in my own field of observation have never justified the supposition that malaria was the exciting cause *; and the facts usually adduced in support of the contrary opinion have seemed to me to admit of a more ready explanation, either in the predisposing influence of malaria, or the exciting influence of the cold, damp air, which in marshy tracts frequently co-exists with malaria. It was to the cold, damp condition of the atmosphere that Pringle attributed both remittent fever and dysentery. He does not allude to malaria, to which since his time both fever and dysentery have been referred. When intermittent and remittent fever co-exist with dysentery, it will probably always appear that the conditions of malaria co-exist with a damp and variable atmosphere. But according to my belief malaria causes the fever †, and the cold damp air the dysentery: hence we can understand why the two affections may sometimes be associated, but also be frequently distinct.

It would be foreign to the objects of this work to enter into a critical examination of the arguments of those who consider malaria to be an exciting cause of dysentery. Indeed, the assumed facts are so generally wanting in precision, that it may be doubted whether practical profit could arise from engaging in the inquiry. Yet allusion may be made to some points which fail to make that impression upon me which they seem to effect upon others.

1. The fact that fevers and dysentery prevail in the same divisions of the Indian army, is not necessarily confirmatory of identity of cause. They who think otherwise forget that a "division" may refer to an extensive tract of country, and may present in different localities considerable variety of climate and of physical feature.

* On the contrary, the 4th Dragoons, who suffered much at Kaira from malarious fever, were little affected with dysentery there. At Belgaum, dysentery is a frequent and fatal disease; malarious fevers not so. Of the dockyard peons, so frequently under treatment in my clinical ward with malarious fevers, only two were received ill with dysentery.

† To prevent misapprehension, I would suggest a reference to Section I., and that part of Section II. which refers to mortality — of the Chapter on Intermittent Fever. It will there appear that full importance is attached to cold and wet as a determining cause of re-attacks in the previously tainted with malaria. My present observation relates to the previously healthy, and expresses the belief, that in these malaria alone excites the fever, but that the co-existing cold and wet, not the malaria, excite the dysentery.

Moreover, in the kind of statements now referred to, mention is not generally made of the months or seasons of the year in which the two diseases have respectively prevailed; hence we are left in ignorance whether the occurrence has been in the same or in a different season. Again, the character of the fever is frequently not stated; for example, Dr. R. Williams, in his work on Morbid Poisons *, places the Presidency division of the Madras army first in his list of instances of the prevalence and identity of cause of paludal fever and dysentery in the same district. Whereas, the fact is, that this division of the Madras army is singularly free from malaria; and of the fevers registered in it, the larger proportion is febricula, and not paludal.

2. Complication of intermittent or remittent fever with dysentery, has been of rare occurrence in my own experience, but it would seem not unfrequently to exist in other provinces of India and in other countries, and is then accepted as evidence that idiopathic dysentery is caused by malaria. In this conclusion, however, I am unable to concur. Elsewhere in this work it will be shown that remittent fever in the natives of Bombay is often complicated with pneumonia, but it has never on this account been inferred that malaria is an exciting cause of idiopathic pneumonia; yet the conclusion would be quite as logical as that which has been drawn with reference to dysentery from analogous premises.

3. When a person, tainted with malaria, becomes affected with dysentery, sometimes the symptomatic febrile phenomena evince a periodic character, and occasionally the dysenteric symptoms show a similar tendency; but in this we have no proof that malaria has been the exciting cause of the dysentery. A similar order of events has been observed in other inflammations, as well as in injuries, in the same kind of constitution. Though a staunch advocate might still insist that malaria may be the exciting cause of these other inflammations also, yet he will hardly maintain that the contused wound or fractured limb — which, equally with dysentery, may be accompanied by symptomatic fever of periodic character — can be thus accounted for.

4. Nor does the alternation of febrile accessions with symptoms of dysentery or diarrhœa — occasionally observed in persons tainted with malaria, and previously affected with intermittent fever — imply that malaria has been the exciting cause of the dysentery. The alternation of dysenteric symptoms with those of chronic

* Volume ii. p. 540.

laryngitis, of pulmonary affections, and of rheumatism, has from time to time come under my observation; but such facts have not been held necessarily to indicate identity of cause of these several affections.

5. Mr. Grant, in his interesting report * on the prevalence of dysentery and diarrhœa in the Himalayan Hill Sanitaria, while he attributes much to the cold moist atmosphere of these stations, yet believes that malaria is also influential as an exciting cause. The chief argument which he adduces in favour of this opinion is, that in other hill stations possessing analogous climates, as regards temperature and moisture, this tendency to dysentery has not been observed. Nainee Tal, Murree, Darjeeling, the Neilgherries, and Mahubuleshwur, are instanced as hill localities which enjoy this immunity. In respect to the four first stations I am not aware whether the experiment has been made of exposing cachectic persons to the influence of their cold, moist atmosphere; but in respect to Mahubuleswhur I know that the result has been similar to that so ably detailed by Mr. Grant, relating to Kussowlie, Subathoo, Simla, and Dugshai.

The sanitary station on the Mahubuleshwur hills was established with the view of benefiting the health of the sick European soldiers of Poona and Bombay. The experiment was made in 1829. Badly selected invalids were sent to the hills at the end of October, or commencement of November, with the following result: — The tendency of dysenteric and hepatic affections to relapse, and of soldiers cachectic from fever, mercury, syphilis, rheumatism, to become affected with dysentery or hepatitis, was so well marked that the scheme was very properly speedily abandoned and has not since been revived.

These facts were necessarily unknown to Mr. Grant, because they are not stated in Mr. Murray's interesting Reports † on the climate of Mahubuleshwur. These reports relate to an after period and to other sanitary objects. My information has been derived from Mr. Walker's official reports, or rather, I should say, that such are the deductions to be drawn from these reports. Mr. Walker was at the time medical officer in charge of the station. When myself acting in that situation from 1833 to 1835, I had an opportunity of consulting the records of the station, and have again very recently enjoyed this privilege through the courtesy of the Medical Board. It is not improbable that my conclusions may be met by statements

* "Indian Annals of Medical Science," No. 1, p. 311.

† "Transactions, Medical and Physical Society of Bombay," Nos. 1, 2, 5, and 7.

of an opposite tendency, but on this point I venture to suggest a caution. It is often forgotten that the characteristics of hill climates vary much at different seasons. The results which I have stated to have occurred at Mahubuleshwur, in November, December, and January, would no doubt have been observed in much less degree in March, April, and May.

In thus venturing to differ in part from the opinions expressed by Mr. Grant, I have not overlooked his remark, that attacks of dysentery or diarrhœa were not confined to persons in broken-down health; but this is merely to say that the exciting cause was adequate to produce the disease, irrespective of peculiar predisposition.

This discussion has been prolonged further than I at first intended or than its practical importance may seem to require. For it may be objected that when so much importance has been attached to malaria as a *predisposing* cause, the difference is rather of words than of facts. But there is surely more than this. The opinion that malaria, *in common* with many other causes, induces cachexia, and that this state gives a susceptibility to dysentery, enforces the importance, with the view of preventing the disease, of protection from the influence of such predisposing causes. While, on the other hand, the opinion that conditions of the atmosphere which abstract heat are the common exciting cause, enforces the importance of protection from their influence by avoiding exposure to them, and by attention to clothing, houses, &c., and this the more especially when we have to deal with cachectic individuals. To state the difference in still more practical terms, the just inference from the principles which have been here advocated is, that the cold season of all hill climates in India is liable to excite dysentery in cachectic individuals irrespective of the presence of the conditions of malaria; whereas the view that malaria is itself the exciting cause of the dysentery must tend to condemn only those hill climates in which the conditions of malaria are apparent.

SECTION IV.—*Symptoms of Dysentery.*

The division of dysentery into several varieties, the allotment of a particular name to each, and the attempt to distinguish the one from the other by symptoms, are not calculated to advance our clinical knowledge of this disease, or to strengthen our hands in its treatment. It is sufficient that, in respect to each case of dysentery, we propose to ourselves the following questions:—Is it recent or advanced? Does it engage much or little, and what part of the mucous membrane of the large intestine? Is it idiopathic, or co-existing with remittent fever? Is it simple, or combined with hepatitis, peritonitis, or other disease? What is the state of constitution; is it sthenic, or likely to be the subject of erysipelatous inflammation; is it asthenic from former disease, deficient food, or elevated temperature; or is it tainted with malaria, scorbutus, struma, syphilis, mercury, or retained excretions? What is the condition of the mucous membrane, — simply reddened, or thickened, or ulcerated, or sloughing?

I must assume that the clinical student of dysentery understands how, by inquiry into the history and by observation, he is to make himself acquainted with the diathesis of his patient; and I shall, therefore, in my description of the symptoms, keep in view chiefly the other practical points to which his attention has just been directed.

Variation in Symptoms. — The severity of the disease in a measure depends on the extent of surface of the mucous membrane of the large intestine, which is involved. The symptoms will also somewhat vary, according as the inflammation is in one part or other of the intestine. It may be chiefly in the cœcum or ascending colon, in the transverse colon, in the descending colon, or in the sigmoid flexure and the rectum. But in the severer acute forms of the disease the greater part of the surface is generally implicated.

Acute form in sthenic Europeans. — The symptoms of acute dysentery as it occurs in sthenic European troops shortly after their arrival in India will first be noticed. The disease in them frequently commences with a relaxed state of the bowels; thin feculent evacuations being passed with some degree of griping and general uneasiness of abdomen. The fact that serious dysentery in India may begin with symptoms differing little from those of an ordinary feculent diarrhœa is practically most important. It inculcates both on patient and physician the lesson of carefully watching such cases, with a view to the prevention of the disease *, or the detection of its earliest symptoms. Not a few instances have come to my knowledge of fatal dysentery having been permitted to develop itself from oversight of this simple rule.

It is probable that at this early stage there is merely increased vascularity of a limited portion of the mucous surface; and that as this extends, and passes into the more advanced stages of thick-

* The importance of watching these symptoms of diarrhœa with reference to cholera has been enforced elsewhere, p. 221.

ening, exudation, and sloughing, the characteristic symptoms of acute dysentery gradually evolve themselves. Thus the feculent diarrhœa may continue for two or three days; then the discharges become more scanty, but the calls to evacuate are more frequent, and attended with more griping pain and some degree of tenesmus. Now the dejections consist sometimes merely of portions of clear mucus more or less tinged with blood; at other times there is mixed with these bloody mucous discharges more or less feculence, generally thin, of various colours, sometimes natural in appearance, at others greenish and gelatinous. Or, instead of clear blood-tinged mucus alone or intermixed with feculence, the evacuations may have a slimy appearance like oil paint of various colours, yellowish, greenish, streaked, or speckled with little patches of blood: such evacuations are in general passed without much tenesmus.

In regard to the *diagnostic value of these different kinds of discharges,* they all indicate that the inflammation has not passed on to its advanced stages. When the evacuations consist of mucus clear or tinged with blood, passed unmixed, in small quantity, and with much tenesmus, it may be inferred that the secretions proceed from the inflamed mucous lining of the rectum and lower part of the colon, and are uncombined with those of the liver and small intestine; and that probably the disease is as yet chiefly confined to the lower part of the bowel.

When, however, the evacuations are more copious, partly of mucus tinged or not with blood, and intermixed with more or less thin feculence, — generally passed with some degree of tenesmus, — the case differs from the first, inasmuch as the secretions from the inflamed mucous lining of the large intestine are accompanied by more or less of the natural contents of the small intestine; and all — in consequence of the increased peristaltic action resulting from the more extensive inflammation of the mucous membrane of the large intestine — are passed rapidly through with tormina, and discharged. We may infer, then, that when the evacuations are of this latter character, a greater extent of the colon has become involved; and if such discharges take place with little or no tenesmus, we may further conclude that as yet the lower part of the bowel is little engaged.

But in applying these suggestions to clinical diagnosis it is necessary to caution the practitioner not to lose sight of the nature of the remedies which have been previously used. It is very evident that in the first supposed case — that in which the disease is chiefly confined to the lower part of the bowel — the action of a purgative will give to the discharges the character related to the second supposed case — that in which the disease has affected a more extensive and higher part of the large intestine. Again, a too free use of opium may give to the discharges of the second the character of those of the first.

In reference to the diagnostic value of the intestinal excreta, one general remark may be prefaced, viz., that I entertain a strong suspicion that much of the dark green, gelatinous, and other varieties of discharges which have been described by various authors, and to which much pathological importance has been attached, are the products of the excessive use of calomel and purgatives and not true symptoms of the disease.

Dysentery in Bombay and Bengal very generally commences with diarrhœa in the manner which has just been described, but sometimes it is otherwise. In the disease, as observed by me in Her Majesty's 40th Regiment, at Belgaum, the bowels were often rather constipated at the commencement, than relaxed, and there was a sense of fulness and uneasiness experienced in the course of the colon, followed after a time by mucous and scanty dejections. It is when the disease originates in this manner that the intermixed feculence may occasionally exhibit a scybalous character.

The further description of the symptoms will equally apply, whether the disease has commenced with diarrhœa or in the manner last alluded to.

Abdominal pain. — Associated with the frequent and morbid discharges, the tormina and tenesmus, there is a sense of uneasiness experienced in some part of the colon; and therefore in all cases of dysentery the abdomen should be carefully examined with the view of ascertaining in what situation this uneasiness is chiefly present. We must not expect to find the acute tenderness of idiopathic peritonitis, but rather a sense of soreness which is however distinctly aggravated by pressure. The extent and situation of this discomfort will indicate the extent and parts of the intestine affected. The degree of the pain will suggest the complication, or not, of general or partial peritonitis, and our suspicion of this will receive confirmation from the co-existence of tenseness or induration * in the neighbourhood of some part of the large intestine.

* In respect to a feeling of induration in some part of the course of the colon, it is necessary to offer this caution. If the abdominal parietes be thin, we may frequently feel the intestine indurated merely from being in a state of contraction. We must be careful not to confound this with induration depending on thickening or other organic

The clinical observer will readily appreciate the importance of symptoms of peritonitis appearing in the course of dysentery when he recollects that this serious complication attends only the worst forms and the advanced stages of this disease, — those in which there is sloughy ulceration of the mucous membrane with threatened perforation of the intestine. (P. 265.)

But in respect to the import of tenderness in the course of the colon as a symptom of dysentery, I must guard myself against being misunderstood. That degree of tenderness, tenseness, and induration related to peritonitis is a condition of an advanced and generally hopeless stage of the disease. In those early stages, however, when precise diagnosis is practically so important, a careful observer will be able to discover some *uneasy* part of the large intestine — caused by inflammation of the other tissues — to which his remedial means may be more particularly applied; but should he fail in detecting this symptom, he is not on that account to attach the less importance to the evidence of presence or severity of the inflammatory action derivable from the character and manner of the discharges alone.

Dysuria and retention of urine are occasional occurrences in the course of acute dysentery. They have been generally attributed to extension of irritation from the rectum to the neck of the bladder. Without denying that this may be the explanation of these symptoms (more particularly of mere irritability of the bladder), in occasional cases, yet the tendency of my own observation has been to regard them in a much more serious light. Retention of urine will very frequently be found co-existing with inflammation of the peritoneal covering of the bladder, — to be, in fact, an illustration of paralysis of the muscular fibre of a hollow organ, consequent on inflammation of its serous covering. (Cases 60, 82.)

Tenesmus. — In the account of the symptoms of dysentery usually given in systematic works, the straining, the frequent calls to evacuate, and the scanty mucous, blood-tinged discharges, are dwelt upon as the very characteristic phenomena of the disease. It is true that when the sigmoid flexure and rectum are the parts chiefly affected these are prominent symptoms. But in Indian dysentery the inflammation is very often principally in parts of the large intestine above the sigmoid flexure, and then, as already explained, the discharges may be more copious, and

change. The state to which I now allude is not morbid, and with careful examination and under this caution ought not to be mistaken for disease. I have observed it most frequently in the left iliac region.

scantiness and tenesmus be symptoms which attract little attention. All the best writers on tropical dysentery confirm this truth, and yet it often fails to correct the contrary erroneous general impression. It is because the fact that inflammation of the mucous membrane of the large intestine — dysentery — may be present without tenesmus or scanty mucous discharges, is so constantly overlooked, that cases of dysentery are very frequently returned as diarrhœa, and thus our statistical data vitiated at their very source.

General symptoms do not assist much in the diagnosis of this disease. The tongue is often white at the commencement, but it exhibits no characteristic appearance and is seldom much coated except in sthenic lately arrived Europeans in whom biliary derangement is also present. In the advanced stages it may become florid and glazed, or present other features related to the state and degree of constitutional disturbance. Symptomatic fever is generally absent at the outset of dysentery, and is often very slight even when a considerable degree of inflammation is present. The co-existence of well-marked febrile phenomena with the early stage of dysentery should always suggest the suspicion that the disease is not simple, but a complication of remittent fever. Then the course of the affection should be very carefully watched with the view of determining this question — a most important one as respects the system of treatment.

Symptoms of advanced stages. — Hitherto in my remarks on the symptoms — with exception of those relating to a co-existing peritonitis — I have had in view those periods of the disease in which the inflammation has not as yet passed on to ulceration or sloughing. The course of dysentery to these more advanced stages and to a fatal issue has now to be traced.

The frequent discharges continue, but they become more watery, brown in colour, streaked with blood, or they contain small floating clots of blood, or white shreddy-looking films, or patches of sloughy tissue. Then the watery fluid becomes still more tinged red, and the fœtor peculiar and very offensive. Febrile exacerbations now become distinct — the skin may be hot and dry, and the pulse irritable, or the skin may be covered with perspiration, and the pulse small and compressible. The tongue becomes coated in the centre and dry, the abdomen not unfrequently full and tense, and before the fatal issue some degree of muttering delirium is sometimes present.

When the dejections are serous, more or less tinged red, contain floating clots and shreds, and possess a strong dysenteric fœtor, we may infer that they have proceeded from an ulcerated and sloughy surface of the mucous coat of the large intestine: they also may be more or less intermixed with the secretions from the mucous lining of the small intestine and the liver.

The disease, as just described, may run its fatal course in from nine to fifteen days. In those cases in which death takes place most quickly it may be assumed that the inflammation has been erysipelatous in character, and has led to extensive gangrene of the mucous membrane. While, on the other hand, in those in which the several stages have been passed through more slowly, we may infer that the morbid state has been thickening, exudation, gangrene, and sloughing of transverse or other shaped patches of the membrane.

Hæmorrhage. — There are still, in relation to the severer and frequently fatal forms of dysentery, other symptoms to allude to. The discharges may contain dark-coloured blood in considerable quantity, constituting that form of the disease to which the name hæmorrhagic has been given. A reference to the detailed cases will show that in some (73, 128,) a considerable quantity of blood has been found in the intestine after death, associated with a state of sloughy ulceration. But the occurrence of considerable hæmorrhage from the bowels in dysentery, is a rare event in Bombay compared with what the experience of Mr. Twining, Dr. Raleigh, Dr. Mouat, and Mr. Hare shows it to be in Bengal. In some cases it would seem to be related to a state of ulceration, to the diathesis, — scorbutic or other, — perhaps to the co-existence of hepatic disease, as cirrhosis; but in others, the hæmorrhage would appear to present itself in the early stages before the advent of ulceration, and to be a transudation dependent on congestion of the mucous membrane, and an altered state of the blood: this state, I apprehend, generally complicates forms of remittent fever, caused by intense malaria, and is probably pathologically distinct from dysentery. It is not an inflammation, but passive congestion tending to hæmorrhage. This distinction is clinically important, for cases with red-tinged serous discharges (that is discharges which in dysentery proceed from a sloughy ulcerated surface, and are of most unfavourable prognosis), are sometimes unexpectedly recovered from. Close inquiry will, however, generally prove that these have not been of dysentery, but simply of congestion; and the diagnosis will chiefly rest on the fact, that in the latter the discharges occur early in the illness, and are associated with more or less of the symptoms of congestive fever.

The dangers of dysentery may further be enhanced by a complication of hepatic disease. But this subject, as already observed, will be treated of, with more advantage, in connection with *Hepatitis.*

I have traced the course of acute dysentery in its more formidable aspects, and must now follow that of the great majority of cases, to their more favourable termination.

The frequent calls to stool, the blood-tinged mucus intermixed with feculence, passed with griping and more or less tenesmus, and attended with abdominal uneasiness, may, under appropriate treatment, progressively decline, and health be restored. Under these circumstances we may infer that the inflammation of the mucous membrane had not advanced beyond the state of redness and turgescence, and that its texture had escaped uninjured.

Chronic form. — Instead of progressive recovery in this manner, the symptoms may continue with, perhaps, alternations of alleviation and exacerbation. The discharges, still frequent, may become gradually more copious, and consist of thin feculence, frequently of pale colour, and frothy, streaked with mucus and blood, or reddish serum, or speckled with small blood clots, films, and shreds, and be passed with some degree of griping, but very generally with little tenesmus. This change is attended with increasing emaciation, and the tongue becomes florid at the tip and edges, with sometimes a glazed appearance. The acute dysentery has passed into a chronic state. Or this chronic condition may take place without having been preceded by the symptoms of the acute degree — the diarrhœa with which I have said dysentery frequently commences, may continue and gradually merge into this chronic form. The reader, with these facts before him, will at once understand that long-standing diarrhœa and chronic dysentery are generally one pathological condition; and that, therefore, a large proportion of hospital disease, returned under the head diarrhœa, is in fact dysentery.

The pathological condition of the mucous membrane in chronic dysentery may consist merely of a state of increased redness of the membrane; or the tissue may also be thickened, and have granular exudation on its free surface. There may be various states and stages of ulceration, more generally, however, of the circular form, and with cicatrisation in different degrees of progress.

It is observed by an able writer *, "The second stage is said to

* "Elements of Medicine." By R. Williams, M.D., vol. ii. p. 553.

commence when pus appears in the stools, but it must be admitted there are cases in which the disease pursues a chronic course, and terminates fatally without any such appearance." When we consider the morbid changes that have taken place in chronic dysentery, the probability of the presence of pus in the intestinal canal, and its ready detection by the microscope, in the evacuations, may be admitted. But that the presence of pus in the discharges of Indian chronic dysentery is frequently suggested to the naked eye of the clinical observer, is at variance with my experience. Indeed, I am certain that in the numerous diaries of dysenteric cases written by me in Bombay hospitals, European and native, such terms as pus, puriform, purulent, applied to the intestinal excreta, will seldom be found.

In Natives. — In describing the symptoms of dysentery, I have not thought it necessary to distinguish the disease as occurring in natives of India from that of Europeans. Cases 54, 55, 56, 67, 69, 70, 75, 76, 80, 89, show that it occurs in the former in forms as severe as in the latter. The general description is equally applicable to both.

Section V. — *Treatment. — General Principles and Indications. —Detailed Remarks on Blood-letting, general and local, Calomel, Mercurial Influence, Ipecacuanha, Purgatives, Diaphoretics, Opium, Chloroform, Astringents, Tonics, Fomentations, Blisters, Enemata, Diet, and Change of Climate in Dysentery.*

General Principles. — The treatment of dysentery must necessarily vary, according to the stage of the inflammation, and the state of the constitution; and neglect of this simple therapeutic principle, has led to needless confusion and uncertainty. Success in the treatment of dysentery depends on the recency of the attack, and the judgment displayed in adjusting the remedies to the state of the constitution.

Early stage. — The indication in the early stage is to prevent the simply reddened and swollen membrane from passing into a state of thickening, ulceration, or gangrene. In effecting this it must be remembered that the amount of antiphlogistic means, which in some states of constitution may be required to prevent disorganisation, will in others be the most certain method of ensuring it. Nor are we to expect in inflammation of the intestinal mucous membrane the speedy and marked effects from remedies which sometimes occur at the commencement of the inflammation of other tissues, but must rest satisfied with steady, progressive amendment; for the contrary expectation is apt to lead to frequent change, and to the continuance of medicines after benefit from them has ceased and injury begun.

Advanced Stages.—After the early stage has passed, and disorganisation of tissue has taken place, it must be borne in mind that restoration to health can only be effected by processes of repair; and that the indication with this view is simply to place and to maintain the affected part, and the system generally, in the conditions most favourable for growth and nutrition. The means used for this purpose differ from those which it is often necessary to adopt at the commencement of the attack, in order to prevent lesion. Hence we cannot safely enter on the treatment of dysentery, unless we regard the period of the disease, and determine whether disorganisation has to be prevented or repaired. But these two conditions do not comprise all the contingencies of practice; for there is a transition stage, in which disorganisation, though in progress, has not yet been completed, and the period of repair has consequently not yet arrived. In this the treatment must partake of the transition character of the morbid action, and consist of a gradual change from the principles of the early to those of the more advanced period of the disease.

In my remarks on the causes of dysentery, much importance was attached to predisposing states of the constitution. It has also been stated that we may not hope to conduct the treatment of the early stages successfully unless we rightly appreciate these conditions of the system; and now I would advert to their importance in that period of the disease when recovery can only be effected through processes of repair. With a view to the restoration of disorganised structures generally, two leading principles command our attention:—1. Asthenic or cachectic states of the system are to be corrected; 2. The parts must not be unduly disturbed. It is true that in the instance of the external surface of the body various local appliances may also be used, but these are of trivial consequence, compared with the two leading indications; and in respect to parts removed from the sphere of our senses, the accurate application of local means becomes impracticable, and the attempt to use them is often of questionable expediency.

These considerations lead to the conclusion that the successful treatment of dysentery must always depend on a just discrimination of its stage, and of the state of the constitution. In the early stage the remedies for inflammation are regulated with reference to the diathesis. In the advanced stage the means conducive to repair are also selected with reference to the diathesis, and in recollection that the time required for effecting restoration — generally considerable — will vary according to the reparative power of the general system.*

When we reflect on the details involved in applying these principles, we can be at no loss in understanding how the treatment of dysentery is often complicated and confused, how it must always be unsatisfactory, and frequently injurious, unless these principles are kept steadily before us, and unless the further doctrine be admitted that in all inflammations of mucous tissue and in all chronic diseases time is a necessary condition of restoration to health.

What are the remedies which, if used with discrimination in the early periods of dysentery, are efficacious, but most of which, if used in the stage of repair, are injurious? Blood-letting, general and local; mercury; purgatives; ipecacuanha; opium.

What are the remedies which, if used with discrimination in the stage of repair, are more or less efficacious, but most † of which, if used at the outset of the disease, are injurious? Astringents; tonics; alteratives; opium.

Then what are the states of constitution which demand consideration, and modification of the details of treatment? The constitution may be sthenic, or in that condition favourable to erysipelatous inflammation; it may be asthenic or cachectic from malaria, scor-

* On the pathology and etiology of dysentery, pp. 237, 273, allusion has been made to a theoretic analogy between inflammation of the skin and of the mucous membrane of the large intestine. The question may be put in respect to treatment. Should future research demonstrate that inflammation of the intestinal mucous lining is various as regards its course and causes—as inflammation of the skin—will it not follow that the principles of treatment now inculcated for dysentery will become inapplicable and require complete revision? The true answer to this question will be found in a reference to the treatment of diseases of the skin. What are the principles applied to these? (*a.*) The prevention of disorganisation in the early stages by sedative means. (*b.*) The favouring of processes of repair in the advanced stages. (*c.*) Above all, the correction of the diathesis on general principles; for it is but in very few instances that we can pretend to a knowledge of means special to particular affections. True, local applications are of subsidiary use, and generally had recourse to with more or less advantage. But it is evident that whatever advances may be made in the pathology of intestinal inflammation, the safe and effective use of local remedies must always be very limited, for the simple reason that the great extent of the structure must always be hid from our sense of sight. The statement of such self-evident propositions would call for some apology to the reader were it not that I am desirous of guarding the practice of medicine in India on all sides from the rash and dreamy therapeutics of which I have seen much and read more.

† I use this qualifying term in reference to opium and ipecacuanha, which may be used under both circumstances.

butus, vitiated atmosphere, struma, syphilis, &c. Asthenic and cachectic states—always difficult to correct—are necessarily more so when an important part of the intestinal canal is the seat of disease; but in order to effect good and to avoid injury in medical practice, we must always keep before the mind a clear view of the whole subject, with all its attendant difficulties.

Having premised these observations on the *principles* of treatment in dysentery, I proceed to explain the *clinical details.*

The leading indications of cure may be stated as follows: —

1. To subdue increased general and local vascular action by blood-letting, general and local. To sustain vascular action, when too depressed, by tonics and stimulants.

2. To favour — by preserving unembarrassed the capillary circulation of all the organs included in the portal circle — the free circulation of the blood in the mucous membrane of the large intestine, with the view of maintaining the integrity of that tissue before inflammatory action has led to organic change; or of favouring the repair of lesions when they have taken place. This is to be chiefly effected by rest*; also by, in the early stages and in robust subjects, increasing the secretions from the liver and the entire tract of the mucous lining of the small intestine; and by, in the advanced stages, checking these very secretions when too profuse.

3. After ulceration or other organic change has resulted, to favour the processes of repair by attention to the state of the tissues implicated, and of the general constitution of the individual affected.

The first question which arises in the treatment of a case of dysentery is, whether the inflammation has terminated in disorganisation, and if so, whether the disorganisation has ceased to extend, and left recovery, if practicable, to be effected only by repair of tissue. In deciding this question, we must, in a great measure, be guided by the duration of the attack, and the character of the symptoms and of the diathesis.

If the disease be of a few days' duration, and the constitution of the patient not broken by previous disease, or long residence in India; if the abdomen be full, but not tense, the dejections frequent and scanty, consisting of mucus more or less tinged with blood and passed with tenesmus; if the tenderness of abdomen be not acute, the tongue white but not much coated, and little, if any, febrile

* The importance of the recumbent position in the treatment of dysentery cannot be too strongly inculcated.

excitement present, then we may hope that disorganisation has not taken place, and may be prevented, and that a cure may soon be effected by appropriate antiphlogistic remedies. In the application of these means, however, we must remember that inflammatory action, once established in a mucous membrane, does not admit of being checked in the speedy manner of which it is susceptible in serous and other tissues.

If, on the other hand, the disease has existed for some time*, it is probable that ulceration or other organic change has taken place, and that recovery cannot be effected unless time be allowed, and the patient be placed in the circumstances most favourable to reparative action. In the treatment of these cases there is much room for discrimination, because there is often difficulty in determining the precise pathological condition, and, consequently, the indication of cure.

I shall attempt to point out the leading distinctive features.

(*a.*) Cases in which the abdomen is distended, tender, and tense; the dejections frequent, scanty, passed with little tenesmus, and consisting of turbid serous fluid, more or less tinged red and of offensive fœtor; the skin coldish and washy, the pulse frequent and compressible; or the skin hot and pungent, the pulse thrilling and irritable, but still compressible, with the tongue moist or dry according as the first or second state of the skin and pulse is present. In such cases, generally of from ten to twenty days' duration, the disease will be found to have already occupied the greater extent of the mucous lining of the large intestine, and to have terminated in sloughing, extensive ulceration, and matting of the omentum over the colon and cæcum. Persons admitted into the European General Hospital in this stage and condition of the disease, have generally been sailors or others of dissipated habits, the residents in low taverns, either altogether neglecting the disease, or still more frequently adopting the vain and delusive course of attempting to check its symptoms by the use of ardent spirits. Cases such as these must, I fear, generally be regarded as hopeless. But though we may regret our inability of being permanently useful, we ought to recollect our ability to do harm. The kind of treatment — antiphlogistic — which, at an earlier stage, would have been beneficial, will under these circumstances, be positively injurious, and must expedite the fatal termination.

(*b.*) Under this head may be included all the variety of cases,

* It is impossible to be more definite because the state of the constitution influences the result.

usually classed as chronic dysentery, of duration from one to two months and upwards, in which ulceration of varying character and extent exists; or, instead of ulceration, thickening of the tissue with or without granular exudation, generally existing in states of constitution more or less deteriorated. It may be that the tone of the constitution has been sufficiently preserved, to make the chief indication of cure the mere removal of sources of irritation, and the placing thereby the injured structures in circumstances most favourable to restoration by the natural actions of the system. In such cases a tonic plan of treatment should be avoided, and a mild antiphlogistic course pursued.

(*c.*) But when the ulceration or other organic change exists in deteriorated states of the constitution, from whatever cause arising, then the cachexia must be chiefly considered under the certainty that, if it can be removed or lessened, the reparation of the disorganised tissues will thereby be most effectually advanced. Just as in external ulcers in similar circumstances it is vain to attempt to heal them by any other means than those which effect an improvement in the general system. When the cachexia, however, has been brought about mainly by the long continuance of the local disease, — the patient having been, in other respects, situated favourably, — then the chances of recovery are small. But in a great many instances other causes of general cachexia will be found to have aided the influence of the disease. For example, medical treatment may have been neglected, or too depressing, the patient may have been badly clothed, housed, or fed, or exposed to unsuitable air or climate: in these circumstances it is reasonable to expect benefit from treatment judiciously tonic, and from the removal of the influences which have operated injuriously.

The remedial means which have been chiefly used with the view of effecting these several indications will now be noticed.

Blood-letting, general and local. — The degree to which increased vascular action, general and local, may be subdued by *blood-letting*, general and local, must be determined in each particular instance by the judgment of the practitioner. The tone of the constitution, the state of the skin and pulse, the degree of abdominal tenderness, the duration of the attack, and the consequent probable condition of the mucous coat, — whether ulcerated or not, and whether complicated with peritonic inflammation, — must be carefully considered.

General blood-letting may be used with advantage within the

first two or three days of the attack in Europeans of good constitution, not long resident in India, and unaffected by the depressing influences of heat, moisture, or malaria, provided the pulse be of good volume and strength, the skin without coldness and moisture, the dejections frequent, scanty, and mucous, and the abdomen more or less uneasy on pressure. The benefit thus likely to result may be maintained and increased by the subsequent application of leeches, and the use of the other means presently to be noticed.

General blood-letting is seldom, if ever, expedient in the treatment of dysentery in natives of India. When the disease occurs in states of constitution asthenic or cachectic, whether in Europeans or natives, and has existed for several days, the proceeding is altogether inadmissible.

In cases in which, from the state of the system, general blood-letting is contra-indicated at the commencement of the attack, recourse may be had to the application of leeches, in numbers of from two * to six dozen, repeated more or less frequently according to circumstances. With the view of determining the part of the abdomen † on which they may be best applied, the situation in which uneasiness on pressure is chiefly experienced shôuld be carefully ascertained. It has been already said that asthenic and cachectic conditions of the system are contra-indications of general blood-letting; and when present in great degree they are equally so of local blood-letting.

Though the benefit derived from the abstraction of blood will generally be proportionate to the recency of the attack, and the consequent probable absence of ulceration or other organic change, still it is not to be inferred that the utility of the measure is exclusively confined to these circumstances. Though, from the duration of the attack and the character of the dejections, there is reason for suspecting the commencement of ulceration; still, if there be abdominal tenderness and much tenesmus, — the state of the pulse, the skin, and general system not distinctly contra-indicating, — we may have recourse to cautious local depletion in the belief, that

* These numbers relate to the Bombay leech, which is small; one dozen not abstracting more than about an ounce and a half of blood. The size of the leech varies much in different parts of India, and must of course always be regarded by the practitioner. In respect to proportioning the local abstraction of blood to stage of disease, and state of constitution, clinical experience and observation can alone teach this.

† On the comparative efficacy of the application of leeches to the abdomen or to the anus, I am unable to offer an opinion. I have been always sufficiently satisfied with their efficacy when applied to the abdomen.

though lesion of the mucous coat exists, there is also present an amount of vascular obstruction of the surrounding portions of the tunic, incompatible with repair, and favourable to an extension of the ulcerative action.

Though important in suitable circumstances, it is not to be supposed that blood-letting is always requisite in the early stage of dysentery in persons of good constitution. Cases frequently occur in which, from the recency of the attack and the mildness of the symptoms, the disease may be readily cured by rest, the removal of lædentia, a mild laxative, an opiate, and abstinence. These will be met with more frequently in natives of India than in Europeans; and in respect to the latter, the caution of not permitting the patient himself to be the judge of the mildness or severity of the attack cannot be too earnestly inculcated. The symptoms should invariably be carefully investigated, and the character of the alvine discharges particularly noted. This is a most important rule of practice, for the mortality from dysentery in India is increased by the patient's ignorance often leading him to make light of his illness, and by the physician's credulity favouring neglect of that complete examination of the case, without which there can be no safety in the management of this serious disease.

The *second* indication of cure, viz., to favour the free circulation of blood in the mucous membrane of the large intestine, by maintaining unembarrassed the capillary circulation of all the organs included in the portal circle, is most important, and to be held in view in succession to the abstraction of blood. *It is the indication which constitutes the chief object of treatment in the majority of cases.*

It may be assumed that when the capillary vessels of any portion of the portal vascular system are congested, and when in consequence the blood does not pass readily through them, then an important step in the removal of this state is to free the entire portal circulation, by augmenting the secretions which proceed from the arterial capillaries of the mucous coat of the whole tract of the intestine, as well as those which depend on the capillary terminations of the portal vein itself. In other words, to increase the secretions from the small intestine and from the liver, is the second indication of cure in the early stages of dysentery.

This principle of treatment is observed in the management of many affections of the lower part of the bowel, arising from deranged circulation, as in hæmorrhoids, and in fistula in ano. It is surely equally applicable in the treatment of dysentery — a deranged state of the circulation of the tissues of a higher portion of the same intestine.

How is this indication to be effected? Many of the remedies generally found efficacious in dysentery, as calomel, blue pill, ipecacuanha, and purgatives, act in this manner; but their influence has often been otherwise explained. By some (Sydenham) they are considered useful, because they eliminate a morbid material from the blood; by others because they assist the discharge of vitiated and acrid intestinal contents. But whichever theory be preferred, this practical fact remains, that the efficacy of these means is related to the recency of the attack and the state of the constitution, — that is, to the inflammation being as yet in great part in the stage of capillary stagnation, and to the quantity of blood in the general system being still sufficient.

On the use of calomel. — In persons whose constitutions are uninjured by former disease or other cause, it forms an important part of the treatment of the early days of the attack, after adequate general or local blood-letting, to give, at bed-time, a ten-grain dose of calomel combined with a grain and a half or two grains of ipecacuanha, and the same quantity of opium, with on the following morning from four drachms to an ounce of castor oil. The state of the tongue — whether coated or not; the character of the dejections — whether scanty or free; and the condition of the abdomen — whether full and resisting, or supple and soft — will indicate the expediency of repeating these means, or abstaining from their further use. When the abdomen is supple and soft, there seldom can be any necessity for full doses of calomel.

Though calomel in these doses is generally only applicable to the first few days of the attack, it occasionally happens that it may be given with advantage in more advanced stages, when the tongue is coated, the discharges pale and scanty, the abdomen full, and the general condition and strength of the patient not much impaired. In fact, in circumstances in which it is reasonable to conclude that the excretions are not free, and the portal circulation in consequence embarrassed.

The object in exhibiting calomel is to increase the secretion of the liver and of the mucous lining of the small intestine, but at the same time to be careful that it does not aggravate the existing inflammation of the large intestine. This latter injurious effect is to be guarded against by avoiding the frequent repetition of the calomel, and by combining it, when used, with opium. This caution is the more necessary when there is good reason for believing that ulceration has taken place; because the irritant action of the calomel is then more certain, and there is, moreover, in a lesion requiring time for its restoration less necessity for attempting to influence the abnormal circulation of the large intestine by a decided and speedy effect on the upper part of the portal circulation.

The treatment of dysentery by large doses of calomel repeated and continued for some time, on the supposition that they exercise a sedative effect * on the inflamed mucous coat, is, I trust, now obsolete in India. It may be assumed that this system, at one time strongly advocated, and generally followed, would not have fallen into universal disuse, unless it had signally failed of success. My own conviction is, that as a general method of treatment it is irrational and injurious.†

Calomel is seldom required in the treatment of dysentery in the natives of India.

Mercurial influence.—Though not related to the indication of cure now under discussion, yet the present is the most appropriate place in which to notice the treatment of dysentery by inducing the constitutional effect of mercury. The use of calomel, with this view, must be kept distinct from the cholagogue action, which has just been considered. It is unnecessary to discuss in detail the mercurial treatment of dysentery, for as a rule of practice, it has been generally and justly abandoned in India.

In theory, perhaps, it may be admitted that deposits of lymph in the sub-mucous tissue of sthenic individuals might be appropriately controlled by mercurial influence. Yet when we reflect, that ulceration and sloughing, consecutive on thickening, are sure to be aggravated by mercury, and further that the disease very often exists in states of constitution in which mercury is hurtful, we must acknowledge that the reasons for not applying this therapeutic principle in dysentery are just and convincing. I can further state, from repeated observation of the fact that individuals under the influence of mercury are very predisposed to dysentery: this is particularly true of the natives of India.

Doubtless the records of medicine abound with reports of dysentery cured after salivation. My earliest clinical acquaintance with

* This question has been already alluded to in my remarks on the use of calomel in remittent fever, p. 136.

† I regret to observe in Haspel's Diseases of Algeria, a distinct leaning to the treatment of disease by scruple doses of calomel, which as a routine system has proved so injurious in India, and in consequence fallen into general and complete disuse.

this disease was in the hospital of Her Majesty's 40th Regiment at Belgaum in the year 1830. The chief means of cure were free blood-letting and mercury. Many recoveries, of course, took place, and, to my inexperience, the treatment seemed efficacious. But the opportunities which have been afforded me, during the thirty years which have since elapsed, have enabled me to correct these erroneous early impressions, and to justify the adverse opinion which I now entertain on the mercurial treatment of dysentery.

On the use of Ipecacuanha. — Of the various remedies recommended in this disease, there is none so generally efficacious and applicable as ipecacuanha alone or combined with blue pill, or, in some cases, with opium, provided it be fairly tried and steadily continued.

This medicine, brought from the Brazils by Piso *, towards the end of the 17th century, was given by him in dysentery in drachm doses in the form of infusion. It was in more or less use throughout the 18th century, and about the middle of the century was much esteemed by Sir John Pringle, who gave it sometimes in scruple doses, at other times in five-grain doses, three or four times at intervals of two or three hours. Mr. Mortimer and other medical officers of the Madras army, upwards of thirty years ago, thought highly of it, and used it freely in scruple doses, combined with powdered gum arabic. Still more lately Mr. Twining advocated its use in doses similar to the smaller ones given by Sir John Pringle. Haspel also combines ipecacuanha in full doses with calomel in the early stages of the disease.†

The efficacy of ipecacuanha in dysentery has been attributed by some to its nauseant action, by others to its diaphoretic effect, and by others, among whom is Sir J. Pringle, to its laxative or purgative effect. It is to this last property that its efficacy seems to me to be due; and it is with this view that I have always used it.

* Waring's Manual of Therapeutics, p. 298.

† Since the publication of the first edition of this work, the use of ipecacuanha, in doses of from ten to ninety grains, has been advocated by Mr. Docker, surgeon of the 7th Fusiliers—(*Lancet*, July 31st, August 14th, 1858)—but he does not seem to have been aware of the extent to which the remedy had been previously used in large doses, both in India and elsewhere. Subsequent to the publication of Mr. Docker's reports, rumours used to reach me at Poona, from Central India, of the wonderful success attending the *new* method of treating dysentery by large doses of ipecacuanha. After what I have at different times written on this subject, I cannot well be charged with undervaluing ipecacuanha in dysentery, in doses related to the severity and stage of the attack; but I regret this returning cycle of indiscriminate use and praise which is sure to lead to injurious reaction,—that invariable result of extreme opinions in medical practice.

In the early stages of *acute* dysentery, after blood-letting general or local, calomel, ipecacuanha, and opium with laxatives, have been used on the principles already laid down, — then the most satisfactory course is to give ipecacuanha in the doses and combinations recommended by the late Mr. Twining, viz., from six to three grains combined with blue pill from five to two grains, and extract of gentian from four to two grains, every third, fourth, sixth, or eighth hour, and to continue it steadily till amendment takes place. The proportion of the ipecacuanha and the frequency of its repetition must depend on the acuteness of the symptoms. The duration of the treatment and the gradual diminution of the dose and of the frequency of its repetition, must be contingent on the rapidity and permanency of the amendment. It must also be kept distinctly in view that, whilst the treatment by ipecacuanha is being pursued, it is often necessary — according as the state of the pulse, or the uneasiness of the abdomen on pressure, may indicate the necessity — to apply leeches; and also — according to the character and scantiness of the evacuations, and the greater or less fulness of the abdomen — to give castor oil, occasionally, in moderate doses.

In dysentery in the natives of India, or in Europeans, when the disease comes under treatment at a more advanced stage or in a cachectic diathesis, it is often necessary at once to commence the treatment in the manner just described, omitting the preliminary exhibition of calomel and opium, and castor oil, as recommended for the earlier stages in good constitutions. We must be careful not to continue the blue pill, in combination, sufficiently long to run any risk of inducing the constitutional effect of mercury: in determining this risk we must be chiefly guided by the state of the constitution. In cachectic individuals the ipecacuanha and extract of gentian should be used without the blue pill from the commencement of the attack.

The addition of opium to the ipecacuanha, blue pill, and extract of gentian, will be considered in my subsequent remarks on the use of opium in this disease.

It is not often that it is necessary to omit the ipecacuanha in consequence of nausea and vomiting. Whether this immunity from the emetic action of the drug proceeds from the effect of the extract of gentian, as supposed by Mr. Twining, or whether from a tolerance induced by the disease, analogous to that of tartar emetic in pneumonia and of opium in tetanus, is of little practical importance. My own impression is that it depends on the latter cause, and that it will generally be found in practice, that when ipecacuanha disagrees, it is either because the disease is very mild — rather threatens than exists — or has been already removed by treatment; or because the dysentery is complicated with, and secondary to, some other serious disease, as abscess in the liver.

The principle on which the efficacy of ipecacuanha and blue pill depends, is, I believe analogous, but less in degree to that assumed of calomel and purgatives. They cause a moderately free secretion from the liver and small intestine, and thus tend to place the mucous coat of the large intestine in the state most favourable for the return of its deranged capillary circulation to a normal condition.

Though approving the use of ipecacuanha in these doses and combinations, the practice here recommended differs in one very essential feature from that advocated by Mr. Twining. I mean the absence of the daily exhibition of a dose of compound powder of jalap. My objection to this system of treatment will be more appropriately stated under the subsequent head.

On the use of purgatives. — To follow the exhibition of calomel and opium, as already advised at the commencement of attacks of *acute* dysentery, with a dose of from one ounce to six drachms of castor oil, is a necessary part of the treatment; and during the use of ipecacuanha and blue pill, to give occasionally smaller doses of castor oil, is also important. The chief indications, under both circumstances, are a scantiness of the dejections, and at the same time a full and puffy abdomen.

There is, however, room for the exercise of considerable discretion in the use of laxatives and purgatives in the treatment of dysentery. Given occasionally in moderate doses in suitable stages of the disease and states of the constitution, they assist very materially— perhaps are absolutely necessary — in keeping up a free exercise of the secretory functions of the upper part of the portal circulation. But, when carried beyond this limit, or when given in advanced periods, or cachectic habits, they not unfrequently increase the inflammation of the mucous coat of the large intestine, and thereby prolong and aggravate the disease. This error is very frequently committed.

At the same time it ought not to be forgotten that injury may result from neglecting the use of purgatives when required, and thereby allowing the contents of the small intestine to accumulate. The following case is an illustration of this: —

91. *Dysentery.—The use of purgatives too much abstained from.—The lower end of the ileum distended from thin feculence.*—John Smith, aged sixteen, admitted on the 23rd April, 1842, ill with dysentery of a few weeks' duration, tender abdomen and frequent scanty stools. Treated by moderate leeching, blister, ipecacuanha, blue pill, and gentian, and opiate enemata; no purgative. Pulse 120. For two days before death, considerable distention of abdomen. Died on the night of the 30th.

Inspection.—Matting of the omentum, ulceration and friable state of the colon. Small intestine distended with air, and the lower part of the ileum full of thin yellow feculence, and somewhat distended thereby..

By regarding fulness of the abdomen in connection with the character of the discharges, and taking care not to confound the former with the state of tension and distention, not unfrequent in the latter stages of bad attacks, and related to peritonitic inflammation or hepatic abscess, little difficulty will be experienced in deciding on the expediency of giving or withholding purgatives in dysentery.

These remarks have had reference chiefly to castor oil, for it is the purgative best suited for the disease. Still, I believe, that the course of treatment recommended by the late Mr. Twining, of a daily dose of compound powder of jalap in association with ipecacuanha, blue pill, and gentian, is applicable during the three or four first days, in some forms of acute dysentery; but that its longer continuance is under any circumstances a very doubtful measure, and under some, as when the tenesmus is very urgent or the secretions not scanty, an injurious one.

This caution in respect to purgatives in dysentery is unquestionably necessary in Bombay, and I believe that it is equally applicable to Bengal. Still it may be useful to remark that the treatment by purgatives, in the manner advocated by Mr. Twining, has appeared to me more useful in dysentery in European troops in the monsoon season in the Deccan than in the island of Bombay. I have also, in former times, used the same treatment with advantage in well-conditioned native troops in the cold season in the Deccan; and more recently (February 1844) at Gharra in Scinde. The latter instance was the more instructive, because this method had proved inapplicable to the disease in the same body of men at Hydrabad in the previous month.

It is important to keep these facts in mind, because in all probability difference of season and of climate may call for modifications in the treatment of dysentery, as in that of other forms of disease. It is not improbable that purgatives ought to be given more freely in drier and colder, than in moister and warmer, climates; but the state and amount of the excretions, and the habit of body ought always to suffice for determining this point of practice in individual cases.

It should, moreover, be remembered that benefit from laxatives is chiefly confined to the outset of the disease, and that nothing can be more faulty than the too frequent system of giving castor oil to every patient admitted with dysentery, as a matter of course, irrespective of his state or the stage of the disease. This routine practice is often hurtful and is altogether at variance with rational therapeutics.

Diaphoretics. — The maintenance of sufficient warmth of the surface of the body, and the avoidance of all risk of its depression, must be carefully attended to in the management of dysentery. But general diaphoresis either caused by internal remedies, or external appliances, as the warm bath, does not, in my opinion, constitute any part of the treatment of dysentery in India. Even were a perspiring state of the skin a positive benefit in this disease, which I very much doubt, still the practical disadvantage would more than counteract the gain; for free perspiration is apt to interfere with the thorough ventilation of the sick room, and to increase the chance of exposure to chills, when the patient is disturbed by the frequent alvine discharges characteristic of the disease.

On the use of opium. — Opium in appropriate combinations and doses is useful in almost every condition of the disease. It may be given with advantage combined with calomel at the commencement, with ipecacuanha, and blue pill in the more advanced stages, and alone or in union with tonics and astringents after the disease has become chronic.

The doubt in regard to the efficacy of opium in dysentery which was partially entertained by Pringle, and more distinctly avowed by Twining and Haspel, may be readily removed by attention to combination and to other points of treatment, as Sydenham well knew and explained.

The mode of action is probably the same under all the circumstances of the disease for which opium is suitable. It controls the increased peristaltic action of the intestine, and allays the distressing sensations caused by it and by the other effects of the inflammation. But, it may be objected, that opium given frequently in free doses represses secretion; and that therefore its use is opposed to an important indication of cure in the early and middle stages of the disease — the maintenance of a moderately free secretion from the small intestine and the liver. To the practice of giving opium alone in these stages this objection is just; but it may be obviated by, in the early stages, combination with calomel, and, afterwards with ipecacuanha and blue pill. Thus two important objects are effected. The irritation of the large intestine is mitigated by opium, whilst secretion is favoured by calomel, ipecacuanha and blue pill; and we lean to one indication or the other by varying the proportions of the ingredients according to the circumstances of particular cases. For example if, in the treatment with ipecacuanha and blue pill, the discharges are free and frequent, the tenesmus distressing, and the abdomen soft and supple, improvement will follow the addition of a grain or a grain and a half of opium to each dose. But, after a time, the adverse action of the opium may begin to appear, the secretions may become scanty, the abdomen rather full, and the tongue somewhat coated. Under these circumstances it will generally be better to omit the opium for a time and continue the ipecacuanha and blue pill, than to give a purgative, and then immediately resume the opium. For the better illustration of this principle extreme cases have been supposed; but between these there are many degrees which must be met by corresponding modifications in the treatment, such as by lessening the quantity of opium rather than by omitting it altogether.

When opium is given alone, or in union with tonics or astringents, in chronic dysentery, with the view of favouring the reparation of ulcers, or repressing excessive secretion, then its efficacy is still more evident, because both the sedative and astringent actions assist in fulfilling the indications of cure. Under these circumstances opium may be used in two or three-grain doses every third, fourth, or sixth hour with great advantage. It alleviates suffering and diminishes evacuation, and thus places the patient in the condition most conducive to his cure. The following case illustrates the good effects of full opiates: —

92. *Good effects of opium in the treatment of some states of dysentery illustrated.*—George Pemball, aged nineteen, of strumous habit, and slight frame, after eight days' illness with dysentery, was admitted into the General Hospital, on the 30th June, 1840. He was leeched two or three times, and blistered. Ipecacuanha, blue pill, and gentian, and anodyne enemata were used. He improved for a few days, and then fell off. About the 15th July he was in a very precarious state. There was much emaciation, the pulse was frequent and small, the tongue was florid, sometimes dry, and sometimes coated. The dejections were frequent and scanty, consisted of mucus and blood, were sometimes yeasty and offensive, and were passed with much tenesmus. From this time the treatment consisted of large opiates, combined with quinine, blue pill, or trisnitrate of bismuth. On the 28th July he began to take three grains of opium, with one each of quinine and blue pill, every third hour. The amendment was now tolerably steady and progressive, and the quantity and frequency of the opiate

was gradually reduced. On the 30th there was slight relapse, when four grains of bismuth and one and a half of opium was used every fourth hour with excellent effect. On 22nd August all medicine was omitted, and he left the hospital on the 24th in tolerable flesh, and with regular bowels. From the 15th he had chicken for dinner.

My remarks on opium have had reference to its exhibition in the form of pill, but I by no means undervalue its use by enema, in the manner usually employed.

Chloroform. — Dr. Lownds * has pointed out the good effect of chloroform, taken internally in a twenty-minim dose, in relieving severe tenesmus in dysentery. Dr. Stovell † also bears testimony to its utility. I have used it in several cases, and its power in allaying the pain consequent on intestinal spasm is undoubted; but I have observed that when repeated several times it is apt to create gastric irritation, indicated by a sense of heat at the epigastrium, and a florid tongue. Chloroform should, therefore, be only used occasionally, to relieve tenesmus or other symptoms of spasm of the muscular fibre of the intestine, when urgent. ‡

We have hitherto been engaged in considering the two first indications of cure (p. 291). The third remains to be noticed.

3. The *third* indication of cure has in view the repair of ulcers of the mucous coat. This, after increased vascular action of the mucous lining has been subdued, must be effected by tonic treatment in its most extensive sense — medicinal, dietetic, climatic — and by restraining the excessive discharges which are apt to exist in old cases in reduced subjects.

On the use of astringents and tonics. — In the advanced stages of dysentery, when ulceration exists, when recovery is only possible by processes of repair, and when the lesion is attended with free discharges from the bowels and a deteriorated state of the constitution, then as already stated the efficacy of opium is very apparent. Under the same circumstances, astringent and tonic remedies are often very beneficial. Of these the most common are acetate of lead, nitrate of bismuth, sulphate of quinine, sulphate of copper, preparations of iron, nitrate of silver, catechu, kino

* "Transactions Medical and Physical Society of Bombay," New Series, No. 3, Appendix, p. iii.

† Ditto, p. 32.

‡ The vapour of chloroform introduced into the rectum, is probably deserving of a more extensive trial than it has yet had in the circumstances for which opiate enemata are usually employed. It might be conveniently applied by means of the simple caoutchouc cylinder and tube, used by Dr. Simpson, for conveying the vapour to the os uteri.

If it be a therapeutic fact as stated by Dr. Simpson, that carbonic acid is anæsthetic and curative of foul ulcers, then applied by the same simple means it may be worthy of trial in chronic dysentery.

hæmatoxylon, pomegranate, Bael fruit, gallic and tannic acids. The metallic salts are, in general given, with varying quantities of opium, and on this combination much of the benefit doubtless depends.

Astringents and tonics, however, have hitherto been used with little discrimination, and further careful observation is necessary to determine the circumstances of the disease for which they are respectively applicable. All that I can attempt on this point is to offer some suggestions on principles and then to state the result of my own experience of particular agents.

Astringents are indicated only in chronic dysentery, and in the hæmorrhagic form of the acute disease. In chronic dysentery, ulcers or other lesions require to be repaired; and, for this, some degree of tone of constitution is favourable. Increased intestinal discharges debilitate the system; therefore we endeavour to restrain them by astringents. This is the simplest and probably the truest explanation of the action of this class of remedies in chronic dysentery; and should the astringent principle be in combination with a tonic principle, then the efficacy of the remedy will be enhanced.

A condition of the body fit for the reparation of lesions can only be brought about and maintained by suitable arrangements of the vital stimuli — food, air, &c. Medicines which favour the action of these stimuli, are named tonics; but they are very subsidiary to the vital stimuli themselves, and must always be used with much care, lest they operate adversely instead of favourably. This caution is especially necessary, in diseases of the alimentary canal; hence in the treatment of chronic dysentery there is risk of injury in unskilful hands from astringents and tonics.

The cachectic states associated with chronic dysentery are various. The special means at our command for the correction of special cachexiæ are limited, but they should be carefully studied with a view to their increase; for it is in this direction that the resources of medical art are most susceptible of improvement in the treatment of chronic dysentery. In illustration of this statement it may be observed that when dysentery is related to malarious cachexia, we may expect the greatest benefit from astringent and tonic preparations of iron, from quinine, and from a combination of vegetable bitter and astringent principles. When there is reason to think that the cachexia is scorbutic, we may turn with confidence to vegetable acids, and to astringent, tonic, and mucilaginous principles in combination with them. It is in this diathesis that the *Bael fruit*, lately again favourably reported of in Bengal, by Mr. Grant and others*, is probably useful.

My experience of the Bael fruit is limited, yet I may venture to entertain the apprehension that unless the states of the disease for which it is appropriate be carefully determined, the good which it is doubtless capable of effecting in suitable cases will be lost to medical practice. I do not suppose that physicians expect to find in the Bael, or any other article of the Materia Medica, a universal remedy for dysentery; but I have had opportunities of learning something of the state of popular credulity in the instance of the Bael, and of noting its tendency to exercise an injurious influence on rational treatment.

Still another remark may be made on such remedies, as pomegranate, Bael fruit, and others whose positive therapeutic properties cannot be great. There is reason to believe that sometimes the benefit is negative. The fact may be lost sight of that these kind of remedies are usually had recourse to after many others have been previously tried, and not unfrequently injuriously continued; and that, therefore, the benefit from the change may proceed from the removal of lædentia, not the application of juvantia. That this suggestion is not fanciful I know from experience. In dysentery in children it often happens that if opiates be unduly continued, the discharges become pasty and scanty, and the general state of the child deteriorates. If under these circumstances the opiates be omitted, and a weak decoction of pomegranate be substituted, speedy improvement may be anticipated. But in these facts, there is not proof of the therapeutic virtue of the pomegranate, but merely evidence of a want of skill in the previous use of the opiates. It is well observed by Cullen that the physician shows as much skill in determining when to leave off a remedy as when to prescribe it. There can be no doubt that a want of appreciation of the injurious effects of previous remedies is a great source of fallacy, in judging the true effects of subsequent ones; and to no disease does this principle apply more forcibly than to dysentery.

Acetate of lead has been little used by me in the treatment of dysentery, because the trials which I have from time to time made have failed to inspire me with confidence. To improve the general state of the constitution is an indication in chronic dysentery, but this result is not to be looked for from a salt of lead, and therefore the continued use of this agent must generally be inexpedient. Acetate of lead has, with a sad want of discrimination, been

* "Indian Annals of Medical Science," No. 3.

occasionally given in the early stage of acute dysentery with injurious consequences.*

Trisnitrate of bismuth, and *quinine*, have been frequently used by me, and often with advantage. But *sulphate of copper* is the remedy of this class which is most immediately and generally useful. It has been given by me in doses of from a grain to two and a half grains, with an equal quantity of opium, every sixth, fourth, or third hour, according to the urgency of the symptoms. The cases for which it has seemed most applicable, are those in which the dejections are very frequent, copious, often frothy, showing that the secretions from the small intestine are in excess, and not retained, for any time, in the large intestine. In the advanced stage of acute attacks with sanious blood-stained discharges — the evident exudation from an extensive, irritable, probably sloughy ulcerated surface — it is very proper to try either the acetate of lead or sulphate of copper, or any other astringent which may hold out the prospect of benefit; — but with a knowledge of the existing pathological conditions, it is vain to expect much advantage from their use.

Nitrate of silver, in doses of one to three grains, combined with opium, has been occasionally tried by me, both in Europeans and natives, but without evidence of its efficacy.

In respect both to the salts of copper and of silver, it may be said that as we cannot point to any particular cachectic state for the correction of which they are appropriate, their use must at present be regarded as empirical, and attended with the occasional risk of harm.

Of the *preparations of iron*, the solution of the persesquinitrate has been the most efficacious in my hands. With the sulphate of iron combined with opium I have been disappointed.

Of the *vegetable astringents*, gallic and tannic acids are the most deserving of confidence in chronic dysentery.

It is very doubtful whether any astringent can be used with much prospect of advantage, unless the tongue be moist and tolerably clean; and though in cases in which the tongue is florid, chapped, and dryish, it may be proper to give them cautiously, — because no other course is open to us, — still it should be done with much watching, and with no sanguine expectation of a good result.

* Opportunities of observation after my return to India have convinced me that this error in practice is much more common than I supposed, when I first expressed this opinion. It is difficult to understand how a system of treatment which evinces both ignorance of the therapeutic action of acetate of lead and of the pathology of acute dysentery can have originated.

In chronic dysentery the evacuations are often pale, sometimes almost of chalky appearance; but this is not an indication of the expediency of mercury, and not a contra-indication of astringents; for it not unfrequently happens that as the dejections decrease in frequency, their colour gradually assumes a more healthy aspect.

Should the bowels show a tendency to become confined under the use of astringent remedies, it is always better to intermit them, and thus avoid the exhibition of a laxative or purgative, which, under these circumstances, is apt to aggravate the disease.

The astringents which have been used with the view of restraining hæmorrhage in the hæmorrhagic form of dysentery, are chiefly the acetate of lead and the vegetable astringents. The most striking effects of this kind which I have witnessed were in the practice of Dr. Leith, from gallic acid and tincture of catechu — eight grains of the former and two drachms of the latter were given every hour and a half alternately, and port wine was at the same time freely used. The case was one of hæmorrhagic dysentery, with adynamic phenomena, in a European officer, and recovery was complete.

Fomentations to the abdomen, carefully used, are often useful in the early stages of acute dysentery, and materially aid the more important measures. The *wet compress* of the hydropathic system frequently proves a convenient mode of applying heat and moisture to the surface of the abdomen. In chronic dysentery the maintenance of an equable temperature of the surface of the abdomen by appropriate clothing, flannel bandages, &c., is an essential part of the treatment.

Blisters. — When symptoms of inflammation continue after local detraction of blood has been sufficiently employed, a large blister is not unfrequently applied to the abdomen; but my belief is, that blisters under these circumstances do little good, and, as they occasion considerable discomfort, I am averse to their use.

When, however, the inflammatory action is limited to particular parts of the intestine, as the cæcum or sigmoid flexure, — indicated by tenderness or induration, — and when, from the stage of the disease, it is probable that ulceration is associated with that inflammatory condition of the surrounding tissue which is favourable to disorganisation, and adverse to repair, — then a blister, of two to three inches square, is often useful in succession to adequate leeching. By this course the derivative advantages of the blister are obtained without the risk of constitutional disturbance.

The liquor lyttæ has seemed to me the most convenient epispastic.

Enemata. — When tenesmus is urgent, and pain at the lower

part of the rectum distressing, the local application of opium by enema, or suppository, often affords great relief. The addition of acetate of lead has not in my experience seemed to increase the efficacy of the opiate enema.

To these uses, and to the occasional exhibition of cold water enemata, my experience of this class of remedies is restricted.

The exhibition of large enemata in the treatment of dysentery, acute and chronic, has been lately urged upon the attention of the profession by Mr. Hare *, of the Bengal Medical Service. In acute dysentery a flexible tube is passed above the sigmoid flexure, and warm water, without limit in quantity, is then slowly injected by a powerful pump, till the patient complains of the distention, and the abdomen becomes visibly enlarged.

In chronic dysentery large enemata (six or seven pints) are used daily, with the view of removing acrid secretions, softly stretching the strictured parts, and applying emollient, astringent, or stimulant lotions to the diseased surface of the intestine.

Though unable to offer an opinion on this system of practice from my own observation, still it is incumbent on me to state the convictions left on my mind from a consideration of the subject.

In respect to large warm water enemata in acute dysentery, I would remark:—1. That, should a case of dysentery present itself in which there is good reason for believing that the large intestine is loaded with scybalous or other feculence, the advantage of removing these contents by a sufficient enema of warm water may not be called in question. But a case of dysentery answering to this description I have never seen, and, if a possible occurrence, it must be certainly so rare as not to call for notice in laying down a method of treatment of this disease. 2. That many cases of dysentery may recover well under rest, abstinence, and large warm water enemata, is not to be doubted; but such cases will recover equally well under rest, abstinence, three or four drachms of castor oil and an opiate, or even without these latter means. Therefore in such the enemata are unnecessary. 3. That the treatment of the severer forms of dysentery, in which thickening soon takes place, or the inflammation is erysipelatous—passing on to gangrene and sloughing, and secondary peritonitis,—can be much advanced by the application of fomentations to the affected mucous surface, is to invest this remedy, in respect to the intestinal tissues, with a therapeutic value which it certainly does not possess, when used in the same degrees and kinds of inflamma-

* "Indian Annals of Medical Science," No. 2, p. 485 and 495.

tion in other textures of the body. 4. That dysentery is caused or kept up mainly by the acrid nature of the secretions is a pathological doctrine from which I altogether dissent. Surely it is not when the secretions from the small intestine are passing copiously into the large intestine, and being discharged, that the symptoms of the disease are most distressing. Is it not rather when the discharges are scanty, and consist of little else than the mucous, bloody, or serous exudations proceeding from the inflamed membrane itself that we are chiefly called upon to palliate pain? and though it may be admitted, that under these circumstances the application of warm water to the intestinal surface may have a soothing effect, yet it cannot, on this account, be advanced to any other than a very subsidiary and occasional place in the treatment of this serious disease. 5. Under any circumstances of dysentery, to distend the intestine, — thus alter the relation of the mucous to the other coats, and do away with the advantage of rest, — is, I apprehend, a proceeding of very doubtful expediency. But when we recollect what pathology teaches us, that there comes a stage, often quickly, and not marked by characteristic symptoms, in which the coats of the intestine become friable, and sloughy apertures are closed up by tender patches of lymph, I would ask, what is likely to be the effect on such an intestine of water injected into it without limit by a powerful pump, till the patient complains of distention and the abdomen becomes visibly enlarged?

In respect to the use of large enemata in chronic dysentery: — 1. All that has been said in relation to the acute form on the removal of acrid secretions and the distention of the gut, applies also to the chronic form. 2. In the treatment of cutaneous ulcers, or those of visible mucous membranes, local applications are undoubtedly useful; yet they are subsidiary to general and constitutional treatment, and to the rest, position, and support, by which the local circulation of the part is favoured. Moreover, the degree of utility accorded to topical remedies is contingent on the ulceration being visible, — that is, on our ability to vary the applications according to circumstances, and to apply them with precision. Keeping these facts in view, and recollecting that ulcers of the large intestine are out of sight, I would ask whether the repeated use of large injections of solutions of sulphate of copper, alum, nitrate of silver, &c., are not as likely to be injurious as beneficial? It may not, I admit, be justifiable on these grounds, to dissuade altogether from the use of these means in chronic dysentery, because in the weakness of our art we must act at times on probabilities;

but I can have no hesitation in recording my opinion that they must at best be very subsidiary, always require to be used with caution and discrimination, and under a full appreciation of the leading importance of constitutional treatment and rest of the affected structure in the management of chronic dysentery.*

On Diet. — The principles which direct the medical treatment of dysentery must guide us in determining the diet appropriate in particular cases and different stages.

So long as the indication of cure is, by antiphlogistic remedies, to prevent disorganisation of the mucous coat, or to check its extension, the diet, as a matter of course, must be very restricted. When, on the other hand, the indication of cure is to favour the reparation of lesions, it must be recollected that the debilitated or deteriorated system cannot effect this without suitable nutriment. It must be supplied of that kind and in that quantity which the digestive organs, in part impaired by disease, are capable of fitting for assimilation. I need hardly observe that with neglect of this essential part of treatment, medicine must be utterly useless.

In arranging the diet for acute cases, in which antiphlogistic

* In medical writing I am most anxious to avoid the semblance of a controversial spirit, from the tendency which it has to obstruct inquiry and true progress, yet I cannot avoid noticing the subjoined passage with which Mr. Hare concludes his paper. To use the vague statistical data of Indian or other hospitals for the determination of questions in therapeutics, is an error which has exercised, and does still exercise, an injurious influence on the practice of medicine. The statistics of disease adequate for this important end do not as yet exist in India, or in any other country, except on a most limited scale, and they will require to be of a nature very different from that of ordinary hospital records.

To base on data altogether insufficient for the purpose an argument for returning to the treatment of dysentery by salivation, is, I think, very much to be deplored. It is advocating, on unsound reasoning, an injurious system of practice. Mr. Hare thus writes:—

"I must remark, in conclusion, on malarious dysentery, that if the above treatment by injections be not adopted, statistical facts of the most undoubted kind prove the necessity of our returning without delay to the salivating system. For the returns of the largest and longest established dysenteric hospital in the world, show, that since mercury has been avoided, the mortality has been double, for many years' continuance, what it was when salivation was sought for, as the first and only object of treatment; and to complete the remarkable proof of the importance of mercury (if my system by quinine and injections be not received), these statistics clearly show, that as mercury has gradually been disused, so the mortality has correspondingly increased. If statistics then, are, as they ought to be, our only guide to rational practice, our path is clear, —we must return to salivation till some more successful method be discovered. But the fact that in treating 346 cases in Calcutta, I had but $4\frac{3}{4}$ per cent. deaths, will, I hope, induce a trial of large injections by others, and thus prevent the necessity of resorting to the more injurious remedy—mercury."

remedies are indicated by the stage of the disease and the state of the constitution, there is no difficulty. Thin farinaceous solutions in small quantity from time to time are the only food that is necessary or safe: and as recovery advances, the change to more nutritive food must be cautiously made.

But when the constitution is asthenic or cachectic, and organic lesion exists, then the adjustment of the diet will require all the judgment and skill of the physician; and, in regulating it, he must be guided by his knowledge of the principles of physiology and pathology, and of the digestibility and nutritive value of different articles of food. Those from which selection may be made are farinaceous solutions and jellies, milk, animal broths and jellies, solid farinacea and animal food. When a scorbutic diathesis is suspected *, then the usual special modification of diet will be necessary: it is in such states that ripe grapes have been given at the Cape of Good Hope and elsewhere with advantage. In the use of wine we must be also regulated by general principles: it will be sometimes useful; but, on the whole, the error of undue use is more frequent than that of abstinence.

The affectation and empiricism of regarding particular articles of food as of universal application must be avoided, and we should keep always before us the golden rule, — when the indication is to restore injured structures by nutrition, — not to overtask the digestive and assimilating powers of the weakened system; and further we must recollect that, in dysentery it is a part of the organs of digestion that is structurally impaired.

On Change of Air and of Climate. — In considering the causes of dysentery, importance was attached to conditions of the atmosphere as predisposing or exciting causes.

If an atmosphere, loaded with moisture, or vitiated by malaria or emanations from decomposing vegetable and animal matter or excess of carbonic acid, favours the onset of the disease, then removal from these influences is essential to success in treatment. But the physician, in applying this principle, will sometimes have to exercise much judgment and discretion, in balancing the advantages of rest and medical care and the disadvantages of local influences, against the evils of the excitement of motion and less careful treatment. On the whole, however, this difficulty will not often arise; for the benefit from rest and careful medical treatment

* I use the term "suspected" because there can be no question that the scorbutic diathesis exists long before its presence is made certain by spongy gums and subcutaneous extravasations.

at the commencement of acute dysentery is so unquestionable, that we are not justified in withholding it unless the evidence of injurious conditions of the locality be very clear. This remark applies to such change of air as involves a journey and the interruption of medical treatment, — not to that merely from one house or room to another; for in this, as in all other diseases, the removal of the sick from confined houses and ground-floor apartments to those that are well ventilated and elevated, is an advantage which should be secured whenever practicable.

It may be laid down, then, as a rule subject to very few exceptions, that, in the management of acute dysentery, rest and watchful medical treatment are to be enjoined; and the excitement and disturbance of travelling and the interruption of medical care strongly dissuaded from.

But to what extent are we to expect benefit from change of climate in chronic dysentery? If the climate, in which the patient resides, is adverse to processes of repair — is not tonic in its general influence—but from malaria, moisture, or continued elevation of temperature, exercises a depressant influence on the vital actions, then removal from such climate is a leading indication of cure.

In selecting a climate suitable for such cases, we must be careful, while we aim at securing a temperate and pure atmosphere, to avoid considerable and sudden reductions of heat, by absolute lowness of temperature, winds, or varying states of atmospheric moisture. Resort to the Hill Sanitaria in India, more particularly in the cold season of the year, is, on these accounts, generally unsuitable in this disease. In removing to other countries, the season of the year and the character of their climate, in respect to these atmospheric conditions, must be carefully considered; and if they cannot be altogether avoided, the risk of injury must, as far as practicable, be obviated by great attention to clothing and avoidance of exposure. A cold moist air is the most injurious.

The means by which the change is to be effected are also very important, for exposure to the excitement of motion, unsuitable food, confined and vitiated air, in the passage from one country to another, are injurious influences, often overlooked, but which the physician must never neglect in recommending change of climate. For example, the efficacy in chronic dysentery of a sea voyage in temperate latitudes, in a comfortable roomy ship, is undoubted. From the diminished alvine and urinary excretion, observed in persons at sea, we may infer that there is a corresponding increase of pulmonary and cutaneous elimination; and that the benefit derivable from a sea voyage, in affections of the bowels, is perhaps in part to be explained by this altered relation of the eliminatory processes, and the fuller influence of oxygen which is involved in it. But this advantage of sea air is in a great measure neutralised in the overland journey from India as now conducted. The invalid has to contend with the adverse influences of the discomfort of the coaling stations, the fatigue and excitement of the journey through Egypt, the unsuitable dietaries, and the overcrowded and badly ventilated cabins. These are all serious evils *, and are sure to operate injuriously on those who journey from India by this route, in any but a state of advanced convalescence.

Section VI. — *Dysentery in Children in India.*

My opportunities of studying the morbid anatomy of dysentery in young children have been limited, and I am unable to say to what extent the sloughy disorganisation, common in the adult, occurs in the early periods of life.

The general description of the symptoms, and the principles laid down in respect to the causes and the treatment, apply equally to all ages.

In regard to the treatment, it may be further observed, that in the child the abstraction of blood is inexpedient, and the necessity of it is best obviated by early and careful watching, and by such judicious use of other means as shall prevent the disease passing to that degree of severity which may require the application of leeches.

Caution in the use of calomel is as applicable to the child as to the adult. It can only be requisite in sthenic children, and then merely at the commencement of the attack, in small doses, combined with ipecacuanha, and not repeated above two or three times. Fomentations or the wet compress are very useful in the acute dysentery of children. The indication for the use of castor oil, in small doses, and the cautions against its abuse, are the same as those laid down in respect to the adult; with perhaps this modification, that a greater degree of alvine excretion is physiological

* I venture on this statement from having been a passenger in 1853, in three of the vessels of the Peninsular and Oriental Company, on the Suez and Calcutta line, and in two between Bombay and Ceylon. Also in 1854 from Bombay to Suez, in one of the Hon. East India Company's vessels: in this the adverse influences complained of were still more apparent. Again from Suez to Bombay in 1856, and Bombay to Suez in 1859, in the Peninsular and Oriental Company's vessels.

during the season of growth, and that this fact should not be lost sight of in using laxatives.

Ipecacuanha, given in the manner already recommended, is fully as valuable a remedy in the treatment of dysentery in the child as in the adult. It may be combined with blue pill and extract of gentian, and be given, rubbed up with a little aromatic water; or the extract of gentian may be dried, and chalk and mercury substituted for the blue pill, and the compound prescribed in the form of powder. If opium be indicated, a suitable proportion of Dover's powder may be added. For a child between two and three years of age, two grains of ipecacuanha will be a suitable dose in the acute disease. It may be increased or lessened according to the constitution of the child, the acuteness of the symptoms, and the tolerance of the remedy. The following case illustrates the efficacy of the ipecacuanha in the treatment of dysentery in childhood:—

93. *Acute dysentery in a child.— Treated with ipecacuanha and blue pill.* — Charles Bowen, a European child, of three years of age, after suffering from dysenteric symptoms for fifteen days, was received into hospital on the 9th December, 1851. The calls to stool were very frequent; the evacuations were scanty, consisted of blood-tinged mucus, and were passed with straining and prolapsus. The skin was dry, and above the natural temperature; the tongue was white; there was no fulness of abdomen, and he did not acknowledge abdominal tenderness. Two grains of ipecacuanha three of extract of gentian, Dover's powder, and blue pill, each one grain, were given every third hour. The hip-bath and fomentations were used, and the diet consisted chiefly of sago. The improvement was rapid: the stools became less frequent, more copious, feculent; passed with less straining and no prolapsus. The Dover's powder was omitted and the medicine was continued at longer intervals. He was discharged well on the 15th.

Opium in the form of Dover's powder, or the compound chalk powder with opium, is also beneficial in the treatment of dysentery in children, and the principles laid down for its use in the adult should be observed, with, however, this additional caution. The astringent effect of opium in the adult is more likely to be adverse in sthenic states of the system when excretion is most active. This principle also applies to the child during the season of growth. The continuous use of opiates is a more common practice in the treatment of dysentery in the child than in the adult; whereas, if the law just stated be correct, it ought to be less so, and to be conducted with more caution.

When the disease becomes chronic in children, we must trust chiefly to vegetable astringents and the preparations of iron, with judicious adjustment of food and of climate, and attention to the state of the skin.

SECTION VII. — *On Gastro-Enteritis.*

This disease — inflammation of the mucous coat of the stomach, of the small intestine, and of the colon — is not uncommon in its chronic form in cachectic individuals, both European and native. It is characterised by some degree of irritability of stomach, chiefly after taking food, accompanied with more or less diarrhœa. The skin is dry, the body is emaciated, the abdomen retracted, and the tongue florid, glazed, and sometimes aphthous at the tip and edges. In fatal cases the mucous membrane of the stomach presents patches of dark, marbled redness, and is often softer than natural. The lower part of the ileum and the colon are the parts of the intestinal canal usually affected. The morbid appearances are vascular patches, sometimes with softening, at others with granular exudation. The solitary glands are often enlarged and prominent, and circular ulcers are occasionally found scattered here and there.

In consequence of the general relation of chronic gastro-enteritis to depraved states of constitution the treatment is perplexing and unsatisfactory. It resolves itself into carefully-regulated diet, attention to the functions of the skin by suitable clothing, the use of opium in small doses, with alkalies, or (according to the diarrhœa) vegetable astringents. Dilute hydrocyanic acid with bi-carbonate of soda, is often very useful in allaying the irritability both of the stomach and of the bowels. An occasional small blister to the epigastrium or right iliac region is also attended with benefit. In selecting a suitable climate, the extremes of heat and cold and much moisture should be avoided.

The practical lesson inculcated by these brief remarks is the great importance of *preventing* the cachectic states on which the occurrence and intractable nature of gastro-enteritis mainly depend.

SECTION VIII. — *On Diarrhœa.*

The term diarrhœa occupies a prominent place in the hospital returns of tropical climates, because it is often used in its etymological, not its pathological sense. It is only correctly applied to increased alvine discharges, dependent on active or passive congestion of some part of the mucous lining of the intestinal canal. The increased evacuations consequent on inflammation of the same tissue, either in its early stages or after it has led to structural change, are inaccurately designated diarrhœa. Yet this name is often given to chronic dysentery, muco-enteritis, and gastro-enteritis; and the returns of disease are in consequence rendered incorrect and untrustworthy. The diagnosis is not difficult; it rests on a careful consideration of the history of the case and of all the attendant symptoms.

Let us now consider the varieties of true diarrhœa.

1. Transient increased feculent discharges, consequent on excess or errors of diet, or exposure to cold, occur in India in the previously healthy, as in all countries, but not so frequently. This form of diarrhœa requires, however, to be watched with care, because, as already explained, both dysentery and cholera often commence with very similar discharges (pp. 221, 281).

2. In Europeans recently arrived, increased discharges, tinged with acrid bile, — bilious diarrhœa, — occasionally occur; but this is a rare form of disease in the seasoned European and in the natives of India.

3. In asthenic or cachectic persons, Europeans or natives, diarrhœa is apt to come on consequent on errors of diet, but much more frequently from cold and wet. The discharges are watery, generally pale, often chalky and yeasty in appearance. We have illustrations of this form of disease in the cold and rainy seasons at hill stations in India, or in the change to colder latitudes at unseasonable periods, or imprudently conducted. In fatal cases, the mucous membrane of the intestine is found pale and attenuated. It is an error to suppose, as many do, that this diarrhœa is symptomatic of hepatic derangement. No doubt the secretion of bile is deficient; but can it be otherwise when the system is anæmic, and an active derivation of the fluids to the intestinal surface is going on.

The indications of cure are a regulated diet, derivation to the skin by a suitable climate and appropriate clothing, the use of astringents, and the kind of tonics best adapted to the particular constitutional state. If there be a series of amendments and relapses, the disease may continue as a diarrhœa for a considerable period, but its tendency always is, under lengthened continuous persistence, to pass into chronic dysentery, muco-enteritis, or gastro-enteritis: hence the reason why in fatal cases the structural lesions of inflammation are often present.

SECTION IX. — *Statistics of Dysentery in the European Hospital, and of Dysentery and Diarrhœa in the Jamsetjee Jejeebhoy Hospital and Byculla Schools at Bombay.**

TABLE XXIV.—*Admissions and Deaths, with Per-centage, from Dysentery, in the European General Hospital at Bombay, for the Five Years from July* 1838 *to June* 1853.

	July 1838 to June 1843.		Monthly Average.		
	Admissions.	Deaths.	Deaths on Admissions.	Admissions on total Admissions.	Deaths on total Deaths.
January . .	78	17	21·8	14·2	39·5
February . .	29	12	41·8	7·0	37·5
March . . .	34	5	11·6	8·3	15·1
April . . .	37	8	21·6	6·3	19·5
May . . .	34	9	26·4	4·0	11·2
June . . .	49	9	18·3	6·2	17·6
July . . .	57	8	14·	7·9	21·6
August . . .	43	7	16·2	7·0	20·0
September . .	33	11	33·3	6·0	21·1
October . .	47	3	6·2	6·5	11·1
November . .	73	6	8·2	10·6	12·7
December . .	93	18	19·3	15·1	27·2
Total . .	616	113	18·3	8·1	20·7

TABLE XXV. — *Admissions and Deaths, with Per-centage, from Dysentery, in the European General Hospital at Bombay, for the Five Years, from* 1844 *to* 1848.

	1844 to 1848.		Monthly Average.		
	Admissions.	Deaths.	Deaths on Admissions.	Admissions on total Admissions.	Deaths on total Deaths.
January . .	51	12	23·5	8·2	26·1
February . .	29	9	31·03	2·6	25·6
March . . .	32	4	12·5	6·6	13·3
April . . .	21	6	28·6	4·1	19·3
May . . .	26	1	3·8	4·5	3·3
June . . .	34	3	8·8	4·7	9·09
July . . .	58	6	10·3	8·5	16·7
August . . .	33	2	6·06	6·0	13·3
September . .	30	4	13·3	6·5	18·2
October . .	18	5	27·7	2·9	13·2
November . .	38	5	13·2	6·8	16·1
December . .	60	14	23·3	11·5	35·0
Total . .	430	71	16·5	6·3	18·4

* For further information on the statistics of dysentery and diarrhœa, the reader is referred to Sections I. and III. of this Chapter.

TABLE XXVI.—*Admissions and Deaths, with Per-centage, from Dysentery, in the European General Hospital at Bombay, for the Five Years from* 1849 *to* 1853.

	1849 to 1853.		Monthly Average.		
	Admissions.	Deaths.	Deaths on Admissions.	Admissions on total Admissions.	Deaths on total Deaths.
January . .	56	17	30·4	12·4	43·7
February . .	23	4	17·4	6·2	22·2
March . . .	27	11	40·9	6·1	32·4
April . . .	37	6	16·3	7·2	24·0
May . . .	30	5	16·7	5·8	20·8
June . . .	37	6	16·3	6·4	20·7
July . . .	46	9	19·6	8·7	27·3
August . . .	41	8	19·5	8·3	21·6
September . .	22	5	22·9	6·2	20·0
October . .	27	8	29·7	6·8	34·8
November . .	47	9	19·2	8·9	30·0
December . .	61	17	27·8	10·03	42·5
Total . .	454	105	23·1	7·8	29·4

TABLE XXVII.—*Admissions and Deaths, with Per-centage, from Dysentery, in the Jamsetjee Jejeebhoy Hospital at Bombay, for the Six Years from* 1848 *to* 1853.

	1848 to 1853.		Monthly Average.		
	Admissions.	Deaths.	Deaths on Admissions.	Admissions on total Admissions.	Deaths on total Deaths.
January . .	120	49	40·8	5·7	10·9
February . .	93	26	27·9	4·9	8·1
March . . .	65	34	52·3	3·02	8·8
April . . .	73	35	47·9	3·4	10·2
May . . .	91	20	21·9	4·1	6·9
June . . .	82	43	52·4	3·8	14·007
July . . .	129	55	42·6	6·3	14·7
August . . .	118	46	38·9	5·9	14·03
September . .	99	44	44·4	4·8	14·1
October . .	75	36	48·0	3·5	10·6
November . .	102	37	36·2	4·7	11·2
December . .	154	49	31·8	6·6	12·3
Total . .	1,201	474	39·4	4·7	11·5

TABLE XXVIII.—*Admissions and Deaths, with Per-centage, from Diarrhœa, in the Jamsetjee Jejeebhoy Hospital at Bombay, for the Six Years from* 1848 *to* 1853.

	1848 to 1853.		Monthly Average.		
	Admissions.	Deaths.	Deaths on Admissions.	Admissions on total Admissions.	Deaths on total Deaths.
January . .	102	41	40·2	4·9	9·1
February . .	65	30	46·2	3·4	9·4
March . . .	57	39	68·4	2·6	10·1
April . . .	73	22	30·1	3·4	6·4
May . . .	83	24	28·9	3·8	8·4
June . . .	93	25	26·8	4·5	8·1
July . . .	122	44	36·4	6·04	11·1
August . . .	110	61	55·5	5·5	18·6
September . .	91	33	36·2	4·4	10·6
October . .	111	40	36·04	5·2	10·03
November . .	93	30	32·1	4·3	9·07
December . .	104	36	34·6	4·5	9·08
Total . .	1,104	425	38·5	4·3	10·3

TABLE XXIX.—*Admissions and Deaths, with Per-centage, from Diarrhœa and Dysentery, in the Byculla Schools, for the Seventeen Years from* 1837 *to* 1853.

	1837 to 1853.		Monthly Average.		
	Admissions.	Deaths.	Deaths on Admissions.		
January . .	95	1	1·05		
February . .	117	3	2·56		
March . . .	142	4	2·8		
April . . .	131	6	4·58		
May . . .	151	2	1·32		
June . . .	213	3	1·4		
July . . .	285	7	2·43		
August . . .	195	9	4·63		
September . .	97	3	3·09		
October . .	83	1	1·2		
November . .	95	2	2·1		
December . .	82	1	1·23		
Total . .	1,686	42	2·49		

CHAP. XV.

ON HEPATITIS.

Section I. — *Comparative Prevalence of Hepatitis.*

The following table shows the ratio of hepatitis to strength in European and Native troops in the three Presidencies: —

* Presidency.	Europeans.			Natives.		
	Per-centage of Admissions to strength.	Per-centage of Deaths to strength.	Per-centage of Deaths to Admissions.	Per-centage of Admissions to strength.	Per-centage of Deaths to strength.	Per-centage of Deaths to Admissions.
Bengal . . .	5·65	0·40	7·16	0·10	·007	7·54
Bombay . . .	7·78	0·41	5·27	0·18	·019	10·28
Madras . . .	7·0	0·29	4·1	0·12	·013	10·07

A judgment may be formed of the comparative prevalence of the disease in India, by observing the ratio in other countries; thus the per-centage of admissions to strength is in —†

Canada	·75	per cent.
Nova Scotia	·82	"
England	84	"
Malta	2·09	"
Cape of Good Hope . . .	2·18	"

Though hepatitis is a more common disease in India than in temperate climates, still it is rare compared with fevers and affections of the bowels, as is proved by the following tabular statement: —

* "Ewart's Vital Statistics," pp. 127, 137.

† *Ib.* p. 125, where there are also further similar facts in respect to other countries.

EUROPEAN TROOPS.

Presidency.	Fevers.		Dysentery and Diarrhœa.		Hepatitis.	
	Per-centage of Admissions to strength.	Per-centage of Deaths to strength.	Per-centage of Admissions to strength.	Per-centage of Deaths to strength.	Per-centage of Admissions to strength.	Per-centage of Deaths to strength.
Bengal . . .	72·64	1·99	30·41	2·02	5·65	0·40
Bombay . . .	61·93	1·37	27·13	1·71	7·78	0·41
Madras . . .	31·62	0·37	23·43	1·24	7·0	0·29

NATIVE TROOPS.

Presidency.	Fevers.		Dysentery and Diarrhœa.		Hepatitis.	
	Per-centage of Admissions to strength.	Per-centage of Deaths to strength.	Per-centage of Admissions to strength.	Per-centage of Deaths to strength.	Per-centage of Admissions to strength.	Per-centage of Deaths to strength.
Bengal . . .	48·50	·528	6·18	·173	0·10	·007
Bombay . . .	41·20	·57	6·57	·196	0·18	·019
Madras . . .	25·04	·30	3·08	·190	0·12	·013

A similar result also appears on examining the returns of the European General Hospital and the Jamsetjee Jejeebhoy Hospital, thus: —

	Fevers.		Dysentery and Diarrhœa.		Hepatitis.	
	Per-centage of Admissions on total Admissions.	Per-centage of Deaths on total Deaths.	Per-centage of Admissions on total Admissions.	Per-centage of Deaths on total Deaths.	Per-centage of Admissions on total Admissions.	Per-centage of Deaths on total Deaths.
European General Hospital . .	19·7	10·3	12·9 *	28·9 *	3·7	7·8
Jamsetjee Jejeebhoy Hospital . .	9·8	7·5	9·0	21·8	1·5	3·0

From these statements we learn that hepatitis, though a common disease in Europeans in India compared with temperate climates, does not nearly equal fever and affections of the bowels in frequency or in the mortality which it occasions. Moreover I believe that hospital returns in India very generally exaggerate

* As my own notes do not supply me with the return of diarrhœa in the European General Hospital, I have incorporated the ratios of dysentery of my own tables with those of diarrhœa of Dr. Stovell's Report, for the ten years from 1846 to 1856.

the proportion of hepatitis. A sense of fulness and weight in the region of the liver from congestion and enlargement consequent on recurring fever, are not unfrequently classed as hepatitis, partly from inaccurate diagnosis, but chiefly because the nosological classification in use has not kept pace with the progress of pathology and does not provide for these distinctions.

Notwithstanding my belief that the frequency of hepatitis in Europeans is over-estimated, I am certain that the statement made by Twining, and generally concurred in by writers on tropical disease, that "acute liver disease terminating in abscess is exceedingly rare among Asiatics," * is erroneous. In six years the deaths, from hepatitis in the Jamsetjee Jejeebhoy Hospital amounted to 125, and the fifty-five cases of hepatic abscess in natives now before me, and partly detailed in the sequel of this chapter, form but a part of those which at different times have come under my observation. The origin of this common error is easily explained. The imperfect statistics of disease in the Indian army have been applied to the general population of the country, which is equivalent to judging of the forms of disease prevalent in England from the hospital returns of the troops serving in that country.

Section II. — *Preliminary Remarks on the nature of the Symptoms of Hepatic Disease.— Arrangement of the Subject.*

In distinguishing the diseases of the liver, we are often unassisted by derangement of its function — that is, by altered conditions of the biliary secretion. In many affections of this organ there is no evidence that the secretion is modified; and though it has been customary to attribute various of the morbid appearances presented by the alvine discharges to a changed state of the bile, and to infer the existence of hepatic disease, yet the proof is frequently insufficient, and the fact that the altered character of the secretions may have been caused by the remedies used is often lost sight of.

It is, therefore, very necessary that the clinical student should avail himself of all other useful sources of information. Above all, it is essential that he should bring to the inquiry a precise knowledge of the anatomical position and relations of the organ, and that this should be constantly present to his mind while he investigates its morbid states.

* Twining, "Diseases of Bengal," vol. i. p. 388.

It is since the practice of percussion has been added to our methods of diagnosis, that great accuracy in respect to the position of the liver has acquired its full value; for by this means we can ascertain during life the normal limits of the organ, and also their increase or decrease. In the normal state there is dulness on percussion from the sixth right rib, downwards to the costal margin. The degree of dulness between the sixth and seventh rib varies according as observation is made under expiration or inspiration. Percussion about the fifth, sixth, and seventh ribs should always be gentle, because as the convex part of the liver rises as high as the level of the fifth rib, strong percussion will indicate dulness higher than the sixth rib, and will prevent us from determining whether the liver is normally, or otherwise, overlapped by the thin part of the lung.*

There are leading features of the intimate structure of the liver which should also be held in remembrance. The arrangement of the portal capillaries, the position of the portal vein, and its branches in the portal canals. The origin of the radicles of the hepatic vein in the lobules, and their relation there to the portal capillaries. The distribution of the hepatic artery. The situation of the origin of the hepatic ducts. The supposed function of the hepatic cells, and their relation to the terminal parts of the ducts. Nor may we forget that by far the larger proportion of the blood flows through the portal vein to serve the purpose of secretion; and that a much smaller portion circulates in the hepatic artery to serve for the nutrition of the solid tissues of the organ, and then to mix with the portal blood, and thereby, also, assist in secretion. The liver is moreover abundantly supplied with lymphatics, and with nerves, chiefly derived from the sympathetic system.

In describing the inflammatory affections of the liver I shall use the terms *Hepatitis* and *Cirrhosis*. *Hepatitis* signifies inflammation of the peritoneal covering of the organ, of its substance, or of both combined. When occurring in the investing membrane, it may be recovered from with, or without, exudation of lymph and consequent adhesion. When occurring in the parenchyma it may be recovered from, and the organ be left

* Though the great importance of careful systematic percussion in the diagnosis of hepatic disease, is undoubted, still I have reason to believe that it is often very imperfectly attended to. It has happened to me on not a few occasions to become cognisant of cases, in which enlargement of the liver was undiscovered, though the exercise of moderate skill in percussion could not have failed to detect it. And on the other hand, I have known instances in which congestion or enlargement was erroneously supposed to exist, simply because this means of diagnosis had been neglected.

sound; or exudation of lymph may take place, and abscess may result.

The symptoms will be distinct or obscure, and the morbid processes will follow a quick or a slow course, and will tend to recovery or structural lesion according to the part and extent of the organ implicated, and the diathesis of the individual affected.

The term *Cirrhosis* is applied to that slow inflammatory action which, invading the fibrous and areolar tissues of the portal canals, and generally caused by spirit-drinking, injures the structure of the liver.

I prefer these terms to "suppurative inflammation," and "adhesive inflammation," because the former, as a substitute for "hepatitis," does not include the cases of peripheral inflammation, and seems to imply that every inflammation of the substance of the liver, not of the character of cirrhosis, necessarily ends in suppuration — a conclusion to which the observer of disease in India is unable to assent. My objection to the term "adhesive inflammation," as restricted to cirrhosis, is, that it would be more correctly applied to those numerous inflammations, primary or secondary, of the peritoneal covering of the liver which lead to exudation of lymph and adhesion of surfaces.

In arranging my remarks on *Hepatitis*, I shall consider—1st, the pathology; 2nd, the causes; 3rd, the symptoms; 4th, the treatment.

SECTION III.— *Pathology.— Preliminary Remarks on the General Pathology of Hepatitis.— Morbid Anatomy of Stage of Vascular Turgescence, of Exudation of Lymph, and Formation of Abscess explained.— The several Courses and Situations of Rupture of Hepatic Abscess.—Abscess Absorption.— Secondary Peritonitis and Formation of circumscribed Purulent Sacs.— Secondary Pleuritis, circumscribed and general Empyema.— Secondary Pericarditis.— General Secondary Peritonitis.— Colour of Pus in Hepatic Abscess.*

Before proceeding to describe the morbid anatomy of hepatitis, I would notice a preliminary pathological question of some interest and importance, but which, so far as I know, has not engaged the attention of previous writers. Which are the capillary vessels of the liver concerned in inflammation? If the pathology of inflammation be correct, viz., that it is an altered state of the nutritive processes of the affected part, depending upon something faulty in one or other of the conditions of normal nutrition, — then the capillaries concerned in inflammation must necessarily be those which circulate, in their normal state, arterial blood for purposes of nutrition. The capillaries of the hepatic artery are the nutrient vessels of the solid structures of the liver, and consequently the only ones which can be directly engaged in the inflammatory processes of those structures.* On the other hand, the portal capillaries circulate venous blood for purposes of secretion, and are not supposed to take any part in the nutrition of the liver; they are therefore not directly engaged in inflammation. This is not merely an unimportant speculation because — Firstly, if we regard the small capacity of the capillaries of the hepatic artery in comparison with those of the portal vein, we have, under the view that the former are those concerned in inflammation, an explanation of the fact that the bulk of the organ is little increased in inflammation compared with congestion — a deranged state in which the capacious portal capillaries are directly implicated. Secondly, this view helps to explain how it happens that the secretory function of the liver is often not deranged in hepatitis. Thirdly, it tends to remove that difficulty which practical writers on hepatitis have experienced in reconciling the results of clinical observation with therapeutic theory. It has been urged that to give mercury with a view to its cholagogue action in hepatitis is opposed to the doctrine that the special stimulants of secreting organs are contra-indicated in the active inflammations of these organs. But this principle — doubtless true when the secreting capillaries and the inflamed capillaries are the same, and both carrying arterial blood, — cannot correctly apply to the liver, if the secreting capillaries and the inflamed capillaries are distinct from each other. Further, if we hold that the capillaries of the hepatic artery finally pass into the portal veins, then to quicken the portal capillary circulation by increasing secretion seems, in theory, a rational method of lessening stagnation in the capillaries of the hepatic artery. These observations are not now made with any view of advocating the mercurial treatment of hepatitis, for this question will be discussed elsewhere; but simply with the object of showing that the question — which are the capillary vessels engaged in the inflammation, is not an idle

* I am aware that it may be urged that the hepatic cells must be classed with the solid structures of the liver, and that (viewing the close analogy between secretion and nutrition) in one sense it may be said that they are nourished by the portal capillaries. But this is apart from the argument, and the usual meaning of nutrition, which, speaking generally, is a process requiring as one of its conditions arterial blood and arterial capillaries.

one, but is intimately related to the therapeutics, as well as to the physical signs, and the symptoms of hepatitis.

In considering the *morbid anatomy* of hepatitis, it is important to remember the great size of the liver, and the consequent fact that inflammation will vary according as it involves a greater or less extent, and one or several parts of the substance or surface.

That inflammation of the capsule of the liver, with but little implication of the parenchyma, may really occur is not to be questioned. We may believe that in some instances recovery takes place and leaves behind no trace of disorder. In other instances, however, adhesions between the opposing peritoneal surfaces, or an opaque and thickened state of the membrane, without appreciable change of the parenchyma, result. Appearances occasionally found after death prove this; but from their rarity we are justified in concluding that inflammation, limited to the periphery of the liver, is not a common form of disease in India. This is the common opinion, and a review of my own cases serves to confirm it. Still the subject is one to which further attention should be directed, for in recorded cases (my own as well as others) positive information is often defective. It is hardly necessary to observe that my present remarks do not apply to the almost universal co-existence, at one period or other, of inflammation of the peritoneal covering with that of the parenchyma: its absence is exceptional, just as in the pleura and lung.

When the substance of the liver is the seat of inflammation, then a period of vascular turgescence, analogous to the first stage of pneumonia, is the first pathological condition. This may be resolved by treatment, or may lead to interstitial exudation of lymph and its ulterior changes. These morbid processes may affect portions of the organ ranging from the size of a pea to that of an orange and upwards; and in number from one to many. It is seldom, if ever, that inflammation of the entire substance of the liver occurs.

Opportunities of studying the post-mortem appearances of the first stage of parenchymatous hepatitis are necessarily limited, for death seldom occurs at this early period of the disease. Still occasional instances of death from some other cause, the first stage of hepatitis being present (Case 6), and the inspection of the parts of the liver immediately surrounding exudations of lymph enable us to ascertain the general appearance of vascular turgescence of the liver. The structure is redder and softer than natural, and blood oozes from it when cut. Rokitansky adds, that it is largely granular.

The large dark-red liver, easily lacerable into a bloody pulp, described by the older writers on tropical disease, and by them regarded as evidence of inflammation, is not the state just described. These were not appearances resulting from inflammation, but were conditions of the organ found in fatal cases of congestive malarious fever in full-blooded Europeans, and caused by accumulation of deteriorated blood in the capacious hepatic venous systems.

Under the continuance of inflammation, however, the morbid process will not long remain in the state of mere vascular turgescence. Interstitial exudation of coagulable lymph of varying extent will soon follow. Still, so long as the lymph maintains the liquid form in which it is first exuded, there is hope of complete recovery by re-absorption and resolution. When, however, the lymph has coagulated in the interstices of the parenchyma, then one of the three following courses will result:—

1. The liquid parts of the exudation may be absorbed, and the solid lymph become organised into fibrous tissue. This termination presupposes a good diathesis, exudation of limited extent, and the return of the surrounding parenchyma to its normal state of capillary circulation. We have evidence, I believe, of this occurrence in the fibrous nodules or patches that are sometimes found in the liver after death. (Cases 83, 84.)

2. The exuded lymph, instead of becoming organised, may reliquefy, be absorbed, and disappear. This termination is likely to occur only in a good diathesis, when the exudation has been of limited extent, is recent, surrounded by tolerably normal structure, has not been circumscribed by an organised layer, and has not been so copious as materially to interfere with the vitality of the tissues amid which it is placed.

3. The lymph changes into pus, the tissues amongst which it has been deposited become softened, liquefy and disappear, and the whole is more or less circumscribed by membrane of low organisation. Hepatic abscess has formed. This termination is favoured by the extent of the structure involved, the severity of the inflammatory action, the copiousness of the exudation, and above all, by the diathesis of the individual affected, and sometimes by the nature of the cause.

This progress from vascular turgescence to the formation of abscess may sometimes be distinctly traced, as I have been enabled to verify in several instances. The following are the appearances which have come under my notice:—

(*a*) A part of the substance of the liver is redder and softer than the surrounding structure. (*b*) Another portion exhibits a similar appearance, but with the addition of a circumscribed part of fawn yellow colour of moderate texture, caused by lymph deposited in the centre of the inflamed tissues. (*c*) In another part, a similar fawn-coloured circumscribed portion, but softer and friable in the centre, indicating that the lymph has begun to change into pus. (*d*) In a more advanced stage, the centre of the deposit becomes broken down, and converted into pus; the parts immediately adjacent to the pus being shreddy and flocculent, those beyond fawn-coloured and firm, bounded by reddened parenchyma gradually passing into healthy structure. (*e*) In a still more advanced stage, the outer layer of lymph becomes organised, in varying degrees, into a membranous investment, and the central parts—lymph and tissue—change more or less completely into pus, varying in character according to the diathesis of the individual. But even in this stage the inner surface of the investing membrane is not unfrequently roughened and flocculent from portions of the vascular or other tissues, which, remaining in a condition more or less organised, form nuclei round which flakes of shreddy lymph become attached.

But the history of the formation of the abscess is not yet completed. More lymph exudes from the inner surface of the investing membrane, and changes into pus. The sac becomes distended, the bulk of the liver increased, and tumefaction takes place in different directions, according to the situation of the abscess. Adhesion of opposing serous surfaces follows; then the circumscribing wall becomes thin on one side by interstitial absorption, and pointing and rupture succeed. Sometimes the tendency to point and to rupture is counteracted by the sac becoming thickened and strengthened in the following manner. The surrounding parenchyma becomes compressed by the increasing sac, and, in consequence, the lobular structure, for two or three lines around, is atrophied and disappears, but the connecting tissue remains. (Case 99.)

The completion of these processes, that is, the formation of an outer organised membrane, the change of the central lymph and tissues into pus, the adhesions, interstitial absorption, and rupture —must depend on the constitution of the individual, the size and number of the abscesses, and the judgment displayed in the medical treatment. In the greater number of hepatic abscesses death takes place while these processes are yet in progress.

In this description of the formation of hepatic abscess, sketched from actual observation, we find nothing different from what occurs in the course of an ordinary phlegmonous abscess in a good constitution: the parts of the lymph most remote from the living tissues—the central—change into pus; those adjacent to the living tissues—the peripheral—become organised into membrane.

Without pretending to assert that this is the only way in which abscesses of the liver are formed, I am very certain that it is the most common. It readily explains why these abscesses are generally not single, and why, when several, they are often in various stages of progress. Though it is no doubt true that large abscesses are sometimes formed by the coalition of several adjoining small ones, still I do not concur with Rokitansky in considering that this is the only mode; for I think there can be no question that a large hepatic abscess has sometimes its origin in a single extensive lymph exudation.

In these remarks reference has not been made to diffuse suppuration of the liver. In truth I have no knowledge of it. The absence of circumscribing tissue may be observed in that stage when, as yet the lymph has not all broken down; but when the change into pus has been nearly completed, there is, according to my observation, always a limitary tissue of some kind.

The cases which follow (94 to 102) will be found to illustrate, in some degree, the remarks which have now been made; also 125, 137, 140, 141, 172.

94. *Abscess in the brain not suspected during life.—Abscess in the liver, with pneumonia of the lowest lobe of the right lung, revealed by symptoms.—Vascular turgescence of liver.*—Thomas Saunders, boiler-maker, aged thirty-six, of stout habit, was admitted into the European General Hospital on the 9th August, 1838. He had arrived lately in India, and had suffered whilst in England from pain of his right side. He had been ill for five days before admission with pain of head, side, and limbs. These symptoms had lessened, but the pain of the right side had increased much the night before admission; it was at the margin of the ribs, was accompanied with cough and impeded full inspiration. After free leeching, the warm bath and purgatives, the side became easy; but the pain continued to recur from time to time, attended with headache and frequent pulse, and hot skin towards evening. He was dull of hearing on admission; his manner was slow and undecided, and his hands tremulous; his spirits were depressed, and the pulse easily excited. The bowels were kept free by mercurial and other medicines; leeches and blisters were applied, and quinine was at different times given. On the 1st September it was thus reported: Is still nervous, but makes no complaint of pain; the pulse is easily excited; there is abnormal fulness of the right hypochondrium. About two inches below the right nipple, laterally and posteriorly below the inferior angle of the scapula, there is dulness on percussion; the respiratory murmur is obscure, with occasional sibilus and crepitation; the latter, smaller behind and rather subcrepitous laterally. On the left side of the chest there is occasionally sibilus, and mucous rhonchus; there is no cough. Subsequently the cough became troublesome, and the pulse frequent, and on the 16th he became drowsy for the first time, then insensible, and died at 7 P.M.

Inspection twelve hours after death.—Head.—In the anterior and middle lobe of the right hemisphere there was an abscess of considerable size, the inner surface having in parts a red fungous appearance; and the surrounding substance of the brain was softened. *Abdomen.* — The substance of the liver was red and softened, and adhered to the ribs and the diaphragm; on separating the latter adhesion a small abscess was discovered, and opposed to it the lung adhered to the diaphragm. The lowest lobe of the right lung was hepatised, and the left lung was congested with blood.

95. *Hepatitis. — Several abscesses in the right lobe. — Nodules in the left lobe. — The mucous coat of the colon ulcerated. — Serous effusion in the head without symptoms.* — John Robinson, aged twenty-six, a seaman, tall and fair, was admitted with symptoms of acute hepatitis on the 7th February, 1840. He stated that he had been ill since the day before admission. He was freely bled at the arm, and very freely leeched, mercury was used internally and externally without inducing ptyalism. On the 12th there began to be evening febrile accessions, which continued. On the 15th there was fulness at the margin of the right ribs with hepatic sound an inch below them and to two inches from the nipple. The fulness of the side increased, he became sallow and emaciated. The dejections were generally light yellow and thin. The breathing became oppressive, and he died on the 22nd.

Inspection. — Head. — There was a thin veil of serum on the convex surface of the brain, and an ounce at the base of the skull. *Chest.*—The lungs were emphysematous, and the liver encroached on the chest to the level of the fourth rib. *Abdomen.*—There were no adhesions between the concavity of the diaphragm and the surface of the liver. In the right lobe of the liver there were several abscesses, each the size of an orange. There was one to the right of the mesial line and superficial; two were at the concave surface of the lobe, and their walls were in close adhesion with the hepatic flexure of the colon. The inner surface of the walls of the abscesses was very flocculent when floated in water. The left lobe filled the left hypochondrium, was of pale colour, and presented whiter defined proportions the size of a pea, like tubercles in appearance, but not so hard in texture. The colon was studded with closely set circular ulcers, some of them sloughy; where the adhesions to the liver were, there the ulcerations had advanced furthest. At the end of the ileum there was granular yellow lymph effused.

96. *Dysentery complicated with delirium tremens. — Milkiness of the arachnoid. — Matting of the omentum over the colon.—Numerous sloughy ulcerations of the mucous coat of the cæcum.—Many abscesses in liver.*—Cornelius Moriarty, aged forty-six, a serjeant in the Grand Arsenal, of dissipated habits, and in hospital at different times with delirium tremens. He was admitted on the 7th November, 1840, with symptoms of hepatitis, complicated with delirium tremens. He died comatose on the 11th.

Inspection five hours after death.—The liver enlarged and mottled yellow, was brittle and hard in texture, and seven or eight small abscesses were detected; the largest was the size of a walnut, the others the size of horse-beans. The smaller ones were occupied with thick adhesive pus, the large one had the appearance of parenchyma infiltrated with purulent matter, but not yet broken down, and the surrounding texture was mottled red and friable. The description of the other morbid appearances is omitted.

97. *Illustrates formation of abscess from breaking down of lymph deposit. — Pus tinged with bile.—The corpuscles granular and broken down.—Surrounding turgescence.*—The liver of a dysenteric patient with abscess was sent to me from the European General Hospital. In the right side of the right lobe there was a part, the size of a large orange, the centre pulpy and broken down; around it, for quarter of an inch, there was a thick layer of buff-coloured structure; around that, for some distance, an engorged part. In one other place there was a yellow-buff portion the size of a bean, without central pulpy state. The rest of the organ was healthy. Hepatic cells were distinct under the microscope. In the central pulpy part the puriform fluid was tinged yellow (bile); examined under the microscope, the biliary tinge was very

marked, and the corpuscles in greater measure had separated into their constituent granules.

98.—*Hepatitis.—Abscesses: in one, breaking down of the parenchyma; in the other, the deposit in the interstitial tissue had not yet broken down into pus.—Mucous coat of the colon dark red, and covered with firm granular exudation.*—Richard Cox, aged forty-six, a seaman of the ship *Tweed*, was admitted on February 4th, 1841. He stated that he had ailed for a week with dry cough, increased during the two days previous to admission, and attended with pain at the lower part of the chest extending to the epigastrium, and attended with pain on pressure. Pulse frequent; skin dry. He was bled once and leeched frequently; took calomel in ten-grain doses. The pain never ceased, though it was relieved. The mouth did not become affected. There was not much purging, but the skin became washy, pulse feeble, countenance collapsed; and he died on the morning of the 12th.

Inspection six hours after death.—Chest.—There were old adhesions of the pulmonary to the costal pleura on both sides. *Abdomen.*—On the lateral part of the right lobe of the liver there was a superficial abscess, containing dark reddish serous fluid; the inner surface of the sac was yellow and flocculent. About the middle of the anterior part of the right lobe there was a somewhat prominent part, which, when incised, showed a yellow substance the size of a walnut, softened in the centre, firmer beyond. The parenchyma of the liver was generally mottled buff. The mucous coat of the colon presented a dark red surface throughout the greater part, covered with a yellow granular firm exudation with frequent traces of ulceration. There was commencement of yellow deposit in one of the kidneys.

99. *Hepatitis.—An abscess lined by firm membrane in the right lobe.—Several nodules in different places of the liver; in some suppuration commencing at the centre.—Traces of ulceration in the colon.—Granular exudation on the mucous coat of the rectum.*—John Richard Pauper, aged twenty-six, an Indo-Briton, was admitted on the 29th January, 1841. He stated that for three weeks he had suffered from pain of the right hypochondrium, increased much during the two days previous to admission. The pain prevented full inspiration and decubitus on the right side. The pulse was badly developed and frequent. He was leeched and blistered, and an attempt was made to affect the system by the moderate exhibition of calomel and opium and mercurial inunction. The pain was much relieved; never, however, completely removed. No fulness at the margin of the ribs occurred. The gums became swollen, but he was never fully under the influence of mercury. On the 1st February dysenteric symptoms appeared for the first time, following a seven-grain dose of calomel, and attended with a good deal of tenesmus till about the 5th. After this, the bowels were moved generally seven or eight times in the twenty-four hours, the dejections being brown and watery. He lost flesh. From the 8th the treatment was chiefly palliative, anodynes with quinine and light nourishment. He died on the 17th. Rigors are not noted as having occurred in any of the reports.

Inspection eighteen hours after death.—Body emaciated. *Head.*—There was a thin veil of serum on the convex surface of the brain. *Chest.*—The right lung was emphysematous, and adhered by tender bands to the diaphragm. The left lung was closely united to the costal pleura. There were no tubercles in the lungs. The heart was healthy. *Abdomen.*—The liver did not extend beyond the ribs. The surface was of buff colour, externally and internally. The lateral part of the right lobe adhered to the concavity of the ribs; and underneath the adhesions there was an abscess the size of an ostrich egg, containing about twenty ounces of thick pus, and lined by a firm cartilaginous membrane: beyond it, for three or four lines, the substance of the liver was cartilaginous and condensed. From the inner surface of the sac loose flocculi depended. Elsewhere, here and there, in both lobes, there were round buff-yellow defined portions from the size of a tare to a horse-bean, some consistent throughout, others with a drop of pus in the centre. The mucous coat of the colon was pale, with traces of ulcers in process of cicatrisation. In the rectum there was granular lymph. The mucous coat of the pyloric end of the stomach was mammillated; at the cardiac end there were dark brown vascular ramifications, but the texture of the coat was sound. The kidneys were healthy.

100. *Hepatitis.—Two large abscesses from degeneration of lymph and tissue.—The liver mottled buff.—The mucous coat of the colon dark grey with red patches, and several ulcers.—The kidneys malformed.*—James M'Martin, aged thirty-eight, of the ship *Ingleborough*, was admitted into hospital on the 2nd February, 1841. He stated that for a fortnight previously he had suffered from dysentery, and had passed blood for several days. There was much tenderness across the abdomen. Pulse 100, irritable. He was bled to sixteen ounces, and freely leeched. The blood was cupped and sizy. During his stay in hospital, the pain was chiefly about the margin of the right ribs, shooting downwards to the iliac region, or backwards, or towards the epigastrium. Latterly there was distinct fulness and tenseness at the margin of the ribs. On the 4th there was a distinct febrile paroxysm with rigors. The dysenteric symptoms were little urgent till the 12th, when a considerable quantity of brick-red puriform matter was dejected, and continued till his death, on the 14th. At first the case was treated as one of dysentery, and ipecacuanha pills were given; but they were rejected, and in consequence omitted. Subsequently an attempt was made to induce mercurial action, but irritation resulted, and it was not persisted in. Latterly wine with quinine and opium were given.

Inspection twenty hours after death.—Chest.—The lungs were emphysematous, but otherwise healthy; no costal or diaphragmatic adhesions. *Abdomen.*—There were two large abscesses in the liver: one, to the right of the gall-bladder, had thin anterior and lateral walls opposed to the abdominal parietes and the concavity of the false ribs, and its lower wall adhered firmly to the hepatic flexure of the colon; but there was no communication with the gut. The other abscess, the size of a large orange, was in the centre of the right lobe. There were no adhesions to the diaphragm. The contents of both abscesses were dark brown, and quite serous. The inner surface of the sacs was flocculent. The rest of the liver had a bright buff mottled appearance. The walls of the colon were not thickened. The mucous coat was dark grey with dark red patches and numerous extensive superficial ulcers. There was a malformation of the kidneys. The two kidneys were connected, and in a horse-shoe form, the convexity downwards, extended across the abdomen, before the vessels and behind the mesentery,—the whole length about ten inches,—the transverse part about one inch and a half broad. Throughout the whole extent the cortical and tubular parts might be traced, but the texture was soft and yellow, and probably altered by disease. There were two ureters following their usual course.

101. *Abscess in the liver.—Sac smooth without flocculi.—Large intestine, with sloughy ulceration of the mucous coat.—Complicated with intermittent fever, which at the commencement was the prominent feature.—Several lymph nodules.*—David Hopkirk, Indian Navy, aged twenty-six, was admitted on the 15th December, 1840, under the head of intermittent fever, and died on the 9th February. He had been ill for three weeks before admission with regular febrile paroxysms. There was also pain, increased on pressure, at the upper part of the abdomen. The chief symptoms during his residence in hospital were the frequent recurrence of this abdominal pain with occasional febrile paroxysms, with rigors at first—tendency to dysenteric symptoms—marked during the last ten days by considerable purging and tenesmus, with gradual loss of flesh. He was never brought fully under the influence of mercury, though calomel was given freely with this intention. He was bled freely, leeched and blistered. There was clavus hystericus at one time, the result probably of the depletory measures.

Inspection eight hours after death.—Body emaciated. *Head.*—Brain pale, with about four drachms of serum at the base of the skull. *Chest.*—The lungs were emphysematous, and there were old adhesions of the right lung to the costal pleura. The heart was healthy. *Abdomen.*—The omentum spread over the intestines adhered to the brim of the pelvis and to the cœcum. In many places the intestine, chiefly the cœcum and sigmoid flexure, was black and friable. The inner surface of the gut throughout presented a ragged sloughy appearance, with hardly a trace of the mucous coat. The lateral part of the right lobe of the liver adhered to the parietes, and at the point of adhesion there was a superficial abscess, the size of an ostrich egg; the sac lined with a firm, smooth membrane. In the parenchyma, and around the abscess, there were several yellow points, the size of a pin's head; and in the centre of the right lobe there was one the size of a horse-bean. The liver was red and firmer than natural. The mesenteric glands were generally enlarged, many of them being larger than an almond. In the kidneys yellow degeneration had advanced considerably; in one it was uniform, in the other it was striated.

102. *Large hepatic abscess, with shreddy flocculent walls and surrounding vascular turgescence.—No intestinal ulceration.*—Shaik Abdoo, forty-three years of age, a Mussulman, servant in a grog-shop, using spirits freely, of somewhat emaciated frame, after ten or twelve days' illness, with pain of right side, cough, and daily double febrile accessions, was admitted into the clinical ward on the 29th November, 1848. There was dry cough, hiccup, tenderness below the right ribs, a yellow coated tongue with florid edges, high-coloured urine, relaxed bowels, and febrile disturbance. There was a sense of induration with dulness in the epigastric region, and below the margin of the right ribs to within about an inch of the umbilicus. These symptoms continued with aggravation of the diarrhœa, and he died on the 8th December. He was treated with leeches over the tender part, followed by a blister, and calomel three grains, ipecacuanha one grain, opium half a grain every fourth hour. Slight fulness and tenderness of the gums on the 4th.

Inspection eleven hours and a half after death.—Chest.—Both lungs collapsed, and were crepitating. *Right lung.*—There were old adhesions between the upper lobe and the costal pleura. The base of the lung adhered to the upper surface of the diaphragm, by recently effused lymph, and the lateral surface of the third lobe to the opposite costal pleura. A portion of this lobe was œdematous. No adhesions of the left lung. The heart and pericardium were healthy. *Abdomen.*—The liver was so much enlarged as to reach on the right and left sides to the level of the tenth and eleventh ribs, and to a point about two inches above the umbilicus. There were tender adhesions between the right lobe and the diaphragm, also between the gall-bladder and the adjacent border of the right lobe of the liver and the colon, as well as between the lower surface of the liver and the duodenum. An abscess occupied the lower and posterior part of the right lobe, and was very superficial at the lateral part, so that the walls, which had contracted adhesions with the opposite parietal peritoneum, gave way and remained adherent to the latter, and seemed to consist only of the visceral peritoneum thickened. The abscess was large, about the size of a cocoa-nut, and contained pus with abundant shreddy-looking flocculi. The portion of the substance of the liver surrounding the abscess was red, and the rest was mottled white and red, and was very firm under the knife. The ascending colon passed obliquely upwards and inwards to the notch in the anterior border of the liver and to the gall-bladder, and thence the transverse part stretched downwards towards the left iliac fossa, close to the anterior superior spinous process of the os ileum, and thence it passed upwards, then downwards, as the descending colon. No disease of the large intestine, except that its mucous membrane was thinner than natural, and softer in parts: it was not ulcerated. The stomach was quite concealed by the liver, and pushed more towards the left side than natural; it was also very contracted, so much so that it appeared no larger than the intestine. Kidneys healthy in structure. Cranium not opened.

Courses followed by Hepatic Abscess.— Having traced the manner in which abscess in the liver is formed, I shall now describe the different directions in which it may point and rupture.

1. Hepatic abscess may open into the lung or sac of the pleura.
2. Into the stomach, or some part of the intestinal canal.
3. Into the pericardium.
4. Into the biliary ducts.
5. Into the cavity of the peritoneum.
6. Externally on the surface.

I shall here notice the first five directions, and leave the sixth to be considered in connection with the question of puncturing hepatic abscess as a part of treatment.

1. *Into the Lung or Sac of the Pleura.*—As the right lobe of the liver is the most common seat, and as abscess is frequently formed not far distant from the convex surface of the organ, a tendency to point towards the diaphragm, and open through it, is not an uncommon occurrence. This, according to my observation, is the direction in which hepatic abscess most frequently opens; more so, even, than on the external surface, unless puncture is had recourse to. Taking 140 cases of hepatic abscess, the notes of which are before me, and which constitute only a part of my experience in this form of disease, I find that 14 or ten per cent. opened into the lung, or sac of the pleura. Dr. Stovell reports that of the cases of hepatitis in the European General Hospital during ten years, abscess opened into the lungs or pleura in 3·837 per cent.* When the abscess has been small, single, not deep, and the constitution tolerably preserved, then there is a fair chance of recovery after communication with the lung. On the other hand, when the abscess is large or not single, and the constitution is either originally bad, or much reduced by disease or injudicious treatment, then a fatal issue, with exhausting hectic fever, is the usual termination.

The most satisfactory results of hepatic abscess communicating with the lung are those reported by Dr. Stovell †, viz., sixteen cases, with nine recoveries. The symptoms presented by the successful cases justify the inference, that the abscess in each had been small

* The reader will not fail to notice that Dr. Stovell's data differ from mine. He gives the ratio to the total admissions of *hepatitis*. I give the ratio of a certain number of cases of *hepatic abscess*.

† "Transactions, Medical and Physical Society," No. 1, Second Series; and again No. 3, Second Series, p. 43.

and single. My own notes do not supply an equal success; for, of the four following cases, the history of three, in which recovery promised, is incomplete.

103. *Abscess in the liver discharged by the lung, followed by convalescence.—Proceeded to England, and died shortly after arrival.—No account of the post mortem appearances.*—Robert ——, aged fifty-one, lieutenant, of the pension list, thirty-two years' service in India, resident in Bombay, a free liver, and the subject of occasional hepatic ailments, was admitted into the General Hospital on the 23rd June, 1842. He complained of occasional uneasiness of the right side, want of appetite, and irregular bowels. On the night of the 4th July he was seized with a fit of coughing, and ejected about six ounces of frothy puriform-looking fluid. He continued till the 17th August expectorating puriform matter, at times of brick-red colour, and occasionally to the extent of several ounces in the course of the day. After the 17th the puriform expectoration ceased, but occasional scanty mucous sputa were ejected. He improved in general health, left the hospital on the 6th September, and proceeded to England by sea; but died shortly after his arrival in that country on the 8th February, 1843; under what circumstances is not known.

104. *Hepatic abscess attributed to blows.—Opening into the lung.—Improvement.—Record as to the issue incomplete.*—Syud Merim, a Mussulman labourer of forty years of age, about two months before his admission into the clinical ward, on the 28th June, 1850, received several blows on the right side of the chest, in a quarrel. He experienced no inconvenience till a month afterwards, when acute pain came on suddenly in the right hypochondrium, with difficulty of breathing. On admission, he was a good deal reduced; the respiration was short and hurried. The ensiform cartilage, the margins of the ribs, and a line drawn from the left tenth rib across the abdomen above the umbilicus, formed the boundaries of a full, resistant, and dull space. The dulness extended upwards to the fourth right rib, and there was bulging below the fifth rib. The decubitus was dorsal, the pulse feeble, the bowels regular, and he suffered from evening febrile accessions. On the 23rd June he expectorated eight ounces of pink-coloured sero-puriform fluid, with some relief to the dyspnœa. There was now more or less expectoration daily, with less febrile disturbance. On the 2nd July the bulging of the right false ribs had nearly disappeared. He continued to improve slowly, but, becoming discontented, he left the hospital on the 8th July; after which date there is no record of his case. He was treated with anodynes and tonics.

105. *Hepatic abscess opening through the lung.—Result of the case not recorded.*—Luxuman Ragoo, a Hindoo blacksmith, of thirty-five years of age, using about three ounces of spirits daily, was admitted into the clinical ward on the 22nd February, 1853. There was some degree of fulness of the lower part of the right side of chest, with sense of induration and dulness for three inches below the right false ribs. The dulness reached upwards to the fifth rib. There was pain, on pressure, below the right false ribs, and in the epigastrium. Decubitus easy on all sides. Had occasional short dry cough. Suffered two months before from occasional febrile accessions. These ceased; but about ten days before admission, while engaged in his ordinary avocations, he suddenly felt uneasiness of the right hypochondrium. For six days the bowels had been relaxed. On the 26th he began to expectorate pinkish muco-puriform sputa. This continued sometimes copiously, and on the 1st March all fulness below the margin of the right ribs had ceased, and dulness did not reach above half an inch below them. Subsequently the cough was still troublesome, but the sputa chiefly consisted of frothy mucus. Throughout this time there was little constitutional disturbance, and the diarrhœa had ceased. The diary of the case closes abruptly on the 6th of March, through carelessness of the clinical clerk, without record of the issue.

106. *Hepatic abscess communicating with the lung.* (?) — *Result not known.* — Isaac Ibrahim, a Mussulman cart-driver, of forty years of age, was admitted into the clinical ward on the 5th November, 1852. He was emaciated. The respiration was short and hurried, and the right side did not move freely. There was complete dulness of the right dorsal and lateral regions, with defective resonance of the scapular, interscapular and mammary, with absence of vocal thrill and respiratory murmur in the two first. There was no induration or dulness below the right ribs, but pain on pressure there. On measurement, the right side of chest exceeded the left by half an inch. He was troubled with cough and expectoration of muco-puriform red-tinged sputa. Bowels relaxed. He said that he had suffered from intermittent fever five months before, which ceased in fifteen days, and was followed by pain below the margin of the right ribs, and of the right shoulder. The cough came on about six weeks before admission, was mild for the first fifteen days, but then became troublesome, and the sputa tinged red. The dysenteric symptoms had existed for a month. Admitted that he had used spirituous liquors pretty freely. He remained in hospital till the 12th November, when he was removed by his friends. During his stay he experienced evening febrile accessions.

Remarks.—The physical signs and symptoms were hardly adequate to determine the diagnosis of hepatic abscess, communicating with the lung; but, coupled with the history, they were probably sufficient.

The common expression, hepatic abscess has opened into the bronchi, is not correct if it be meant to imply that direct communication has taken place between the abscess and a large bronchial tube. In fatal cases it will be generally found that adhesions have formed between the diaphragm and the concave base of the right lung on the one side, and the convex surface of the liver on the other; and that a ragged excavation exists in the lower part of the lung communicating with the abscess in the liver. Occasionally an opening into the sac of the pleura is observed, as well as into the lung; and sometimes it is only into the pleura, causing empyema.

Of ten cases before me, the six following are narrated in illustration of these remarks: —

107. *Dysentery.* — *Secondary hepatic abscess forming obscurely.* — *Opening into the lung.*—*No ulceration of the intestine.* — Rustom Khan, a worker in tin, a Mussulman, of thirty-five years of age, reduced in flesh, not using spirits, was, after twelve days' illness, admitted into the clinical ward on the 21st December, 1851. He suffered from dysenteric symptoms, without abdominal fulness or induration, or febrile excitement. After the 29th there were occasional accessions of fever, commencing with chills and terminating with sweating. The dysenteric symptoms continued, but in less degree; and on the 29th January there was pain of the right shoulder for the first time, and on the 30th, below the margin of the right ribs, on full inspiration, but without dulness. There was apparent fulness of the right side of the chest, from the nipple to the margin of the ribs, but dulness did not reach above the fifth rib. The right side of abdomen was more resistant than the left, respiration was short and hurried, the pain of shoulder and side continued, and on the 5th February there was dulness and induration for half an inch below the ribs. On the 8th there was troublesome cough, and extension of the dulness an inch below the ribs. The febrile accessions had become less, and the dysenteric symptoms were almost gone. On the 18th the right side, at

the nipple, measured an inch more than the left. On the 23rd five ounces of pinkish puriform sputa were expectorated; this continued more or less with occasional recurrence of dysentery till the 19th April, when he died. The urine was frequently tested, but showed no trace of albumen.

Inspection twenty hours after death. —*Abdomen.* — The cavity of the abdomen contained a pint of limpid serous fluid. On removing the enlarged liver, with the right lung which adhered firmly to the diaphragm, a large abscess, the size of an ostrich egg, containing about a pint and a half of healthy pus, was found in the substance of the right lobe. The walls lined by thin fibrous membrane were formed inferiorly, and on the left side, by the parenchyma of the liver; on the right, superiorly, by the diaphragm, but at the right edge of the superior wall, for the space of about two and a half inches in circumference, the diaphragm was absorbed and destroyed, and the pus lay in contact with the substance of the inferior lobe of the right lung, which was also absorbed, forming a slight excavation, having a surface, red, soft, and irregular, but not lined by adventitious membrane, nor communicating with a large bronchial tube. The left lobe of the liver was healthy. Both kidneys were pale, but healthy. The mucous lining of the large intestine presented here and there patches of redness; otherwise it, and the other coats were healthy. Peyer's glands, solitary and agminated, were slightly enlarged, but not ulcerated. The coats of the small intestine were thin and pale. The other viscera were healthy. *Chest.* — Both cavities of the chest contained about a pint of clear serous fluid. The left lung was healthy. The two upper lobes of the right lung were soft and crepitating; but the inferior lobe which adhered firmly posteriorly to the pericardium and to the diaphragm, though in its upper half healthy, was towards its base red, dense, and very œdematous.

108. *Large hepatic abscess with brick-red pus.* — *Smaller one opening into lung.* — *Brick-red sputa.* — *No diarrhœa till just before death.* — *Intestines not examined.* — *A spirit drinker.*—Kalloo, a Mussulman sailor, a native of Calcutta, twenty-six years of age, in bad condition, was admitted, after twenty days' illness attributed to excessive spirit-drinking, into the clinical ward on 18th April, 1849. The respiration was thoracic, and chiefly with the left side. There was dulness of the right side of the chest, from the fourth rib to the margin. The abdomen was generally soft, with exception of induration without prominence, for two and a half inches below the right ribs, with pain on pressure, augmented by cough and full inspiration. There was febrile heat, and frequent small pulse; but the tongue was moist and nearly clean. He stated that his illness commenced with fever, ushered in with chills, and that after seven days there was pain of the right hypochondriac region, with a marked evening exacerbation of fever, sometimes terminating in sweating. Cough, pain of right side, and hectic fever persisted, and on the 23rd there was crepitus anteriorly above the third right rib, and below it dulness and absence of breath sounds. After the 27th the mucous sputa became tinged of a brick-red colour, and were sometimes copious. The urine, generally free, ranged from 1004 to 1016 in density, and showed no trace of albumen. There was no diarrhœa till three days before death, on the 7th May. He was treated with anodynes, quinine, and mineral acids, and a small blister was applied above the right nipple when the crepitus was detected, sponging the side with nitro-muriatic lotion having been previously used.

Inspection seven hours after death.—*Abdomen.*—A large abscess containing upwards of two pints of reddish-coloured thick pus, occupied the outer side of the right lobe of the liver. It projected from the concave surface towards the colon. The liver adhered firmly to the lateral abdominal parietes and to the diaphragm, and these parts formed the external lateral wall of the abscess. Another small abscess the size of a hen's egg, occupied the upper convex surface of the right lobe, separated from the upper wall of the large abscess by a layer of compressed parenchyma, about an inch in thickness. This small abscess opened through the diaphragm, by a free orifice with rounded edges, into a sac, the size of an orange, in the base of the third lobe of the right lung. At the anterior and lateral part of this sac, about the level of the fifth and sixth ribs, there was a gangrenous opening into the cavity of the pleura, which was filled with grey serous, fetid pus; and the pleura, in contact with the effusion, had a greyish gangrenous look, and was covered with flakes of friable lymph. The upper and middle lobes of the right lung were compressed against the mediastinum by the pleuritic effusion. Both kidneys, when divested of their capsules, presented a red and yellow mottled appearance.

109. *Hepatic abscess opening through the lung.— Causing pleuritis and effusion.— Also presenting externally, but not opened.*—Goohee ——, a Mussulman sailor of stout frame, a native of Calcutta, thirty-eight years of age, and for twenty years engaged in voyages to all parts of the world, and habitually using spirits freely, was after a month's illness admitted into the clinical ward on the 6th August, 1850. The respiration was short and hurried, and the lower part of the right side of chest moved imperfectly. Occasional crepitus was audible in the lower part of right mammary region, but there was no abnormal dulness. The abdomen was full, resistant below the margin of the right ribs, with dulness, but no distinct induration, for three inches below the ribs. He had dull pain of the right hypochondrium, increased by full inspiration and pressure below the ribs, occasional cough, with frothy mucous sputa. The bowels were rather slow. Morning and evening chills but no febrile heat were complained of, and the tongue was moist and almost clean. While at sea he had been attacked with fever, followed in three days with acute pain of right side, and attributed to wet. The fever, he said, left him, but the pain persisted. After admission, evening febrile accessions, with night sweats, were noticed, and the bowels began to be relaxed. On the 29th August there was indistinct fluctuation between the seventh and eighth right ribs, an inch and a half external to a vertical line dropped from the nipple. The fluctuating point became more distinct and prominent, and there was general bulging of the lower right chest. The cough had persisted with mucous sputa, but on the 26th September the sputa became more copious, pinkish, and muco-puriform; on the 27th eighteen ounces were expectorated. The fulness, tenseness, and fluctuation disappeared, and the hectic fever lessened. From this to 10th October there was relation between the quantity of the sputa and the uneasiness and tenseness of the side, and the absence or presence of fluctuation. On the 10th October severe pain of the right side of chest was complained of, and on the 14th that side ceased to move in respiration. The diarrhœa, more or less present during his residence in hospital, increased. Exhaustion and dyspnœa became aggravated, and he died on 20th October.

The treatment previous to the 29th August consisted in the application of small blisters to the right side, the use of quinine, combined with ipecacuanha and opium, and occasionally blue pill. Afterwards anodynes, tonics, and stimulants, with suitable nourishment, were the means used.

Inspection twelve hours after death.—Chest.—On removing the sternum, a fluctuating sac was seen to the right of the mediastinum formed of partially organised lymph. It was somewhat pyriform in shape, in contact, anteriorly, with the ribs and their cartilages, posteriorly, with the anterior surface of the third lobe of the right lung, and rested, inferiorly, upon the diaphragm which was here normal in structure. On laying open the sac a large quantity of limpid serous fluid was found mixed with flakes of fibrine; and it was further divided into two or three sacculi by bands of friable lymph. When traced upwards, this sac was found to be separated by a layer of lymph from another large one from which, on being opened, a few bubbles of gas escaped. This second sac contained a large collection of fluid (about a pint) seropurulent in character; it involved almost the whole of the right pleura, compressed the two upper lobes of the lung against the mediastinum, and passed behind the third lobe, as far as the diaphragm, — being, however, separated from the lateral, anterior, and inferior surfaces of this lobe by the firm connections which these parts of the lobe had formed with the costal pleura and diaphragm. On cutting into the third lobe, a ragged and irregular cavity was seen, which, laterally, approached very nearly to the surface, and was torn open on the lung being separated from its adhesions to the costal pleura, and here it had probably communicated with the sac of the pleura, and led to empyema. Inferiorly, this cavity communicated through the diaphragm with a circumscribed excavation, about the size of a large orange, situated in the upper and lateral part of the right lobe of the liver, lined by a membrane with irregular surface, and extending from the sixth to the tenth rib. The abscess in the liver communicated externally, at the most prominent part of the swelling noticed in the side during the lifetime of the patient, through the intercostal space between the seventh and eighth ribs. The intercostal muscles were in this situation in a gangrenous state, and the contents of the abscess were infiltrated into the surrounding areola tissue for the distance of an inch around. The abscess contained a few ounces of sero-sanguineous pus, similar in character to the matter expectorated. In other respects, the liver was normal, both in size and structure; it projected about two inches below the right false ribs. The left lung was healthy and free from adhesions. The intestines were discoloured externally, but were not examined internally. The kidneys were healthy. The heart was not examined.

110. *Hepatitis, ending in abscess discharged through the lung.—An abscess in the third lobe of the right lung, communicating freely through the diaphragm with the abscess in the liver.—Mucous coat of the large intestine ulcerated.—Many of the ulcers cicatrised.* — John Shea, aged twenty-eight, was admitted into hospital on the 22nd November, 1840, in a moribund state, and died eight hours after admission. He had been sent from the sloop *Clive*, off Aden, and had been first taken ill with hepatitis on the 6th August; had improved, but the disease recurred severely on the 23rd of the same month. There had been severe pain increased by decubitus on the left side, and pressure upwards. On the 6th October, he was suddenly seized with expectoration of pus, which continued with diarrhœa till the period of his death.

Inspection twelve hours after death. — *Head.* — Nothing worthy of note. *Chest.* — Neither lung collapsed. The posterior part of the left one was very œdematous, the anterior emphysematous with a few tubercles disseminated. The right lung adhered to the costal pleura, and to the diaphragm by tender lymph; there were a few tubercles in the upper lobe. The rest of the lung was very œdematous, but chiefly the third lobe, which was also in parts hepatised. At the anterior part of the base of the third lobe, there was a cavity the size of an orange, with a ragged and flocculent inner surface, which communicated through the diaphragm with an abscess in the upper part of the right lobe of the liver, about the size of a small orange, superficial, and lined with a firm membrane with irregular flocculent surface. The rest of the liver was healthy, and not mottled. On the surface of the heart there were many white pearly spots; but the organ was sound. *Abdomen.*—There were a few ounces of serum in the cavity. The stomach, much distended, occupied the whole space between the umbilicus and ribs; its mucous coat was pale and sound in texture. The colon, covered by the stomach, was contracted, and had formed no unnatural adhesions. The mucous coat was reddened in parts, and there were a few small circular ulcers, with the cicatrices of many others, chiefly distinguished by their dark grey colour, their depression below the rest of the surface, and closer connection to the subjacent tunics. The edges of some of the ulcers were puckered, but those of the greater number were rounded, and not thickened. The kidneys and spleen were healthy.

111. *Two Hepatic abscesses. — One opening into the lung, with expectoration of deep bile-tinged puriform sputa.*—An Indo-Portuguese, of twenty-six years of age, was admitted into the Jamsetjee Jejeebhoy Hospital, on the 8th January, 1848, ill with symptoms of hepatitis for six weeks. He stated, that three days before admission,

he began to expectorate sputa of bloody appearance and intensely bitter taste. After admission, the sputa consisted of ordinary pus; but on the 9th they became of deep yellow colour, thick and glairy, easily expectorated, and in great quantity, and the swelling of the right side, much less than on admission, extended downwards to a line drawn transversely from the umbilicus. The abdomen was swollen, and pain was felt to the right of the epigastrium under the cartilages of the false ribs. He said that it had before extended over great part of the right side of the chest. Dejections whitish. Died rather suddenly on the night of the 17th.

Inspection. — *Abdomen.* — Opaque pinkish or chocolate-coloured fluid, with flocculi of lymph, was found in great abundance in the abdomen. The peritoneum of paries and viscera was of red colour. A large abscess in the left lobe of the liver pressed on the stomach, having at its upper part the substance of the liver extended over it, but this gradually thinned away, and at the lower part, the wall was formed of the thickened peritoneal covering. Another large abscess occupied the lower part of the right lobe of the liver. Both these abscesses contained pus, very slightly tinted of a greenish yellow, and that in the abscess of the left lobe was more abundant and thinner; both had ragged walls. There were adhesions to the stomach and duodenum. The capsule of Glisson was thickened. The gall-bladder contained only a little viscid mucus of a greenish colour. At the upper part of the right lobe there was adhesion to the diaphragm, and corresponding thereto the right lung was also adherent. On separating the adhesion of the lung, a cavity was opened which extended into a small abscess in the liver with thick firm lining of adventitious membrane. The neighbouring portion of the liver was much gorged with blood, and the cavity extended upwards into the lower part of the lung; its walls there being very ragged and uneven, and the surrounding portion of the lung was hepatised and gorged with blood. The portion of this common abscess which was in the liver contained only thick whitish pus; while that which was in the lung contained pus of deep yellow or greenish yellow, and its ragged walls were deeply stained of the same colour, and on pressing the abscess before opening it, deep yellow fluid was made to flow upwards through the divided bronchial tubes.

Remarks. — Dr. Leith was present with me at the inspection of this case. To him I am indebted for the note of the appearances observed, and for the information that he had not long before witnessed a somewhat similar case of bile-tinged sputa in the hospital of the Bombay police corps.

112. *Abscess in the liver opening through the diaphragm into the sac of the pleura and causing purulent effusion there.*—James Oakhum, aged thirty-two, a feeble man of reduced and emaciated habit, was admitted into the European General Hospital on the 27th September, 1843. He stated that he had been under treatment for eight days, suffering from pain of the right side, first under the clavicle, subsequently at the margin of the right ribs, and that he had been leeched and blistered. On admission, the skin was hot and dry, and the tongue florid at the tip. On the 28th he complained of pain at the margin of the right ribs, impeding full inspiration; and laterally and posteriorly there was perfect dulness and inaudible respiratory murmur. Evening febrile exacerbation, and occasional diarrhœa, but seldom any complaint of pain of the side were present till the 3rd October, when in addition he began to be troubled with cough, accompanied on the 4th with expectoration of thin puriform fluid. The cough, the puriform sputa, the dulness of the right side, the febrile symptoms, the occasional diarrhœa continued, accompanied with progressive emaciation and collapse, and latterly short and oppressed breathing, till the morning of the 12th October, when he died.

Inspection eleven hours after death.—The body was much emaciated. *Chest.*—On the right side, from the fourth rib downwards, anteriorly, the lung adhered to the costal pleura, and to the diaphragm; but there was no adhesion of the posterior part of the lung. At the posterior part of the right side of the chest, and also the anterior above the level of the fourth rib, there were about two pints of faint reddish-coloured puriform fluid. This effusion communicated through the diaphragm behind the lung, with an abscess in the upper and posterior part of the right lobe of the liver, larger than an orange. The lung was compressed, but healthy in texture. The left lung was healthy. The abdominal viscera were not particularly examined, but the intestines were healthy externally.

I have met with cases in which the symptoms of hepatic abscess had been well marked, and the occurrence of puriform expectoration suggested that communication had taken place between the abscess and the lung, and yet examination after death failed to verify it. Three cases of this nature are before me. In the two first an opening was carefully looked for, but not found; and the condition of the lung was not such as to account for the character of the sputa. In the third the sufficiency of the examination is doubtful, and the base of the right lung was hepatised. From such cases it may be surmised that when interstitial absorption is in progress in the wall of an abscess, between the liver and the lung, and the tissues are becoming soft and succulent, the thinner contents of the sac may perhaps pass through by imbibition before the occurrence of actual rupture. At all events, this question may be proposed for future inquiry to solve.

2. *Hepatic Abscess opening into the Stomach or Intestine.* — Five cases, 3·57 per cent. of this termination have come under my notice. Dr. Stovell's ratio to the admissions from hepatitis is 0·451. Of my five cases three recovered. In two the abscess was supposed to have opened into the colon, in one into the stomach and colon. In one of the fatal cases the situation and marked decrease of the swelling favoured the belief that an abscess had opened into the stomach; but neither vomiting nor purulent dejections occurred; yet, after death, the diagnosis was proved to be correct, for communication existed between the abscess and the stomach. In this case the pus must have oozed slowly into the stomach, and thence passed in small quantity at a time through the intestinal canal, probably in an altered form. In the other an opening into the colon was found after death, but the account of the symptoms during life had been incomplete.

It is a common belief that the discharge of hepatic abscess into the alimentary canal is not rare; and that it is always clearly indicated by the sensations of the patient and by free vomiting or dejection of pus. My experience, however, does not confirm this opinion. In two of my cases (113, 115) the pus must have drained so slowly into the canal as not to affect the appearance of the discharges, though its presence had been carefully looked for. In other two (116, 117) pus was present; and in my remaining case (114) there was no record of the symptoms. I am satisfied that there has been much loose observation and inaccurate record on this subject; and that too much weight has been generally accorded to the statement of the patient. At all events, in two or three instances in which this supposed occurrence has been reported to me, the evidence has failed to convince me.

The following are the five cases to which I have adverted: —

113. *Abscess in the left lobe of the liver opening into the stomach.—No vomiting.—No detection of pus in the intestinal discharges.—No intestinal ulceration.*—Ibrahim Mahomed, a Mussulman water-carrier, of thirty years of age, using spirits, and at one time opium, habitually, was admitted into the clinical ward on the 30th June, 1853. He was emaciated, countenance anxious, pulse small. In the epigastric region there was a painful swelling, the size of a cocoa-nut, prominent, soft, indistinctly fluctuating, not pointing, but somewhat tense. Decubitus on the back, or either side. Three months before, a small swelling appeared in the situation of the present large one, and gradually increased; it was not very painful, and not attended with fever. He had suffered from fever before the swelling was noticed; but then there was no pain in the region of the liver. His bowels had been regular, and there had not been any vomiting. On the 3rd July the size and prominence of the swelling were less, the bowels had been four times opened, and the discharges were reported to be dark coloured. From the 4th to the 15th there was no recurrence of diarrhœa, the evacuations were feculent, and still the swelling lessened. Its prominence was gone on the 12th. On the 16th again diarrhœa, with discharges described as thin, feculent, and of buff yellow. The swelling was now gone, and dulness did not extend more than two inches below the ensiform cartilage. There had been no vomiting. From this time there were occasional dysenteric symptoms, occasional slight febrile accessions, and a failing pulse; then, on the 2nd August, copious intestinal discharges; and death on the 4th. Treated with anodynes and tonics. The urine gave no traces of albumen.

Inspection twelve hours after death.—Chest.—The anterior surface of the lungs was pale, spongy, and somewhat emphysematous at the edges. No adhesions. *Heart.*—The walls of the left ventricle were thickened, and the cavity small. *Abdomen.*—The external surface of the liver was of dark red colour. The liver extended to about two inches below the ensiform cartilage, and about two and a half inches below the margins of the right false ribs. There were not any adhesions between it and the diaphragm, but the concave surface of the left lobe adhered firmly to the smaller curvature of the stomach, and to the pancreas. On separating the adhesions to the pancreas, an opening about the size of a rupee, with dark grey edges, was apparent in the liver. The opening conducted into an empty sac, about the size of a large orange, situated in the inferior surface of the left lobe. This sac was lined by a firm membranous layer, with irregular surface; it also communicated, by an opening sufficiently large to admit an ordinary blow-pipe, with the stomach close to its pyloric end. The substance of the liver, for about half an inch beyond the upper wall of the sac, was of dark grey colour, indurated and condensed. The inferior wall of the sac was about a quarter of an inch thick, partly fibrous and partly condensed substance of the liver. The substance of the right lobe of the liver was healthy. *Stomach.*—Much distended, and containing about a pint and a half of light-coloured yellow turbid fluid with white floating flakes, which, examined under the microscope, showed no pus globules. *Intestines.*—In general pale, except at the end of the ileum and rectum; in both these situations a blush of redness was seen, and the membrane was softer than natural. *Kidneys.*—Right one healthy. Left one somewhat lobulated, of pale buff colour, externally and internally; cortical substance encroached considerably on the tubular portion, which in places was very indistinct.

114. *An abscess of the liver communicating with the colon.—Others in process of repair by absorption.*—An old man was admitted into the Jamsetjee Jejeebhoy Hospital with fulness below the margin of the right ribs, indicating the existence of hepatic abscess. Before death the fulness had lessened considerably, but how caused was not understood.

Inspection after death.—Towards the thin edge of the right lobe of the liver there was an abscess the size of an orange, having the concave surface adherent to the right kidney for its lower wall. It communicated by an opening the size of a goose-quill with the hepatic flexure of the colon. The mucous membrane around the opening was free of disease. The walls of the abscess were almost cartilaginous in density. The substance of the liver was very firm, and here and there were yellow dense circumscribed deposits the size of a horse-bean and upwards in size. They were tubercular-looking in appearance; and in one, the size of a walnut, the contents were soft and putty-like. The contents of both were examined under the microscope. The dense tubercular-like matter consisted of small granules. In the less consistent there were also granules; but some of them had, in many places, aggregated into distinct corpuscles: it seemed as if the breaking down of the pus corpuscles, and the escape of their contained granules, had not proceeded to the same extent. These, then, had been abscesses, and were in process of repair by absorption. There was Bright's disease of the kidney in this case.*

115. *Hepatic abscess, recovered from, by probable opening into the colon.*—Mahomed Jaffer, a Mussulman, forty-five years of age, a painter, using spirits occasionally, and the subject, a year before the date of the present case, of hepatic symptoms, was admitted into the clinical ward on the 5th December, 1853. He was reduced, the countenance was anxious, skin hot, pulse frequent, small and sinking. The respiration was somewhat hurried. Below the margin of the right ribs and the ensiform cartilage, there was resistance, tenderness, and dulness, bounded below by a line drawn from the eighth left rib, curving to about half an inch above the umbilicus, and extending to the eighth rib on the right side. Decubitus easiest on the back and right side. The tenderness on pressure was considerable; fever and pain of abdomen had come on simultaneously twenty days before admission. The fever was remittent, with midday exacerbation and evening remission. On the 13th December there was epigastric fulness with indistinct fluctuation. Now there was abatement of fever; but he had troublesome cough with frothy mucous sputa. On the 24th, while turning in bed, he experienced a peculiar sensation in the swelling, as if something had given away, and on examination it was found to be considerably diminished. No diarrhœa, no trace of pus in the evacuations. There was now gradual slow decrease of the swelling, with occasional febrile recurrences; and he was discharged on the 15th February, 1854, with a small induration perceptible an inch and a half above the umbilicus, not painful, but with dulness, continuous upwards with that of the liver. He was treated chiefly with quinine and anodynes, then dilute nitric acid, and occasional laxatives, and warm water application to the epigastrium.

---

* About the same time, somewhat similar appearances were brought to my notice in a preparation sent to me from the European General Hospital. In this the membranous sac was distinct, the contents being partly pulpy, partly tough, and presenting an appearance of layers. It was in the cirrhosed liver of an emaciated sailor, who died of ascites. In this case there was also granular degeneration of the kidney.

116. *Hepatic abscess.—Opening into the colon (?)—Recovery.*—Camajee Yellojee, aged forty-eight, a Jew of intemperate habits, was admitted into hospital on the 6th March, 1837. There was tenderness below the margin of the right ribs, which he said had existed for a month. On the 7th, purging during the night reported; evacuations not seen: but a pale-coloured stool passed on the 7th consisted chiefly of pus, as proved by the microscope. After this there was no further appearance of pus.

117. *Hepatic abscess.—Opening into the colon and stomach (?)—Recovery.*—Pestonjee Dadabhoy, aged twenty, an intemperate Parsee buggy driver, was admitted into hospital on the 18th January, 1857, with symptoms of acute hepatitis. Fulness at the epigastrium indicated the formation of abscess. On the 27th there was vomiting. The ejected matters were not kept, but the epigastric fulness became very sensibly diminished; and on the 28th, about two ounces of unmixed pus were passed by stool. Afterwards there was no more vomiting, and no further traces of pus in the dejections. He left the hospital on the 22nd March, improved in flesh, and with no signs of hepatic enlargement.

3. *Hepatic Abscess opening into the Pericardium*—is very rare. Rokitansky and Graves each report a case. There is one recorded by Mr. Fowler.* Mr. Leahy, a very intelligent apothecary of the Bombay establishment, gave me the notes of a case observed by him at Peshawur in the Bombay Fusileer Regiment; in it there were two abscesses, one communicating with the right lung, the other with the pericardium. I have never witnessed this termination of hepatic abscess.

4. *Hepatic Abscess opening into the Biliary Duct.*—It is stated in systematic works that this is the most favourable course for hepatic abscess to follow; but surely this assertion rests on theoretic grounds. The only case, with which I am acquainted, proving that hepatic abscess sometimes communicates with the ducts, and may be discharged by this channel, is recorded by Dr. Leith in the following words:—"The case of a foot-artilleryman, sent from Bombay with abscess of the liver, who died in the hospital, is worthy of notice, although he does not come properly within the subject of this report. The tumefaction in the side gradually disappeared; and after his death the abscess was found nearly empty, and two hepatic ducts communicating with it were found carrying pus to the duodenum." †

5. *Hepatic Abscess opening into the Cavity of the Peritoneum.*—My cases do afford distinct evidence of rupture of hepatic abscess into the sac of the peritoneum: in two it was probable, but was not positively established.

Contents of Abscess removed by Absorption.—The different

* "Transactions of the Medical and Physical Society of Bombay," Second Series, No. 2, p. 305.

† "Transactions of the Medical and Physical Society of Bombay," No. 4, p. 57.

directions in which hepatic abscess may discharge its contents have been described, and we have found that, in a small proportion of the cases, recovery results. But it is not only by this course that hepatic abscess may be recovered from. Cases sometimes occur in which the existence of abscess has been undoubted, and the fluctuating swelling has gradually lessened and finally disappeared without any appreciable discharge.* The inference that in such cases the removal of the pus has been effected by absorption, is confirmed by appearances occasionally found after death. The process is probably of this nature: first, normal capillary circulation in the tissues around, then absorption of the liquor puris, with consequent shriveling and breaking up of the corpuscles into their constituent granules — an encysted putty-like or cretaceous residuum being left. Three cases (118—120) which I shall presently narrate, and case 114, will serve to illustrate this process of absorption, which is fully recognised by Rokitansky. Case 121 was probably recovered from by absorption.

118. *Two hepatic abscesses in process of absorption. — Death from cholera. — Painful decubitus on right side explained by situation of one of the abscesses. — Ulceration of colon.* — Annajee, a Hindoo labourer, of thirty-two years of age, accustomed to the moderate use of spirits, and of six grains of opium daily, after eight days' illness was admitted into the clinical ward on the 10th of December, 1850, not reduced by sickness. The respiration was somewhat hurried and oppressed, but occasional bronchitic rales were the only signs of pulmonic disease. The abdomen was full and somewhat resistant. On the right side, dulness on percussion reached from the sixth rib to a line drawn obliquely from the left eighth costal cartilage to the point of the last right rib. Between this line and the margin of the ribs, there was distinct induration, and pain increased by pressure. Decubitus dorsal, and on the left side, but causing pain and distress of breathing on the right. There was febrile disturbance, a tremulous tongue, and regular bowels. The local symptoms had been present eight days, and the febrile five. On the 23rd he complained of pain of the right shoulder. Under the use of cautious leeching, small blisters and quinine, combined with ipecacuanha and blue pill, the induration and dulness below the margin of the right rib had almost disappeared by the 29th. But the pain of right shoulder continued, and the cough was more troublesome, with increase of bronchitic rales. The urine was frequently examined: it was generally free, somewhat turbid, and without albumen. On the 7th January the induration was gone, and the dulness extended about an inch below the ribs; the pain of shoulder had ceased, and the cough was less troublesome. Had recurrence of febrile disturbance on the 13th. Symptoms of cholera came on on the 15th, and he died on the morning of the 16th. There were slight dysenteric symptoms on the 18th and 19th December.

Inspection six hours after death.—Abdomen.—On opening the cavity, the thin edge of the right lobe of the liver was seen projecting to the extent of about an inch beneath the ensiform cartilage and the cartilage of the eighth and ninth ribs of the

* I have not thought it necessary to consider the question of the elimination of the contents of hepatic abscess by the kidney. I think with those who believe that the transfer of entire pus corpuscles from the liver to the urine, through the blood and secreting processes, is physiologically impossible.

right side. There were firm adhesions of the most prominent part of the convex surface of the right lobe to the under surface of the diaphragm, and a good deal of difficulty was experienced in removing the organ from the abdominal cavity. On incising the right lobe of the liver at the site of the adhesions, corresponding in situation to the bodies of the seventh and eight right ribs, there was a small abscess the size of a pigeon's egg, with firm membranous walls, and containing healthy pus. Between the cavity of the abscess and the diaphragm only a thin layer of the parenchyma intervened. A little above and to the left of this there was another abscess the size of an olive, also bounded by a membranous cyst and containing yellow putty-like substance, which was amorphic and granular, with here and there a corpuscle. The rest of the liver was healthy. The small intestine was distended with gas, and the large one was contracted. At the end of the ileum the mucous membrane presented enlarged glands, and small superficial ulcers were observed in the sigmoid flexure and the upper part of the rectum. Otherwise the coats of both the small and large intestines were healthy. Spleen of smaller size than natural. The kidneys were healthy. *Chest.*—There were firm adhesions of both lungs to the costal pleuræ, and of the base of the right lung to the convex surface of the diaphragm. The pulmonary tissue was in part crepitating, and in part woolly to the feel, and when incised presented a pale appearance, intermixed with numerous black specks. The heart was healthy.

119. *Four hepatic abscesses.—General peritonitis, but no evidence of abscess rupture.—Two of the abscesses in process of cure by absorption.*—Dajee Gungajee, a Hindoo buggy driver, of thirty-three years of age, using spirits habitually, was admitted into the clinical ward on the 4th of December, 1851. The countenance was anxious, the respiration short, and thoracic; the abdomen was tense, tender, and somewhat tympanitic; the decubitus was dorsal, and the thighs flexed; the skin was coldish, and the pulse thready. The tongue was coated white on the sides, but florid at the tip and centre. His illness commenced seven days before with fever, followed by uneasiness below the right false ribs, which gradually extended over the abdomen, and three days ago attained its present severity. Under the application of a blister to the abdomen, the use of quinine and opium, wine and ammonia, he lingered till the 9th December. He had received a blow on the right side of his chest two months before the present attack.

Inspection nineteen hours after death.—Chest.—There were some old adhesions between the base of the right lung and the diaphragm. The substance of both the lungs was healthy. The heart of natural size and normal. Slight firm deposit on the lining membrane of the ascending aorta. *Abdomen.*—There was about a pint of red-tinged serum in the cavity of the abdomen. The intestines were distended, and presented streaks of redness on the peritoneal surface, and flakes of lymph existed between the convolutions as well as between the lateral parietes and the ascending colon. The liver, much enlarged, extended three inches below the margin of the right false costal cartilages, and across to those of the opposite side. Extensive lymph effusion existed between the left lobe of the liver and the anterior parietes. The concave surface of the liver was firmly adherent to the transverse colon, to the stomach at its pyloric extremity and to the duodenum, by a thick layer of lymph. There were also firm adhesions between the convex surface of the liver and the diaphragm, and the posterior wall of the abdomen. On separating the adhesions between the concave surface of the liver, stomach, and duodenum, the walls of an abscess in the liver gave way about an inch to the left of the gall-bladder which was firmly adherent to the colon. The abscess was about the size of a large orange, and yellow flaky matter was attached to the inner surface of the membranous cyst which enclosed it. In the centre of the right lobe of the liver was another abscess the size of a cocoa-nut, not communicating with the one on the concave surface, but just above it;

it contained thick flocculent pus, enclosed by a thin membranous layer. At the posterior edge of the right lobe there was another abscess distinct from the two above described. It was about the size of a hen's egg, and contained thick putty-like pus; the walls were of thickened membrane more organised. In the left lobe towards its concave surface there was included, in a still thicker membranous sac, a fourth collection of still more consistent and putty-like contents; it was the size of a walnut. The concave surface of the liver immediately over the cyst had a somewhat depressed and puckered appearance. The substance of the right lobe of the liver presented generally a dark red colour, and was not softened; the left lobe was of pale colour, and more lacerable. The putty-like contents of the third and fourth abscesses, submitted to the microscope, presented no trace of pus corpuscles, but consisted of small granular matter, with an oil globule here and there. The spleen was much smaller than natural. The right kidney congested and lobulated; the left somewhat pale. The mucous membrane of the stomach presented variegated patches of redness, best marked at the lesser curvature.

120. *Hepatic abscess in process of cure by absorption.*—Hybattee Sinday, aged forty-nine, a water-carrier, was admitted into hospital under Dr. Ballingall's care, on the 16th April, 1857. He was emaciated, affected with phthisis and diarrhœa. He died on the 28th.

Inspection.—There were tubercles in both lungs, with cavities in the upper lobes. About the middle of the liver, posteriorly, there was a single abscess-sac about the size of a small apple, filled with putty-like matter. The walls were thick and firmly organised. The gall-bladder was full of dark-coloured concretions. The solitary glands of the large intestine were distinct, and there were sloughy ulcers here and there.

121. *Hepatic abscess.—Absorption.—Recovery.*—Narayen Nuthoo, aged twenty-four, admitted 25th November, 1857. A prominent fluctuating circumscribed swelling in the epigastric region, reached to the umbilicus. It was suspected to be hydatid. But after a fortnight it gradually lessened and finally consisted merely of slight induration three inches below the ensiform cartilage—without prominence or fluctuation. The bowels were relaxed for three or four days, but the evacuations were not seen and they were not coincident with the decrease of the swelling.

Secondary partial peritonitis.—Circumscribed Puriform Sacs.—It has been already stated (pp. 327 and 329) that secondary inflammation of the peritoneal covering of the liver, in the course of hepatic abscess, with consequent adhesion, is the rule. In occasional cases, there is absence of peritonitic inflammation. But in other cases there is another kind of deviation: in this the secondary peritonitis has not led to adhesion at all points, but a portion of the lymph changing into pus has formed a circumscribed sac between the liver and the opposed surface. The most common situation is between the liver and the diaphragm; but it may also occur in relation with the concave surface of the organ. Sometimes the sac communicates with the hepatic abscess: more frequently, however, it is merely superimposed.

A collection of pus, however, may form in close proximity to the liver, independent of hepatic abscess, as is shown in the two following cases (122, 123). The first was communicated to me by Mr. Plumptre, the medical officer in charge of the Sanitarium at

Poorundhur. On the 29th December, 1858, I saw the case on the occasion of my visit to the station—and never doubting that it was abscess of the left lobe, recommended that it should be punctured in a few days.

122. *Purulent sac, between the liver and the diaphragm, communicating with the left lung.—No hepatic abscess.*—A private in the 3rd Dragoon Guards, aged thirty-two, of 12 years' service, and ten months in India, after dysentery, reputed colic, and dyspepsia, was sent from Kirkee to Poorundhur on 22nd September, 1858. He had pain of epigastrium extending to the left hypochondrium. No enlargement. The symptoms were considered to be dyspeptic, and he was discharged free of pain on the 8th November. He was re-admitted on the 26th November, with return of pain and suspected enlargement of the left lobe of the liver. Discharged on 11th December. Re-admitted on the 20th. There was now distinct swelling at the left side of the epigastrium with dulness for three inches around. On the 29th it was prominent, obscurely fluctuating and tending to point. It was opened with a bistoury on the 4th January. Red-tinged pus discharged freely, and was always increased after eating. There was hectic fever and increasing emaciation. On the 7th February he expectorated with little effort a considerable quantity of greenish yellow pus. Up to the 23rd February the puncture looked healthy, but now the edges became gangrenous. On the 25th the abdomen was tense, distended, and tender, the features anxious, the pulse 110, and somewhat sharp. He died on the 1st March.

Inspection fourteen hours after death.—Body emaciated. There were six pints of sero-pus in the abdomen. The intestines were distended, and their surface smeared with flakes of friable lymph. A large purulent sac existed between the liver and the diaphragm. It communicated with the punctured wound, also with the left lung, which which was consolidated at its base and firmly adherent to the diaphragm. No direct communication with the cavity of the peritoneum was discovered, The substance of the left lobe was not implicated. The liver was enlarged and of nutmeg appearance. The diaphragm was adherent to the surface of the left lobe at the circumference of the sac.

123. *Amputation of the right hand, followed by general bad health, and chronic hepatitis.—A purulent sac between the liver and the ribs filled with fœtid pus.—Hepatisation of the lower part of the right lung.*—Gresham Stewart, aged thirty-one, gunner's mate Honourable Company's steamer *Cleopatra.* On the 29th of July, 1842, the right arm was amputated above the wrist in consequence of a severe injury received while incautiously extracting the charge of a gun. The operation was performed immediately after the accident. On the 8th August he was admitted into the European General Hospital. Union had not taken place and the stump presented a sloughy appearance. He, by degrees, however, improved, and was discharged well on the 5th October. He was re-admitted on the 5th November, sallow and reduced, with feeble pulse, complaining of occasional shooting pain of the right hypochondrium, and at times suffering from diarrhœa. He continued labouring under these symptoms, more or less till towards the end of January, when the pain of the right hypochondrium increased and became more constant, with coated tongue and sharpish pulse. On the 10th February, it was reported that there was distinct hard swelling of several inches in circumference over the lateral part of the right false ribs, commencing about the sixth rib and extending to the tenth. There was no preceptible fluctuation. During the night of the 11th, there was hæmoptysis to a considerable extent, succeeded the following day by cough with rusty-coloured sputa, at times in considerable quantity. Under these symptoms, much harassed by cough, he lingered, and died on the 27th February, very much emaciated.

Inspection twelve hours after death.—The body much emaciated. *Abdomen.*—Between the liver and the ribs there was a sac containing fœtid dark-coloured pus; the walls of the sac being sloughy and ragged. [This purulent sac was opposed to the site of the tumefaction during life, but there was no purulent effusion between the ribs and the integuments, nor had the pus made a way through the intercostal muscles.] The peritoneal surface of the liver was in one or two places abraded, but the substance of the organ was not implicated. There was no communication between the abscess and the sac of the pleura, or the lungs. *Chest.*—The right lung adhered to the costal pleura and to the diaphragm, and was in the first stage of hepatisation, giving out frothy blood-coloured serum when pressed. There was a considerable quantity of serum in the pericardium. The other viscera, though attenuated, were healthy.

That purulent collections may occur consequent upon ordinary secondary peritonitis, and independent of hepatic abscess, is proved by the cases just narrated. The occurrence may be held to indicate a depraved diathesis. There is moreover a practical lesson in these circumscribed sacs. They teach us to be cautious in attributing a pointing fluctuating swelling in the right intercostal spaces below the seventh, and in the epigastrium, to the presence of hepatic abscess: it may be caused by a collection of pus between the liver and the diaphragm.

Cases 124 to 127 are of secondary partial puriform peritonitis in connection with hepatic abscess; also 160, 161, 168, 172.

124. *Abscess in the liver.—Also one external and circumscribed communicating with former.—Dark red colour of mucous surface of large intestine, which contained much clotted blood.*—Serjeant O. M——, of Her Majesty's 40th Regiment, aged thirty-two, was admitted into hospital at Belgaum, on the 21st June, 1830. This man was a hard drinker, and was said to have been ill with dysentery fourteen days before admission. There was much purging with severe tenesmus and griping. The dejections were scanty, mucous and bloody, then became red, watery, and fœtid, and for the last two days before his death consisted entirely of grumous, dark-coloured blood. Tenderness of abdomen moderate. He sunk gradually, and died July 2nd.

Inspection.—On opening the abdomen a superficial abscess presented itself; situated on the superior surface of the thin edge of the right lobe of the liver, having for its walls, posteriorly, the liver, anteriorly, the abdominal parietes, inferiorly, the colon extremely distended and adhering to the margin of the liver. The abscess dipped down between the ascending colon and the concave surface of the liver, and then communicated with another abscess, which occupied the whole interior of the right lobe of the liver; and below it terminated in a large collection of pus, situated behind the caput cœcum. The cœcum and ascending colon were internally of dark red colour, and filled with clotted blood; and in parts of the colon the peritoneal was the only tunic left. The liver was light coloured, and adhered to the right side and to the diaphragm. Adhesions existed between the right lung and diaphragm, opposite to those of the liver.

125. *Hepatic abscess bounded by a firm sac.—A circumscribed sac in the peritoneal cavity over the edge of the liver.—Substance of the liver mottled red and white.*—Thomas Conolly, aged forty, of slight habit, a seaman, admitted on the 24th March, 1841. He stated that he had suffered from acute pain of the right hypochondrium at the margin of the ribs, for four days, attended with frequent purging. The pain was acute, preventing full inspiration, and extending downwards in the direction of the right iliac region. Pulse 100, sharpish, but easily compressed. Skin moist. Tongue

coated in the centre, and florid at the tip. He was bled to sixteen ounces and freely leeched: he bore the depletion badly. The pain continued unabated, and frequent vomiting was superadded. On the 28th, there was fulness and tenseness extending from the right iliac fossa to the margin of the ribs and reaching as far as the umbilicus. The left side was supple. He died at midnight of the 30th. At the beginning, two full doses of calomel with opium were given; it was then omitted and camphor mixture with spiritus ammoniæ aromaticus and wine substituted.

Inspection seven hours after death.—Head.—The brain was firm, and there was a thin veil of serum beneath the arachnoid membrane at the interspaces of the convolutions. *Chest.*—The lungs did not collapse, in consequence of their emphysematous state. *Abdomen.*—The omentum adhered in places to the intestines and also to the edge (partly overlapping it) of the right lobe of the liver. There was a portion of the substance of the liver, the size of a large orange at the thin part of the right lobe, of white colour, in parts tolerably firm, in others pulpy, in others breaking down into pus,—bounded by a firm sac, from which the white part could be scraped; and over that portion of the liver there was a circumscribed abscess bounded by the abdominal parietes, the omentum, and liver. The substance of the liver generally was mottled red and white. The colon was contracted, with ulcers, here and there, on its mucous coat.

126. *Abscess in the liver communicating with purulent deposit in the right iliac region.—Habitual constipation.—The sigmoid flexure of the colon much contracted.*—A gentleman, aged about forty-six, of full habit, and subject to occasional attacks of gout and rheumatic swelling of the joints, after a residence of twenty-seven years in India, at the end of 1832 (previous to which time, though subject to constipation, he had never suffered from acute visceral disease), was attacked with inflammation of the bowels attended with constipation, and requiring much general and local depletion for its removal. After convalescence he went to the Cape of Good Hope, resided there one year, and returned to Bombay at the commencement of 1835. About two months before I saw him, consequent on exposure to cold, and irregularities of diet, diarrhœa supervened, alternating with occasional constipation, and scybalous discharges. When he came under my care on the 17th April, 1835, he was much reduced from his usual fulness. The expression of countenance was languid and anxious. The tongue was florid. The bowels were relaxed, the dejections being of dark-green colour, watery, and offensive. There was tenderness on pressure of the right iliac region. On the 27th April, occasional drowsiness was for the first time observed, and there was increasing weakness. Death took place at noon of the 2nd May, having been preceded by vomiting of inky coloured fluid.

Inspection four hours after death.—Abdomen.—The parietes of the cavity and the omentum were loaded with fat. The stomach was filled with dark inky coloured fluid, but, with the exception of softening of some points of the mucous coat, was healthy. There was a collection of pus in the right iliac region, circumscribed by part of the concave surface of the liver, the fundus of the gall-bladder, a matted portion of the omentum, the ascending colon, and the right kidney. It communicated with an extensive, but very superficial abscess, on the inferior surface of the liver, to the right of the lobulus Spigelii. The descending colon was contracted, and the sigmoid flexure was of about the diameter of a swan's quill. The mucous lining of the cœcum and ascending colon was thickened, and presented black mottled patches with the traces of cicatrices. All the coats of the descending colon and of the sigmoid flexure were thickened, but there was no puckered irregularity of the inner surface. The small intestine was filled with dark green viscous contents.

127. *A circumscribed sac between the liver and the ribs.—An abscess in the substance of the right lobe.—The mucous coat of the colon studded with circular ulcers.*—George Bignel, of moderate habit, aged twenty-eight years, and nine months resident in India

for three days before admission into hospital on the 2nd January, 1840, had suffered from pain of the right side, shooting to the shoulder, and impeding full inspiration. He was twice freely bled and very freely leeched and blistered; and on the 8th, 9th, and 10th, he was mildly under the influence of mercury. He did not convalesce in a satisfactory manner, and on the 29th there was recurrence of the pain of the side, and the liver was distinctly felt two inches below the ribs. The fulness below the ribs became subsequently more distinct, and there was hepatic sound almost to the nipple. He suffered frequently from pain of the side, became emaciated, subject to hectic and diarrhœa, with a tongue florid at the tip. He died on the 26th February.

Inspection.—Head.—There was an ounce of serum at the base of the skull and a veil of serum between the arachnoid and pia mater on the convex surface of the brain. *Chest.*—There were old adhesions of the right lung to the diaphragm and posterior parietes, and firm adhesions of the liver to the concavity of the ribs. There was a circumscribed purulent sac between the surface of the liver and the ribs. The liver extended three inches below the margin of the ribs, and in the upper part of the right lobe there was an abscess, the size of a hen's egg, with flocculent walls. The mucous coat of the stomach was of red-brown colour, but sound in texture. The mucous coat of the large intestine presented a surface of closely set circular ulcers, in places running into each other, and giving a honey-combed appearance to the membrane; in places the margins of the ulcers were of bright red colour, and were generally softened in texture.

Secondary Pleuritis, leading to General or Circumscribed Empyema.—It has just been shown that secondary inflammation of the hepatic peritoneum may lead to the formation of a purulent sac instead of adhesions. A reference to the cases quoted in different parts of this chapter will show that secondary diaphragmatic peritonitis, is very frequently associated with secondary diaphragmatic pleuritis, leading to adhesion between the base of the right lung and the diaphragm. But just as in the peritoneum, we may have in the pleura a similar deviation from this rule. Instead of adhesions taking place, or sometimes in association with them, the lymph changes into pus, and general or circumscribed empyema is the consequence. It is important to know that there may be empyema co-existing with hepatic abscess, not caused by communication, but merely by extension of inflammatory action through the diaphragm,—in individuals prone to the suppurative process. It appears, then, that empyema, from communication, or independent of it, is not an unfrequent complication, and it sometimes renders the diagnosis of hepatic abscess obscure: the signs of the empyema may be attributed to the encroachment of the liver on the chest; or, if rightly interpreted, they may throw a doubt over the previous diagnosis of hepatic disease.

It is not, however, only in the pleura that we have evidence of the extension of inflammation from one diaphragmatic surface to the other. It may also occur, but much more rarely, in the *pericardium*. Of this I have met with two instances (131, 132).

In one the relation of the pericarditis to hepatic abscess was well shown. These two cases, and three (128 to 130) illustrative of my remarks on empyema, are here submitted. The latter may be considered in connection with cases 170, 171, which exemplify the same morbid state.

128. *Abscess in the liver.* — *Empyema of the right pleura.* — *Symptoms not well marked.* — *Dejection of a pint of clotted blood before death.* — *Mucous coat of the colon dark red with ulceration.* — Richard Dunstan, aged thirty-nine, two years in India, was admitted on the 16th January, 1841. He was reduced in flesh, having been ill for several days, and having taken no food. He complained chiefly of uneasiness at the epigastrium not amounting to pain, nor increased by pressure, full inspiration or decubitus on either side. Skin moist. Pulse 112, feeble, and easily compressed. He continued languid, depressed, with collapsed and anxious countenance, feeble and quick pulse, tongue sometimes dry in the centre, sometimes brownish, bowels generally scantily moved, but on the 23rd there was passed by stool more than a pint of clotted blood. He died early the following morning.

Inspection eight hours after death. — *Chest.* — The heart and left lung were healthy. Adhesions connected the third lobe of the right lung to the diaphragm, and there were about thirty ounces of sero-purulent fluid in the right sac of the pleura. Flakes of lymph lined the costal pleura and parts of the pulmonary pleura. *Abdomen.* — The liver filled both hypochondria, the right lobe adhered to the diaphragm, and in that lobe there were two abscesses of considerable size. The left lobe was healthy in texture. There were patches of vascularity here and there in the stomach. The colon contained dark claret-red slimy contents; the mucous coat had, throughout, a reddish tint, and presented several patches of ulceration.

129. *Abscess in the liver.* — *Effusion of four pints of serum, with lymph, in the right pleura.* — *Ulcerated colon.* — *No coma.* — *Serum between the pia mater and arachnoid, and two or three ounces at the base of the skull.* — James Roberts, aged twenty-nine, a gunner, of feeble habit, was under treatment for acute hepatitis, from the 30th April to the 16th May, 1839. He was bled and leeched freely, took calomel and opium, but not to ptyalism, and he was discharged well. Was re-admitted into hospital on the 5th June, affected with diarrhœa, which, under much variety of treatment, continued more or less troublesome. On the 3rd July, distinct hardness and tumefaction between the margin of the right ribs and the crest of the os ilium, was first noted. Blisters were frequently applied without benefit. He continued to lose ground. Became more emaciated and sallow, and on the 3rd August, it is noted for the first and only time, that he had been much troubled with cough during the previous night. The sinking increased, and he died at 3 P.M. of the 24th.

Inspection fifteen hours after death. — No evident tumefaction of either side of the abdomen or chest. *Head.* — The membranes were exsanguine. The convex surface of the brain was veiled with a thin layer of serum, and there were between two and three ounces at the base of the skull. *Chest.* — The right sac of the pleura contained about three or four pints of clear fluid serum at the upper part, thickened with flocculi of lymph at the posterior and lower parts. The costal and pulmonary pleuræ were coated with adherent flocculi of lymph. The lung was condensed against the mediastinum. There was about half a pint of serum in the left pleura, and about three ounces in the cavity of the pericardium. The left lung and the heart were healthy. *Abdomen.* — The right lobe of the liver extended for three inches below the margin of the right ribs; and the edge of the lobe, to the right of the gall-bladder, was occupied by an abscess, the size of a large orange with dense fibrous walls. The hepatic flexure of the colon and part of the omentum were matted to the walls of this abscess. Close to the diaphragm there was another abscess in the right lobe, and there were adhesions of the convex surface of that lobe to the diaphragm. The rest of the surface of the liver was mottled white. The mucous coat of the cœcum was studded with small follicular ulcerations, some of them cicatrising. The rest of the mucous coat of the colon was nearly healthy. Stomach healthy. The kidneys were both rather enlarged. The left of buff colour, with the tubular and cortical parts not well defined. The right one was nearly natural in texture, with buff streaks of the cortical part. There was about a pint of serum in the cavity of the abdomen.

Remark.—The record shows a want of attention to the physical signs, as the existence of the pleuritic effusion does not seem to have been detected.

130. *A small purulent sac circumscribed in part by the base of the right lung and by the diaphragm, and extending to the fissure between the second and third lobes of the right lung, mistaken for hepatic abscess.*—Serjeant James Deans, aged twenty-nine, of feeble habit. From November 1842 to April 1843, was almost continuously under treatment in the Artillery Hospital, suffering from dysentery, attended at times with much abdominal tenderness. From the 5th to the 21st December, he was again under treatment for a similar complaint. On the 29th January, 1844, he was re-admitted with febrile symptoms attended with cough, pain of chest and frothy expectoration. These symptoms continued with more or less alleviation, and the sputa at times assumed a globular appearance with rusty tinge, till the 7th February, when he was transferred from the Artillery to the European General Hospital. The cough continued troublesome, there was occasional hectic fever; the expectoration became more copious and puriform in character with a reddish tinge, more or less deep. A mucous rale was heard over the chest. He continued under these symptoms, gradually losing strength, and latterly suffering from a complication of dysenteric symptoms, and died on the 31st March.

Inspection six hours after death.—The body much emaciated. *Chest.*—The left lung was healthy and collapsed completely. The right one adhered in parts to the costal pleura and very generally to the diaphragm. The upper lobe was collapsed. Between the base of the lung and the diaphragm, and also in the fissure between the second and third lobe, there was a circumscribed sac containing about six ounces of thick pus, and the portions of the lung adjacent to it were indurated and hepatised. There was no communication through the diaphragm. *Abdomen.*—Old adhesions connected the omentum in several places to the abdominal parietes. The liver was much enlarged, grey, and indurated, and extended to the crest of the os ilium, but was without any abscess.

131. *Hepatitis.—Abscess in the liver.—Five pints of pus in the sac of the right pleura.—A layer of lymph on the surface of the heart and inner surface of the pericardium.—General peritonitis, with effusion of lymph and sero-purulent fluid.*—Stephen Cain, a pensioner, aged fifty, of broken habit, after eight days' illness was admitted into hospital on the 24th January, 1840. He complained of pain of the right side, shooting from the margin of the ribs to the shoulder. On the 4th February there was tenseness, fulness, and hardness, at the margin of the right ribs, and the pulse was feeble. The feebleness of the pulse continued. On the 7th the breathing was somewhat oppressed, and there was general painful distention of the abdomen. He died on the 14th February.

Inspection.—There was an ounce of serum at the base of the skull. *Chest.*—There were five pints of pus in the sac of the right pleura. The inner surface of the pericardium and outer of the heart, were red and roughened by a thin layer of firm granular lymph. There was commencing disease of the aorta above the valves, but no hypertrophy of the heart. *Abdomen.*—The liver projected two or three inches beyond the margin of the ribs, and there was an abscess about the size of an orange, and circumscribed, chiefly between the diaphragm and the upper surface of the liver. The peritoneal surface of the intestines was dark red. The convolutions were united by flakes of lymph, and sero-purulent fluid was effused among them. The mucous coat of the stomach was of dark leaden grey colour.

132. *Pericarditis.— The inner surface of the pericardium and the outer side of the heart covered with a thick layer of irregular lymph.—Also effusion of serum and displacement of the liver, partly caused by the distended pericardium.— Abscess of the liver.*— John Devair, aged twenty-five, seaman, was admitted on the 12th November, 1840. He stated that he had been ill for two months and a half; that his complaint began with pain of the abdomen, shooting from the hypogastrium and the left side, thence through the chest. These symptoms were not attended with diarrhœa, constipation or difficulty of micturition; but his statement was confused. He passed a restless night, and on the 13th, the epigastrium was tense, resisting, and painful on pressure; and on percussion, the sound was dull almost to the umbilicus, also midway between the crest of the os ilium of the right side and false ribs, and extended into the hypochondrium. The breathing was a good deal oppressed; the skin above natural temperature; pulse 120, feeble and compressible; tongue pretty clean. Anteriorly, on the right side of the chest and below the nipple, the sound was clear on percussion. On the left there was much dulness about the cardiac region, extending to the arch of the left false ribs and to the sternum; no bulging. On the 20th the uneasiness of the chest and dyspnœa were increased, and he had suffered from rigors; the pulse was 100, very irregular, unequal, with occasional intermission; the abdomen full and tense. Between the left nipple and the sternum the action of the heart was perceptibly increased; and there was a very distinct fremissement, more distinct at that situation than at the apex of the heart. There was now almost constant orthopnœa; pulse very feeble. On the 23rd the fremissement had ceased. He died on the night of the 24th.

Inspection ten hours after death.—Body not much emaciated. *Chest.*—The pericardium completely occupied the anterior part of the chest and extended into the right side for some distance; its transverse diameter was fully ten inches, and it reached from the top of the sternum to the diaphragm, to which muscle it adhered firmly, as also to the inner aspect of both lungs. There were about twenty-two ounces of clear serum in the cavity of the pericardium. The inner surface of the pericardium was lined throughout with a layer of lymph, a line in thickness, with a rough reticulated inner surface of dark red colour; this layer could be peeled from the pericardium with tolerable facility. The outer surface of the heart was coated with a similar layer of lymph, more firmly adherent, however, and presenting a more irregular and reticulated external surface; where the greatest irregularity existed (chiefly at the posterior part) thick bands of firm but friable lymph, about an inch or more in length, extended between the pericardium and the heart. The heart itself and the vessels were healthy. The lungs, with the exception of some old adhesions and some slight œdema, were also healthy, and there was trifling serous effusion in the right cavity of the pleura. *Abdomen.*—The transverse colon, much distended with air, occupied the umbilical region. The liver, displaced by the distended pericardium, extended four inches below the sternum, and about three below the last right false rib. There was an abscess in the left lobe of the liver, lined with a firm membrane with flocculent surface; it was the size of an orange, and was adherent to the diaphragm where opposed to the adhesions of the pericardium. The stomach was healthy. The cortical part of both kidneys was streaked white and red, and these organs were considerably enlarged.

Secondary General Peritonitis.— Secondary general peritonitis is not unfrequent in the advanced stages of hepatic abscess. It occurred in 10 per cent. of the cases at present under review. Its access is generally marked by symptoms sufficiently distinct; and flaky lymph or sero-purulent effusion is found after death. It has been already stated that the opening of an abscess into the cavity of the peritoneum is rare; and there can be no doubt that in the majority of instances general peritonitis is not due to a direct cause of this kind, but is merely additional evidence of the tendency of secondary inflammations to arise in the course of hepatic abscess, and, by the form which they assume, to indicate the degree of cachexia present.

The four cases which follow are of this nature. On this point of pathology reference may be further made to cases 140, 172, 185.

133. *General peritonitis.—Abscess of the liver following head symptoms.—Serous effusion in the head with thickening of the arachnoid membrane.—The kidneys had undergone yellow degeneration.* — Garrott Dunn, aged thirty-eight, of spare habit, was admitted into the European General Hospital, on the 6th August, 1838. He was deaf, and could not give a distinct account of himself. He articulated indistinctly. Complained of vertigo with a constant singing noise in his ears. He was bled from the arm, and cupped on the back of the neck, his head was shaved, and his bowels were freely acted upon by purgative medicine. He continued with more or less of these symptoms till the 17th October. Throughout this period, the deafness was constant, the vertigo and noise occasional. He was cupped, leeched, and blistered several times. Aperient medicine was from time to time exhibited. The action of mercury was induced mildly on the system. The decoction of sarsaparilla was also given, first with the hydriodate of potass, and then with corrosive sublimate. The head symptoms at one time presented a periodic tendency, and quinine was exhibited. No benefit resulted from these different courses of treatment, and on the 17th October, in addition to the former symptoms, tenderness of the abdomen was complained of attended with diarrhœa. Leeches were applied, and anodynes and absorbents given. On the 25th there was distinct fulness to the right of the epigastrium, accompanied with tenderness. Under these symptoms he gradually sunk, and died on the 8th November.

Inspection twelve hours after death.—Body emaciated. *Head.*—There was increased turgescence of the vessels of the pia mater on the upper surface of the brain and over the posterior lobes. There was also opaque thickening of the arachnoid membrane in many places, chiefly at the dipping down between the hemispheres of the brain. There was about an ounce and a half of serum in the ventricles, and a considerable quantity at the base of the skull. The substance of the brain was quite firm and natural in all parts. *Chest.*—The lungs were healthy. A thin layer of old lymph for the extent of an inch in diameter was attached to the serous covering of the heart. *Abdomen.*—There was a small quantity of sero-purulent fluid in the cavity of the abdomen. The intestines were distended with gas, and adhered in places by flakes of lymph to the abdominal parietes. The whole of the peritoneal covering of the right lobe of the liver was covered with flakes of lymph, and there were flakes between the stomach and liver, and a close matting of the edge of the left lobe to the colon; that intestine was also closely embraced by the omentum. In the left lobe of the liver, at the point of adhesion to the colon (the site where there had been fulness and pain before death), there was an abscess the size of an orange. The substance of the right lobe was healthy. In places of the mucous lining of the colon, there was dark grey discoloration. In others a thinning of the coats, chiefly to all appearances induced by the removal of the free surface of the mucous tunic. In the descending colon and sigmoid flexure, there were a few round ulcers, and some dark grey cicatrices. The mucous lining of the stomach was covered with adhesive mucus, was dark grey at the cardiac end, marbled dark red at the pyloric, but was neither softened nor thickened. The cortical substance of both kidneys had undergone yellow degeneration to a considerable extent.

134. *General peritonitis. — Matting of the omentum over the cæcum. —Round ulcers in the colon, and an abscess in the liver.*—Antone Lopes, aged forty-two, a Portuguese seaman, who had arrived from Goa about two months before his admission into the European General Hospital, on the 22nd January, 1839. On admission into hospital, his countenance was sallow and anxious. The abdomen was somewhat distended, and tense, with tenderness over the cœcum. The tongue was expanded and little furred. The pulse was feeble. He stated that he had been affected with dysenteric symptoms for about twenty days, that the purging, at first considerable, had decreased, and that the pain had increased, during the two or three days before admission. On the 23rd there was a distinct defined hardness felt over the cœcum. He gradually and slowly lost ground, and died on the 7th February. The tumour at the site of the cœcum continued distinct, till the 2nd of February, when the fulness and tenderness of the abdomen became more general. At first, leeches were applied to the abdomen, and at three different times a blister was applied. For the first two or three days, blue pill or calomel were given with ipecacuanha and opium, and afterwards sulphate of quinine with a small quantity of hydrargyrum cum creta with opium and ipecacuanha. Then the ipecacuanha and mercury were left off, and the quinine was given with opium and aromatic confection.

Inspection five hours after death.—Body emaciated. Abdomen moderately distended. *Head.*—About an ounce and a half of serum in the cavity. *Abdomen.*—The omentum crossed from the ninth or tenth left false rib, adhered to the anterior parietes, passed obliquely to the hollow of the right os ilium, and thus divided the cavity into two parts. The upper contained about a pint of pus in a circumscribed sac lined with false membrane, and covering the projecting edge of the liver, the stomach, and part of the omentum. The lower division contained about two pints of clear serum with flakes of lymph. There was vascularity of the peritoneal covering of the small intestine and much matting of the convolutions in the pelvis, and to the bladder. The cœcum was matted firmly to the omentum and to the hollow of the os ilium, and tore readily on attempting to separate it. The descending colon was covered with flakes of lymph. There were round isolated ulcerations, the size of a sixpence here and there, in the colon. The liver was much enlarged and contained a large abscess in the right lobe lined with firm membrane; the parenchyma was of dark red colour, and mottled white. The mucous lining of the stomach was thickened. The left kidney had partly undergone yellow granular degeneration; the right one was not examined. *Chest.* — The thoracic viscera were healthy.

135. *General peritonitis, with sero-purulent effusion and abscess in the liver.*—James Harrison, aged thirty-three, of slight habit, a sub-conductor in the Ordnance Department, was admitted into the European General Hospital on February 25th, 1839. He had served thirteen years in India, had suffered from dysentery whilst at Deesa in 1829, and was under treatment in the General Hospital for fever about ten months before the present date. On admission he stated that some days previously he had experienced uneasiness at the epigastrium, for which he was leeched and took medicines. Since the day before admission, there had been pain and much tenderness of the right iliac region, with sense of induration and dulness, extending from two inches above the crest of the os ilium, to the margin of the right false ribs, and to within two inches of the umbilicus. Pulse 88, small, sharpish. The tongue was pretty clean. Features sharp and anxious. He vomited the day before admission, but not since. One hundred leeches were applied to the abdomen, a warm bath ordered, and calomel with ipecacuanha and opium given. On the following day (26th), the pain continued; pulse 84, weak. A large blister was applied to the abdomen. At the evening visit there was no febrile exacerbation, the bowels had been four times moved by the castor oil, and the evacuations were yellow and watery. The pulse small and feeble. Calomel three grains, quinine two, and opium one, in the form of pill, were

ordered at bed-time. From this time, the pain of the abdomen was more or less complained of, and on the fourth, the distention had considerably increased. The pulse was generally from 80 to 88, feeble and often thready; the skin was cold and damp; the tongue was moist and without fur, and two or three watery yellow evacuations were in general passed daily. The treatment consisted of quinine in combination with hydrargyrum cum creta and half a grain of opium thrice daily. He died on the night of the 5th March.

Inspection eight hours after death.—Body not much emaciated. *Abdomen.*—Was moderately distended and tense. The omentum, vascular and thickened was matted over the transverse colon, the edge of the liver, and the cœcum. It also adhered firmly to the hollow of the os ilium. There was general redness over the peritoneal coat of the bowels, with flakes of lymph. There were about three pints of sero-purulent fluid in the cavity of the peritoneum, chiefly between the right lobe of the liver and the ribs, and in the iliac and pelvic regions. The liver was of natural size, mottled and of pale fawn colour, except in the neighbourhood of two or three small abscesses in the right lobe, where the mottling was dark red. The coats of the cœcum and colon were not thickened; their mucous coat was of dark grey colour, but not ulcerated. The stomach was healthy. In the left kidney the distinction of cortical and tubular portion was not well defined; the right kidney was healthy. The thoracic viscera were healthy. *Head.*—At the base of the skull there was an ounce of serum.

136. *Probably small superficial abscess of under surface of lobulus Spigelii, leading to a puriform sac in gastro-hepatic omentum, and this by rupture to general peritonitis.*—*Jaundice.*—Ingan Khan, a Mussulman butler, using spirits in moderate quantity, of forty years of age, and in reduced condition, was admitted into the clinical ward on the 19th October, 1850. The respiration was somewhat hurried, partly abdominal and partly thoracic. There was some degree of general fulness of the abdomen, and a line drawn from the point of the right ninth rib to within two inches of the umbilicus, and then obliquely upwards to the eighth left rib, formed the lower limit of a distinctly full and almost circumscribed induration, of which the thoracic margin was the upper boundary; this space was dull on percussion, painful on pressure, deep inspiration, and coughing. There was some yellowness of the conjunctivæ, febrile disturbance, a coated tongue, constipated bowels, and high-coloured urine. The illness was of twenty days' duration, and commenced with febrile symptoms. These recurred every evening with chills, and terminated with sweating. Suffering much as on admission, he continued under treatment till the 29th October, when, in consequence of alleviation of the epigastric uneasiness, he was urgent for his discharge. He was re-admitted on the 1st November with anxious countenance, hurried and short respiration, and small frequent pulse, and skin about the natural temperature. There was epigastric tenderness, and some degree of general abdominal fulness; but the epigastric induration was scarcely perceptible, and the dulness was limited below by a line curving from the cartilage of the eighth right rib to that of the seventh left rib. On the 2nd the symptoms of general peritonitis were fully marked. He died on the morning of the 3rd. The urine was frequently examined, but gave no signs of albumen. He was treated chiefly with moderate leeching, small blisters, laxatives, quinine, diaphoretics, and anodynes.

Inspection eight hours after death.—*Abdomen.*—About two pints of straw-coloured serum were contained in the cavity of the peritoneum. The intestines were generally distended with flatus; their peritoneal surface presented a dusky hue chiefly where the convolutions were in contact, with flakes of lymph here and there. The lymphy effusion was abundant on the convex surface of the liver, which seemed somewhat compressed, and adhered to the diaphragm by friable bands. The thin edge of a part of the concave surface of the left lobe of the liver was firmly adherent to the stomach, the transverse colon, and the hepatic flexure. Easily separable adhesions also existed between the right lobe of the liver, the fundus of the gall-bladder, and the lateral part of the diaphragm. The omentum was matted over the ascending colon, and reached as far as the right abdominal ring. On separating the adhesions between the concave surface of the liver and the stomach, a thick layer of friable lymph was seen on the surface of the latter and on the duodenum, with a few ounces of sero-pus, which seemed to proceed from a sac, chiefly formed in the gastro-hepatic omentum. One part of its wall was in relation with the inferior surface of the lobulus Spigelii. This lobe was compressed, its tissue of a dark-red colour, mottled, and presenting near the surface, and in relation with the wall of the sac, two or three purulent deposits, each the size of a small bean. The transverse or portal fissure, with the large blood-vessels and duct, were not involved. No other traces of abscess were detected in any other part of the liver, which was of normal size, and extended from the level of the fifth to the ninth rib. When incised in various directions, its surface presented an olive-green colour, and was somewhat indurated, seemingly from a state of commencing cirrhosis. The upper surface of the right lobe was much puckered. The mucous membrane of the stomach was covered with a large quantity of pultaceous mucus, but its texture was in every respect healthy. The mucous membrane of the duodenum presented a dark-red colour, but it also was normal in structure. *Chest.*—The lungs collapsed freely. Old adhesions connected in places the costal to the pulmonary pleura on both sides.

These details show that circumscribed collections of pus in relation with the peritoneum and pleura, also puriform general peritonitis, are not uncommon events in the course of hepatic abscess. This result is probably dependent on the cachectic condition of the individuals affected. But here the question may be proposed, whether these complications are due to particular forms of cachexia? If so, and if we have diagnostic symptoms of these cachexiæ, it is evident that we shall be in possession of knowledge likely to bear on prognosis and treatment. Is this tendency to suppurative inflammation related to the cachexia of malaria, scorbutus, struma, mercury, intemperate spirit drinking, syphilis, prolonged elevation of temperature, habitual residence in a vitiated atmosphere, or to that which co-exists, as cause or effect, with Bright's disease of the kidney? My own observations are insufficient to elucidate these important practical questions; but it is very probable that further investigation will establish a relation between these forms of secondary inflammation and the cachexia of Bright's disease. On referring to my cases, with a view of testing the likelihood of this suggestion, I am disappointed by finding them so frequently defective. Many of them were recorded at a time when attention had not as yet been generally directed to this important part of pathology. Yet imperfect as they are, granular degeneration of the kidney is noted in six of the eighteen cases, and in the remaining twelve the state of the kidney is not described.

Character of the contents of Hepatic Abscesses. — In the cases detailed in these pages the appearance presented by the pus in hepatic abscesses is so generally stated, that I should have thought it unnecessary to allude to the subject more particularly. But there are statements made on this point by Rokitansky and Budd, differing so materially from the results of my own experience, that it would be an omission on my part not to advert to them.

Rokitansky says: "A large abscess of long standing, invariably contains pus mixed with a considerable amount of bile, which arises from the communication established between the cavity and larger gall ducts." *

We are not told of the number of cases on which this general statement is grounded; nor whether the presence of bile was determined from the general colour of the pus, or by the microscope or by chemical tests. Assuming from the expression, "considerable amount of bile," that the inference has been drawn from the colour as appearing to the naked eye, I find myself unable to assent to the assertion of this eminent pathologist.

There are before me 98 cases in which the morbid appearances of hepatic abscess are described, and ten others in which the contents were artificially discharged. They were all observed and noted by myself, but of only four (97, 111, 137, 141) is a bile-tinged state of the pus recorded; and I can hardly think that so notable a character, if existing, would in 104 cases have failed to attract my attention. I place the more confidence in my own observations, because since becoming aware of the opinion of Rokitansky, and feeling how opposed it was to my previous belief, I have spoken with several of my professional friends, whose experience in this form of disease has been considerable, and have hitherto found that their conclusions coincide with my own. The statement of the able German pathologist cannot therefore be considered applicable to hepatic abscess in India, as hitherto observed.

In Dr. Budd's work on Diseases of the Liver are the following remarks: —

"Many of the old writers describe the pus of abscess of the liver as being generally red or claret-coloured, but this statement is incorrect. In all the abscesses of the liver that I have examined, the pus was white or yellowish, just like that of a phlegmon. The error of those who have described it as being reddish, resulted, perhaps, from their having met with a case in which the abscess opened into the lung, and in which the pus, in its passage through the lung, became mixed with blood and broken-down pulmonary tissue. They describe the matter *expectorated*, and not the matter contained in the abscess. It is not very uncommon for an abscess of the liver to open into the lung. Several instances of this kind have fallen under my own notice, and in all of them the matter expectorated was a dirty red or brownish pus. The reddish

* "Pathological Anatomy," Sydenham Society, vol. ii. p. 132.

colour of the pus was acquired on its passage through the lung. The matter in the abscess was yellowish or white." *

Cases 108, 149, 161, 165, confirm the statement of the old writers, that the pus in hepatic abscess is sometimes of a red colour, and do not accord with the opinion above expressed by Dr. Budd.

Haspell having observed a pink colour of the contents in two of his three successful cases of puncture of hepatic abscess, has inferred that this colour is a condition of the early stage of the abscess, and that when present in punctured abscess it justifies a favourable prognosis. These inferences, deduced from very limited data, are not supported by my cases 161, 165.

Inflammation of the Portal or Hepatic Vein -- is a pathological state of interest and importance; but it is one with which I have little practical acquaintance. Of portal phlebitis I have not met with a case, and have only seen the morbid appearances in one of hepatic phlebitis. In this case there was abscess, and the branches of the hepatic vein in its neighbourhood were dilated, contained pus, and their coats were somewhat thickened.

SECTION IV. — *Etiology of Hepatitis. — Exciting Causes. — External Cold, elevated Temperature, Intemperance, Mechanical Causes. — Importance of Predisposing Causes stated. — The Complication of Hepatic Abscess and Dysentery considered in reference to the Pyœmic Theory of the Causation of Hepatic Abscess.*

In the etiology of dysentery, much importance was attached to those conditions of the atmosphere which reduce the temperature of the surface of the body, as an exciting cause. The same view may be taken of the etiology of hepatitis. Dysentery was found to prevail most in the cold months, November, December, January; next in June, July, and August; and then in February and March.

On comparing the proportional admissions from hepatitis per cent. of the total hospital admissions with those from dysentery †, the following differences may be noted: — 1. The admissions from dysentery are fully twice as numerous as those from hepatitis; 2. The months of February and March are those of greatest prevalence

* "On Diseases of the Liver," Second Edition, p. 98.

† Pages 274 and 362.

of hepatitis, then follow November, December, January. The hot months, April and May, as well as September and October, take precedence of the monsoon months, June, July, August, which latter, in the instance of dysentery, stood next to the cold months.

Why the admissions from hepatitis in February and March have in both hospitals exceeded those of the three preceding colder months, I am unable to explain, but probably more extended data will show that it is accidental. The fact, however, does not affect the conclusion, that external cold is a common exciting cause of the disease. It is not improbable, when we bear in mind the advanced stages of disease at which admissions take place into general hospitals, more especially at seaports, that a scrutiny of the admissions of February and March would prove that a proportion of them had commenced in the months which preceded.

The admissions of dysentery were fewest in the hot months April and May *; but we find that the admissions of hepatitis in these months came next to the cold months, and took precedence of the rainy months. Without attaching undue importance to limited and partial statistics, it may be remarked that these results tend to confirm the generally admitted impression, that elevated temperature has more influence in the causation of hepatitis than of dysentery. To this subject I shall presently more particularly advert.

Proportional Admissions from Hepatitis in different Seasons.

	European General Hospital.	Jamsetjee Jejeebhoy Hospital.
February, and March,—transition from cold months	4·8	2·0
November, December, January,—cold months	3·8	1·7
April and May,—hot months	3·4	1·6
September, October,—transition from rains	3·2	1·0
June, July, August,—rainy months	2·9	1·4
Annual proportion	3·7	1·5

When explaining the causes of dysentery I dwelt at considerable length on the importance of a right appreciation of predisposing conditions as favouring the action of the exciting cause. The principles then inculcated are equally applicable to hepatitis.

* This remark is only strictly applicable to the European General Hospital; for in the Jamsetjee Jejeebhoy Hospital the admissions from dysentery in April and May took precedence of those of February and March.

Whether, of the various kinds of cachexia alluded to as predisposing to dysentery, there are some rather than others which predispose to hepatitis, is a question for future inquiry to determine; but allusion may be made to one or two points relating to it. There is nothing before me to show that there is any particular connection between hepatic abscess and the tubercular diathesis. Tubercles in the lungs were found only in one of the cases of hepatic abscess. Tubercles in the liver were noticed in only three cases — one (48) of melanosis of the colon, the other two of tubercular phthisis.

The evidence that intemperance in drinking exercises a peculiar influence in causing hepatitis is by no means conclusive. That a considerable proportion of both European and native hospital admissions from hepatitis are of intemperate individuals is undoubted; but this fact is equally true of other forms of disease. That the cachexia engendered by spirit drinking and the exposure to cold and wet consequent on the direct effect of intoxication, are often operative in inducing disease, is also not to be questioned; but there is nothing in my notes or my impressions to convince me that these are more frequent causes of hepatitis than of dysentery. Spirit drinking as a special cause of cirrhosis is not called in question, but this is a form of disease common to the spirit drinker in all countries, and almost exclusively confined to his class. That hepatitis, on the other hand, in its severest forms, is not an unusual event in persons of temperate habits, — is a statement which experience in India will generally confirm.

Is hepatitis, with a liability to suppuration, peculiarly related to cachexia engendered by the prolonged influence of elevated temperature? I believe that it is so. It is very probable that future research will show that the exhausted and enfeebled by continued heat, and its associated debilitating conditions, are very prone to hepatitis, and that in such individuals the inflammation is very frequently excited by exposure to external cold — I mean to such depression of temperature as suffices to influence bodies whose power of generating heat is low.

But there is another question to propose in regard to heat. Is it ever the *exciting* cause of hepatitis, as it assuredly sometimes is of cerebral disease? The occurrence in the hot months of the year of hepatitis in plethoric Europeans, lately arrived in India, with excreting functions deranged by free living, is probably sometimes best explained on the supposition that tropical heat is occasionally an exciting cause of hepatitis.

Cases 166, 171, and two others not detailed, show that *mechanical causes* are not to be overlooked in the etiology of hepatitis.

In my remarks on jaundice as a complication of remittent fever, a case (38) is detailed, in which a lumbricus was found in the hepatic duct. In the case which follows, a lumbricus * was found in the centre of an hepatic abscess. These circumstances are sufficient to justify the idea that hepatitis may be sometimes caused by *entozoa*. The fact that dracunculi have also been detected in the liver may countenance the probability that the lumbricus is not the only entozoon which may act in this manner.

137. *Large abscess in right lobe, flocculent walls, communicating with a branch of the hepatic vein.—Lumbricus in the abscess.—Pus orange coloured.—No ulceration of large intestine.—Jaundice.*—Hurree Gomajee, a Hindoo cart-driver, of thirty-five years of age, and using spirits to the extent of three ounces daily, was admitted into the clinical ward on the 9th January, 1853. He was much reduced. The conjunctivæ were tinged yellow, and there was slight œdema of both feet. The respiration was short and hurried, the pulse small and compressible, and the tongue florid at the tip and edges. An indistinctly fluctuating swelling occupied the epigastrium, bounded inferiorly by a curved line from the tenth left rib to the eleventh right rib, crossing the umbilicus. It was painful. He stated that fifteen days before he was injured on the back by a log of wood; that two days afterwards, pain of the right hypochondrium, with febrile symptoms, set in; and that the swelling appeared six days before admission. The pulse became feebler, the dyspnœa increased, and he died on the 12th with very slight diarrhœa. The urine gave no signs of albumen.

Inspection four hours after death.—All the white tissues were tinged yellow.—*Chest.*—There were old adhesions between the costal and pulmonary pleura of the right side. The lungs were crepitating and spongy. Opaque patches were found on the external surface of the heart; the cavity of the left ventricle was somewhat smaller than natural. Valves healthy. *Abdomen.*—No traces of peritonitis were observed except some adhesions which existed between the concave surface of the liver and transverse colon, and also with the kidney of the right side. Adhesions were also found between the convex surface of the liver and the diaphragm. The liver extended as low as the tenth rib on the left side, and the last rib on the right side, and occupied the whole of the abdomen above these points; it was of dark mottled red colour externally. On making an incision, an abscess was found occupying almost the entire right lobe. It contained about two pints of orange-coloured sero-pus, and a large quantity of pulpy flocculent matter was loosely adherent to the walls of the abscess. A lumbricus was found in the abscess. The small portion of the right lobe left around the abscess was of red colour. On incising the left lobe, thin pus was seen to flow freely from a large branch of the hepatic vein, which could be traced to the abscess, with which it communicated. The substance of the left lobe, free of abscess, was mottled red and white. The stomach was contracted. The mucous surface was rugous, and dotted red here and there. There was some degree of increased vascularity of the mucous lining of the rectum, with commencing granular deposit on the mucous surface. No trace of ulceration anywhere. The kidneys were healthy.

* There is an excellent specimen of lumbrici in the biliary ducts in the Museum at Fort Pitt, Chatham. I have also seen another in the Museum of Comparative Anatomy at the Jardin des Plantes at Paris; and no doubt many others might readily be found.

The co-existence of hepatic abscess and ulceration of the mucous membrane of the large intestine, is treated by me, in connection with the etiology of hepatitis in consequence of the explanation of this event, lately proposed by Dr. Budd. His opinion is that a very frequent, if not the exclusive, cause of inflammation of the liver—not cirrhosis—is the transmission to the organ of pus or vitiated secretions from an ulcerated intestinal surface. This doctrine necessarily implies the termination in abscess of every inflammation thus arising. In other words, it rejects the termination of hepatitis by resolution.

On these views I shall simply observe that, if we acknowledge *pyœmia* as a pathological condition, we must allow that the *occasional* occurrence of hepatic abscess, in the manner supposed, is sufficiently probable. As a *general* proposition, however, it is at variance with the results of clinical research in India, as the following remarks will, I believe, sufficiently prove:—

1. Fatal dysentery with ulceration but without hepatic abscess is a common occurrence in India. Fifty cases are now before me and many of them have been cited in this work. Intestinal ulceration without hepatic abscess is almost invariable in European countries. Recovery from dysentery, in which ulceration had probably been present, is not unfrequent in India. These facts, which show a very large amount of intestinal ulceration without hepatic abscess, are not consistent with the idea that abscess of the liver, when existing, is always, or most commonly, the sequence of the direct transmission to the organ, of the morbid matter of intestinal ulcers. If this doctrine were true, ulceration of the intestines and abscess of the liver would be much more frequently co-existent.

2. Primary uncomplicated hepatitis is not an unusual disease in India. Restricting my inquiry to the five years of my service in the European General Hospital, I find that, of the total admissions of hepatitis, 318, or 86 per cent. recovered; and this is a result incompatible with the pyœmic origin of hepatitis. This statement may be met by the objection that the numbers are probably incorrect, from mistakes in diagnosis and the inclusion of cases of cirrhosis. But making every allowance for this, it cannot be supposed that the error was committed in all the successful cases, but avoided in the 14 per cent. of fatal ones.

3. There are now before me, twenty-one fatal cases of hepatic abscess without ulceration of the intestine. Setting aside all other arguments, these positive facts are conclusive against the theory that pyœmia from intestinal ulcers is the exclusive cause of hepatic

abscess. Six of these cases (138 to 143) will presently be narrated; and seven others (107, 113, 135, 137, 162, 166, 168) are elsewhere detailed.

4. There is good reason for believing that the records of pathology misrepresent the natural proportion of intestinal ulceration and hepatic abscess. I have long entertained the opinion that mercurial and other purgatives, too frequently repeated in hepatitis, materially favour the access of muco-enteritis and subsequent ulceration. This suspicion is confirmed by the fact, that of my twenty-one cases of abscess without ulceration, sixteen occurred in natives admitted into hospital in advanced stages and not previously treated with mercurial and other purgatives.

138. *A large abscess in the liver.—No dysenteric symptoms.—No ulceration.—No projection of liver below the ribs.*—John Williams, a seaman, aged twenty-eight, was admitted into hospital on the 20th May, 1838, with acute pain at the scrobiculus cordis, increased by pressure, attended with febrile excitement, and on the 22nd, extending to the right hypochondrium, and affected by deep inspiration and decubitus on the left side. On the 30th he had rigors, followed by febrile excitement, and subsequent hectic. There was no enlargement below the edge of the right false ribs, but there was a perceptible though not great bulging of the ribs, and a want of depression of the intercostal spaces, with dulness to the axilla. Latterly there was much irritability of stomach, but nothing ejected except ingesta and the mucous secretions. Throughout the whole period of illness there were no symptoms of dysentery or diarrhœa. On the contrary, laxatives were often required; and generally, and more especially latterly, the evacuations were formed, and perfectly natural. He died September 5th.

Inspection fifteen hours after death.—Body much emaciated; perceptible bulging of the right hypochondrium and filling up of the intercostal spaces. *Chest.*—The lungs were collapsed and crepitating. There was no effusion into the chest. Tender adhesions existed between the upper surface of the diaphragm and base of the right lung. The liver had pushed the diaphragm to the level of the second rib, at the most convex part of its arc; and its curve touched the ribs at the level of the upper part of the fourth. The left side of the chest was natural. *Abdomen.*—The liver adhered to the abdominal parietes at the margin of the false ribs, but did not project beyond it. The entire right lobe adhered to the diaphragm, and was completely occupied by a large abscess, containing serous fluid at its upper surface and pus below, in all about four pounds. The sac was lined by a firm cartilaginous membrane, to which yellow flocculi adhered. The thin layer of parenchyma interposed between the peritoneal covering and the lining membrane of the sac was dense and fibrous, and nowhere above half an inch in thickness. The left lobe was mottled. The gall-bladder contained some bile. The stomach and intestines were almost natural. There was a good deal of congestion of the mucous coat of the depending parts of the small intestine, and also of the cœcum; but the texture was quite sound. The colon was partially occupied with formed and perfectly natural feculence. The kidneys were healthy.

139. *Hepatitis.—Abscess in the right lobe.—Mucous coat of the large intestine dark red without ulceration.*—Thomas Hall, aged thirty-two, private in Her Majesty's 15th Hussars, was admitted into hospital on the 9th January, 1840. He stated that he had suffered more or less from pain of the right side for three weeks before admission. On the 13th there was dulness two inches below the margin of the right ribs, but not extending into the epigastrium; it subsequently reached as high as the nipple. He died on the 15th March.

Inspection.—Head.—There was a thin veil of serum on the convex surface of the brain, and an ounce at the base of the skull. *Chest.*—The lungs were collapsed. *Abdomen.*—The liver reached to the level of the third rib, and there were tender adhesions between the right lung and the diaphragm. It also extended two inches below the margin of the ribs, and there were adhesions to the diaphragm and concavity of the ribs. An abscess containing three pints of thick pus occupied the right lobe, and the upper wall consisted merely of the diaphragm and the peritoneal coating of the liver. The rest of the liver was mottled. The cardiac end of the stomach was mottled red. The mucous coat of the large intestine was dark red and dark grey in parts, but not ulcerated.

140. *Chronic pneumonia of upper part of left lung.—Secondary hepatitis and abscess, with flocculent walls, and peritonitic inflammation.—No intestinal ulceration.*—Huree Mydhur, forty years of age, a Hindoo sailor, was admitted, after a month's illness, into the clinical ward on the 27th June, 1848. He had cough, with muco-puriform expectoration, and he pointed to the left subclavian and mammary regions as the seat of pain, and there defective respiratory movement was evident. There was also dulness on percussion, subcrepitus and bronchial sounds. He continued under observation till the 17th July, when he died. There was more or less hectic fever, and frequent cough with sputa, sometimes brick-red and puriform. On the 9th there was delirium. On the 10th, fulness of the epigastric region, and dulness to within an inch of the umbilicus, and uneasiness on pressure there. He gradually lost strength, but there was no diarrhœa. From admission up to the 13th, a cautious endeavour to affect the system with mercury was made, but without success. It was during this mercurial course that the hepatic symptoms appeared.

Inspection.—The lung of the right side was crepitating and healthy. The left lung adhered firmly to the lateral part of the parietes of the chest, and was separated with difficulty. In the lateral part of the upper lobe, separated by a thin wall from the pleura, there was an excavation of two or three inches in length, the evident result of gangrene of that part of the lung. The inner surface of the excavation was irregular, of dark grey and black colour; and the boundary was dense and membranous. The rest of the upper lobe was in a state of grey induration, and the upper part of the second lobe was red and indurated, but in some parts still permeable to air. The mucous membrane of the bronchial tubes was dark red. There were three or four ounces of serum in the pericardium. The heart healthy. *Abdomen.*—General friable adhesions of lymph over the entire peritoneal surface, with purulent effusion amongst them. The liver mottled white in its texture. Two large abscesses existed in the right lobe, with flocculent shreds adherent to their inner surfaces. The concave surface of the liver adhered by thick layers of lymph to the stomach and colon, and, on separating these, the lower wall of the largest abscess readily gave way; it was supported by these other viscera. The mucous coat of the large intestine was healthy.

141. *Three abscesses in different stages of progress.—Pus bile-tinged.—General peritonitis without rupture.—No ulceration of the intestines.*—Sagoo Beekia, a Hindoo cultivator, thirty-five years of age, and of temperate habits, was admitted into the clinical ward on the 15th January, 1854. He was in good condition. The respiration was short and hurried, and chiefly thoracic. There was cough and mucous expectoration, and crepitus was audible in the right dorsal region. A swelling dull to percussion occupied the space between the margin of the ribs, and a line drawn from the tenth left rib across the umbilicus to the last right rib. The dulness reached upwards to the right fifth rib. The tongue was florid at the tip and edges. The pulse was small. Decubitus was easiest on the right side. The bowels were reported regular. He stated that, a month before, he became affected with fever, ushered in with chills, which left him about six days before admission, when the swelling and pain of the epigastrium began to appear. On the 18th and 19th the bowels were relaxed, and

febrile accessions were noted. He died on the 20th of January. The occurrence of general peritonitis was not distinctly marked.

Inspection three hours after death.—There was about a pint and a half of serum in the cavity of the abdomen. The serum was tinged yellow, and mixed with abundant flakes of lymph. There were also yellow flakes effused on the surface of the peritoneum, chiefly that covering the liver. The liver extended across the abdomen from the eighth left rib to the crest of the right ilium. The convexity of the right lobe extended as high as the fourth rib. There were firm adhesions and exudation of lymph between the convex surface of the liver and the diaphragm. On incising the liver, an abscess about the size of a cocoa-nut was found at the upper part of the right lobe. It was separated from the diaphragm by a thin layer of the substance of the liver. The abscess contained pus, in part thick and pulpy, and the walls were lined by a thin membrane, which presented a flocculent appearance when floated in water. In the lower part of the right lobe there was another abscess the size of a mango, separated from the upper one by a layer of the substance of the liver, about a quarter of an inch thick. The walls of this abscess were similar to those of the other. The rest of the substance of the right lobe was of a dark red colour. At the upper part of the left lobe there was a third abscess, about the size of a mango, containing yellow-coloured pus (tinged with bile). The walls were lined by a thicker and firmer membrane than those of the other abscesses, and less flocculent when floated in water. The remainder of the substance of the left lobe was not so dark-coloured as that of the right. Emphysematous bullæ the size of a pigeon's egg occupied the thin edge of the left lung. There were adhesions between the left lung and pericardium; also between it and the walls of the chest. Slight adhesions existed between the base of the right lung and the diaphragm. There was emphysema of the middle and third lobes. There were white opaque patches on the surface of the heart, but the structure and valves were healthy. The cœcum was of dark red colour. There was no thickening or ulceration of the mucous membrane of the large intestine, nor of any part of the small intestine. Kidneys healthy. Spleen healthy.

142. *Hepatic abscess.—No ulceration of the intestine.*—Shaik Ibrahim, aged twenty-five, after two months' illness, was admitted on the 3rd May, 1857. He was emaciated, and complained only of purging. There was no fulness of the right side noticed during life. He died on the 9th.

Inspection.—An abscess the size of a cocoa-nut existed in the right lobe of the liver. There were firm adhesions to the diaphragm. There was caries of the ninth and tenth ribs, and a sloughy state of the tissues external to them. No trace of ulceration in any part of the intestinal canal.

143. *Hepatic abscess.—No intestinal ulceration.*—Deen Mahomed, aged forty, was admitted into the clinical ward on the 22nd October, 1857, with well marked hepatic abscess. Bowels confined. Secondary peritonitis came on, and he died on the 9th November.

Inspection.—One large encysted abscess occupied the right lobe of the liver. There was no trace of ulceration of the mucous membrane of large or small intestines, but redness with slight granular exudation in places.

The co-existence of hepatic abscess and intestinal ulceration may be classed in the following manner:—

1. Cases in which hepatitis has been primary, with secondary ulceration, generally not coming on till suppuration has well advanced.

2. Cases in which dysentery has been primary, with hepatic

secondary abscess, occurring generally in advanced stages of the dysentery.

3. Cases in which dysentery and hepatitis have been coincident, but, in general, not well marked, and with the symptoms of the dysentery, not unfrequently for a time, giving place to those of the hepatitis. This form, however, is rare compared with the other two, and will be more particularly noticed in connection with the symptomatology of hepatitis.

Primary hepatitis ending in abscess and attended by secondary dysentery is not difficult to understand, when we bear in mind the frequency, nay almost the universality, with which the hectic stage of phthisis pulmonalis, and of other forms of extensive suppurative disease, are associated with intestinal ulceration: this event occurring in the hectic stage of suppuration of the liver is merely an illustration of this general law, and nothing more.* In my notes of fatal cases of hepatic abscess with ulcerated intestine, there are seven in which this sequence is evident.

Primary dysentery followed by secondary hepatic abscess, is the only form of this complication which affords support to the pyœmic theory. But that pyœmia is the ordinary cause even of this is not for the following reasons a logical deduction from the facts:—(*a*) Dysenteric ulceration, without hepatic abscess, is common. (*b*) Intestinal ulceration is almost universal in the advanced stage of phthisis pulmonalis, and is always unassociated with hepatic abscess. (*c*) There is no reason for believing that particular climates favour pyœmia. (*d*) There is much that is common in the predisposing and exciting causes of dysentery and hepatitis. (*e*) It may be frequently observed that individuals, in whom hepatitis occurs secondary on dysentery, have previously suffered from hepatic disease. (*f*) It is a well-known pathological law that, in the progress of primary inflammations, there is a predisposition to secondary inflammations, and that these generally prefer an organ weakened by previous disease, or by the influence of other predisposing causes. (*g*) The liver and large intestine are associated in function. It might therefore be reasonably anticipated that they would also be occasionally associated in their pathological conditions.

* This statement is not to be met by the argument that the ulceration of the intestines in phthisis is tubercular, and consequently merely a further development of the diathesis. That such is the character of the ulceration in a proportion of cases may not be questioned, but the result of my observation of phthisis in India leads me to believe that in the majority of cases in that country the ulceration of the large intestine does not differ in character from that frequently observed in dysentery.

A consideration of these facts leads me to the conclusion that hepatic abscess, occurring in the course of dysentery, is, for the most part, simply an instance of a secondary inflammation arising in an organ predisposed by previous disease or other influences, and is not caused by pyœmia. The abscess was, apparently, the result of secondary hepatitis, in nine of my cases.

In respect to those cases in which dysentery and hepatitis appear to be coincident, I would merely observe that when we recollect how much there is common in the causes of these two affections, the wonder is that this original co-existence is not very frequent instead of being rare.

Section V.—*Symptoms of Hepatitis.—Early Stages.—Pain, Respiratory Movements.—Physical Signs.—Altered Secretion, Jaundice.—Constitutional Disturbance.—Suppuration.—Course of Hepatic Abscess.*

The size, situation, and relations of the liver, the constitution of the patient, and the duration of the attack, should always be borne in mind in investigating the symptoms of hepatitis. It should also be remembered that the inflammation may affect varying extents of the organ, as well as one part, or several, of its surface or substance,—separate or combined.

In the early stages of acute hepatitis *pain* will vary in degree, according as the inflammation affects the peritoneal covering or is confined to the parenchyma. In the former case it will be distinct and often acute. In the latter dull—a sense of weight and uneasiness rather than pain—and apt to be obscure, when only limited portions of the organ are engaged, and when the constitution is asthenic. The pain will be increased, occasionally indeed only appreciable, by pressure, full inspiration, and turning to the left side. Sometimes in obscure cases uneasiness, not otherwise detected, may be elicited by meeting the liver, as it descends under full inspiration, by gentle pressure, upwards, with the hand placed on the anterior surface of the abdomen below the margin of the right ribs.

Pain will vary in situation according to the part of the liver affected. It may exist at the posterior, lateral, or anterior parts of the arch of the right ribs below the sixth; at the margin of the right ribs from the seventh to the last, or at the epigastrium just below the ensiform cartilage. But pain from the sixth to the eighth or ninth rib, may be caused by pleuritis or pneumonia: in this diagnosis, auscultation will materially assist us. It is not often that primary pleuritis or pneumonia is so limited in extent; but should partial friction murmur, or crepitus, indicate that these affections exist, then it may be inferred that the liver is not implicated, because the co-existence of hepatitis and pleuritis or pneumonia, common enough in the advanced stages of the first-named disease, is rare at its commencement.

Care must be further taken not to confound costal pain, related to muscular or fibrous tissue and rheumatic diathesis, with the pain of internal inflammation. The history of the patient, and a consideration of the other symptoms, should protect us from an error of this kind.

Pain below the margin of the right ribs may proceed from the colon, the duodenum, the biliary ducts or gall-bladder, and here again a judicious review of the associated symptoms must guide the diagnosis.

If the clinical student remembers what has been said (p. 327), on the infrequency in India, of inflammation of the periphery, compared with that of the substance of the liver, he must already have arrived at the conclusion, that pain is often not a prominent symptom of hepatitis.

What is the value of *pain of the right shoulder* as a symptom of hepatitis? It is present in a small proportion of cases, but absent in the majority. When present it gives additional emphasis to the other symptoms, but its absence in no respect detracts from their import.

We are often materially assisted in detecting inflammation of the liver, by carefully attending to the movements of the lower part of the right side of the chest and of the same side of the abdomen, under inspiration. Defective movement of the lower right chest, and of the abdominal wall below the right costal margin, in the absence of thoracic disease, suggests the existence of hepatitis, as might be anticipated, when we recollect the great extent of the hepatic surface, in relation with the diaphragm, and the movements impressed upon it by the contractions of this muscle. But while importance is thus attached to these partial imperfect inspiratory movements, it must not be forgotten that the inflammation may be so limited and so deep as to be removed from the influence of the pressure of the diaphragm. Therefore normal respiration does not necessarily imply the absence of hepatitis.

Nor may we overlook the relations of the concave surface of the liver to the stomach, and the explanation which this affords of the occasional occurrence of vomiting. But this symptom is more frequently observed in the advanced than in the early stages of hepatitis.

Do physical signs assist us in the diagnosis of the early stage of hepatitis?

At the commencement of inflammatory action there is always an increased quantity of blood in the affected capillaries, and when this derangement is of an organ well supplied with blood, augmented bulk must be a necessary consequence.

If there be *general* inflammation of the substance of the liver, the size of the organ will be increased, and a sense of weight and tension in the hepatic region, usually aggravated by turning to the left side, will be complained of.

Enlargement of the liver may be ascertained by careful manual examination, below the margin of the right ribs. There, the edge of the organ may be felt, and this result will be favoured by causing the patient to incline towards the left side, while we gently raise the liver, with the left hand placed on the inferior dorsal region, towards the right hand applied below the margin of the ribs. But if hepatitis exists pain may materially interfere with accurate palpation. This, however, is of little consequence, for the lower as well as the upper limit of the organ may be more accurately determined by gentle percussion. Clinical physicians doubtless differ in their estimate of these two methods of investigation. My own preference is for percussion made gently and from below upwards as respects the lower limit, and from above downwards as respects the upper limit. It is hardly necessary to add, that both in palpation and percussion regard must be had to the condition of the contents of the adjacent hollow viscera.

Enlargement is, however, not so common a sign of the early stage of hepatitis as casual reflection might suggest. The capacity of the capillaries of the hepatic artery — those concerned in inflammation — is small compared with that of the portal capillaries; therefore enlargement of the liver from capillary turgescence is a more probable sequence of fulness of the portal vein than of the hepatic artery. Portal capillary turgescence is not hepatic inflammation, but hepatic congestion; therefore augmented size of the liver, quickly appearing, is more likely to arise from the latter than from the former; moreover, *general* inflammation is rare, but the conditions which favour general congestion are of common occurrence: they are disease of the heart and of the lungs, also the deteriorated blood, and deranged balance of circulation in malarious fevers.

A liver, tense and enlarged by congestion, is often also tender on pressure; therefore, on the detection of enlargement, we must carefully inquire for the other symptoms of inflammation, and for the conditions which favour congestion; also whether the patient has previously been the subject of hepatic enlargement from recurring fever, or from malarious or other cachexia. The result of this inquiry will decide the diagnosis.

This question of diagnosis from enlargement rests on the hypothesis of *general* hepatitis, but as the inflammation is commonly limited in extent, it follows, that hepatitis, in its early stages, is frequently unattended by enlargement.

Mr. Twining believed that deep-seated hepatic inflammation was generally indicated by a peculiar tense state of the upper part of the right rectus muscle. Subsequent observers have not confirmed this opinion. That the muscular fibres of the anterior abdominal walls often spasmodically contract to keep off the pressure of the hand from a tender organ beneath, is true; and the tension or resistance thereby occasioned,—whether occurring at the margin of the right ribs, or elsewhere,—is often a valuable sign of subjacent inflammation. But that this sign has any special relation to deep-seated hepatic inflammation is not in accordance with my experience.

Do *altered states of the biliary secretion*, as evidenced by the condition of the alvine discharges, assist us in the diagnosis of hepatitis? Most certainly not. Clinical research is on this point in keeping with physiology and pathology. If the bile be secreted from the portal capillaries, if hepatitis be a derangement of the capillaries of the hepatic artery, and generally only of a small portion of them — then the reasonable inference is, that hepatitis is not unlikely to be attended with a normal state of the biliary secretion. Observation of the disease proves the accuracy of this conclusion. In hepatitis the secretion may be normal; or it may be excessive or defective.

The bile is secreted by the portal capillaries. Pathology teaches us that the circulation in these is often deranged, and suggests that altered secretion is more likely to be related to deranged circulation of the portal vein than of the hepatic artery; and that when it occurs in hepatitis it is not a symptom of it, but of co-existing portal derangement. Both observation and theory justify the statement that the state of the biliary secretion is of little value as a symptom of hepatitis.

Jaundice is mentioned as a symptom of hepatitis in systematic works on disease; and considerable prominence has been given to it, even in a recent able special treatise on the diseases of the liver. But, as regards India, the statement is erroneous. In that country jaundice is very seldom present in hepatitis; and its absence or presence is of no account in determining the diagnosis. In evidence of the accuracy of this statement, I need only refer to the numerous cases of hepatic abscess now before me. There are only five in which jaundice has been noted, and in them the explanation is sometimes supplied by such events as the presence of a lumbricus in the abscess (137), or the pressure of pus in the neighbourhood of the common and hepatic ducts * (136).

Pain, enlargement, deranged secretion of the liver, and modified function of adjacent organs, in their relation to the symptomatology of commencing hepatitis, have been considered; but we have yet to inquire whether general or constitutional symptoms are of importance.

The local symptoms which have been described may be preceded by a sense of chilliness, to be followed by *heat of skin and frequency of pulse;* and some degree of this febrile disturbance generally continues throughout the course of the disease. The pulse is more or less full, the tongue more or less coated, and the bowels are generally confined. The degree of these symptoms has reference to the state of the constitution, being more marked in the sthenic than in the asthenic.

It was stated that not unfrequently dysentery may exist without much febrile disturbance. The same fact is true of hepatitis, more especially when the central parts of the organ are the seat of the inflammation; and it is very probable when the morbid action is of limited extent and the diathesis asthenic.

It has been already explained (p. 278), that when inflammation attacks individuals, — European or native, — who have been exposed, for some time, to the influence of malarious climates, the symptomatic fever frequently assumes a remittent form. This remark applies to hepatitis as well as to other inflammations; but the fact has been more frequently noted by me in natives than in Europeans.

Such, then, are the symptoms on which we may rely for the

* I do not, in connection with hepatitis, make prominent allusion to a dark, dingy appearance of the skin not unfrequently observed in Europeans suffering from acute disease in India, and which may be held to indicate an inadequate elimination of bile; because, though occasionally present in hepatitis, it is not confined to that disease, and can hardly be considered a symptom of it. When observed, however, it necessarily directs our attention to the condition of the liver and its functions.

diagnosis of acute hepatitis in its early stages. They are sometimes, it appears, sufficiently distinct and expressive; but at other times, unfortunately, vague and unsatisfactory. This obscurity, moreover, is most apt to attend inflammation of that part of the organ, and in that kind of constitution, in which suppuration is likely to occur.

Though, then, the diagnosis of hepatitis may be occasionally doubtful, still I entertain the belief that too much prominence has been given to this feature by practical writers. My conviction is, that with a careful inquiry into symptoms, local and general, the observation of the diathesis, and a just attention to the previous history as respects former disease and exposure to predisposing and exciting causes, hepatic abscess, unsuspected or undetected during life, ought to be a much rarer event than is generally supposed. The contrary opinion has a manifest tendency to encourage careless investigation.

When hepatitis occurs in individuals of good diathesis, is seen early, and is met by judicious treatment, the symptoms, local and general, will, for the most part, gradually disappear, and the individual be restored to health.

In many cases, however, in consequence of bad diathesis, or advanced stages, or other causes, recovery does not take place, in some suppuration occurs, and *hepatic abscess is formed.* It is of importance to be able early to detect this result and to note its progress, because principles of treatment different from those suitable to the antecedent stages are indicated. There can be no doubt that tardiness in detecting suppuration and in modifying the treatment accordingly has led to undue mortality from hepatic abscess.

I proceed now to describe *the symptoms which indicate that hepatic inflammation has terminated in suppuration.* When the pain or other symptoms of hepatitis have continued with little or no abatement, there may appear after some time — eight or twelve days — increased fulness of the lower right false ribs, or fulness or tenseness below their margin or in the epigastrium, attended with increased dulness on percussion. Or the signs may point to enlargement upwards. There may be short dry cough, the respiration may be short and thoracic, and dulness on percussion may extend above the normal limit. Or in some cases the signs of increase both upwards and downwards may be combined. When such phenomena occur in succession to well-marked symptoms of acute hepatitis, there can be no doubt that abscess has formed.

But this distinct transition of the inflammation into abscess is not the usual course. Some degree of alleviation, consequent, perhaps, on the treatment employed, is more common: the pain may cease, or be very much lessened, and the febrile excitement may pass away; but emaciation increases, and a constant sense of languor is experienced. This state may continue for some days. Then occasional chills * may be complained of, or some degree of febrile excitement may be apparent towards evening, slight at first, perhaps overlooked, but soon increasing in degree, and assuming the character of hectic, with a tongue florid at the tip and edges, or tending to be apthous. With all this constitutional disturbance, there may, as yet, be no return of local symptoms — no signs of enlarging liver; but, notwithstanding this, slowly-developed hectic fever, consecutive on previous symptoms of hepatitis, affords almost conclusive evidence that suppuration is in progress, and will shortly be proved by the positive signs of hepatic abscess. Some degree of uneasiness and sense of weight will, however, be usually experienced in the region of the liver; or a feeling of oppression at the lower part of the chest, attended with dry cough. Sometimes, at this stage, acute pain of the right side comes on suddenly, caused either by tension from the increasing contents of the abscess, or by sudden recrudescence of the inflammation; and now, if the previous symptoms have not been carefully noted, and the right diagnosis formed, a serious error may be committed. This sudden access of acute pain may be interpreted as indicating the onset of primary acute hepatitis; and injudiciously active treatment may, in consequence, be adopted.

The disease still advancing, the physical signs of considerable enlargement, gradually appear. If in the direction downwards, it will be indicated by fulness and hardness and dulness at the margin of the right ribs, and for some distance below them; if the left lobe is the seat, the fulness and dulness will be in the epigastrium. If, on the other hand, the enlargement be towards the chest, there will be cough, impaired movement of the lower part of the right chest, and increasing dulness above the sixth rib.

With these physical signs of enlarging liver, and symptoms of deranged function of adjacent organs, there will be increasing emaciation, continuance of hectic fever, and at times acute pain of

* In respect to the occurrence of rigors, in the course of hepatitis, I would remark that when distinct they afford strong suspicion, but not certain evidence, of suppuration; for I have known them present in cases in which abscess did not result. On the whole, the symptom is not of much value, and the observer will be in continual error if he allows their absence to influence his diagnosis.

the side. Then, at this stage, dysenteric symptoms, chronic in character, generally appear; or, to express it otherwise, secondary inflammation of the mucous membrane of the large intestine, usually passing on to ulceration, is apt to arise.

The hepatic abscess has been traced to a stage in which its existence is no longer doubtful, and its still further progress has to be described. But before doing so, I am desirous of also following to the stage at which we have now arrived —1, abscess not preceded by well-marked symptoms of hepatitis, — the obscure cases to which reference has been made on several occasions; 2, abscess secondary on dysentery; 3, those cases in which dysentery and hepatitis have been coincident, but the symptoms of both have been badly developed, and the issue has been in hepatic abscess.

1. We have just learnt that hepatic abscess is sometimes developed in this manner, viz., the symptoms of hepatitis are more or less, it may be entirely, removed, and are succeeded by certain phenomena, which, viewed in connection with the fact of previous symptoms of hepatitis, justify the conviction that suppuration has taken place. But hepatic abscess may occur, unpreceded by distinct symptoms of hepatitis, and the question now is, by what means, under these circumstances, may we detect or infer its presence. We fix our attention on the symptoms which are so expressive in succession to those of marked hepatitis, viz., loss of flesh, sense of languor and debility, florid tongue, occasional chills, evening flushings of heat gradually passing into hectic fever. Should these occur in an individual of sallow complexion, cachectic from elevated temperature, mercurial courses, mental anxieties; or the subject, at former times, of attacks of hepatitis, or of deranged bowels with pale discharges, and not addicted to the intemperate use of spirits, or certainly tainted with malaria, then we may entertain a strong suspicion that we have to deal with an obscure hepatitis passing into suppuration. In the instance of the spirit drinker, we must keep in view the probability of cirrhosis. In the instance of the tainted with malaria, we must consider the probability of this influence, being a sufficient explanation of the symptoms.

The chief difficulty, however, will be experienced in those occasional cases in which the abscess forms slowly *, is small,

* An interesting case of long existing abscess is given by Dr. Budd, at p. 169 of his work, second edition.

Dr. Maclean, of the Madras army, in a very valuable paper on the "Abuse of Mercury in Hepatic Disease," in the third number of the "Indian Annals of Medicine," also quotes a case of obscure and old hepatic abscess. Careful perusal of the cases

deep, becomes encysted, and quiescent, or has partially undergone absorption. For such may endure for months, it may be years, and give, only occasionally, and at long intervals, obscure indication of its presence. Still, even in these rare instances, the feeble general health and the character of the occasional derangements, viewed in connection with the previous history, may generally serve to excite our apprehension in respect to the condition of the liver.

I find in my notes the following case illustrative of the general tenor of these remarks on the symptoms of obscurely forming hepatic abscess. Several years ago I attended a delicate European female, with acute hepatitis. She recovered under the cautious use of leeching, and gentle mercurial influence. Subsequently she became pregnant, and was delivered at the full period. She nursed for several months, but was obliged to discontinue. Then, as I learnt, she suffered from occasional febrile accessions, and relaxed bowels, and became emaciated, but made no complaint of pain in the region of the liver. This state continued, with occasional abatement, but no suspicion of serious organic disease was entertained. The symptoms were thought to depend on debility from lactation. I now incidentally saw her, as a friend rather than professionally, between six and seven o'clock in the evening, and was much struck with the great emaciation, the hot dry skin, the feeble frequent pulse, and very florid tongue. I made no examination of the side. Three or four days afterwards she died suddenly; hepatic abscess had burst into the sac of the peritoneum.

2. Let us next notice the cases of hepatic abscess which are distinctly secondary on dysentery. The disease, we may suppose, has been correctly viewed as dysentery, it has attained to such degree of progress, that ulceration has probably resulted; or, not unfrequently, the symptoms indicate that improvement has commenced, but it is not steady, the emaciation and languor being greater in degree than the amount of the dysenteric symptoms can satisfactorily explain. If, under these circumstances of dysentery, an evening febrile accession, with increasing floridity of tongue, is detected, then there are good grounds for suspecting that abscess has either formed, or is forming in the liver, to become evident, in due course, by the usual physical signs. A large proportion of such cases will be found to be of individuals predisposed to hepatitis by former disease, or by those influences which have been already several times mentioned, and the recognition of which, under the

narrated in this chapter will discover several in which the course of the abscess was very slow.

circumstances now adverted to, will tend to confirm the diagnosis of hepatic abscess.

3. But it is not to the advanced stages of dysentery that a co-existing hepatitis with tendency to terminate in abscess is confined. It sometimes happens that the dysenteric symptoms have been present for a few days only, have not been severe, perhaps neglected; then the symptoms of hepatitis creep on slowly and obscurely, and as they become confirmed, the dysenteric symptoms may disappear, or continue in a subdued form. Here we have an illustration either of the two diseases originating at the same time under the influence of the same causes, or of a primary disease, slight in degree, giving place to the greater development of a secondary one. This relation of hepatic abscess to dysentery is very rare compared with that in which the hepatitis is a feature of the advanced stages of dysentery. But it is very important—its gravity is apt to be overlooked. It is not confined to the cachectic and old resident, but has been witnessed by me only in Europeans. I have the impression that it will probably be found to be related to the predisposing influence of depressed vital actions consequent on malaria, mental anxiety, or other similar causes. This form of disease is well illustrated by the following case:—

144. *Slight dysenteric symptoms of some days' duration, followed by febrile symptoms.—Those of hepatic inflammation coming on obscurely, and ending in abscess.*—Mr. H——, a gentleman, about thirty-five years of age, who had been resident some years in Bombay, at the beginning of July 1847, suffered from occasional dysenteric symptoms. He passed small quantities of blood-tinged mucus. This, however, had abated much, without treatment. I saw him first on the 16th July. There was not any febrile disturbance, no uneasiness on pressure of the abdomen, and the scanty discharges did not take place more frequently than twice or thrice in the twenty-four hours, but he passed sleepless nights. On the 17th slight uneasiness of the right side of the abdomen was first complained of, and on the 18th there was a febrile accession, which recurred with greater severity on the evening of the 19th, with uneasy epigastrium, occasional retching, a coated tongue, and a dingy yellowish tinge of the skin. The dysenteric symptoms had ceased. There was now fever, with morning remission and evening exacerbation; and on the 22nd there was considerable pain below the right ribs, on turning to the left side, and on full inspiration; and on the 23rd there was general fulness of the lower right ribs, but the liver was not detected below them. On the 24th, after pain suddenly and severely felt below the right ribs and over the abdomen generally, relieved by sinapisms and anodynes, a distinct defined hardness midway between the ribs and iliac fossa became perceptible. There was now abatement of the febrile disturbance, cessation of the dysenteric symptoms, and quiescence of the hepatic; and he was sent early in August to the Cape of Good Hope, in a comfortable ship. He died shortly after arrival there of hepatic abscess. He was treated with free leeching, calomel, ipecacuanha and opiates, with quinine during the febrile remissions.

Having described the different circumstances under which suppuration in the liver may become developed, I return to the history at that stage when, however originating, the existence of abscess has become certain; and proceed to follow it to its several issues.

In a large proportion of cases, death takes place in consequence of the exhausting effects of hectic fever, and co-existing diarrhœa, without rupture of the abscess. This is the course when there are many abscesses scattered about the substance of the liver, or when one or two large abscesses exist deep in the parenchyma of the right lobe. The fatal termination is, no doubt, in instances, hastened by the too long-continued use of antiphlogistic remedies, intestinal irritants, or injudicious operative proceedings. In these circumstances of hepatic abscess, the prognosis is necessarily most unfavourable, but it forms no part of the art of medicine to add to the danger by unseasonable interference.

The abscess may advance to the external surface, fluctuate distinctly, and point at the margin of the right ribs, the epigastrium, or an intercostal space. If life be prolonged, rupture will take place, and the likelihood of a successful result will depend on the state of the constitution, on the abscess being single or not, being seated in the thin parts of the organ or extending to its deeper structures, and on its being associated, or not, with dysentery. But the natural course in cases of this kind has been frequently modified by surgical interference, and our data are therefore rendered imperfect. The question of the puncture of hepatic abscess will be considered as part of the treatment.

Hepatic abscess may extend in the proximity of the diaphragm, and pleuritis and pneumonia of the base of the right lung may be excited. This may be indicated by, in addition to cough and defective respiratory movement, friction murmur, or crepitus. This event is most likely to occur when the abscess is large.

A "hepatic compression rhonchus" has been described by Dr. Walshe, as present in enlargement of the liver, and is attributed by him to expansion of the lower portion of the lung previously compressed. It has been inferred, that this sign may serve to assist in the diagnosis of abscess when pressing upwards, and causing compression of the lung. I am unacquainted with this sign, and though I may not question the accuracy of Dr. Walshe's observation, or the justness of his explanation*, yet I may doubt its applicability without great caution to hepatic abscess; for here there is a great

* I may observe, that my knowledge of Dr. Walshe's opinion is derived from an interesting inquiry into the "Statistics and Pathology of Abscess in the Liver," lately published by Mr. E. J. Waring, Residency Surgeon at Travancore, and the able author of a "Manual of Practical Therapeutics."

probability that, by less practised ears, the rhonchus may be confounded with friction murmur, and thus the existence of pleuritis be overlooked. I am the more confident in this opinion, because my late much valued friend, Dr. Malcolmson, committed this error, in the year 1838. In a paper published in the 21st volume of the Transactions of the Medico-Chirurgical Society, he describes a sound between "a crepitous rattle and a bleating," and he attributed it to compression of the thin edge of the lung; but it is evident from the description of the appearances after death, that the sound heard had been a friction murmur. "At the spot where the sound was heard, there was a slight adhesion of the thin margin of the lung to the sixth and seventh ribs."

When the pleuritic inflammation has terminated, as occasionally happens, in circumscribed or general effusion, then there may be doubt whether the dulness, absence of vocal thrill, and other signs of displacement and compression of the lung, are due to empyema, or simply to enlargement of the liver. Perhaps this difficulty ought only to be experienced in cases which come under notice at this advanced stage, and in which there has not been the opportunity of observing the early symptoms, and thus ascertaining the previous existence of. hepatitis. If the following case had occurred in a hospital in Europe, there would have been little hesitation in at once determining it to be one of right pleuritic effusion; but admitted into a hospital in India, in which hepatic abscess encroaching on the chest, sometimes associated with empyema, is not an unfrequent event, there was room for the doubt which was experienced, and which is expressed in the heading of the statement.

145. *Diagnosis doubtful: whether right pleuritic effusion, or large hepatic abscess, or both conjoined.*—Shaik Chand, twenty-one years of age, a Mussulman butler, of emaciated frame, and with anxious countenance, addicted to the moderate use of spirits, was admitted into the clinical ward on the 13th November, 1852. The respiration was short, hurried, and chiefly thoracic, and the movement of the right side of the chest was defective. The right dorsal, lateral, and mammary regions were completely, the scapular and interscapular slightly, dull on percussion. In these dull situations, bronchial respiration was audible, and vocal thrill altogether absent. In the subclavian resonant region the respiration was puerile. The præcordial dulness commencing at the second left rib, was bounded internally by the left sternal border, and below was continuous with the hepatic dulness. The heart's apex beat between the fourth and fifth left ribs, half an inch below and external to the nipple. The right side across the nipple exceeded the left by one inch. Below the margin of the right ribs, there was sense of induration, with dulness, continuous with the thoracic dulness. A curved line from the point of the right twelfth rib, to that of the tenth left rib, and passing about an inch above the umbilicus, formed the lower limit of this indurated and dull space. Decubitus easiest on the back, most difficult on the left side. Complained of pain of the right side, and occasional cough. Stated that five months before he had suffered from intermittent fever, and been cured. It recurred, how-

ever, six weeks before admission, followed by cough. The induration below the ribs had been first noticed fifteen days ago. He continued under observation, suffering from febrile accessions, dyspnœa, some increase in the size of the right side of chest, till the 23rd, when he was removed by his friends. The urine had given no trace of albumen.

I add another instructive case, in which the error in diagnosis was committed, probably in consequence of adhesions preventing the descent of the liver, and the great extension upwards of the abscess preventing marked lateral bulging.

146. *Hepatic abscess mistaken for pleuritic effusion.*—Pascoal Kyttan, aged forty, was admitted into hospital on the 28th February, 1857, after ten days' illness. There was hurried respiration, febrile heat, feeble pulse, tenderness below the right ribs, with dulness for an inch, defective movement of the right side of chest, dulness of lateral, infra-scapular and lower scapular regions with defective breath sounds, occasional crepitus and feeble vocal thrill; also slight general fulness of the right infra-mammary and infra-axillary regions. He continued suffering from evening febrile exacerbations, more or less dyspnœa, sometimes pain of right side of chest. Crepitus was heard, from time to time, and friction murmur was on one occasion suspected in the infra-scapular regions. He died on the 2nd March.

Inspection.—The right lobe of the liver was throughout its entire surface firmly adherent to the diaphragm. It did not project above an inch below the ribs. It was converted into a large abscess sac, the upper wall of which for a considerable extent consisted chiefly of the diaphragm, which ascended to the third rib. The gall-bladder, full of bile, was part of the lower wall. There was pretty firm adhesion of the diaphragm to the base of the lung; but no engorgement or solidification of the lung there or elsewhere; it crepitated throughout. The left lung was also healthy. The left lobe of the liver was healthy, and was pushed over to the curve of the left ribs. There was streaked vascularity of the mucous membrane of the colon, with two or three superficial ulcers with granular exudation in the cœcum and rectum.

Hepatic abscess may point at the diaphragm, rupture, and communicate with the lung. (*a*) If the abscess has been large and has opened into a bronchial tube of some size, a considerable quantity of pus may be quickly expectorated, and if the constitution has been good, recovery may take place; but communication with the lung in this manner is of rare occurrence. (*b*) The abscess may be small, and, on opening into the substance of the lung, may excite, in some degree, inflammation in the tissues adjacent, then muco-puriform sputa, generally tinged red, will be expectorated in moderate quantity, for varying periods, and if the constitution has been good and the abscess single, there will be a fair chance of restoration to health. The majority of recovered cases of abscess communicating with the lung are of this nature. (*c*) The abscess may be large and open into the substance of the lung, excite inflammation, softening, liquefaction of tissue, and lead to the formation of a ragged cavity, of varying size, in the base of the lung, and continuous with the sac in the liver. The sputa then will be muco-puriform or sero-puriform, often in considerable quantity, generally of red or brown tint, very rarely bile-tinged, and expectorated with harassing cough. A fatal result will take place in periods longer or shorter, according to the diathesis. In such cases careful auscultation should detect the presence of cavernous sounds in the base of the lung.

In "Notes on Hepatitis," as observed by me in the European General Hospital, presented to the Bombay Medical and Physical Society in May 1845, and published in No. VI. of their "Transactions," I find the following remark relative to the opening of hepatic abscess into the lung :—

"This expectoration of brick-red puriform fluid I am disposed to consider as pathognomonic of abscess in the liver opening into the lungs, because there is not any disease of the lungs in which we can conceive, as a result, the co-existence of pus intimately intermixed with blood; the one, pus, being the result of an advanced stage of inflammatory action; the other, blood, the result of an early stage of the same action. But when we suppose that the pus comes from the liver, and the blood from the lung irritated by the foreign body, the co-existence is sufficiently intelligible."

Dr. Budd, in his "Treatise on Diseases of the Liver," * published in June 1845, writing of the opening of hepatic abscess into the lung, thus expresses himself: —

"When this happens, it is marked by very characteristic symptoms, by a new train of stethoscopic phenomena, which it is perhaps unnecessary to detail, and by the sudden expectoration of a dirty red or brownish puriform matter. The peculiar colour of this matter, which has been already noticed, arises from the pus, in its passage through the lung, becoming mixed with blood and broken down pulmonary tissue. There is no matter like it expectorated in any disease of the lung itself; and I believe that its appearing is pathognomonic of abscess of the liver, or at least of abscess perforating the lung. I observed it in several instances in the *Dreadnought*, and more than once was led by it to detect an abscess in the liver, of which I had previously no suspicion."

Here, then, are two observers, remote from each other, unacquainted with each other's researches, making at the same time, and very nearly in the same words, the same observation relative to a symptom of disease; yet both were certainly in error in regard to the exclusive light in which they viewed the symptom.

The kind of sputa, which I have described in my remarks on pneumonia, under the designation of red-tinged muco-puriform sputa, observed in states of asthenic pneumonia, is not to be distinguished from that which I formerly considered to be pathognomonic of hepatic abscess having opened into the lung. Confiding in my former investigations, I, in more instances than one, committed an error in diagnosis, after my transference from the European to the Jamsetjee Jejeebhoy Hospital brought me for the first time into practical acquaintance with asthenic forms of pneumonia.

* First edition, page 88.

The diagnosis between asthenic pneumonia and communicating hepatic abscess, when undue importance is not attached to this character of the sputum, may, no doubt, in the majority of cases, be satisfactorily made out; but yet not in all, as the following cases will serve to illustrate:—

147. *Asthenic pneumonia mistaken for communicating hepatic abscess.*—Dhoondee Pelajee, a Hindoo mason, fifty years of age, was after twenty days' illness, admitted into hospital, on the 24th January, 1846, affected with fever, anxiety, dyspnœa, and pain across the lower and anterior part of the chest. There were bronchitic rales, with crepitus and bronchial respiration in the posterior part of the right side of the chest. The disease was considered to be pneumonia. But on the 26th the pain extended from the right nipple to two inches beyond the margin of the right ribs; and there was dulness on percussion throughout this extent. The sputa were of brick-red colour, and in detached masses. The opinion was then entertained that there was abscess of the liver, which had opened into the lung, and that the pneumonia was secondary. He died on the 30th January. The liver extended an inch beyond the margin of the ribs; it had formed slight adhesions with the diaphragm, was congested with blood, but without abscess or other disease of structure. The right lung adhered to the diaphragm and the ribs by tender adhesions; the lower lobe was in a state of red induration.

148. *Whether asthenic pneumonia or communicating hepatic abscess—doubtful.*—Allawoodeen, a Mussulman weaver, thirty-seven years of age, was admitted into the clinical ward on the 27th December, 1850. He had been ill four months. He was emaciated; his respiration was short and hurried; there was dulness, with some slight bulging of the lower part of right side of the chest. There was defectiveness there of vocal thrill, and absence of sound under the stethoscope. There was tenderness below the margin of the right ribs. He had constant troublesome short cough, expectorated red-tinged opaque mucus, and suffered from hectic. The illness had commenced with pain of the right side of chest and margin of the ribs four months before admission; the cough and expectoration had existed for six weeks. The sputa became muco-puriform, and tinged red. About a month after admission there were signs of a cavity at the lower angle of the right scapula, and dysenteric symptoms came on. He was removed from the hospital in a moribund state. This case was entered Pneumonia in the hospital returns, but I am very doubtful of the accuracy of the diagnosis that was then formed. I believe now that hepatic abscess had opened into the lung.

Abscess may open into the stomach or intestinal canal, the peritoneum or pericardium, but I have not under this head any remarks to make in addition to those already offered on the pathology of these events (pp. 342, 345).

SECTION VI.—*Treatment of Early Stages.—Blood-letting, general and local.—Mercurial and other Purgatives.—Mercurial Influence.—Blisters.—Treatment when Abscess is forming and is perfected.—Question of Puncture considered.—Change of Climate.*

I shall first describe the treatment of the early stages of acute hepatitis, and then that which is applicable after suppuration has taken place. Several of the remedies which have been noticed in the chapters on fever and dysentery will again come under review; but I shall not deem it necessary to reiterate principles which have been already fully explained.

Success in the treatment of hepatitis, as in all inflammatory diseases, depends on the recency of the attack, and the diathesis of the patient — whether favourable to resolution or to disorganisation.

General Blood-letting.—When the period of the attack renders it probable that the inflammation has not passed the stage of vascular turgescence or commencing exudation —when the general aspect of the patient, the rate, fulness, and firmness of the pulse, and increased temperature of the skin, indicate febrile disturbance with sufficiency of blood and excessive action of a heart of adequate power — then general blood-letting should be had recourse to.

Vascular turgescence will always be increased when the blood not deficient in quantity is impelled by a heart of adequate power and excited action; and this evil may be best controlled by general blood-letting.

But it is only in the early stage of hepatitis in Europeans not long resident in India, and uninjured by the depressing influences of malaria, elevated temperature and intemperance — or in the sthenic natives of the more temperate regions of India—that we may expect the conditions which are usually benefited by general blood-letting. Moreover, we must be careful that even in suitable cases this remedy is not used in an injurious degree.

It is the most prompt and therefore the best means of reducing excessive action of the heart, co-existing with sufficiency of blood. But when the action has been reduced, and the blood diminished in quantity, the utility of general blood-letting ends; and from this time, if persisted in, it becomes injurious, by favouring the change of exuded lymph into pus, and lessening the chance of subsequent repair. The useful application of general blood-letting is chiefly limited to the stage of vascular turgescence. If it be used in the stage of exudation (exception being made in favour of those occasional cases in which the conditions indicating its expediency are still present), it will generally prove ultimately injurious. It is impossible to be more precise, or to lay down rules as to whether the quantity of blood abstracted should be sixteen, twenty, or thirty ounces, or whether it should be repeated or not; but there can be no question, that the excessive blood-letting advocated by some (especially Mr. Twining) is altogether at variance with the principles which I have been endeavouring to inculcate.

When these remarks are regarded in connection with those on the pathology, etiology, and symptoms of hepatitis, the conclusion must be evident, that general blood-letting is a remedy not frequently required in the treatment of this disease as it presents itself to the practitioner in India.*

Local blood-letting, chiefly by leeches, is of more general application. It is valuable in succession to general blood-letting, and also in those cases for which general blood-letting is unsuitable. The number used and the frequency of repetition must depend on the size of the leech, the stage of the disease, the severity of the symptoms, and the character of the diathesis. Though local blood-letting is also most beneficial in the early stages of vascular turgescence; still it is of value after exudations have taken place — even after their degeneration has commenced — for it acts favourably on the surrounding turgescent parts. It must always be remembered that exuded lymph will not become absorbed — will not go through the other processes that may be most favourable to restoration — unless the capillary circulation immediately surrounding it be in a tolerably normal state. In using leeches, however, in these more advanced stages of inflammation, especial regard must be had to the state of the constitution; for if there be doubt of its ability to bear further loss of blood without injury, we must desist, and call to our aid other means of derivation.

As remedies subsidiary to blood-letting and useful in the same stage as well as subsequently, fomentations frequently applied, or the warm water compress with bandage and appliances to prevent evaporation, may be mentioned.

Mercurial and other Purgatives. — The principle on which the action of calomel and of other purgatives is useful, in certain conditions of the early stages of dysentery, has been explained at some length. They favour, by increasing secretion, the free movement of the blood in the portal capillaries and the mucous lining of the small intestine; and thus tend to relieve stagnation of blood in the capillaries of the large intestine. These remedies form also an important part of treatment in the early stages of

* It can hardly be necessary to say, that this observation is to be understood as applying to medical practice in India in the aggregate. The proportion of cases calling for general blood-letting in the practice of different individuals, will vary according to the field in which it is followed. I really fear that I may be charged with tediousness in the reiteration of this principle; but I have seen so much neglect of its observance in the course of my service, that excess of caution may well be pardoned.

certain conditions of hepatitis; and their efficacy is explainable on the same principle. The blood of the arterial capillaries of the liver, equally with that of the mucous membrane of the large intestine, is passed into the portal capillaries; and, consequently, free circulation in the latter must equally tend to lessen stagnation in the capillaries of the hepatic artery. Therefore the frequently-quoted remark of Abercrombie — "If the liver be supposed to be in a state of torpor, mercury is given to excite it; if in a state of acute inflammation, mercury is given to moderate the inflammation and reduce the action," conveys to my mind no expression of inconsistency.

Consecutive on general blood-letting, or the early application of leeches, it is generally useful to give ten grains of calomel and one of opium, with so much ipecacuanha as the stomach is tolerant of, and in four or five hours afterwards, a moderate dose of castor oil, or compound jalap powder. The necessity of repeating these means will bear relation to the sthenic state of the system, the recency of the attack, the presence of congestion of the portal capillaries, and a deranged state of the biliary secretion. The symptoms of portal congestion are: — (*a*) A yellow-coated tongue, without irritation of the mucous lining of the mouth to account for it. (*b*) Scanty alvine discharges, dark or pale. (*c*) General fulness of the upper part of the abdomen, with, it may be, the physical signs of hepatic enlargement. (*d*) A dingy state of the skin and scanty high-coloured urine.

Calomel and other purgatives are used, not to exercise any direct effect on the inflamed capillaries, but to remove a co-existing congestion of the portal capillaries, which must tend to prevent a return to normal circulation in the capillaries of the hepatic artery. This combined derangement is likely to be present, in such degree as to require these remedies, only in the early stages of hepatitis and in systems well supplied with blood. In advanced stages, in previously healthy individuals, and in cachectic constitutions in all stages, these means are contra-indicated, because a tendency to dysentery is a characteristic feature of cachexia as well as of an advanced stage of hepatitis; and there is no more certain exciting cause of it, in these states, than calomel and purgatives. When under these latter circumstances there is suspicion of portal stagnation, or other indication for the use of eliminants, then small doses of blue pill in combination with ipecacuanha, or the extract of taraxacum with an alkali, and the external application of nitro-muriatic acid should be resorted to.

Ipecacuanha is very beneficial in hepatitis, given to the degree that may be practicable; but there is not that tolerance which is a characteristic feature of dysentery. So true is this that when a dysenteric patient is intolerant of ipecacuanha, we should make it a rule to investigate closely the condition of the liver.

In combining opium with calomel, the quantity must be regulated by the tendency, or not, to gastric or enteric irritation.

Quiescence in the recumbent posture, and a very restricted diet, are essential adjuvants in the management of the early stages of acute hepatitis.

By steadily observing this system of treatment we may hope, in persons of good diathesis, to cure the disease by resolution in a considerable proportion of cases in which it has not advanced beyond vascular turgescence or commencing exudation. But to ensure this result an important caution is necessary. We must be careful not to commit the error of thinking that the removal of the inflammation and the cessation of the symptoms are always, or even generally, coincident events. The deranged capillaries return slowly to their normal state, and, probably, do not commonly attain it till some time after the symptoms have disappeared. The latter event is in all likelihood rather coincident with the period when the onward progress of diseased action has been checked, and return to a healthy state has fairly commenced. Relapse is apt to occur, and is often traceable to the error just adverted to. When the disease has clearly existed recovery must still be regarded as incomplete till several days have elapsed since the removal of pain and febrile disturbance; and during this period the patient should be confined to bed, the diet should still be most carefully regulated, and any derangement of the secretions be corrected by gentle means.

But the attack may be only moderated, not removed, by the means of treatment recommended; and the conclusion, that exudation and coagulation of lymph are taking place is forced upon us. Or the case may have come under treatment at that stage which renders it probable that this event had already occurred. What are the resources of our art under these circumstances? Let us recollect what pathology has taught us, — (*a*) That plastic lymph exuded and coagulated may become organised into fibrous tissue, and thus cause more or less permanent organic injury. This is an occasional but rare result of hepatitis. (*b*) Plastic lymph exuded and coagulated, instead of becoming organised, may speedily re-liquefy, and be absorbed, and thus complete recovery may result. But this event necessarily implies a nearly normal state of the capillary circulation, and of the quantity and quality of the blood, in the surrounding tissues. To effect this termination is the object of treatment in this stage of hepatitis, and we have good reason for believing that it is not unfrequently attended with success. (*c*) Plastic lymph may be exuded in such quantity, and so remote from normal structure, that its organisation into tissue, or its removal by absorption, is impracticable; it necessarily, in part, becomes converted into pus, and abscess is formed. Or, aplastic lymph may be exuded. It is inorganisable, and has no tendency to be absorbed, partly from its excessive quantity and bad quality, partly because the capillaries around are unfit to absorb. It changes into pus, and in this manner also abscess is formed. Both these results are common in hepatitis.

It would seem, then, that it is only under the second contingency (*b*) that there is still the opportunity of complete restoration. The question may be thus put. Lymph not in excessive quantity having exuded and coagulated, and efficient means for controlling the surrounding deranged capillary circulation having been used — do we possess remedies calculated to favour the fusion and absorption necessary to recovery? The answer is, the mild constitutional influence of *mercury* is believed, and probably with truth, to possess this power.

But, does this admission not suggest that mercury may also be beneficial when, from abnormal condition of surrounding parts, excessive quantity or bad quality of lymph, pus is formed, but is not absorbed? Certainly not, for when exuded lymph tends to change into pus, the action of mercury will favour this tendency, that is, promote suppuration and the formation of abscess.

If these pathological and therapeutic doctrines approximate to the truth, then we are provided with a principle of treatment of hepatitis by induction of mercurial influence, viz.: — When the disease, in a good diathesis, is at that stage in which the exudation of lymph is likely to be going on, mercurial influence is indicated. If, on the other hand, the diathesis is bad, or there is reason to believe that suppuration has already taken place, mercurial influence is contra-indicated.

It is evident then that mercury can only be used with advantage in hepatitis when, by careful observation and inquiry, the stage of the disease and the diathesis of the patient have been ascertained with tolerable accuracy. The opinion at one time generally entertained, that mercury exercises some special power in hepatic inflammation, is unsupported by clinical experience. This erroneous doctrine is perhaps, in part, to be traced to inattention to the distinction between the cholagogue and the constitutional action of this agent: the nature and application of the former have already been explained, and my present remarks are to be understood as having exclusive reference to the latter.

Instead of thinking that the constitutional influence of mercury has a special value in hepatitis, I believe, for the following reasons, that more caution and discrimination are required in its application in this disease than in the other membranous or parenchymatous inflammations, in the treatment of which it is generally used.

1. There is no organ so prone in India as the liver to become the seat of suppuration, and the constitutional states which favour this result of inflammation and frequently cause it, are certainly aggravated by mercury.

2. The opinion that gentle ptyalism may prevent hepatic abscess, can only be true in those cases for which mercury is indicated in accordance with the principles just explained. That suppuration, after mercurial influence, has not been an unusual occurrence in the treatment of hepatitis, has been amply proved by the clinical experience of myself and others. The statement made long since, and repeated by Annesley and others, that, hepatic abscess, when present, prevents the constitutional action of mercury, probably rests on very insufficient evidence, for it is difficult to believe that the experiments necessary to determine the question have been frequently made. I have myself no practical acquaintance with the use of mercury in the treatment of hepatic abscess.

3. The cases before me, more particularly those of sick officers, show a marked predisposition in those who have been the frequent subjects of mercurial influence to suffer from uneasiness in the region of the liver, and to be affected with pale alvine discharges, languor, &c. Under these circumstances, the liver is undoubtedly liable to become the seat of sub-acute inflammation from ordinary exciting causes, as cold. This statement accords with the observation made by Graves *, that enlargement of the liver is sometimes a feature of mercurial cachexia.

I now return to details of practice. If the symptoms of acute hepatitis treated from the outset in a good constitution are not speedily and decidedly removed by blood-letting, mercurial and other purgatives, rest and appropriate diet, then mercurial influence with the continuance of other suitable measures, is indicated,

* "Clinical Lectures," vol. i. p. 448.

and it may be best induced by from two to four grains of calomel, with a quarter or half a grain of opium, and a grain of ipecacuanha, when tolerated, every third, fourth, sixth, or eighth hour; so regulating the dose as not to interfere with sleep, or to produce more effect than distinct swelling of the gums with slight ptyalism.

When, however, the case has first came under notice after two or three days' illness, mercury may be expedient from the very commencement of the treatment.

Should, on the other hand, the disease be first submitted to our care at such stages, and with such symptoms, as render the existence of suppuration probable, then, whatever may be the character of the diathesis, mercury is contra-indicated. And this is equally the case, if, whatever the stage of the disease, the appearance of the patient, or the history, denote a previous cachexia. When the contra-indication depends on cachexia, then we may inquire whether other alterative deobstruents, as liquor potassæ or the iodide of potassium, are likely to be advantageous. On this point I am unable to speak with confidence: liquor potassæ has seemed to me of use in some cases.

To find an agent which improves the plasticity of the lymph and the general nutritive processes, and to abstain from mercury—which has an opposite action — are the points to which attention should be chiefly directed in the treatment of hepatitis in cachectic constitutions.

Blisters.—Sooner or later in all cases of persisting hepatitis there comes a stage when we are no longer justified in attempting to lessen vascular turgescence by the derivative action of leeches; and then we must avail ourselves of those other means which act similarly without causing much evacuation from the blood, as dry cupping, rubefacients, epispastics.

If a normal capillary circulation in the parts adjacent to exuded lymph be a necessary condition of absorption— or of the organisation of the limitary layer — when absorption is impracticable — the reduction of vascular turgescence by derivation is an indication not confined to the early stages of hepatitis, but extends also to the more advanced periods, and is then to be effected by the class of remedies now under notice. Of these, the cantharides blister is the most generally used. But a very large one is inexpedient.* One from

* There is a caution relative to large blisters to which it may be useful to allude. There is a risk that cutaneous and subcutaneous fulness, from serous infiltration consequent on the irritation of a blister, when at and below the margin of the ribs, may

three to four inches square, placed over the affected part of the liver, is preferable. The use of blisters may be commenced when the stage for leeches has passed. Blisters cease to be beneficial and begin to be injurious when abscess has fully formed, and is advancing to the nearest surface. The reason is plain. At this stage some degree of inflammation favours the interstitial absorption and the adhesions necessary to the safety of the remaining chance of recovery. Nothing can be more irrational than the application of a large blister over the right hypochondrium, tumid from hepatic abscess, yet I have witnessed this.

My remarks have been confined to blisters, but dry cupping, sinapisms, turpentine oil, iodine paint, and tartar emetic ointment, all act on the same principle, though less efficaciously.

Let us now suppose that the treatment has been unsuccessful, and that abscess has formed. Recovery may still take place by one or other of the courses described in my notice of the pathology and symptoms; and we must now consider what are the means which best conduce to this end, and what are those which tend to prevent it.

Mercurial and all other depressing remedies must be at once abandoned. There may be a transition stage when antiphlogistics are contra-indicated, but in which, from the character of the febrile disturbance, tonic remedies and regimen may be doubtful: in this, opiates or other anodynes, with mild diaphoretics or other gentle eliminants, may be temporarily employed. Then we may gradually pass to the use of tonics—as quinine with dilute sulphuric acid, or nitric acid, with a bitter infusion,—while the opiate is continued at bed-time. The diet should also be improved, by addition of light puddings, milk, animal broths, jellies, and eggs, adjusted to the condition of the digestive organs and the assimilating powers. Wine or beer, when they do not excite the pulse or irritate the gastro-enteric linings, are also necessary.

I have already expressed my belief that the injudicious continuance of mercurial and other purgatives in the advanced stages of hepatitis is, in part, the cause of the frequent co-existence of intestinal ulceration. These remedies must be altogether omitted; and should eliminants be indicated, we must trust to taraxacum, alkalies*, nitric acid, and the external use of nitro-muriatic acid.

be mistaken for the sign of enlargement of the liver, and lead to an erroneous impression of the progress of the disease.

* Of hydrochlorate of ammonia, used with this view by German physicians, I have no experience, but the Indian practitioner will do well to try it.

When the abscess has opened into the lung, anodynes, tonics, and support, regulated to meet the requirements of particular cases, are the means of treatment. When the abscess has opened into the alimentary canal, similar remedies must be given, and intestinal irritants be carefully abstained from. When the abscess has opened into the sac of the peritoneum, the pleura, or pericardium, and inflammation of these serous tissues has been excited, or when general peritonitis has arisen, in the more common manner, independent of rupture, then, though the issue is in general too surely fatal, we may prolong life and palliate suffering by giving opium, in doses of from one to two grains every third or fourth hour, in the manner recommended by Dr. Stokes of Dublin.

When the abscess tends towards the external surface, then, in addition to the means advised in the other courses, we may endeavour to lessen discomfort by warm water applications, or cataplasms. When fluctuation has become apparent, the question of *puncturing the abscess* falls to be considered. I shall best explain myself on this point of practice, by stating the amount, results, and deductions of my own experience.

Puncture of Hepatic Abscess.—The notes of twenty-four cases in which I have witnessed the puncture of hepatic abscess are before me. Of these, eight may be classed as successful, and sixteen as unsuccessful.

Of the eight favourable cases, there was complete recovery in five; the history was incomplete, but restoration probable, in two; there was recovery from the punctured abscess, but death a year afterwards from a second abscess, in one. In all these cases the abscess pointed at the epigastrium, or at the margin of the right ribs, above the level of the ninth. They were all of moderate size, and, from their position, it may be inferred that they had formed in the thin part of the left lobe, or in the thin edge of the right lobe. We may further, from the fact of recovery, conclude that in each instance the abscess had been single.

These eight cases, 149 to 156, are here detailed.

149. *Hepatic abscess pointing at the epigastrium and successfully punctured.— Trocar used.*—Cassim Mahomed, a Mussulman butcher, aged fifty, was admitted into the Jamsetjee Jejeebhoy Hospital, on the 23rd August, 1848. There was a prominent swelling in the epigastric region, chiefly in the mesial line and towards the right side; it was soft with obscure fluctuation without discoloration of the skin, or tension, and the right side of the chest was resonant on percussion as low as the sixth rib. He stated that about a year before admission he had received a blow on the epigastrium, that the swelling made its appearance some time afterwards, and had gradually increased to its present size. He continued under observation till the 1st of September, not suffering from febrile accessions, when the swelling, which was much in the same

state as on admission, was punctured by a trocar, and about four ounces of red-coloured pus were discharged. On the 2nd, one ounce, and on the 3rd, three ounces more of reddish pus escaped from the puncture. He continued without fever, the discharge gradually lessening, and left the hospital on the 13th September, when the discharge had ceased, the wound had healed, and there was only a sense of thickening perceptible in the situation of the swelling.

150. *Hepatic abscess pointing at the epigastrium, punctured successfully.*—Gungajee Saccaram, a Hindoo, aged twenty-five, after a month's illness was admitted into the Jamsetjee Jejeebhoy Hospital on the 18th April, 1846. There was a prominent tumour in the centre of the epigastrium, tense, and apparently superficial. There was no tenseness at the margin of the right rib, and no dulness on percussion; there was slight heat of skin. The abscess was punctured, and some dark grey-coloured pus discharged. On the 19th the swelling had become considerably reduced, but there was still a good deal of discharge of thick pus tinged with blood. On the 22nd there was very little discharge, no tension, but considerable hardness around the puncture, and the tongue continued coated, but there were no febrile accessions. On the 27th the fulness and hardness had decreased much, but there was still slight discharge. On the 12th May he left the hospital, the fulness and hardness and puriform discharge having disappeared.

151. *Hepatic abscess pointing between the eighth right rib and umbilicus, successfully punctured.*—Through the kindness of Dr. Arbuckle I had the opportunity of seeing, about the year 1850, an English medical gentleman affected with hepatic abscess. It pointed about three inches below the margin of the right ribs, in about a line drawn vertically from the cartilage of the eighth rib. The abscess was opened, and recovery took place. This gentleman died about two years afterwards, but with what symptoms there is no record in my notes.

152. *Hepatic abscess punctured.—Recovery.*—Krushnah Poonjajee, a Hindoo cart-driver, of thirty years of age, a spirit drinker, was admitted into the clinical ward, on the 11th January, 1853. He was much reduced, and his countenance was anxious. A prominent swelling reached from the margin of the right false ribs and the ensiform cartilage to half an inch below the umbilicus. It was dull, and the dulness passed upwards to the level of the fifth rib. The swelling was painful, distinctly fluctuating, and at its lower part there was a small circular opening from which purulent discharge issued. Two months and a half before he had suffered from febrile accessions, and pain below the margin of the right false ribs. In fifteen days afterwards a small swelling below the margin of the ribs was noticed. It had gradually increased, and the opening with discharge of three ounces of pus took place the night before admission. He had suffered from frequent accessions of fever, commencing with chills, but not from bowel affection. The opening was enlarged with a bistoury, and two pints of brick-red pus discharged. The discharge continued profuse till the 20th, then gradually lessened, and the wound finally closed, and he was discharged well on the 4th March. Recovery was somewhat retarded by dysentery at the end of January and early part of February.

Remark.—This case occurred in my absence, when Dr. Forbes Watson had charge of the clinical ward.

153. *Hepatic abscess, punctured at the point of the right ninth rib.—Recovery.*—Nursingah, a Hindoo labourer, of thirty-five years of age, suffered three months and a half, before admission into the clinical ward, from daily accessions of fever, followed in fifteen days by pain of right hypochondrium, which had continued till the time of his admission, on the 15th September, 1851. He was in the habit of occasionally using spirits. On admission he was reduced in flesh. The respiration was somewhat hurried. There was some degree of fulness of the right hypochondrium, and dulness from the fifth rib to two inches below the margin of the right false ribs, where an

induration was perceptible, somewhat conical, and obscurely fluctuating at the point of the ninth rib. The pain was increased by decubitus on either side, and deep inspiration. There was not any cough. There was slight heat of skin, and the bowels were regular. The fluctuation having become more distinct, on the 20th September a puncture was made at the point of the ninth rib, with a straight bistoury; twenty ounces of healthy-looking pus were discharged, and a similar quantity on the evening of the same day; and again ten ounces on the 26th. From that time till the 19th February, 1852, there was daily slight reddish-tinged discharge. Then it ceased, the wound closed, and he was discharged well on the 15th March, when abnormal dulness below the ribs no longer existed. Treated with tonics, wine and support.*

154. *Hepatic abscess pointing between the right ninth rib and umbilicus, punctured.—Case not followed to the close, but in all probability successful.*—Fakeer Mahomed, a Mussulman Lascar, aged forty, addicted to the use of spirituous liquors, was admitted into the Jamsetjee Jejeebhoy Hospital on the 17th April. Below the margin of the right false ribs there was a distinctly circumscribed swelling, reaching from the cartilage of the seventh rib to within two inches of the umbilicus, and in a transverse direction from the ninth rib to the linea alba, painful on pressure and on full inspiration. He stated that the swelling had first appeared about two months before admission, and had gradually increased, during which time he had also been affected with irregular febrile accessions. The swelling became slowly more prominent; and on the 26th May, when fluctuation was distinct, an opening was made with a bistoury, and about six ounces of pus evacuated, and slight discharge continued for several successive days. On the 4th July another distinct fluctuating point, close to the former orifice was opened, and an ounce of pus discharged. Discharge from these orifices continued in quantity daily from a drachm or two to an ounce. About the 25th July the swelling again began to increase and to be painful; and on the 29th, while coughing, the orifice of the abscess, which had closed, again opened, and about seven ounces of pus were discharged. The tumour again subsided, and a slight daily discharge took place. During his residence in hospital he had frequently febrile accessions, and on two or three occasions dysenteric symptoms were present for several successive days. He had not lost in strength since his admission, and there was a fair prospect of recovery when this note was taken. There is no further record of the case.

155. *Hepatic abscess pointing at the epigastrium, punctured.—Result not known; probably successful.*—Shaik Mahomed, a Mussulman butler, about thirty years of age, of intemperate habits, was admitted into the Native General Hospital on the 4th March, 1845. There was a prominent pointed swelling towards the left side of the epigastrium, with considerable surrounding indurated swelling, said to have appeared twenty days before admission, but preceded for two months by fever. On the 24th the tumour was opened, and about eight or ten ounces of pus were discharged. He continued in hospital till the 6th May, with more or less discharge from the abscess, and frequent recurrences of fever. When he left the hospital the discharge had ceased, and the swelling was very much lessened, not painful, and the febrile accessions no longer recurred. He was readmitted into the hospital on the 2nd June with return of swelling of side and discharge from the opening. He remained in the hospital for five days, and then left it; and since then he has not been heard of. This case did not come under my observation till about the middle of April, about twenty days after the abscess had been opened.

* This patient was again in hospital in April 1857, with slight fever. He stated that after he left the hospital, in 1852, he returned to his native place in the Deccan, remained there well for three years, then came back to Bombay, and in good health followed his occupation of labourer till eight days before his second admission, when he became affected with slight fever and jaundice, but no hepatic pain or dulness. The cicatrix from the puncture was distinct at the point of the ninth rib.

156. *Chronic hepatic abscesses: one was punctured and healed, but there was no adhesion to the abdominal wall at site of puncture found after death.—Ulceration of colon, but dysentery clearly secondary.—Second abscess, and death.*—Essoo Govinda, a Hindoo labourer of sixty years of age, of emaciated frame, and using spirits freely, was admitted into the clinical ward on the 9th December, 1848. An indurated painful swelling occupied the epigastric and umbilical regions. It was indistinctly circumscribed, but its lower part was plainly felt about three inches below the margin of the right false ribs. There was no fever. He was treated with bitter infusions, mineral acids, taraxacum, iodine, and iron. The swelling was sponged with nitro-muriatic acid lotion, a small blister was applied, and latterly iodine ointment. He was discharged on the 24th January, 1849, with the swelling lessened, free of pain, but still quite distinct. He returned to his village and to his usual occupations. A year afterwards the swelling being, as he reported, in the same state as on his discharge from hospital, was opened with a lancet by a native hakeen, and a pint of pus discharged. It healed quickly. He was readmitted into the clinical ward on the 25th December, 1850. There was general fulness of abdomen, and a curved line from the ninth left to the tenth right rib marked the lower boundary of an indurated enlargement dull on percussion. There was a small puckered cicatrix caused by the puncture, about an inch below the point of the eighth right rib. He had been affected with dysentery for about six weeks. Under these he sank, and died on the 28th December, three days after admission.

Inspection seven hours after death.—Body emaciated. Abdomen somewhat full, but not tympanitic. *Abdomen.*—There were about five ounces of serous fluid in the sac of the peritoneum. Both the small and large intestines were contracted. The liver projected about three inches below the ensiform cartilage, and for some distance below the eighth and ninth costal cartilages of the left side, and the eighth, ninth and tenth ones of the right. Below the point of the tenth costal cartilage of the right side, on the convex surface of the liver near its free margin, corresponding in situation to the fundus of the gall-bladder, there was seen a small puckered cicatrix. There was no adhesion of this or of any other part of the convex surface of the projecting portion of the liver to the abdominal parietes, and the small puckered cicatrix observed on the surface of the latter did not correspond to that on the liver, but was an inch and a half above and internal to it. There were firm adhesions between the posterior part of the convex surface of the right lobe of the liver and the under surface of the diaphragm, also between the concave one and the upper extremity of the right kidney and the hepatic flexure of the colon. On incising the liver in the situation of the cicatrix, a white and fibrous appearance four lines in extent was seen. At the place of adhesion of the right kidney, with the under surface of the right lobe, and in the substance of the latter, there was an abscess of the size of a large orange, extending half way up the lobe, and containing healthy pus. It was bounded by a membranous sac, the inner surface of which was free from floating flocculi. The whole of the right lobe, and especially that part of it surrounding the abscess, was red and mottled. The left lobe was pale, and of natural size. No communication was found between the hepatic flexure of the colon and the cavity of the abscess, or between the latter and the right kidney. The mucous membrane of the ascending transverse, and a part of the descending colon, was of a dark grey colour generally, with small circular ulcers here and there. The walls of the small intestine were thin and pale, and the mucous membrane extensively corrugated, but nowhere was any ulceration seen. The right kidney, when incised, presented a healthy appearance, and there was no purulent cavity or infiltration at its upper end. *Chest.*—There were firm adhesions of both lungs to the costal pleuræ, and of the base of the right one to the convex surface of the diaphragm. The structure of both was spongy and crepitating, of white colour and intermixed with numerous dark specks. About two ounces of serous fluid in the pericardium. Heart of natural size, but with a somewhat greater quantity of fat than usual over its surface. Head not examined.*

Of the sixteen fatal cases, there was, in thirteen, gangrene of the structures around the puncture, more extensive generally in the tissues subjacent, than in the skin itself, thus showing that the progress of the gangrene had been from within outwards. Of these thirteen cases fatal with gangrene, the opening had been made in an intercostal space in five, and below the last rib in one. In these six cases the abscess had been either in the thick part of the right lobe, or there had been a sac between the liver and diaphragm†, or both combined. In the remaining seven cases the opening had been made at or near the epigastric region; and on comparing these with the successful ones punctured at the same situation, it appears that in those fatal with gangrene the abscess was large, or not single, or pointed rather at the concave than the convex surface of the liver, so that some thickness of parenchyma had to be cut through before the sac could be reached: or the constitution was very cachectic.

The thirteen following cases are those in which gangrene took place:—

157. *Abscess in the liver pointing between the right seventh and eighth ribs.—Opening into the lung and also externally.—Gangrene of the integuments around the orifice, also of the intercostal muscles, and caries of a rib.*—William Harris, aged twenty-three, was in hospital in September 1841, with hepatitis. Discharged on the 17th, re-admitted on the 10th October, with return. The disease ran into abscess, and about the 28th there was expectoration of brick-red sputa, which continued. There was tumefaction between the right seventh and eighth ribs with fluctuation, and an opening was made there on the 15th December. Brick-red puriform discharge and air passed from the wound. He gradually lost ground and died on the 1st February.

Inspection six hours after death.—The orifice between the seventh and eighth ribs not far from their junction with the cartilage was enlarged from sphacelus. The parts underneath the integument were in a state of gangrene, and for about the extent of two inches between the seventh and eighth ribs the intercostal muscles had been destroyed. The seventh rib, for about two inches in length, was carious, and in consequence was fractured near its junction to the cartilage. The abscess in the liver was very superficial, bounded by the convex part of the right lobe, the diaphragm and the ribs. The base of the third lobe of the right lung adhered to the diaphragm; part of it was condensed and at its anterior point there was communication with the abscess in the liver, and an excavation in the substance of the lung the size of a walnut. There were old adhesions of the surface of the liver; also of the

* We may not doubt the fact of abscess having been opened in this case and cured. The question arises, Was there absence of adhesion when the abscess was opened, or may we suppose that, consequent on the cure of the abscess, adhesions previously existing, but now no longer required, were gradually removed by atrophy? The latter is, I think, the probable view, and it is countenanced by the want of correspondence found after death between the external and the internal cicatrices.

† Case 122 may be added to these.

omentum to the abdominal parietes. *Chest.*—No effusion into the sac of the pleura and the greater part of both lungs were collapsed and crepitating.

158. *Hepatic abscess punctured over the last right false rib.—Gangrene and sloughing around the wound.—Death.—No inspection.*—Mr. ———, apothecary on the Bombay establishment, aged about thirty-four; after an attack of fever, suffered from acute hepatitis early in June 1843. He was freely depleted, and the constitutional effect of mercury was induced. There was a recurrence of the attack, and he was again similarly treated; but fulness of the right side, with pain, continued, and he had become much reduced. In this state he was sent from Surat to Bombay, and came under my care in the European General Hospital, on the 22nd August. He complained of constant pain of the right side, and there was circumscribed tumefaction over the last false rib. On the 30th August there was an opening made in the swelling and a considerable quantity of pus, at times tinged with blood, was discharged. On the 14th September commencing sphacelation of the soft parts around the orifice of the abscess was first remarked, and on the 16th the sphacelated portion was in diameter about an inch and a half, the orifice being in the centre. He died on the 19th September. There was not any examination of the body made after death.

159. *Large hepatic abscess punctured. — Death from exhaustion, with sloughing of the wound. — No examination after death.*—Shaik Mahomed, a Mussulman, of twenty-one years of age, not addicted to the use of spirits, a native of Bengal, and following for a period of six years the occupation of stoker in a steam-boat, about a year before his admission on the 13th March, 1850, into the clinical ward, had suffered from quartan fever, when he relinquished his usual employment. Twenty-five days before admission he had been attacked with sudden sharp pain of the right side of the abdomen, followed by fever. On admission the respiration was short, hurried, and chiefly thoracic and the decubitus was dorsal. There was occasional troublesome dry cough, and much pain of the right hypochondrium, aggravated by pressure, coughing, and any movement of the body. There was general fulness and prominence of the right hypochondrium, with tenseness and sense of induration below the margin of the right false ribs. Dulness reached from the right nipple to midway between the last false rib and the crest of the ilium, and extended obliquely across the abdomen to the point of the left ninth rib. Fluctuation was perceptible opposite the point of the last right rib. The impulse of the heart was increased and its apex beat in the intercostal space between the fourth and fifth rib directly below the left nipple. There was heat of skin, and a pulse frequent and compressible. The bowels were reported to be regular and the urine scanty and high coloured. The fluctuation was more distinct on the 2nd October, and an opening was made with a straight bistoury between the eleventh and twelfth rib. He died exhausted on the 24th. The edges of the wound showed a sloughy appearance after the 16th. After the operation, the tenseness and pain were lessened, the respiration became freer, and the cough less; but there were evening febrile accessions, with night sweats, more or less relaxation of the bowels, increasing emaciation and failing pulse. The discharge of seventy-two ounces of pus, sometimes tinged red, is recorded, but subsequent to the last quantity noted, there was a constant draining from the wound. The treatment consisted of anodynes, mineral acids, astringents, and support with milk, chicken-broth, eggs, and wine. Examination of the body after death was not permitted.

160. *Superficial abscess of right extremity of the liver leading to circumscribed sac between the organ and lateral abdominal walls.—Punctured between the tenth and eleventh rib.—Sloughy state of wound, necrosis of rib, and death from hectic fever.*—Mahangoo, thirty years of age, a Hindoo washerman, using spirits, was, after two months' illness, admitted in a reduced state into the clinical ward, on the 24th June, 1850. The respiration was slightly hurried. In the right hypochondrium there was a hard circumscribed painful swelling, covered by the six lower ribs, which bulged outwards over it.

The abdomen was generally soft and retracted; but an indurated edge was felt for about an inch below the ninth, tenth, and eleventh right ribs. He was anæmic and without febrile disturbance, or enteric irritation. Stated that the pain of side, first felt two months before when engaged in his occupation, had gradually increased, and that the swelling first attracted his attention seven days before admission. There had been no fever. Febrile accessions, however, were noted while he was under observation. On the 29th the upper part of the swelling was distinctly fluctuating, and it was opened with a bistoury on the 3rd July. Exhausted with hectic, and continued red-tinged discharge, but without diarrhœa, he died on the 11th August. The wound was puffy on the 23rd July, and sloughy on the 4th August. The urine gave no signs of albumen. The treatment consisted of anodynes, quinine, and sulphuric acid, and support.

Inspection ten hours after death. — Immediately below the end of the tenth rib was an opening of about the size of a dollar. The surrounding parts were dark, sloughy, and bounded by a dark blue line, about four inches in circumference; and, on looking into the opening, the eleventh rib was observed hanging bare at the bottom of it. *Chest.* — The left lung was collapsed, and its structure soft and crepitating. Numerous firm adhesions existed between the right lung and the costal parietes, partially also to the diaphragm: its substance was healthy. There was about an ounce and a half of clear watery fluid in the sac of the pericardium. On the posterior surface of the right ventricle of the heart there was a white patch the size of half a rupee. *Abdomen.* — There was an oval cavity of about the size of a large orange, apparently bounded internally by the omentum, externally, by the diaphragm, corresponding to the last four lower ribs, and the lateral abdominal parietes for about three inches below the margin of the right false ribs. Superiorly, the cavity was found to communicate freely and to be continuous with a large excavation about one inch and a half in depth, and eight in circumference, situated at the right extremity of the liver. This excavation was defined by a dark bluish line. The liver extended from the eleventh rib on the right side to the middle of the seventh, left. On cutting deeper into the substance of the liver, near to the abscess, two or three spots of yellowish-white colour, apparently from effusion of lymph, were observed. The other portions of the liver were healthy. That part of the wall of the abscess in which the substance of the liver was not involved, was much thickened, and on cutting into it, soft pulpy matter was found to ooze out on pressure. There were adhesions between the convex surface of the liver and the diaphragm, as well as between the concave surface and the pylorus. The stomach was contracted, and its coats were somewhat thickened. The transverse colon was much distended. The kidneys healthy.

161. *Abscess in the liver punctured.—Carious ribs projecting into the abscess.— At first superficial and leading to circumscribed sac between liver and diaphragm. — Also empyema of right pleural sac without communication.*—Cumblin Rowjee, aged twenty, a Maratha labourer, emaciated; after two months' illness, was admitted 5th May, 1852. Pulse small, breathing short and hurried. A distinct prominent, uncircumscribed, fluctuating swelling, neither tense, red, nor hot, existed on the right side of the chest from the sixth rib downwards. In the epigastric region there was abnormal dulness, and an indurated edge was felt to within an inch of the umbilicus, and extending from the tenth or eleventh right to the ninth left false rib. There was slight cough, not communicating impulse to the swelling. The feet and legs became œdematous. Dyspnœa increased. The swelling became more prominent and pointing. It was punctured on the 13th May between the eighth and ninth rib, and four pints of brick-coloured pus were discharged. On the 16th commencing gangrene around the opening was observed. A slough larger than a rupee formed. He died on the 22nd.

Inspection twenty hours after death. — *Chest.* — There were fifty ounces of sero-purulent fluid in the right pleural sac; flakes of lymph coated the costal pleura, and the lung was condensed from compression. There was no communication between the chest and abdomen. The left lung and heart were healthy. *Abdomen.* — The liver descended lower than natural. Firm adhesions connected its upper surface for a considerable extent, and there was a sloughy state of the tissues of the parietes corresponding to these adhesions, and to the opening by which the contents of the abscess had been discharged. The eighth and ninth ribs had separated by caries at their cartilaginous junctions, and having started inwards projected into the cavity of an abscess in the liver. The cartilages of these ribs were found in their normal position. A similar process had commenced at the cartilaginous junction of the tenth rib, but separation had not taken place. The surface of the liver in this situation for the diameter of five inches, adherent by lymph at its margin, was somewhat depressed below the level of the healthy portion, had flakes of lymph attached to it, and felt rough and fibrous to the touch: in its centre was the opening of the abscess, which was about the size of a large hen's egg. The opening corresponded to the space between the eighth and ninth ribs, through which the abscess had pointed. A considerable extent of the surrounding tissue of the liver was dense and fibrous. There was commencing Bright's disease of both kidneys.

162. *Two large hepatic abscesses. — One deep, the other a sac between the surface of the liver and abdominal walls originating probably in rupture of a small superficial abscess, there being lymph nodules in the part of the liver adjoining. — This abscess punctured. — Sloughing.—No ulceration of intestine.*—Housayree, a Hindoo washerman, of forty-five years of age, using spirituous liquors, was in a much reduced state, admitted into the clinical ward on the 13th February, 1851. The respiration was somewhat short and hurried. There was dulness on percussion of the chest, below the nipple on the right side; and crepitus was detected in the right mammary region, and in both dorsal and lateral regions. Occupying the right of the abdomen there was a large, oblong, tense, painful, distinctly fluctuating swelling; it reached from the margin of the right ribs to the crest of the os ilium. A vertical line, an inch to the right of the umbilicus, formed its internal limit, and one three inches behind the posterior spinous process of the os ilium, its external and posterior one. The skin covering the swelling was red, tense, shining, and pitted on pressure. The rest of the abdomen was slightly full and soft. The feet were œdematous. He suffered from cough, and the bowels were confined. The pulse was frequent and small. His illness was of six weeks' duration, and commenced with fever, remittent in type, and attended with cough. Twelve days before admission a small swelling was noticed under the margin of the right ribs, which gradually increased, but it had not been preceded by pain. On the 17th an opening was made into the abscess in front of the point of the right last rib. The discharge was profuse, followed by relief and diminution of febrile disturbance. On the 18th indication of gangrene at the puncture commenced, and slowly extended to a diameter of two inches. He sunk without diarrhœa, and died on the 23rd.

Inspection twenty-nine hours after death.—*Chest.*—The right lung did not collapse freely. The base was firmly adherent to the diaphragm. Its texture was somewhat firmer, and it did not crepitate freely, but there was no hepatisation in any part. No effusion into the sac of the right pleura. Left lung freely collapsed and crepitating. A few old adhesions existed between the lung and the costal pleura at the anterior and middle parts. No effusion into the sac of the pleura. *Abdomen.*—At the situation of the opening made with the bistoury, the liver was adherent to the walls of abdomen by very thick layers of lymph, softened by admixture with pus. Here the collection of matter seemed chiefly to have been between the walls of the abdomen and the surface of the liver. In this situation the substance of the organ seemed compressed, but in places superficial lymph-nodules were observed. A considerable part of the right lobe of the liver had contracted tender adhesions with the walls of the abdomen and the diaphragm. In the upper part of the right lobe there was a large abscess the size of an ostrich egg approaching to, but quite unconnected with, the abscess that was opened. The rest of the liver was healthy. Flakes of lymph were effused on different parts of the small intestine, and in places formed a thin membranous layer. The large intestine, as well as the lower part of the ileum, were laid open. The mucous membrane not ulcerated, was healthy but pale. Kidneys healthy.

163. *Hepatic abscess punctured at the epigastrium.— Gangrene and sphacelation around the orifice. — Death. — No inspection.* — Rustum Rasid, a Persian Parsee, aged fifty, after twenty days' illness, was admitted into the Jamsetjee Jejeebhoy Hospital, on the 16th July, 1845. He complained chiefly of dyspeptic symptoms, and his disease was looked upon as dyspepsia. On the 31st he was affected with febrile symptoms, and there was a good deal of tenderness at the left side of the epigastric region, and a slight degree of induration was perceived there, which at first was believed to depend on enlargement of the spleen, but with its increase and extension in the direction of the mesial line, it became evident that it was connected with the left lobe of the liver. Febrile accessions recurred from time to time; leeches and counter-irritants were used, and an attempt was made to induce the constitutional effect of mercury by the cautious exhibition of calomel and opium, but without success. On the 31st August fluctuation became perceptible in the tumour at the epigastrium. On the 2nd September it was still more distinct, and an opening was made. Several ounces of thick pus were evacuated; and on the succeeding days there was daily a slight discharge. On the 4th there was considerable tenderness around the opening, and he complained much of the pain of the swelling on the 7th. On the 9th, for an inch round the orifice, the integument had become discoloured, and the epidermis was separating. On the 10th the sphacelus was complete. On the 18th the line of demarcation was distinct, and the sphacelated portion was about three inches in diameter. There was daily hectic fever, and increasing exhaustion, and he died on the 25th. The sphacelated portion had not separated. No examination of the body after death permitted.

164. *Hepatic abscess pointing at the epigastrium, punctured.—Extensive sphacelus around the opening.—Death.*—Geenah Ambah, forty years of age, a Hindoo, was admitted into the Bandora Dispensary, near Bombay, on the 4th May, 1852. There was a prominent distinctly fluctuating and tense swelling between the margin of the right ribs, the ensiform cartilage, and an inch and a half above the umbilicus. He had been attacked with pain in that situation, and fever three months before. The abscess was opened by Mr. Gomez, the officer in charge of the dispensary, and two and a half pints of pus were discharged. He continued under treatment till the 14th July, when he had improved in flesh, and the discharge was very slight. He was now lost sight of, and again appeared at the Jamsetjee Jejeebhoy Hospital on the 18th August. There was some fulness below the ensiform cartilage, the skin was of dusky-red colour, and there was an ulcerated opening. No fever. The ulceration extended, and became sloughy and excavated. He became emaciated, affected with diarrhœa, and died on the 25th September.

Inspection (by Mr. Carvalho) *eighteen hours after death.*—Body emaciated. Occupying the epigastric region, and extending over a space about twelve or thirteen inches in circumference, there was a sloughy gangrenous surface; at the central part of which there was an opening the size of a rupee. The sloughing was superficial, and did not affect the muscular tissue. On cutting through the abdominal walls, and reflecting the flap of the skin, the cavity of an abscess was exposed immediately below the ensiform cartilage. It lay just to the left of the suspensory ligament, and was about the size of half an orange. Superiorly it corresponded to the central tendinous portion of the diaphragm to which it was firmly adherent; and anteriorly was in the greater part covered by, and adherent to, the lower part of the sternum which there constituted a portion of its anterior wall. The surface exposed was of a dark blue colour—gangrenous. The depth of the abscess was about a quarter of an inch, and the surrounding walls were hard, almost cartilaginous. The lobe (left) in which the abscess had been situated, was much reduced in size; its structure was a good deal indurated, and when incised it was found to be of a reddish-colour around the abscess. The liver was smaller than natural, rather hard in texture, firmly adherent by its right lobe to the diaphragm and abdominal wall; and the adjacent portion of the colon was firmly united to its concave or under surface. There was only one abscess. The gall-bladder was contracted. The kidneys were healthy. The intestines were not examined. *Chest.*—There were old adhesions, chiefly of the right lung to the costal pleura and diaphragm. The posterior part of both lungs, and the second and third lobes of the right, were redder than natural, somewhat indurated, and gave out frothy serum when incised. The heart was healthy.

165. *A single abscess at the thin edge of the left lobe of liver existing for five months, punctured.—Gangrene of the orifice.—Dysenteric symptoms latterly.—Ulceration of mucous membrane of the colon.*—Antonio Francis, a native Christian, a sailor, of thirty-four years of age, was under treatment in hospital for a swelling in the epigastric region from the 17th May to the 15th June, 1849, when he was discharged relieved of pain, but with persistence of the swelling. He was readmitted on the 5th October, in reduced condition. The respiration was chiefly thoracic, but there were not any signs of pulmonary disease. The abdomen for the most part was soft, but immediately above the umbilicus, and ascending to midway between it and the ensiform cartilage, there was a circumscribed prominent swelling tender to the touch without fluctuation, slightly pulsating, but without murmur under the stethoscope on any part of its surface, and with clear sound on percussion between it and the margin of the right ribs. The bowels were regular. He suffered from evening febrile accessions. The swelling became more prominent, and fluctuation was distinct on the 16th, when the abscess was opened, and seven ounces of pinkish-coloured pus were discharged. The febrile accessions recurred, dysenteric symptoms set in on the 26th, and he died on the 18th November.

Inspection three hours after death.—Abdomen.—The opening made into the abscess was on a level with the ninth rib, and a probe passed readily through it into the sac. On removing the skin over it, there was found a sloughy state of the parts around the opening for about an inch and a half in diameter. The peritoneum was chiefly adherent to the abdominal wall over the abscess sac, which was about the size of a small orange, and occupied the very edge of the left lobe of the liver. It was empty. The serous covering of the left lobe of the liver had in general an opaque appearance. The liver was not enlarged. The small intestines were much distended with gaseous contents, and a portion of them was displaced upwards. They presented externally, in part a dark red, and in part a dark leaden grey colour; but no patches of lymph were observed. The transverse colon contained dark grey adhesive matter, and adhered closely to the sac; but there was no communication between them. Its mucous surface was of dark red colour—presented a rugous appearance, with several variously sized circular ulcers, some apparently cicatrised, and others in an active state of ulceration. No further examination was permitted.

166. *Two hepatic abscesses: one punctured, with increase of febrile symptoms: attributed to fist blows.—Habits temperate.—Diarrhœa, with redness of mucous membrane of colon.—No ulceration.—Commencing gangrene at the opening in the abscess.*—Dooluh Dewsell, a Hindoo carpenter, twenty-seven years of age, in good condition, and reporting himself to be of temperate habits, was admitted, after twelve days' illness, into the clinical ward of the Jamsetjee Jejeebhoy Hospital on the 13th July, 1849. The respiration was short, hurried, chiefly thoracic, and bronchitic rales were audible in different parts of the chest. The abdomen was full, somewhat tense, and tender on pressure—chiefly so, however, at the upper part, where an indurated fulness was perceptible, extending below the right false ribs, occupying the epigastrium and part of the left hypochondrium, and reaching almost to the umbilicus. It was some-

what prominent in the epigastric region. The decubitus was chiefly dorsal. During the first six days of his illness the symptoms had not attracted his attention much, but then they increased in severity, and were attended with febrile disturbance. They were attributed to fist blows, received in endeavouring to separate two individuals who were fighting. He was under observation thirteen days. The hepatic symptoms persisted; the fever had marked evening exacerbations. There was occasional vomiting and relaxed bowels. The prominence at the epigastrium increased, and fluctuation was indistinct on the 18th. He died on the 25th. After leeching and a ten-grain dose of calomel, with opium, four-grain doses of quinine were given, with blue pill, at intervals during the remissions, and with the effect of lessening the exacerbation. On the 23rd the abscess was opened with a bistoury. There was a good deal of bleeding from the wound at the time, and free discharge on that day, and on the 25th; but there was increase of fever and diarrhœa, a failing pulse, and collapse of features. The result was clearly hastened by the operation.

Inspection fourteen hours after death.—The costal cartilages and cellular tissue were slightly tinged yellow. *Chest.*—Lungs collapsed and crepitating. The third lobe of the right lung was compressed almost flat against the posterior wall of chest. Heart natural. *Abdomen.*—Between the skin and subjacent structures around the opening in the abscess, there was a boggy state of the tissue, caused by infiltration of dark red serum. Stomach and intestines distended with gas. The liver extended considerably beyond the margin of ribs, and for a space about four or five inches in diameter, adhered firmly to the parietes. The omentum was also matted there. The thin edge and a portion of the inferior surface of the left lobe of the liver had adhered firmly to the anterior surface of the stomach. The abscess, the size of a cocoa-nut, occupied a great portion of the left side of the right lobe, and to a considerable extent the substance of the left. It contained about half a pint of thick flocculent pus, and some white firm bands were seen crossing it. Its walls presented a rough and irregular appearance. The anterior part, the thinnest, was separated from the abdominal parietes by a portion of liver about a quarter of an inch thick. A thin small portion of its upper wall intervened between the abscess and the diaphragm, but was free from adhesions to that muscle. On separating the liver from the stomach, the surface of the latter was found adherent to the wall of another abscess, the size of a large orange. Its walls were entire, with the internal surface irregular: it was filled with sero-puriform matter. The two abscesses were separated from one another by a thin portion of the substance of the liver. The large intestine was laid open, the mucous surface was discoloured red, but no ulceration was detected anywhere. Kidneys healthy.

167. *Hepatic abscess pointing at the epigastrium, punctured.—Sloughing around the wound.—Death.*—Early in the year 1854, I saw, in company with Dr. Miller, of Bombay, a case of hepatitis in a European artificer. The symptoms were well marked; abscess formed. The tumefaction was chiefly in the epigastrium. Fluctuation became distinct, and after tendency to pointing had become apparent, the abscess was opened with a bistoury, and considerable discharge of pus followed and continued for the two or three succeeding days. Then a sloughy state of the edges of the puncture took place and extended, and the patient died. These notes I write from recollection, as I have no written memoranda of the case. I do not know whether the body was examined after death.

168. *Cirrhosis of Liver.—Abscess in thin edge of liver, punctured.—Purulent sac between liver and diaphragm.—Ulceration of large intestine.—Death.*—Lingoo, a Hindoo labourer, of thirty-six years of age, addicted to the habitual use of spirits, was admitted on the 2nd July, 1852, into the clinical ward. He was a good deal emaciated, and the respiration was somewhat thoracic. Close to the ensiform cartilage, and extending about half an inch to the right of the mesial line, there was a swelling,

the size of a large orange, somewhat conical, with its apex slightly reddened and fluctuating. It varied somewhat in position, according as decubitus was on the right or left side, and became somewhat depending and more prominent in the sitting and standing positions. It was free of pulsation. There was no dulness on percussion around it, except at its upper and right side, where the dulness was continuous with that of the liver. It was tender on pressure. No cough or vomiting. Decubitus easiest on the right side. Bowels relaxed. He had first observed the swelling three months before, when it was the size of an egg. Suffered from dysenteric symptoms about six weeks before admission, and from irregular febrile accessions for fifteen days. Pulse feeble, tongue coated in the centre, and florid at the tip and edges. The abscess was opened on the 27th, and eight ounces of thick pus were discharged. With continuing discharge, relaxed bowels, nightly hectic fever, and sloughy ulcerated state of the punctured wound, he gradually lost ground, and died on the 7th August. He was treated with quinine, opium, nourishment, and wine.

Inspection twenty-one hours after death.—Body much emaciated. *Chest.*—The lungs were collapsed, and in appearance perfectly healthy. The lower part of the base of the right lung was found attached to the corresponding portion of the diaphragm by firm adhesions. There was, however, no condensation of the lung. The heart was healthy. *Abdomen.*—The intestines presented, externally, a healthy appearance. The mucous membrane of the descending colon, sigmoid flexure, and a part of the rectum, was somewhat thickened, and numerous small circular ulcers existed here and there. The liver did not extend below the margins of the ribs. It was much smaller than natural, dense and contracted. Its surface was corrugated, and studded with small yellow projections, each about the size of a pin's head. It was firmly adherent to the abdominal parietes, a little below and internal to the margin of the cartilage of the left tenth rib, corresponding to the external opening in the skin. The exposed part of the right lobe was likewise adherent to the adjoining parietes; and at the lower margin, a little above the gall-bladder, the surrounding adhesions formed a small sac, containing a small quantity of serum. The diaphragm was firmly attached to the upper surface; and to the right, about opposite the middle of the seventh rib, it was separated from the liver by a sac, the size of an orange, containing a quantity of glairy, tenacious pus. At the parts corresponding to the puncture, two small abscesses, each about the size of a small filbert, separated from each other by a thin septum, were found; their walls were dense and fibrous. A section of the liver presented a surface studded with minute granules. The lower part of the liver, the pancreas, and duodenum, were adherent together by dense fibrous tissue. The gall-bladder was filled with light-coloured greenish fluid. The kidneys were healthy. The spleen was a little smaller than natural.

169.—*Hepatic abscess in epigastric region, punctured; very little discharge.—Dysentery.—Death.—No examination.*—Raga Saiboo, a Hindoo bricklayer of twenty-five years of age, using spirits occasionally, was admitted in an emaciated state into the clinical ward on the 1st October, 1852. At the epigastric region, in the middle line between the ensiform cartilage and the umbilicus, there was a prominent fluctuating swelling about the size of a large orange, painful on pressure, dull on percussion, and immovable. Respiration hurried and chiefly thoracic, pulse small, bowels relaxed. Six weeks before, while at work, was seized with shivering, followed by fever and pain at the site of the swelling, which when first noticed was small; it gradually increased. The actual cautery was applied ten days before admission, and had left an eschar about the size of half a rupee. The dysenteric symptoms were of fifteen days' duration. The swelling was opened with a bistoury to the left of the eschar, but only blood was discharged, and on the 4th about an ounce of unhealthy pus. The swelling did not lessen much, the discharge was slight, the eschar separated, and was followed by sloughy ulceration, which extended to the puncture. The diarrhœa continued. He was removed on the 13th October in a moribund state by his friends. He was treated with quinine, opium, and wine.

In the three cases, fatal without gangrene, the abscess had been large and punctured at the margin of the right ribs. In two there was complication of pleuritic effusion, and in one several abscesses, with general peritonitis. These cases are now submitted. (170 to 172.)

170. *Abscess partly of right and of left lobe, punctured.—Death from secondary dysentery.—Ulceration of large intestine.—Effusion in both pleural sacs.*—Luximan Luckman, aged thirty-five, a Hindoo labourer, using spirits habitually, but in moderate quantity, was admitted into the clinical ward on the 19th December, 1853. He was emaciated, and the respiration was somewhat short and hurried, and chiefly thoracic. The pulse was small and frequent, the bowels regular. Between a curved line drawn from the eighth left rib,—passing quarter of an inch above the umbilicus to the ninth right rib,—and the margin of the right ribs, there was induration with constant pain, increased by pressure and cough. The space noted was also dull on percussion, and the dulness extended upwards to the fifth rib. Decubitus was easiest on the left side. The tongue was moist, and somewhat coated in the centre. Fifteen days before admission he had felt pain of the right hypochondrium, followed by febrile symptoms, characterised by evening accessions, commencing with chills, and terminating with slight sweating. Slight swelling first appeared seven days after the commencement of the attack. On the 28th the swelling became more prominent and indistinctly fluctuating; and on the 30th, the fluctuation being distinct, a puncture was made with a bistoury, and seven ounces of red-tinged serous fluid with floating lymph-flakes were evacuated. He was at this time also troubled with hiccup. From this date the discharge continued, gradually, however, lessening with subsidence of the swelling, and no appearance of sloughing of the puncture. On the 12th January dysenteric symptoms began, and continued more or less till his death on the 20th February. The urine gave no traces of albumen. He was treated with tonics, opiates, gallic acid, suitable nourishment, and wine.

Inspection eight hours after death.—External appearances:—Body very much emaciated and free from rigor mortis. A little to the right side of the median line, and about an inch below the ensiform cartilage, there was a small opening, through which thin yellowish discharge oozed. *Chest.*—Neither lung was collapsed. There were about ten ounces of turbid serum in the right pleural sac, and about six ounces in the left. There were firm adhesions at the upper and back parts of the right lung; also some tender ones at the lower part anteriorly. There were no adhesions between the base of this lung and the diaphragm; nor any between the left lung and the parietes of the chest. The external surface of the whole of the right lung, and the anterior surface of the left lung were pale, dry-looking, and woolly to the feel. The anterior parts of both lungs were emphysematous, but the posterior parts were healthy and crepitating. On incising both lungs in different parts, frothy serum oozed out from some portions, but nothing further abnormal was detected. There were about three ounces of clear serum in the sac of the pericardium. The heart was smaller than natural, but healthy. *Abdomen.*—No traces of general peritonitis present. The liver was somewhat larger than natural; it reached an inch below the margin of the right false ribs, and above as high as the fifth rib. The thin margin of the liver, with a portion of the anterior surface, formed firm adhesions with the anterior parietes of the abdomen to the extent of about three inches in diameter. These adhesions were around the puncture. The convex surface of the right lobe of the liver was adherent to the diaphragm in parts, and the concave surface was firmly adherent to the transverse colon, part of the duodenum, and the pyloric end of the stomach. On enlarging the artificial opening, the abscess was found to occupy part of the left, and part of the right lobe of the liver, and was the size of a common orange. Its contents consisted of thin, puriform, orange-coloured matter. On removing the contents, the walls of the abscess were found to be hard and somewhat cartilaginous. At the lower part of the abscess the substance of the liver was of darkish red colour; but the remaining portions of the organ were healthy. The intestines were grey-coloured externally. The transverse colon and the duodenum adhered to the concave surface of the liver; but there was no communication between the abscess and either of these hollow viscera. There was some degree of vascularity of the mucous membrane of the rectum, and of the transverse and descending colon, and there were about ten or fifteen circular ulcers in the rectum, each the size of a large pin's head. The mucous membrane of the ileum and jejunum was also slightly vascular here and there; but no ulcer was anywhere detected. The left kidney was somewhat larger than the right, and its cortical portion encroached slightly on the tubular portion. The right kidney seemed to be healthy.—The spleen was of natural size and healthy.

171. *Pleuritic effusion.—Abscess in the liver punctured.—Attributed to a blow.—Death the day after the abscess was opened. No examination.*—Wittoo Bappoo, a Hindoo cart-driver of thirty-two years of age, was under treatment from the 21st December, 1851, to the 14th January, 1852, when he was transferred to the clinical ward. The symptoms had indicated the presence of pneumonia and hepatitis, for which he had been cupped, taken antimony, and been brought under the influence of mercury with temporary advantage. From the 4th January, however, there had been more complaint of cough and pain of different parts of the right side of the chest, followed by complete dulness on percussion of that side, and absence of vocal thrill; and such continued to be the state of the chest on admission into the clinical ward, when, also, the circumference of the right side was found to be half an inch greater than that of the left. There were fulness, sense of induration and dulness below the margin of the right false ribs, bounded by a line curving from the point of the right tenth rib to that of the left eighth. There was occasional cough, and decubitus was easiest on the right side. There was some degree of febrile heat, and the gums were still tender from the mercury. The swelling below the right ribs became gradually more prominent; and on the 27th January there was another oval swelling detected above the umbilicus. On the 6th February there was fluctuation of both swellings. On the 7th the one below the right ribs was opened at the point of the eighth rib, and twelve ounces of pus discharged, with diminution of both swellings. He died on the 8th. The urine had been frequently examined, but gave no traces of albumen. He attributed his illness to a blow on the right hypochondrium from the cross-beam of a bullock-cart. Examination of the body not permitted.

172. *Large abscess of right lobe of liver opened with trocar.—Several abscesses in left lobe in different stages.—Also nodules of lymph.*—Emam Bukus, aged about forty, was admitted into the Native General Hospital on the 13th January, 1845. He suffered from febrile symptoms, and pain of the right hypochondrium of six days' duration. By means of leeches, a blister, and mercurials, not, however, carried to the extent of affecting the system, the pain of the side was much relieved, but an evening febrile accession persisted. On the 27th his breathing became short, the countenance anxious, and there was slight fulness of the right hypochondrium apparent. On the 1st February the fulness of the side was distinct and somewhat prominent, and sense of fluctuation was perceptible. The abscess was opened by a trocar below the edge of the false ribs, and twelve ounces of thick pus were discharged; and on the 3rd and 4th there was a further discharge of several ounces of pus following re-introduction of the canula, which had been removed. After the operation there was increased anxiety of countenance; the breathing became shorter and more oppressed; the febrile accessions continued to recur, and he died on the evening of the 5th. There were not at any time symptoms of dysentery or diarrhœa.

Inspection eight hours after death.—Abdomen.—In the cavity of the abdomen, amongst the convolutions of the intestines, there was about a pint of sero-puriform fluid. The peritoneal surface of the small intestine and of the colon presented a deep blush of redness; and thin flakes of friable lymph were effused generally on the surface, and caused adhesions of the convolutions. The liver adhered firmly to the abdominal parietes for some distance around the orifice made by the trocar, which had penetrated a large abscess occupying the lower and anterior lateral part of the right lobe. The inner surface of the sac was lined by thick sloughy-looking shreds. Between the diaphragm and the convex surface of the right lobe there was a circumscribed sac containing about half a pint of sero-puriform fluid, similar in appearance to that contained in the abdominal cavity. The abscess in the liver seemed to communicate with this sac; but no communication could be traced between it and the cavity of the abdomen. In the left lobe there were two or three small abscesses, ranging in size from a walnut to a goose's egg. One or two yellow circumscribed portions were also observed, caused by interstitial effusion of lymph—the condition which so generally precedes the formation of abscess.

My opinions on this question of practice have been formed chiefly on the facts now detailed, because observers who have hitherto written with authority on this subject have done so on still more limited experience. Annesley had witnessed only five cases of puncture of hepatic abscess; of these two recovered. Malcolmson five, all fatal. Stovell* five, with four deaths. Haspel seven, with four deaths. Again, in many of the scattered records of hepatic abscess, including cases in which puncture had been practised, the situation of the swelling and of the opening is not mentioned. Such cases are of no value in determining this practical question.

My cases show that when the abscess is not very large, is single†, situated in the thin part of the left lobe, or thin edge of the right, and is allowed to point at the epigastrium, or margin of the right ribs above the ninth, then puncture with a bistoury or lancet will very generally be attended with success. This result will be materially favoured by previous careful treatment and by the absence of dysentery or other complication.

The two successful cases quoted by Annesley were of this simple nature; and no doubt it was on them that this author grounded his just opinion, that hepatic abscess ought not to be punctured till distinct pointing and inflammatory blush on the skin have taken place. A successful case alluded to by Twining, two narrated by

* Dr. Stovell, in his subsequent decennial report, gives seven cases with six deaths.

† We may form a judgment as to the size of the abscess, and its being single or not, by careful percussion in all directions; and it is of much importance that this means of acquiring precise knowledge of the size of the liver be not neglected in such cases. By inattention to this rule prognosis becomes needlessly vague and uncertain.

Haspel, one by Stovell, and one by Arnott*, are also confirmatory of the inference drawn from my own successful cases. But I would go still further, and say there is nothing decisive on record to prove that success has as yet attended the puncture of hepatic abscess under any other circumstances than those which have just been stated.

This degree of success, however, does not assert much in favour of surgical interference; for it is most probable that in such cases a favourable termination would equally have resulted from non-interference and spontaneous rupture. Dr. Budd has advocated the latter course in such cases. The common surgical rule of puncturing when there is distinct pointing and inflammatory blush, seems to me the preferable course; but at best it is a difference of little moment in practice.

Gangrene of the tissues around the wound took place in 13 of my 16 fatal cases.

This event was first noticed by Mr. Cæsar Hawkins†, but he considered his cases to be malignant disease not hepatic abscess. Dr. Malcolmson, of the Madras Medical Service‡, corrected Mr. Hawkins's erroneous inference, and quoted two cases of hepatic abscess opened and followed by gangrene. This result of puncture of hepatic abscess, so familiar to myself and to others, and so important in reference to practice, is not even alluded to by any other writer with whose works I am acquainted.

Malcolmson attributed the gangrene to the lowered vitality of the thinned and diseased tissues, and recommended the early opening of the abscess as the best means of preventing it; but this explanation, and the practical inference from it, are only partially correct.

I have elsewhere (p. 328) fully described the usual process by which abscess is formed in the liver; and I have called attention to the fact, that when the abscess is large, some time must elapse before the shreddy flocculent debris of the structure of the organ, adherent to the inner surface of the sac, can liquefy and disappear. If an abscess in this state be opened and air admitted, then putrefaction of these devitalised tissues must be the consequence, and the weakened structures around becoming contaminated will readily pass into gangrene. It is in this manner that, in many instances, the liability to gangrene after puncture may be best explained. In

* "Transactions, Medical and Physical Society of Bombay," No. 1, New Series.

† "Transactions, Medico-Chirurgical Society," vol. xviii.

‡ *Ibid.*, vol. xxi., and "Edinburgh Medical and Surgical Journal," vol. li.

such cases the error has not been delay. On the contrary, the abscess has been prematurely opened in violation of a sound surgical principle which directs that the operation should be postponed till *concoction* is completed.

Yet, under some circumstances, there is truth in Malcolmson's opinion that the gangrene may be due to lowered vitality from thinning of the tissues, and defect of nutrition; and that in these the error of delaying the opening the abscess has generally been committed.

The cases which have been detailed seem to me to point to a practical rule in this apparent difficulty.

In the five cases in which the puncture was made in an intercostal space, the gangrene of the soft parts and the carious or necrosed state of the ribs, was caused by the combined influence of inflammatory action, and the increasing pressure of the pus over an extensive surface. If surgical interference under these circumstances is to be of any avail, then it must be had recourse to, early — so soon as bulging of the side and obscure fluctuation indicate the presence of fluid. And we may act in this manner with less apprehension of bad effects from putrefying tissues, because a reference to the cases will show that the pus is collected chiefly between the liver and the parietes, and that when it communicates, the abscess is generally superficial and not likely to have much flocculent debris adherent to its walls.

In seven of the cases fatal with gangrene, the opening had been made at the epigastrium or near the margin of the right ribs. From a consideration of these in connection with those fatal without puncture, it may be inferred that when the liver occupies the epigastrium, reaches to within an inch of the umbilicus, extends two inches and more below the margin of the right ribs, becomes gradually prominent in these situations, and in time gives a sense of diffuse fluctuation, we have to do with large abscess in the thick substance of the organ. This is the condition of hepatic abscess in which there is much likelihood of parenchymatous debris requiring *concoction*, and in which there is danger of gangrene and irritative fever consequent on putrefaction from premature puncture. In these cases we should delay, and this course may be followed with the less hesitation, for there is, in these circumstances, little risk of gangrene from mere thinning of the tissues.

But, I have expressed my belief that success has, hitherto, only attended the puncture of small, distinctly pointing abscesses, situated in the thin parts of the liver; and the question naturally suggests itself, whether the operation ought to be confined to these conditions, and altogether abandoned in the kind of cases which are at present under review. My past experience would prompt an affirmative reply; but we must not hastily conclude that the resources of our art are thus limited.

From the cases narrated it is evident, that when a free opening is made with a bistoury, or large trocar, the large abscess emptied, and air admitted, death is not thereby prevented, but, on the contrary, is frequently hastened. Therefore if good is to be effected by surgery in such cases, it must be by a different kind of operative proceeding. The modification in the operation of puncturing the chest in pleuritic effusions, advocated by Dr. H. M. Hughes and Mr. Edward Cock*, might be extended to the opening of large hepatic abscesses. The slow and gradual evacuation of the pus by repeated puncture at suitable intervals with a small trocar, combined with the careful exclusion of the atmospheric air, is worthy of trial. The objection that the thick part of the contents of the sac will not be evacuated by this method is not of much weight, for we may believe that it may remain as a residuum, and be subjected to those changes which take place in the cure by absorption.

The following, then, are my conclusions on the question of puncturing hepatic abscess.

1. When the swelling is not larger than an orange, and points conically at the epigastrium, or below the margin of the right ribs, we should wait till an inflammatory blush appears on the skin, and then open the abscess with a bistoury, sufficiently freely to admit of the ready discharge of the contents without pressure. The case should afterwards be treated in accordance with ordinary surgical principles. If the abscess has been single, and the constitution not very much impaired, success will frequently attend this proceeding.

2. When there is general bulging of the right ribs below the seventh, with distinct fluctuation and pointing at an intercostal space, it is immaterial whether a puncture be made or spontaneous rupture take place. In both circumstances there will be gangrene, from thinning, of the soft tissues, and probably caries or necrosis of one or more ribs.

3. When the liver occupies the epigastrium, reaches to within an inch of the umbilicus, extends two inches and more below the

* "Guy's Hospital Reports," Second Series, vol. ii. p. 48. Mr. Cock uses a trocar of one-twelfth of an inch in diameter.

margin of the right ribs, becomes gradually prominent in these situations, and after a time obscurely fluctuating, then premature puncture either freely with a bistoury or a large trocar, will lead to irritative fever and gangrene of the soft tissues around the opening from within outwards, due to the putrefaction, from admission of air, of the devitalised tissues adherent to the inner wall of the sac.

4. If there be general bulging of the right ribs below the seventh, fulness of the intercostal spaces, and obscure fluctuation, then puncture may be made with a small trocar, in the manner advocated by Mr. Cock in respect to pleuritic effusion. As delay in these circumstances is inexpedient, an exploring needle may be used in doubtful cases.

5. When prominent extensive swelling at the epigastrium, or below the right ribs, with diffuse sense of fluctuation, indicates the existence of large abscess in the thick part of the liver, we should allow sufficient time for maturation; and then, when fluctuation has become distinct, we may puncture with a small trocar, observing the same principles in respect to gradual evacuation, repetition of the operation, and careful exclusion of air. While, however, we lay down the rule of waiting a suitable time for the maturation of the abscess, we must take care not to delay so long as to give time for the formation of very dense unyielding walls,—an obstacle to success which has been justly pointed out by Dr. Budd.

The three first conclusions are based on clinical observation, but the fourth and fifth are suggestions grounded on sufficient experience of the failure of other procedures.

Further, it must always be remembered, that the probability of success, under all circumstances, will depend on the state of the constitution, and the *conservative* care with which the medical treatment has been conducted throughout, and the absence of dysentery or other serious complication.

We must, moreover, be careful that the object of surgical interference be justly appreciated, for there is a tendency in many minds, to over-estimate its value, and therefore to apply it unsuitably. In the small distinctly pointing abscess, it is of little consequence whether we puncture or trust to spontaneous rupture. In the large and deep abscess, we know that restoration cannot take place unless the contents of the abscess are discharged, and that spontaneous rupture is unlikely, till such destruction of parts and exhaustion by hectic fever have ensued as to render recovery impossible; therefore, when the local conditions are appropriate, and the general strength still sufficient, the operation is proposed as a reasonable measure. When, however, before local conditions are suitable, great prostration of strength has come on, puncture is an injudicious proceeding: it cannot possibly be of service, but will probably increase the prostration, hasten the fatal issue, and discredit the healing art.

There are still some points to notice in reference to this question of practice. When the abscess is not single, then the chances of recovery after puncture are very materially lessened, and the frequent co-existence of several abscesses in the liver has been urged as an argument against the operation. In 76 of my fatal cases examined after death, the abscess was single in 27; and if to these are added my 8 cases of successful puncture, it will give 35 single in a total of 84. In other words, 41·6 per cent. Mr. Waring's * deductions from more extensive data are still more favourable, viz. of single abscess 62·105 per cent.

From these facts, it may be concluded, that the other conditions being favourable, we may act in the hope that the abscess may be single, and not be swayed by doubts to the contrary.

Incertitude of the existence of adhesions, between the surface of the liver at the seat of abscess and the abdominal walls, has also been a difficulty with many in this operation. My own observation would lead me to say, that too much has been made of this objection, for it certainly has not been confirmatory of the remark made by Mr. Twining, viz.:—"It is surprising how often suppuration of the liver occurs without any adhesion of its peritoneal coat to adjacent parts, although the abscess be near the surface."

I find in my notes only three cases of this nature: of these 173 and 180 are the most striking. The absence of adhesion in hepatic abscess has with me been very exceptional, and in none of the cases could the question of puncture have practically arisen; and I further incline to the opinion that the cases of non-adhesion quoted by other writers may all be included in the same category.

Moreover, if in practice we use the bistoury only when there is distinct pointing and inflammatory blush, and the small trocar under the other circumstances when puncture is determined on, we incur no risk. In the first case we are sure that adhesions exist. In the possible exceptional instances of the second,

* "An Inquiry into the Statistics and Pathology of Abscess in the Liver," p. 18.

the use of a trocar and the partial evacuation of the abscess remove the danger of effusion into the peritoneal sac. I therefore attach no value to the suggestion made by Graves and others, of preliminary proceedings undertaken with the view of ensuring adhesion.

173. *Large abscess in the right lobe.—The liver free of abnormal adhesions.—The cicatrices of former ulcers in the colon.—Jaundice.—Enlarged glands in the course of the ducts.*—To the kindness of Dr. Bird, at a time prior to my appointment to the European General Hospital, I was indebted for the opportunity of witnessing the following case:—

A sailor from the *Rattlesnake*, who had been upwards of twenty years at sea and much in hot latitudes, and lately affected with dysentery, succeeded by symptoms of hepatic disease, was admitted into the European General Hospital in January 1836. He was jaundiced, and there was much pain and fulness of the right hypochondrium. As the disease progressed the edge of the liver was distinctly felt some distance below the ribs. He died.

On examination a large abscess occupied almost entirely the right lobe of the liver, and forced its thin edge much below its natural situation. The internal surface of the abscess was lined with irregular, thick lymph, and the surrounding parenchyma of the organ was dark red and friable. There were not any peritoneal adhesions to the diaphragm or elsewhere, and none of the base of the right lung to the diaphragm. The gall-bladder was much distended with bile and tense, and the site of the ducts was occupied by numerous enlarged glands, some the size of an olive. The mucous lining of the stomach at the pyloric end was of dark slate grey colour, but without softening. There had been considerable vomiting during life. The colon was normal externally, and without peritoneal adhesions. The coats were thin, and in many places there were the distinct cicatrices of former ulcers, and the whole surface had a metallic lustre, caused by tenacious light grey not abundant contents. There was not any further disease detected.

The risk of wounding a distended gall-bladder has also been urged as a difficulty in the practice of puncturing hepatic abscess. The error would seem on more than one occasion to have been committed, therefore extreme caution may very properly be enjoined. Still I do not think that apprehension of this danger will often be experienced in practice in India. Considerable distention of the gall-bladder is not of frequent occurrence, at least, I have only met with five instances of it (42, 43, 173, 186, 187), and in only the two last was it evident during life. The signs of hepatic abscess, when advanced to the stage justifying puncture, are moreover so well marked as to afford little room for error.

There is still another observation to make on this subject. Dr. Budd remarks: "In India it seems now to be a common practice to thrust a long exploring needle into the liver where the presence of abscess is suspected; and, now and then, perhaps the disease may be cured in this way." Then follow some very just reflections condemnatory of this practice. I desire to put the medical service of India right with the profession on this point.

About twenty years ago, Dr. Murray, Inspector-General of Her Majesty's Hospitals, recommended the proceeding in question on theoretic grounds, for his previous practical knowledge of hepatic abscess had been very limited. The practice was for a time followed by some of those who came within the sphere of his official influence, and its vague and unsatisfactory records are to be found in the Madras Medical Journal. It was never introduced into the Bombay Presidency, and from personal inquiry, I feel myself justified in saying, that it has now no existence in the sister presidencies, and has almost ceased to be remembered. Under these circumstances it is unnecessary to examine critically Dr. Murray's peculiar doctrines. I will only add, in the words with which Dr. Stovell concludes his very able comments on hepatic abscess*: "For my own part, I must confess, I cannot conceive the existence of any case which could require, or even justify, the adoption of such a measure."

Cure by Absorption.—Recovery from hepatic abscess by discharge of the contents spontaneously, or by artificial opening, and subsequent granulation and cicatrisation has been considered in detail; but we must not overlook the probability of cure, by absorption of the liquid parts of the pus, and the formation of a small cyst of putty-like or cretaceous residuum. Five cases in which this process was distinct, have come under my observation (p. 345); but I entertain the belief, that it is more common, especially in small abscesses, than is at present supposed, and that it would be a still more frequent result if, on the suspicion of suppuration, every attention were given to the conservation of the constitution and of a normal capillary circulation in the unaffected parts of the organ.

On Change of Climate.—The principles respecting change of climate in dysentery are equally applicable to hepatitis, and need not be repeated (p. 312).

In persons whose constitutions are deteriorated by long residence in India, and who are subject to hepatic inflammation, there should be no hesitation in recommending, at a suitable time as respects the disease, and at the appropriate season, change to a more temperate climate.

If the presence of hepatic abscess be suspected, and the strength be still such as to encourage hopes of recovery by processes of repair, this result will undoubtedly be favoured by change to a

* "Transactions, Medical and Physical Society of Bombay," No. 1, New Series, p. 188.

more temperate and tonic climate. But the measure must be so conducted as to avoid the risk of recurrence of acute inflammation from the excitement of travelling or sudden reductions of temperature; while at the same time the advantages of appropriate regimen and medical treatment are secured. If this principle be just, then, a lengthened sea-voyage in a comfortable ship to more temperate latitudes, is the only kind of change that affords the prospect of benefit. A journey to an elevated hill-station, or the discomforts and excitements of the overland route, destroy the remaining chances of recovery and ought to be invariably discouraged.

When the existence of hepatic abscess is undoubted, and prostration considerable, then change of any kind is injurious. The fatigue of movement, the disappointed hope, and the absence of that careful nursing which solaces the close of exhausting disease, will increase the suffering, add to the prostration, and hasten death. This, indeed, may seem a proposition so self-evident as hardly to merit notice; yet, I say it advisedly and from personal knowledge, there is much popular delusion on this point, and not unfrequently great professional weakness in ministering to it.

SECTION VII.—*Hepatitis in Females and in Children.*

FEMALES.—The statistics* of the Bengal and Madras Presidencies show that hepatitis is much rarer in European women than men. The per-centage to strength in the former is 1·95, and in the latter, 4·3. There is no record of the proportion in Bombay.

Though the symptoms in women correspond with the description which has already been given, yet an error in diagnosis, against which the practitioner should be on his guard, is not unfrequently committed.

That acute pain, related to the hysteric diathesis and simulating acute inflammatory disease, may be present in the female is a familiar fact. When we bear in mind the inroads that are made on female health in India by child-bearing, and lactation, in addition to climatic influences; and that this lowered condition of health favours the development of hysteric phenomena, we can have no difficulty in believing that acute pain in the hepatic region in anæmic females in India has often been injudiciously treated as hepatitis. But such mistakes ought not to occur; for the history, the diathesis, the presence of other hysteric phenomena, the absence of febrile symptoms, the very acuteness of the pain, and

* Ewart's "Vital Statistics," p. 129.

its relation to attention being fixed on it or removed from it, are sufficient to prevent them.

CHILDREN.—The ratio of hepatitis in children is in Bengal 0·05, and in Madras, 0·3 per cent. of strength; and the returns of the Byculla Schools prove the rarity of the disease in Bombay at the same period of life: the admissions in 17 years were 9, and 1 death, in a strength of from 250 to 300 children. I have no practical knowledge of hepatitis in childhood. The case of hepatic abscess in a Parsee child of ten years of age, reported * by Dr. Miller, is the youngest with which I am acquainted.

SECTION VIII.—*Occasional Difficulties and Errors of Diagnosis.*

I conclude my observations on hepatitis by quoting two cases,—one reported by Mr. Impey †, the other by Dr. R. H. Hunter. They illustrate well the difficulties that may occasionally beset the diagnosis of hepatitis.

* 174. *Aneurism of the abdominal aorta.—Acute pain of right hypochondrium and shoulder.—The edge of the liver distinct.—Treated four times for disease of the liver.*—I abridge Mr. Impey's case:—

John Hudson was admitted into hospital on the 30th of October, complaining of acute tenderness of the right hypochondrium. The pain affected the right shoulder, and was most felt by decubitus on the right side. The edge of the liver was distinctly felt. There was little febrile disturbance. The pain subsequently extended towards the right groin. He continued to suffer without relief till the 23rd of November, when he was found in a state of pulseless collapse, and died shortly afterwards. He had been a temperate man, but latterly had used opium in considerable quantity. He was treated with local blood-letting, counter-irritation, and purgatives.

Inspection four hours after death.—Abdomen.—The liver and intestines were in a normal state. An aneurism of the abdominal aorta, of oblong shape, and the size of a cricket ball, occupied with concentric layers of fibrine, was found resting on the border and sides of the last dorsal and three superior lumbar vertebræ. The aneurism had burst at its most prominent part below the right renal artery; and blood was extensively diffused under the peritoneum. The bodies of the second, third, and fourth lumbar vertebræ were corroded to the depth of half an inch.

The case reported by Dr. R. H. Hunter ‡ of Her Majesty's Second Regiment is of interest. At one time the patient was supposed to have hepatitis running on to abscess; at another, hepatic abscess conjoined with dysentery; at another, tumour over the aorta; and at one time aneurism of the aorta.

* 175. *A tumour, situated between the edge of the liver and the transverse colon.*—"Private Matthew Sellard was first admitted on the 11th of June with diarrhœa, accompanied with pain on pressure in the hypogastric region, for which he was leeched, and took medicines, chiefly absorbents and opiates, with occasional laxatives; and so

* "Transactions of the Medical and Physical Society of Bombay," No. 10. p. 303.
† *Ibid.* No. 7, p. 177. ‡ *Ibid.* No. 3, p. 134.

far recovered, as to be able to return to his duty on the 14th of the following month. On the 19th, was again admitted with similar complaints. The pain on pressure was now in the epigastric region, where a firm circumscribed tumour was very perceptible, yielding a sharp, heaving impulse. Soon after, he became subject to occasional vomiting, and at last his symptoms assumed a decided hepatic and dysenteric character; under which he rapidly sunk. Died on the 21st September, at 3 A.M.—Autopsy; 11 A.M. Liver enlarged and of a very pale yellow colour, very soft and lacerable, having from its free edge hanging, and firmly attached to the transverse colon, an encysted tumour the size of a large egg, filled with soft brain-like matter, and its cyst lined with gritty osseous plates and spikes. The colon, particularly, in its transverse arch, was extensively thickened and ulcerated."

SECTION IX.—*Statistics of Hepatitis in the European General Hospital and the Jamsetjee Jeejebhoy Hospital, at Bombay.*

We may conclude that cases of cirrhosis are also included in these Tables. The great mortality under the head Chronic Hepatitis in the Jamsetjee Jejeebhoy Hospital shows that a large proportion of the admissions must have been of hepatic abscess.

The proportion of admissions to total admissions is 3·7 in the European General Hospital, and in 1·5 in the Jamsetjee Jejeebhoy Hospital. The rate of mortality is 14·1 in the former, and 34 per cent. in the latter. The comparative admissions in different seasons have been already stated, p. 362.

In the European troops of the Bombay Presidency * the ratio of attacks of hepatitis to the strength is about 7·4 per cent.; the proportion of deaths to treated, 5·7, and of deaths to aggregate mortality, 9·5.

In the European troops of the Madras Presidency † the ratio of hepatitis to strength is 7·178, and of deaths to treated, 4·009.

In the native troops of the Madras Presidency the ratio of admissions to strength is 0·143 and of deaths to treated, 11·917.

Here, again, as in respect to dysentery, there is a higher rate of mortality from hepatitis in the native than in the European troops of the Madras army. The remark made on this feature of dysentery, p. 237, is equally applicable to this disease.

* Mr. Webb's Medical Statistics.

† "Mortality and Chief Diseases of the Troops under the Madras Government," by Lieut.-Col. W. H. Sykes, F.R.S. Journal of the Statistical Society of London, May 1851. The statistics of hepatitis have been already stated (p. 321) from Dr. Ewart's tables—but still I leave these figures, as in the first edition, drawn from other sources. They very nearly correspond.

TABLE XXX.—*Admissions and Deaths, with Per-centage, from Hepatitis, Acute and Chronic, in the European General Hospital at Bombay, for the Five Years from* 1838 *to* 1843.

	1838 to 1843.		Monthly Average.		
	Admissions.	Deaths.	Deaths on Admissions.	Admissions on total Admissions.	Deaths on total Deaths.
January . .	45	6	13·5	8·2	14·0
February . .	39	11	28·2	7·0	34·3
March . . .	36	3	8·3	7·1	9·0
April . . .	41	5	12·1	7·0	12·2
May . . .	25	2	8·0	2·9	2·4
June . . .	31	3	9·6	3·9	5·9
July . . .	23	—	—	3·2	—
August . . .	24	2	8·3	3·9	5·4
September . .	23	9	39·1	4·2	25·7
October . .	22	1	4·5	3·0	1·9
November . .	25	5	20·0	3·6	18·5
December . .	36	5	13·9	5·8	10·6
Total . .	370	52	14·0	4·8	11·6

TABLE XXXI.—*Admissions and Deaths, with Per-centage, from Hepatitis, Acute and Chronic, in the European General Hospital at Bombay, for the Five Years from* 1844 *to* 1848.

	1844 to 1848.		Average.		
	Admissions.	Deaths.	Deaths on Admissions.	Admissions on total Admissions.	Deaths on total Deaths.
January . .	15	2	13·3	2·4	4·3
February . .	15	3	20·0	2·9	8·6
March . . .	15	1	6·6	3·1	3·3
April . . .	10	1	10·0	1·9	3·2
May . . .	18	2	11·1	3·1	6·6
June . . .	11	2	18·2	1·5	6·06
July . . .	7	1	14·3	1·03	2·8
August . . .	17	—	—	3·1	—
September . .	16	4	25·0	3·5	18·2
October . .	13	4	30·8	2·1	10·6
November . .	13	2	15·4	2·3	6·4
December . .	19	1	5·2	3·6	2·5
Total . .	169	23	13·6	2·5	5·9

TABLE XXXII.—*Admissions and Deaths, with Per-centage, from Hepatitis Acute and Chronic, in the European General Hospital at Bombay, for the Five Years from* 1849 *to* 1853.

	1849 to 1853.		Monthly Average.		
	Admissions.	Deaths.	Deaths on Admissions.	Admissions on total Admissions.	Deaths on total Deaths.
January . .	17	4	23·5	3·8	10·2
February . .	15	2	13·3	4·1	11·1
March . . .	13	2	15·4	2·9	5·9
April . . .	15	2	13·3	2·9	8·0
May . . .	14	1	7·1	2·7	4·2
June . . .	13	2	15·4	2·3	6·9
July . . .	12	1	8·3	2·2	3·0
August . .	20	2	10·0	4·05	5·3
September . .	14	5	35·7	3·9	20·0
October . .	13	1	7·7	3·3	4·3
November . .	11	—	—	2·2	—
December . .	15	5	53·3	2·5	12·5
Total . .	172	27	15·7	2·9	7·5

TABLE XXXIII.—*Admissions and Deaths, with Per-centage, from Acute Hepatic Affections, in the Jamsetjee Jejeebhoy Hospital at Bombay, for the Six Years from* 1848 *to* 1853.

	1848 to 1853.		Monthly Average.		
	Admissions.	Deaths.	Deaths on Admissions.	Admissions on total Admissions.	Deaths on total Deaths.
January . .	24	1	4·2	1·15	0·2
February . .	32	2	6·3	1·7	0·7
March . . .	20	1	5·0	0·9	0·3
April . . .	18	—	—	0·9	—
May . . .	12	—	—	0·6	—
June . . .	11	1	9·1	0·5	0·3
July . . .	11	—	—	0·6	—
August . . .	23	8	34·8	1·2	2·4
September . .	7	2	28·6	0·28	0·6
October . .	5	—	—	0·2	—
November . .	19	4	21·0	0·9	1·2
December . .	26	4	15·4	1·1	1·01
Total . .	208	23	11·06	0·8	0·6

TABLE XXXIV.—*Admissions and Deaths, with Per-centage, from Chronic Hepatic Affections, in the Jamsetjee Jejeebhoy Hospital at Bombay, of the Six Years from* 1848 *to* 1853.

	1848 to 1853.		Monthly Average.		
	Admissions.	Deaths.	Deaths on Admissions.	Admissions on total Admissions.	Deaths on total Deaths.
January . .	27	17	63·0	1·3	3·8
February . .	16	16	100·0	0·8	5·0
March . . .	13	9	69·2	0·6	2·3
April . . .	18	7	38·9	0·9	2·4
May . . .	22	12	54·5	1·01	4·2
June . . .	18	4	22·2	0·9	1·3
July . . .	7	3	42·8	0·3	0·9
August . . .	21	13	61·9	1·1	4·0
September . .	19	7	36·8	0·9	2·2
October . .	11	3	27·2	0·5	0·9
November . .	15	5	33·3	0·7	1·5
December . .	11	6	54·5	0·5	1·5
Total . .	198	102	51·5	0·8	2·5

CHAP. XVI.

ON CIRRHOSIS, CONGESTION, LARDACEOUS AND FATTY ENLARGEMENT, CANCER AND HYDATID OF THE LIVER. — AFFECTIONS OF THE BILIARY DUCTS AND GALL-BLADDER. — BILIARY CALCULI. — JAUNDICE. — INCREASED AND DEFECTIVE SECRETION OF BILE.

THE subjects of this chapter will be treated very briefly, for they are now well understood, and described in systematic works.

SECTION I. — *Cirrhosis.* — *Pathology.* — *Symptoms.* — *Treatment.* — *Complication with Hepatic Abscess.*

This disease is common in India, as in other countries, in the classes addicted to the habitual free use of spirits. It consists of chronic inflammation of the areolar tissue of the portal canals, even to their smallest ramifications, followed by exudation of lymph which becomes slowly organised into contractile fibrous tissue. This process leads to a diminution of the calibre of the branches of the portal vein, the hepatic artery and duct, with probably obliteration of some of their smaller divisions. From this, atrophy of the lobular structure of the liver results, and the diminished flow of blood through the portal vein favours congestion of the capillaries of the mucous membrane of the alimentary canal, hence hæmorrhages, also of the peritoneal capillaries, hence ascites.

The exudation in the early stages, before organisation, contraction, and lobular atrophy have taken place, may cause enlargement of the liver and its extension below the margin of the ribs. With progressing organisation the lymph contracts, the lobules become atrophied, and the size of the organ is often very considerably diminished. The liver now becomes hard and tough, and when cut shows a surface variegated with white streaks, and sometimes presents the appearance of little globular nodules, the size of a pea, imbedded in a capsule of fibrous tissue. The external surface becomes irregular and tuberculated in appearance — a state caused, it is believed, by the contractile organisation of the lymph exuded in the proximity of the capsule. The colour of the liver in cirrhosis varies according to the quantity and quality of the retained bile. It may be of pale buff colour, or of bright yellow, or of an olive-green tint. These statements will be found to be verified by cases * detailed in this work.

It is further important to recollect that this condition of the liver exists in a very depraved diathesis, the result of the habits which induce the local disease, and of the imperfect purification of the blood, arising from structural unfitness of an important excretory organ.

The *symptoms* are more or less uneasiness or pain of the hepatic region, with some degree of febrile disturbance, in the early stages. In the more advanced periods, the diagnosis chiefly depends on the deranged digestive functions, the sallow complexion, the increasing emaciation, the intemperate habits, and finally the ascites, or the gastric or intestinal hæmorrhage.

Considering the circumstances in which cirrhosis occurs, the *treatment* is necessarily unsatisfactory. When the early symptoms are present, a modified antiphlogistic treatment by leeches, small blisters, and moderate mercurial and other eliminants, will be of benefit, but there can be no prospect of permanent improvement unless the habit of spirit drinking be abandoned.

When the cachectic diathesis, always present in some degree in this disease, is regarded, there can be little hesitation in determining that the constitutional action of mercury is contra-indicated This conclusion may perhaps be occasionally questionable at the commencement, but as the disease advances there can be no room for doubt; and on the whole we shall act wisely by making the rule absolute. In the advanced stages there is little to be done beyond adjusting the regimen to the ability of the impaired organs, aiding the eliminating power of the liver by taraxacum, hydrochlorate of ammonia, nitric acid, and the external use of nitro-muriatic acid; checking the hæmorrhages by suitable astringents, and favouring the removal of ascites by varying arrangements of diuretics and the external application of iodine lotions.

The two following cases illustrate several of the features of this disease:—

176. *Cirrhosis, with enlargement.—Ascites and jaundice.*—Samuel John Adams, a native Christian, of twenty-five years of age, using spirits habitually, was admitted in an emaciated state into the clinical ward, on the 23rd July, 1849. The respiration

* Cases 61, 176 to 181.

was short and hurried. The abdomen was tense, swollen, bulging laterally, and distinctly fluctuating; dulness on percussion reached to the right fifth rib, and fourth left rib, anteriorly, and to the angle of the scapulæ, posteriorly. The sounds of the heart were normal, but least heard between the third and fourth ribs, midway between the sternum and left nipple. There was œdema of the lower extremities. The pulse was small. The tongue moist, but coated yellow in the centre, and florid at the tip and edges. There was faint yellowness of the conjunctivæ, and the bowels were relaxed. He stated that the jaundice had been present for three months, that irregular febrile symptoms had come on fifteen days before admission, were succeeded by the ascites, and this by the anasarca. The diarrhœa increased after his admission, and he died on the 27th. The urine gave no traces of albumen, and its quantity had increased under the use of diuretics.

Inspection ten hours after death.—All the tissues were tinged yellow. The abdomen was swollen, and the lower extremities were œdematous. *Chest.*—The lungs collapsed, were soft and crepitating, and without adhesions. There was neither pleuritic nor pericardial effusion. The base of the heart reached to the second costal cartilage, and its apex was opposite to the fourth intercostal space from pressure upwards by the abdominal fluid. The structure of the heart was normal. *Abdomen.*—There were about six * pints of yellow turbid serum in the peritoneal sac. The omentum was somewhat thickened. The liver, chiefly its left lobe, was considerably enlarged, its surface was very irregular and lobulated, and was of olive-green colour. It reached transversely to the ribs of the left side, and upwards on both sides to the upper margin of the fifth rib. The gall-bladder was empty, and its structure was indurated. The kidneys were somewhat enlarged, but there was no trace of yellow degeneration. The spleen was much enlarged, somewhat firm in structure. The whole tract of the intestinal canal was laid open. The sub-mucous tissue was, in places, œdematous; but with the exception of patches of dark red discolouration of the mucous membrane of the cœcum and some enlargement of the follicles there, there was no other disease.

177. *Ascites.—Liver small and indurated.—Cirrhosis.—Considerable effusion of serum in the head.*—Patrick McDonald, aged forty-eight, a serjeant on the pension list, a tall spare man, was admitted 23rd July, 1838, into the European General Hospital. He had been twenty-eight years in India, and about four years ago suffered from jaundice. On admission the abdomen was distended, fluctuation was distinct, and the legs and feet were œdematous. His illness had commenced in the beginning of June, with anasarca of the legs. The urine was scanty and not coagulable. The treatment in the first instance consisted in the exhibition of diuretics of different kinds and in different modes of combination—calomel with squills, colchicum wine, tincture of squills, tincture of digitalis, nitrous ether, and the different neutral diuretic salts combined latterly with some bitter infusion, or a solution of quinine; an occasional purgative was also exhibited. Under this treatment, at first the urine increased much in quantity, and the swelling of the abdomen and the anasarca of the limbs decreased; the alvine evacuations were never pale or deficent in bile. The diuretics now lost their effect, the fluid re-accumulated; he was tapped about the 19th October; again on the 2nd November, and thirty-five pints of of straw-coloured serum were drawn off; again on the 12th November, and twenty-one pints; on the 13th December, twenty-six pints; on the 31st December, twenty-three pints; on the 7th January, twelve pints; and on the 4th February, twenty-three pints of slightly turbid serum were drawn off. Throughout this period, the medical treatment was merely palliative and tonic, with an occasional endeavour to re-excite the action of the kidneys. He ultimately became occasionally delirious, and died on the 11th February.

Inspection four hours after death.—Body emaciated. *Head.*—There were about two

* The MS. is not distinctly legible in regard to the quautity of the serum, and that stated above is therefore not positively given.

ounces of serum between the arachnoid membrane and pia mater, on the convex surface of the brain, and at the base of the skull, and six drachms in the ventricles. *Chest.*—The lungs collapsed and were healthy; the heart was healthy; and there was no fluid in the cavity of the pleura. *Abdomen.*—Eight pints of whey-coloured serum were contained in the cavity. The stomach was much dilated, and occupied the left hypochondrium, the epigastrium, and part of the right hypochondrium. The transverse colon was also much dilated. The peritoneal surface of the greater part of the small intestine had a close-set pearly covering* in irregular patches, about the thickness of silver paper, easily peeled from the peritoneal lining, and extending in a continuous but thinner layer over the mesentery. The peritoneal coat was thinner, not pearly, not easily separable from the tunics, and clearly distinguishable. The liver was about half its natural size, and adhered by long areolar bands to the side; its texture was much indurated, pale buff, like cow's udder, with many pale yellow granules scattered throughout. There was a small quantity of bile in the gall-bladder. The spleen was dense, its peritoneal coat was thickened and pearly. The mucous lining of the stomach was of natural texture, but marbled red at the cardiac end and thinned at the pyloric. The contents of the small intestine were tinged with bile. The mucous coat of the sigmoid flexure of the colon was vascular. Where the transverse colon was dilated, there were no rugæ, but these were numerous and in all directions where the dilatation ceased. The tubular and cortical parts of the kidneys were not so distinctly defined as usual, but these organs were otherwise healthy.

It is generally stated that cirrhosis of the liver and hepatic abscess do not occur together. This is doubtless correct of European countries, but it is not so of India, where the co-existence of the affections is not very unusual. I quote four cases illustrative of this remark:—

178. *Abscess in the liver.—Cirrhosis.—Sloughy perforations of large intestine, but no thickening of its coats noted.*—Private M. R——, aged twenty-seven, of Her Majesty's 40th Regiment, was admitted into hospital, at Belgaum, on the 19th July, 1830. He had been six months in India, and never in hospital before; but had, for some days before admission, suffered from pain of abdomen and deranged bowels. On admission, there was tenderness of abdomen, hot skin, full pulse, dejections frequent and morbid. On the 6th August he had slight pain of right side, but it was gone on the following day. Died August 11th.

Inspection.—The liver was of natural size. Its whole surface was rough, granular, and covered with healthy peritoneum. The internal structure was occupied by numerous small abscesses, the size of a hen's egg, and containing thin green watery pus. The parenchyma of the liver, when cut, presented a surface of light gamboge, yellow colour; and was found to consist of numerous small nodules, each about the size of a pea, and confined to a distinct capsule, from which it could readily be picked out.

* I must call attention to the thin pearly layer that invested the peritoneum in this case. I am doubtful whether it is to an appearance of this kind or not that Dr. Budd alludes at p. 139 of his treatise, as induced by peritonitis. It seems to me that a more likely explanation of the appearance described in this case may be suggested. In the normal state of the peritoneum, a very slight epithelial investment suffices for protective purposes; but when serum has for a long time been in contact with the peritoneal surface, then further protection is required, and epithelial hypertrophy may ensue. I would look upon this thin layer as a thickened epithelium. This is a point, however, in respect to which there should not be doubt, for the microscope will readily resolve it.

It was in these capsules that suppuration seemed to have commenced. The liver adhered to the concave surface, and the right lung to the convex surface of the diaphragm. The gall-bladder was full of dark bile. The omentum covered the whole surface of the small intestine, and, where not inflamed, was thinner than natural, as if stretched. Fleshy and thickened at the points of adhesion, the omentum adhered to the cœcum and descending colon; and when pulled away from the latter situation, it was found that the coats of one side of the descending colon had been completely removed, and the loss supplied by the omentum and the abdominal parietes. The sigmoid flexure formed two or three folds in the cavity of the pelvis, and at the angle of each fold the coats of the intestine were destroyed on one side, for the extent of the size of a dollar, the loss being supplied by the opposite side of the folds and by the omentum. The urinary bladder formed the wall of one perforation the size of a dollar.

179. *Abscess in liver with cirrhosis, notwithstanding ptyalism.—Displacement of colon.—Adhesion of it to the left side of diaphragm.— Sloughy ulceration of large intestine, without thickening.*—Private W. H——, of Her Majesty's 40th Regiment, aged forty-three, after one day's illness, was admitted into hospital, at Belgaum, on the 22nd July, 1830. There was much tenderness across the lower part of the epigastric region, and the dejections were frequent. He was freely bled and leeched, and the pain left him; the dejections became bilious and no longer contained blood. On the 25th, ptyalism. 28th, medicines omitted. The dejections were natural, and he seemed to be convalescent. From the 1st of August to the 10th, the dejections continued feculent and formed, with occasionally, however, some drops of reddish mucus passed with tenesmus. On the 10th the purging returned, the tenesmus increased, the dejections became morbid, and the abdomen tender. From this time all the symptoms became aggravated. Ptyalism could not be again induced, and he died, on the 26th August.

Inspection.—The omentum was shrivelled up and laid upon the transverse colon. This intestine, throughout its course, adhered to the abdominal parietes, and to the great curvature of the stomach, following its cardiac extremity, and adhering to the left side of the diaphragm. On the right side the transverse colon adhered to the concave surface of the liver, and firmly to the gall-bladder. The coats of the bowel were thinned, and in some places perforated: the gall-bladder, for example, formed the wall of a perforation. The ascending and descending colon ulcerated internally, were of rather contracted calibre, and adhered firmly to the parietes of the abdomen. When these adhesions were separated in some places, the contents of the bowel escaped. The peritoneal surface of the small intestine was of a dark red colour with here and there patches of effused lymph. The left lobe of the liver was small, hard, and carneous. The right lobe not so hard, was mottled and contained many small abscesses in its structure, none of them, however, larger than a horse-bean. There was not any adhesion of the external surface of the liver, but in some places there were depressed and puckered cicatrices. The coats of the different vessels in the substance of the liver seemed thickened, and felt cartilaginous and hard under the scalpel. The gall-bladder contained thin watery bile. The lung on the left side adhered to the diaphragm, opposite to the adhesions formed between that muscle and the colon.

180. *Abscess in liver, notwithstanding ptyalism.—Cirrhosis.—Cæcum and ascending colon thickened and ulcerated.*—Private B. A——, aged twenty-one, was admitted into hospital at Belgaum, on the 1st August, 1830, affected with griping and passing mucous dejections. On the 3rd, when the gums were tender, the dejections became bilious and feculent, and continued so till August 17th, with however irregular action of the bowels and occasional griping, but without tenderness of abdomen, or febrile excitement. On the 17th, blood was observed in the alvine discharges. From this date the symptoms became aggravated. The dejections, however, retained their bilious

colour, though there was no intermixture of blood and vitiated mucus. No ptyalism. Died September 8th.

Inspection. — The liver, without adhesions, was of slate colour externally, somewhat enlarged, and extended beyond the cartilages of the ribs. Near the thin edge of the left lobe there was an abscess, yellow, elevated above the surface, about the size of a hen's egg, and containing thick pus. The liver was hard in structure. The gall-bladder was full of dark bile, and had formed firm adhesions with the colon and the pyloric portion of the duodenum. There was less peritoneal inflammation than is generally met with. The omentum was vascular, but had contracted few adhesions. The caput cœcum and ascending colon were distended, hard, and thickened. The former was drawn upwards from its usual situation in the iliac fossa. The mucous membrane of the larger intestine was ulcerated, but nowhere was there any trace of perforation.

181. *Dysentery complicated with delirium tremens. — Abscess and cirrhosis of the liver.* — Denis L. Donahen, aged twenty-eight, a man of stout frame but of dissipated habits, aften ten or twelve days' illness with dysentery, was admitted into the European General Hospital on the 11th December, 1842. There was heat of skin, full and frequent pulse, and considerable tenderness about the cœcum. He was bled to twelve ounces, had fifty leeches applied to the abdomen, and took calomel with a full opiate. The following day he was tremulous, and the dysenteric symptoms continued. On the 14th he was in a state of delirium tremens, and there was distinct induration at the site of the cœcum. On the 15th the symptoms of delirium tremens had passed away but the dysentery continued. He was treated chiefly with free opiates without amendment; and on the 29th, to the dysenteric symptoms was added occasional uneasiness of the right hypochondrium shooting to the shoulder. This state persisted with occasional febrile symptoms, collapsing features and declining strength, and he died on the 4th January.

Inspection ten hours after death. — Abdomen.—The omentum adhered firmly to the cœcum, and the transverse colon was rather contracted. The liver was in a state of cirrhosis, and several small abscesses projected from its convex surface, and there was a larger one, at the thin edge of the liver, of which the walls were in part formed by the omentum.

SECTION II.—*Congestion of the Liver.—Œdema.*

The facts which it is important to remember in regard to this pathological state are, the three degrees of congestion described by Mr. Kiernan: the first confined to the hepatic vein, the second implicating the portal capillaries in part, the third involving all the portal capillaries. Thus the varieties of mottling frequently observed on the incised surface of the liver are caused.

The two first of these degrees are liable to be produced by cardiac or pulmonary disease obstructing the ready return of the venous blood to the heart.

Consequent on the altered balance of the circulation and the deteriorated blood in malarious fever, congestion of the portal capillaries, leading to enlargement of the organ and derangement of function, is apt to occur. This pathological state has been already alluded to in connection with the subject of fever, and the caution has been given not to mistake this condition co-existing with fever, for hepatitis.*

It is a favourite theory with some, that blood vitiated by the absorption of matters from the intestinal canal is a common cause, and affords a ready explanation of certain biliary derangements. That, consequent upon blood altered in quality being conveyed to a secreting structure, the processes between that blood and the cells—in other words, secretion—may be impaired and capillary congestion result, is accordant with present physiological doctrine. But † that the food of the middle and upper classes of society, taken in excess, is liable to generate an immense variety of noxious matter, capable of absorption by osmotic force, is surely a statement unsupported by sufficient proof.

In ordinary digestion the assimilable portion of the food is absorbed in the upper parts of the alimentary canal, while its fœcal residuum with the excreta from the surface of, or poured into, the intestinal canal, are passed onwards for rejection. When delayed in the large intestine, that portion of the contents which is absorbable by osmotic force is removed and the density of the residual mass is increased, while the fluid part which has been absorbed is carried to the portal blood; but no evil results, simply because that which is noxious has been left behind, and that which has been absorbed is innocuous.

Why should it be otherwise in the instance of excess? Then the undue quantity of fœcal residuum is hurried through the canal and speedily ejected. Instead of there being greater likelihood under these circumstances of absorption into the portal blood of

* "Congestion of the liver" is at present a common phrase often however used, very vaguely, and without any attempt to ascertain by percussion, whether the organ is enlarged or not. Increased size of the liver is a condition of its congestion, and unless this exists, the assertion that there is congestion of the liver is hardly justifiable.

A persistent, enlarged and friable state, caused by congestion or other change of the large parenchymatous viscera—the liver and spleen—of the abdomen is also important in reference to questions of medical jurisprudence. For example, rupture of an enlarged spleen and speedy death by hæmorrhage, caused by slight and apparently inadequate external injuries, is not a very unusual occurrence in India. Four such cases are recorded by Mr. Heddle, in the 1st volume, "Medical and Physical Society's Transactions," Bombay. The only instance which has come under my own observation was that of police constable, who had strained himself in playing cricket. He was admitted into the European General Hospital on the 1st February, 1840, with uneasy, full abdomen and oppressed breathing, and died on the following day. After death the cavity of the abdomen was found to contain four imperial pints of dark-coloured blood, in part coagulated, which had proceeded from a laceration, an inch and a half in length, on the inner surface of the spleen.

† Dr. Budd, "Diseases of the Liver," second edition, p. 61.

the so-called noxious matters, there must be less, for they are delayed a much shorter time in relation with the structures which are supposed to absorb. That excess in eating and drinking deranges the digestive functions, those of the liver included, is very true; but that this effect is usually caused by the direct transmission of noxious matters of food, by the portal blood, from the intestine to the liver, is for the reasons just assigned, an improbable theory.

Œdema of the Liver — is a pathological state with which I was unacquainted till I met with the following case. This condition is not noticed by Rokitansky, and the only mention of it to which I am at present able to refer, is in the Library of Medicine.* There it is said that œdema of the liver, uncombined with inflammation, has often been observed; but by whom is not stated.

182. *Remittent fever, œdema of the liver.*—Cassim Ibrahim, aged thirty-six, admitted after ten days' illness, on the 6th February, 1857. The skin was hot and dry, the breathing hurried, general tremors, sordes on the lips, the tongue dry and florid, the pulse frequent and small, no abnormal cardiac sounds. The exhaustion increased, and he died in twenty-four hours.

Inspection fifteen hours after death. — The white tissues were tinged yellow. No abnormal vascularity or effusion in the head. The lungs healthy, with exception of considerable œdema, and dark redness of the bronchial mucous membrane. The heart was healthy. The liver, of dark olive colour, reached two inches below the right ribs, and touched the point of the eighth left rib. It weighed four pounds four ounces, and when cut, and gently pressed, serous fluid oozed freely from the surfaces, six ounces were collected. The parenchyma broke down readily under the finger. The incised surfaces presented a dark olive colour, with brown intermixture, but not the mottled redness of congestion. There was commencing Bright's disease of both kidneys. The mucous membrane of the stomach and intestines was, with exception of mottled redness of the former, healthy.

Section III. — *Lardaceous and Fatty Liver. — Cancer, and Hydatid Formations.*

Lardaceous Liver. — This state, termed by Dr. Budd scrofulous enlargement of the liver, found in scrofulous, syphilitic, and mercurial cachexia, is, I believe, very similar to that caused by malaria. I have already, when treating of hepatic enlargement consecutive on intermittent fever, stated my own limited information on this subject, and what seem to me the chief desiderata in its further investigation.

Fatty Degeneration of the Liver. — The etiology and pathology of this morbid state in India are subjects for future inquiry; for

* Vol. iv. p. 180.

it is probably more common than recorded facts have yet proved it to be. This, and all allied processes which imply perversion of nutrition, of great interest in all countries, are particularly so in India, where, for reasons elsewhere adverted to (p. 154), the tendency to degenerative action, is, in all likelihood largely developed. The reader will find a full exposition of the present state of pathological knowledge on scrofulous enlargement and fatty degeneration of the liver in Dr. Budd's work.*

Cancer of the Liver. — Judging from the considerable space allotted to descriptions of this morbid state in works on the pathology of the liver, it would seem that it is not of unfrequent occurrence in European countries.

It is certainly rare in India, and therefore, clinically speaking, it is undesirable that it should fill a prominent place in the mind of the practitioner in that country.

The following is the only case which has come under my observation:—

183. *Treated for supposed dyspeptic symptoms.—Numerous cancerous tubera disseminated throughout the liver.—One had opened into the stomach.*—Chayia Raggia, a Hindoo fisherman, of fifty years of age, a resident of Caranja near Bombay, and using spirituous liquours habitually, was, not much reduced in flesh, admitted into the clinical ward, on the 11th July, 1849, under the head "Dyspepsia." The abdomen was flaccid, and without induration. The tongue was clean and moist. He complained of pain at the epigastrium extending up the sternum coming on in paroxysms three or four times in the day, generally, he thought, when the stomach was empty. The paroxysms were attended with flatulence and a sense of burning and acidity of stomach which were relieved by firm pressure, and also, he said, by the use of spirits. He had suffered more or less from these symptoms for four years. During his stay in hospital the urine was frequently examined, but gave no indications of albumen. He continued under treatment till the 29th July, when he was discharged relieved. He returned to the hospital several times, and was treated for his dyspeptic symptoms as they were termed. The last admission was on the 24th November, 1850. There was pain at the epigastrium, with distinct induration extending in a direction below the margin of the right ribs. The alvine discharges were clay coloured. On the 10th December there was vomiting of dark-coloured fluid, under which he sank and died.

Inspection twelve hours after death.—The liver enlarged, chiefly the right lobe. From different parts of both the convex and concave surfaces there projected in relief circumscribed white elevations of various size, from a pea to an olive. These, when cut into, were found to be white, indurated, circumscribed tubera. There were also numerous similar nodules in different parts of the substance of the liver in size from a pea to a small orange. Some of the large ones were softened at their centres into a pulpy matter, almost of the consistence and colour of pus, which under the microscope exhibited the granular cellular appearance of the encephaloid cells. The intercurrent portions of the liver were natural in appearance and consistence. The concave surface of the left lobe adhered to the surface of the stomach near to the pylorus, and the

* For further remarks on fatty degeneration of the liver and fatty liver, see note, page 9.

inner surface of the stomach at the site of adhesion presented a cup-like depression involving the substance of the liver, the evident consequence of the opening of a tuber into the stomach. Both kidneys, on removing the capsule, presented a buff mottled, somewhat granular appearance, and on incision the cortical portion was pale buff, and encroached on the tubular. There was some degree of hypertrophy of the left ventricle of the heart, and some thickening of the mitral valve.

Hydatid formations in the liver are also rare in India. I have met with only three cases. Two occurred in natives, and in both, echinococci were present in great abundance. The subject of one of these two cases was a negro sailor, a native of Muscat, admitted into the clinical ward with fulness of the right false ribs, and a dull prominent swelling reaching to the eighth left rib, and to near the umbilicus. There was also fever and dysentery. The history was imperfect, but from the hepatic enlargement, the fever and dysentery — the diagnosis was hepatic abscess. He died ten days after admission, and after death a large hydatid sac was found in the right lobe of the liver, containing five pints of clear colourless fluid with floating acephalocysts and echinococci; and numerous nodules of lymph deposit, some softening into pus, were scattered throughout the left lobe. There was sloughy ulceration of the large intestine. The diagnosis was therefore correct, though in complete, and the inference from the enlargement erroneous.

The third case is detailed below — it occurred before the attention of the profession had been called to the general presence of echinococci in the hydatid sac. The subject of it was a soldier of the 15th Hussars, lately arrived from Europe — so that the hydatid in this case as well as that in the Muscat sailor were not of Indian origin.

184. *Phthisis pulmonalis.—Lungs tuberculated, hydatid sac in the abdomen, also in the liver.—Peritoneum studded with miliary transparent tubercles.*—Edward Collingridge, Her Majesty's 15th Hussars, aged twenty-two, had been troubled with a pectoral affection during the voyage, and was admitted into the European General Hospital, on the 10th November, 1839. He was pale, sallow, and had frequent dry cough. Tubercular deposition in the lungs was suspected. On the 3rd December the abdomen was tense and full, with sense of fluctuation. There was constant hectic fever with increasing emaciation, and he died on the 2nd January.

Inspection twelve hours after death. — Body much emaciated. *Head.*—There was a thin veil of serum between the archnoid and pia mater on the convex surface of the brain. The substance of the brain was soft. *Chest.*—There was a pint of serum in the sac of each pleura. The anterior part of the lungs was emphysematous, and miliary tubercles were disseminated throughout. The posterior part of the upper lobe, and almost the whole of the lower lobe of the right lung, were impermeable from tubercular infiltration; in places there were tubercular masses, the size of a pigeon's egg, but generally it was intermixed with the red parenchyma, and presented the variegated appearance (when incised) of shell marbles, in which red and white are the predominating colours. The posterior part of the left lung was œdematous, but there was little tubercular infiltration. The heart was healthy. *Abdomen.*—The intestines were displaced, and the central part of the abdominal cavity was occupied by a hydatid sac which completely filled the pelvis, rose over the promontory of the sacrum, and reached to the margin of the left lobe of the liver. This sac was filled with many pints of hydatids, transparent and clear, ranging from a marble in size to a large orange; there was also a great quantity of yellow membranous shreds, the evident teguments of dead hydatids. In the left lobe of the liver were two sacs, each the size of a small orange, also filled with hydatids. The intestines were of a dark leaden colour, and generally contracted. The mesentery, and much of the peritoneal surface of the intestines, and also the omentum, were studded closely with miliary tubercles, about the size of a mustard seed; and to these the small red ramifications of vessels very frequently extended. The stomach was small. The kidneys healthy. The examination was not further pursued.

SECTION IV. — *Inflammation of the Gall-Bladder and Biliary Ducts. — Distention of the Gall-Bladder.—Biliary Calculi.*

My observations supply very little information on these affections. The cases of jaundice complicating remittent fever, detailed at page 98, do not countenance the idea of inflammation of the mucous lining of the biliary ducts being a common cause of jaundice; and if I may judge from my own experience, inflammation of these structures, as well as of the gall-bladder, is not of frequent occurrence.

A case (185) of inflammation * of the gall-bladder, associated with abscess in the liver, is subjoined; also two cases of distention of the gall-bladder, previously referred to.† In association with the two last cases, 42 and 43 may also be considered.

185. *Hepatitis.—Abscess.—Inflammation of the external and internal surface of the gall-bladder.— Sudden collapse, continuing with varying symptoms for several days.—* John McInnes, aged thirty-three, had been employed as an engineer. After ten days' illness with hepatitis, he was admitted into the European General Hospital on the 12th April, 1841, with the disease unsubdued. On the 20th there was unexpected collapse with vomiting. He continued, till his death on the 30th, with occasional vomiting, hiccup, pulse frequent, and failing in strength. Latterly abdomen full, with pain shifting from place to place.

Inspection.—There were two abscesses in the right lobe of the liver. There was a small quantity of sero-purulent effusion in the abdomen, with tender adhesions of the convolutions of the intestine to each other, and firm adhesion of the liver to the concavity of the ribs. The gall-bladder was moderately distended, its peritoneal surface was of bright red colour, and adhered to the colon; the lining membrane was also of bright red colour, and the contents consisted of tenacious mucus in places almost

---

* I find, in my notes of fatal cases of officers, one of a stout corpulent man of thirty-four years of age, who suffered frequently from pain of the hepatic region, and clay-coloured evacuations. After six weeks' illness with these symptoms, treated freely with general and local blood-letting and calomel, he died exhausted. The liver was found much enlarged, mottled, and readily lacerable. The gall-bladder was small, and filled with calculi, from a pigeon's egg to a pea in size, but without bile; the mucous membrane was red and livid, with sphacelated patches.

† Page 413.

membranous in character; a probe passed through the duct met with resistance. The mucous coat of the stomach was lined with adhesive mucus, and presented a rosy tint, but was unchanged in structure.

186. *Fever, with jaundice.—Gall-bladder distended, seemingly from inflammation of the common duct.—Little improvement from treatment.*—Jamsetjee Sapoorjce, a Parsee carpenter, of fifty-five years of age, following his occupation in the Government dock-yard, and habitually using spirits, was admitted into hospital, on the 24th June, 1852, ill with intermittent fever, complicated with jaundice. On the 2nd July, a pyriform indistinctly fluctuating swelling was observed below the margin of the 10th right rib. It was about an inch and a half in length and an inch in breadth, and was dull on percussion, but not painful. There was pain increased by pressure at the margins of the seventh and eighth ribs, also felt in a direction inwards from them. There was no swelling or abdormal dulness elsewhere. The alvine discharges were pale, and the urine tinged with bile. Leeches and small blisters were applied over the tender part. Quinine combined with taraxacum and rhubarb or aloes was given, also alkalies and diuretics; but he benefited little by the treatment, and left the hospital on the 8th September, with the swelling unchanged.

187. *The gall-bladder, distended, reached to the umbilicus.— Gastritis.— Colon contracted.*—A negro cook, of fifty years of age, a native of the island of Cayenne, resident for some years in France, and latterly in Jamaica, had suffered at different times from illnesses, the nature of which he could not clearly explain; they seemed, however, to have affected chiefly the abdominal viscera. This individual arrived in Bombay about the middle of December 1835, and complained occasionally of irregular action of the bowels, and the tongue was generally thickly coated. These complaints, though relieved by the exhibition of mercurial purgatives, recurred towards the end of December, and were attended with pain of the margin of the right false ribs, relieved by leeches. From the 1st January to the 20th he suffered more or less from irritability of stomach, irregular and torpid action of the bowels, frequently colicky pain, but without distention or tenderness of the abdomen. The tongue was thickly coated, the pulse was natural, the skin was scaly and dry, but of natural appearance. Various purgatives with anti-spasmodics, anodynes, enemata, &c., were freely used. On the 20th the matter vomited was dark-coloured and offensive; there was tenderness round the umbilicus, and pressure there induced vomiting. From this time the irritability of stomach became distressing; vomiting was excited by speaking, and by all ingesta; the matters ejected were watery, fœtid, and sometimes tinged with blood. There was trifling pain of the epigastrium; the pulse became rapid, and feeble, and the skin morbidly hot; there was subsultus tendinum and low delirium; the abdomen was collapsed, and the action of the bowels irregular; and during the last days of life there was occasional tenesmus. He died on the 28th of January.

Inspection five hours after death.—Abdomen.—The lower part of the thorax was contracted, so that the liver and stomach were pushed more towards the umbilicus than is natural. The gall-bladder was distended, and extended two inches beyond the edge of the liver; it passed over the hepatic flexure of the colon, and was opposed to the right edge of the umbilicus; the gall-ducts were natural. The stomach was moderately distended, the mucous lining of the cardiac end was dotted red and softened; that of the body and pyloric end thickened, and presenting a mammillated surface. The small intestine was empty, pale, and contracted. The large intestine was throughout of small calibre, with frequent and considerable contractions, chiefly in the transverse and descending portions; but there was no thickening of the coats; the prevailing tint of the inner surface was dark grey, occasionally merging into streaks of grey black, with here and there dark red patches. There was in places softening of the mucous coat, and cicatrices of former ulcers were apparent, but the traces of the most recent inflammatory action were in the sigmoid flexure of the colon, and the commencement of the rectum.

Biliary calculi have seldom come under my notice in post mortem examinations in India, and I cannot bring to my recollection above three or four cases of individuals suffering from the symptoms characteristic of obstruction of the ducts from this cause.

These results accord with Dr. Budd's experience in the Dreadnought Hospital among men returned from India. But he justly adds, and the remark applies in part to my own field of inquiry, "It is, however, not fair to judge from these men, who were sailors and had probably great immunity from gall-stones, on account merely of their seafaring life." To this may be added that they were also, for the most part, men at a period of life of acknowledged little liability to this affection.

Dr. Budd states that gall-stones are common in the cancerous diathesis. Judging from my own experience, as well as inquiry from others, both cancerous degeneration and biliary calculi are rare in India compared with other countries.

It may be, that the circumstance of my pathological investigations having been chiefly carried on among males, is another reason why biliary calculi have not frequently come under my notice.

If the proclivity of the female sex to the formation of gall-stones be due to the sedentary life which they lead, the affection ought to be common among those females in India who lead secluded lives. My opportunities of witnessing disease in these classes in Bombay have not been unfrequent, yet I cannot call to my recollection a single case of jaundice or of other symptoms that could be attributed to the passage of gall-stones.

The inference to be drawn from these remarks is, that there is still room for further research on the formation of biliary calculi in India.

SECTION V.—*Jaundice.—Pathology.— Causes.—Treatment.*

Though this symptom of hepatic disease has been, from its prominent character, long familiar to medical men, we are still imperfectly acquainted with its proximate causes. These, as at present believed, may be stated to be —

1. Obstruction of the hepatic or common duct by viscid mucus or gall-stones, and by external pressure of enlarged lymphatic glands, the head of the pancreas, gravid uterus, loaded colon, or other mechanical influences of a similar nature. When obstruction

has continued for some time, the hepatic cells become destroyed, their place being taken by granular amorphous matter; and the liver, losing its firmness, becomes soft, flaccid, and pulpy. When the obstruction has become permanent, death takes place by a slow process of exhaustion and emaciation. Jaundice under these circumstances is caused by re-absorption of bile.

2. Destruction of the hepatic cells, independent of obstruction in the ducts. This is the yellow atrophy of Rokitansky. It is characterised by reduced size and a flaccid, pulpy state of the liver, with absence of the nucleated cells. It is attributed to causes affecting the blood-mass as the poison of fever, of serpents, &c. The course is sometimes rapid, attended with adynamic febrile phenomena, delirium, and coma.* This state of the liver has been treated of at some length by Dr. Budd, and he countenances the idea that it may at times affect the organ partially, follow a slower course, and terminate in recovery. The jaundice thus arising is generally believed to be the consequence of suppressed secretion.

3. Congestion is another proximate cause of jaundice, perhaps partly by absorption, partly by suppression.

The notes of forty-five cases in which jaundice had been present are before me: of these, twenty-seven have been already adverted to as complicating remittent fever (p. 98); thirteen were entered as simple jaundice, but from the attendant pyrexial symptoms eight of them might have been more correctly classed with the

* This form of jaundice has also been fully considered by Frerichs in his "Klinik der Leber Krankheiten." The greater prevalence of this severe and generally fatal form, in females, is shown by facts referred to both by Budd and Frerichs. The former alludes to eleven cases of which eight were females; the latter to thirty-one cases of which twenty-two were females. Frerichs further mentions that one half of the twenty-two females were pregnant.

In twenty-eight of Frerichs' cases, death took place in the first week in 13; in the second week in 6; in the third in 5, and in the fourth in 4. In twenty-three carefully observed, the spleen was enlarged from congestion in 19, normal in 3, and small in one. The ages of the thirty-one cases were—

6 . . .	from	10 to 20
20 . . .	,,	20 ,, 30
3 . . .	,,	30 ,, 40
2 . . .	,,	40 ,, 60

Of eleven cases referred to by Budd, the ages were—

3 . . .	,,	10 to 20
3 . . .	,,	20 ,, 30
1 . . .	,,	30 ,, 40
4 . . .	,,	40 ,, 60

Of the four, between 40 and 60 — two were males, and the third male was between 20 and 30.

twenty-seven febrile cases. The five remaining cases were of hepatic abscess. Ten of the febrile cases * and the five of hepatic abscess proved fatal.

My investigations do not support the opinion that obstruction of the ducts by inflammation of their lining membrane is a common cause of jaundice, for the traces of inflammation have not been found in any of the fatal cases; and it is fair to infer that this state was not generally present in the successful ones, even though pain at the right costal margin had been complained of. In only three cases was there satisfactory evidence of mechanical obstruction of the hepatic or common duct: the cause in two † was a lumbricus; in the third ‡, not fatal, it was possibly biliary calculus, and this is my only case which can be fairly related to this obstructing cause. In seven § there was enlargement of the lymphatic glands in the course of the common duct, but it is very doubtful whether, in these cases, it was sufficient to cause obstruction by pressure: at all events, distention of the ducts behind was noticed in only one.‖

In six ¶ of the fatal cases, inflammation of the mucous membrane of the duodenum was observed, and it is reasonable to infer that it may also have been present in a proportion of the recovered cases characterised by tenderness at the margin of the right ribs.

I am unable to explain the relation which duodenitis bears to jaundice. It may be that they are only coincident sequences of one antecedent. As already stated, the usual theory of extension of inflammation from the duodenum to the common duct is not supported by my cases. May it be that from a protective sympathy (if I may be allowed the expression), the bile is prevented from coming in contact with the inflamed surface of the duodenum?

In none of my fatal cases was yellow atrophy of the liver noticed. It is true that the microscope was used in only three instances, but in the others the appearances of the organ, as described, do not accord with those characteristic of this lesion. It is moreover fair to infer that yellow atrophy was also absent in all the recovered cases, though in some of them drowsiness and tendency to coma had been well marked

The opinion entertained by Dr. Budd, that some cases of jaundice may be accounted for on the supposition of the existence of a partial yellow atrophy, and that of recovered cases some may be of this nature, does not seem to me very probable; because, 1. The

* Cases 36—45. † 38, 137. ‡ 186. § 36—39, 42, 44, 173. ‖ 36.
¶ 36, 37, 40, 42, 43, 45.

suspended function of only portions of the liver is generally insufficient to occasion jaundice, as is proved by the rarity of its occurrence in hepatitis. 2. A general blood-cause is not likely to operate partially. 3. As regards the recovered cases the inference, from a review of the whole subject, is against the supposition.

Such, then, are my reasons for concluding that there is still room for further careful investigation of the proximate causes of jaundice, and that much which has been written on the subject is merely hypothetical.*

The exciting and predisposing causes of jaundice are also a subject of much interest. Three of my cases occurred in the guards of an opium convoy, proceeding from Marwar to Bombay, exposed to fatigue and to elevated temperature. They are a class of people frequently addicted to the habitual use of opium.

* The precise constituents of the bile,—whether only the pigment, or the acids also,—present in the blood and urine in jaundice, are not yet determined. I am indebted to Dr. Parkes for the following statement on the present state of this question as regards the urine.

"The changes in opinion respecting the presence or absence of the bile acids in icteric urine have been considerable, and even now the subject is very obscure.

"Before the experiments of Strecker had elucidated the composition of the bile, Thenard and Orfila believed they had found the so-called 'resinous bodies' in the urine. Subsequently, however, it seemed to be acknowledged that though the bile acids could be sometimes found, this was uncommon, and that they were generally absent in the urine of icterus (Lehmann; Gorup-Besanez; Scherer). It has been therefore surmised either that these acids are destroyed in the system or that in icterus the liver ceases to form them, although it continues to produce pigment. Frerichs and Staedeler (*a*) however advanced a most remarkable hypothesis, viz. that in jaundice the *bile acids are converted into bile pigment.* Into their reasons for advocating such a conversion it is not necessary now to enter, as they do not seem to have won many adherents. The fact on which their hypothesis was based (viz. the deficiency of bile acids, and the presence of bile pigment in the icteric urine), has been disputed by Kühne (*b*), who by the employment of another method believes he has succeeded in proving that bile acids, or rather their derivatives (choloidinic acidi or dyslisin?) can really be found in the urine. If Kühne's experiments can be relied upon, they would imply that the formation of glycin (and perhaps of taurin) in the liver is impeded in jaundice, but that cholic acid is still formed, and that there is no conversion of bile acid into pigment. Kühne believes he has shown that benzoic acid does not form hippuric acid in cases of jaundice, owing, he presumes, to the absence of glycin.

"Still more lately, Folwarczny (*c*) has repeated Kühne's experiments, and does not confirm them. In four cases of jaundice he examined the urine in the same manner as Kühne, and found no bile acid. He also gave benzoic acid and found hippuric acid in the urine, as in health. The question is then yet doubtful and a stricter investigation is still required."

(*a*.) Müller's Archiv. 1856, p. 55.
(*b*.) Virchow's Archiv. für Path. Anat. x. p. 310.
(*c*.) Wien Zeitschrift: 1859. Neue Folge ii. p. 15.

Fatigue, heat, opium-eating, — are these common predisposing or exciting causes of jaundice?

The Bombay Fusileer Regiment, after many months' active service in the field, which terminated with the dispersion of Shere Sing's army, were encamped, at the end of March 1849, in front of the Khybur Hills, near Jumrood. They remained under canvas till the 7th of May. The ground was badly selected, being partly on the banks and partly in the bed of a mountain torrent which divided the hospital from the rest of the lines, and which, on more than one occasion, nearly swamped the whole of the sick and completely cut off all access to them. The tents were crowded one upon another, and the place soon became filthy in the extreme, and very offensive. The slime deposited by each subsiding flood, and the dead, putrid, and unburied camels, deposited all around, produced the most offensive odours and a plague of flies, which effectually prevented rest of any kind or anywhere from sunrise to sunset, or the enjoyment of a single meal. Fortunately during this time the weather had not been very hot. Dr. Arnott, from whose interesting report * of the Fusileer Regiment this description is taken, thus continues: —

"The effects on the men of change from the active, regular and excited life of a campaign, to the sedentary, inactive life and looser habits of a standing camp, soon became apparent in their diminished relish for their meals, their predisposition to indigestion, jaundice, and in the prevalence of nausea and vomiting after meals, which, during the time we lay at Jumrood, affected nearly every man and officer of our regiment, and, indeed, I believe almost every man of the force. The complaint, for complaint it was, and a very annoying one too, though not dangerous, I admit, I could not account for in a manner satisfactory to myself. The natives, as they always do, attributed it to swallowing flies, and some became converts to this opinion; they no doubt did soil and corrupt every article of diet or whatever else was left for the shortest period exposed; and if anything could give one an idea of the third plague inflicted on the land of Egypt in days of old, it was here realised in perfection. Many attributed the complaint to the presence of antimony in the water, as it is found in the hills from which the streams issue, but none could be detected in it; and I considered that the real cause lay in the new life and habits we had entered upon. The disease was characterised by no peculiar symptoms besides those mentioned. There was nausea most frequently in the middle of, or immediately after, a meal, suddenly followed by vomiting, till the whole contents of the stomach were ejected; and the feeling of nausea continued for some time afterwards, but gradually subsided, very probably to return again, however, at the following meal.

"In the matter ejected there was seldom anything either bilious or acid, and the bowels were in a natural state, or perhaps rather confined. This state of things might occur once, or might recur frequently, and then the men would apply at the hospital for an emetic or a dose of physic, but seldom to be admitted. From not being able to retain anything on the stomach, and consequently from want of due sustenance, the men felt languid and low-spirited, but no other permanently bad effects resulted from it; and

* "Transactions, Bombay Medical and Physical Society," 1st Series, No. 10, p. 28.

after we moved back towards Peshawur, on the 7th May, there was scarcely a case of it.

"*Icterus.*—Subsequently to this disease, and, as it appeared to me, proceeding from the same causes, cases of jaundice became very frequent, amounting in the nine months we lay at Peshawur to no fewer than thirty-four admissions against two in the corresponding period of the previous year. They were characterised by the usual appearances of yellowness of the skin and eyes, high-coloured urine, obstipation, and clay-coloured stools, want of appetite, languor, &c. An emetic was almost uniformly given on admission; cathartics daily, and most frequently mercury was given to ptyalism. Under this treatment they all did well, though occasionally a considerable degree of debility remained for some time afterwards, which was treated with aperient bitters, alkaline medicines, tonics, and mild nutrient diet."

The European troops employed in the expedition to the Persian Gulf, in 1857, suffered, at Mohamarah and Bushire, in the month of April, from nausea and vomiting, just as the Fusileers did at Jumrood. The 14th Dragoons returned from Persia to Kirkee towards the end of May, and in the month of June ten cases of jaundice were admitted into hospital. Of the men selected as healthy in the first week of June to accompany a force to Aurungabad, four became affected with jaundice. The disease yielded readily to treatment.

Treatment.—The uncertain state of the pathology of jaundice necessarily affects the treatment.

A preliminary question before commencing the treatment of jaundice, is, whether we have to do with a liver previously healthy, or affected with congestion, cirrhosis, or other organic change.

Whenever tenderness at the margin of the ribs is present, we may infer the existence of congestion of the liver, or inflammation of the duodenum or adjacent structures, and conclude that these conditions are related, in some way or other, to the jaundice; and that their removal by leeches and counter-irritation ought to be a leading indication of cure.

To increase excretion from the intestinal surface is also an object to be held in view, and it may be effected by such means as aloes, rhubarb, and saline cathartics; used, however, with caution, in order that inflammation of the duodenum, or adjacent structures, when present, may not be increased, and that in cachectic individuals dysenteric symptoms may not be excited.

The expediency of the cholagogue action of mercury is an important question in the treatment, and from the obscurity which involves the proximate cause of jaundice, it is often difficult to determine. If the existence of a mechanical obstructing cause be suspected, then to stimulate the secreting action of the liver must be injurious. If there be a general destruction of the hepatic cells, is mercury likely to reconstruct them? If we accept the theory of a partial cell destruction, then will mercury, if given, not rather affect the healthy cells and leave the destroyed ones uninfluenced?

These are perplexing questions, and all that we can do in practice is to follow those principles which under the circumstances seem to be most reasonable. So long as symptoms of gastro-enteric inflammation are present we must use mercurials very cautiously, and trust chiefly to local depletion and counter-irritation, the combination of taraxacum with alkalies and ipecacuanha, and mild saline purgatives, as the potassio-tartrate of soda.

When the inflammatory symptoms have been removed, and the jaundice persists unchanged, or when evidences of inflammation have not been present, and the constitution is not much impaired, then two or three grains of calomel, or of blue-pill, or chalk and mercury, may be occasionally combined with aloes or rhubarb.

To give large doses of calomel forms no part of the treatment of jaundice, unless we except the early stages of occasional cases in plethoric Europeans, in whom there is good reason for suspecting a congested and stagnant condition of the portal circulation.

The error, to which I have already on several occasions alluded, of confounding the cholagogue action with the constitutional effect of mercury, has been frequently committed in the treatment of jaundice. The induction of mercurial influence in this disease is unsupported by any rational argument with which I am acquainted.

When that state of constitution in which, on general principles, we abstain from the use of mercurial remedies, co-exists with jaundice, we may use some of the other milder means which are believed to exercise a similar action on the liver, as taraxacum, alkalies, hydrochlorate of ammonia, nitric acid internally, and nitro-muriatic acid externally.

It should be further remembered, as previously stated in reference to jaundice complicating remittent fever, that saline diuretics are often given with great advantage; and, as a rule of practice in this disease, it should also be recollected that time is required for the removal of the bile from the blood, and that we may err by too great haste or too active interference.

SECTION VI.—*On Increased and Defective Secretion of Bile.*

Increased Secretion.—That bilious diarrhœa and cholera may attack Europeans not long resident in India, after injudicious exposure and excesses in eating and drinking, is true, but that they are common affections under any other circumstances is not confirmed by experience.*

Excess of biliary secretion is a rare disorder in the European who lives with ordinary prudence in India, and in the native it is hardly ever observed. The chief importance of bilious cholera is the risk of confounding it with epidemic cholera. The diagnosis of the two affections has been stated in general terms at p. 213. The mistake is not likely to occur to a careful inquirer. The pathology of bilious cholera is very simple. From excess of the constituents of bile in the blood, and active determination of blood in the portal capillaries, an undue quantity of bile is secreted, and as a necessary consequence is speedily ejected.

The leading indication of treatment is to palliate the discomfort by diluents, to allay the vomiting by effervescing draughts, with a few minims of tincture of opium, and the external use of sinapisms, and to watch for symptoms of prostration, and then give opium more freely, as well as stimulants. After the primary symptoms have ceased, gastro-enteritis may follow, and require to be treated on ordinary principles, by leeches, alkalies, ipecacuanha, opium, and perhaps mild mercurials.

The question whether, at the commencement, the discharge of bile ought to be increased or not by the cholagogue action of mercury, will arise. If the subject be a robust European, if the tongue be much coated, and there is tendency to jaundice, or uneasiness of the hepatic region, with signs of enlargement of the liver, then it will be of advantage to give ten grains of calomel with a grain of opium, to be repeated or not, according to circumstances; and the effervescing draught may be made slightly aperient by the addition of small doses of the potassio-tartrate of soda, or other saline cathartic.

* Subsequently to the expression of this opinion, the following statement of Dr. Marshall came under my notice:—

"It may be observed, that the cholera morbus of the systematic writers, a complaint which is supposed to arise from an inordinate secretion of bile, very rarely occurs in Ceylon, either among European residents or the indigenous inhabitants." — *Notes on the Medical Topography and prevailing Diseases of Ceylon*, p. 145, by Henry Marshall, Staff-Surgeon to the Forces.

Defect of biliary secretion, characterised by clay-coloured alvine discharges,—a state to which the name torpor of the liver has been given,—is sufficiently common in India.

Torpor of the liver is an unsuitable term, for it expresses a pathological theory which is probably erroneous, and suggests a system of treatment which is often injurious.

The symptoms are white-coloured alvine discharges, often formed and not passed with more than usual frequency, a sense of languor, depression and anorexia, and a pale but little coated, tongue, without jaundice. This derangement occurs for the most part in adults, cachectic and anæmic from malarious influence, prolonged exposure to elevated temperature, abuse of mercurial or other depressant remedies. Mental anxiety is in these states of constitution sometimes the exciting cause. Anæmic children are also liable to this affection, and in Bombay it is observed in them more towards the close of the hot season than at any other period of the year.

That this condition proceeds from torpor of the liver is an improbable theory. There is absence of bile in the intestinal canal, but also absence of it in the blood (jaundice). The just inference from these facts, is, not that the liver, specially, is inactive, but that the metamorphosis of waste tissue into the excreta of bile is not duly carried on in the blood. All the attendant phenomena point to languid general assimilation and excretion, and the leading indication of cure is, not to stimulate the liver by cholagogue remedies, but to lessen the cachectic state by appropriate regimen and tonics.

While holding these opinions on the pathology of this affection*, I would caution against neglect in inquiring into the state of the liver; for a pre-existing defect of the organ, congestive or organic, will necessarily favour a more early development of the symptoms, and when existing ought to receive due consideration in the treatment.

We shall best treat this derangement by a suitable adjustment of diet, of which animal food should form a part. In two cases the use of strong coffee two or three times in the day, seemed to be beneficial, and in one it restored the secretions to a healthy state,

* Anæmic European children, sent at the close of the hot season of Bombay to Poona at the commencement of the rains, or to Mahubuleshwur at the end of October, are very apt, unless there be great attention to the temperature and action of the skin, to be affected with clay-coloured alvine discharges. Under these circumstances the presence of some degree of congestion of the liver is a probable event, and should always be looked for.

after various preparations of taraxacum had been freely used and failed. It is worthy of further trial, but the coffee must be genuine and fresh. Should observation confirm this impression, the result will probably be explained on Liebig's theory of the identity of caffeine and the principle of bile. Along with appropriate regimen, such remedies as quinine, bitter infusions, iron in small doses, or dilute nitric acid should be used. Change to a more temperate climate will be of benefit, but considerable and sudden reductions of temperature should be avoided. Under all circumstances external cold or damp must be guarded against by suitable clothing.

If deficiency of bile be truly related to anæmic or cachectic states, then it may be predicted that under a rational sanitary system and better therapeutic principles, it will cease to be familiar, as now, to the practitioner in India.

Though the use of cholagogue remedies has not been distinctly admitted, yet reflection will suggest that the milder members of the class may occasionally be beneficial. It is reasonable to suppose that even with an improving condition of the blood, the hepatic cells, in consequence of suspension of function, may evince a want of readiness in assuming it again, and that special remedies may be useful under these circumstances. Whether this theory be just or not, still I believe that the inference drawn from it is practically correct, viz., that though any but the most guarded use of mercurials is sure to be injurious, we may always look for benefit from such means as taraxacum, coffee, and the external application of diluted nitro-muriatic acid by sponging or stupes.

Children with deficiency of biliary secretion are very predisposed to dysentery; but in this fact there is probably nothing more than an illustration of the general predisposing influence of anæmic and cachectic states.

CHAP. XVII.

ON PERITONITIS, ILEUS AND COLIC.

SECTION I.—*Peritonitis.—Pathology.—Plastic and sero-puriform Exudations related to Diathesis.—Chronic Tubercular.—Chronic not Tubercular, and not Consecutive on Acute.—Treatment.*

IN the chapters on Dysentery and Hepatitis it has been shown that acute general peritonitis, secondary on the advanced stage of dysentery, or the formation of hepatic abscess—but independent of perforation or rupture,—is not an uncommon event in the course of those diseases in India, and is, in all probability, favoured by constitutional states. A secondary partial protective peritonitis is likewise not unfrequent.

But *acute idiopathic general peritonitis* in a sthenic diathesis, independent of traumatic causes, is a rare form of disease in India, as in other countries. In the notes of my own practice there is not a single illustrative case. On examining my memoranda of fatal cases of sick officers, I find seven of peritonitis, which is in the ratio of 2·25 per cent. of the deaths from all causes. But of these seven there are only three which can be regarded as idiopathic and sthenic. Two of them occurred in officers consequent on exposure to cold after fatigue in the heat of the day. The third was caused by excesses in eating.

It is of interest to note carefully all fatal cases of *traumatic* general peritonitis, for they may demonstrate the morbid changes which result from this inflammation in persons of good diathesis, and afford more precise knowledge than we can otherwise obtain, of the length of time requisite for their development. Much interest also attaches to those slighter wounds, which though penetrating the abdomen—as proved by slight visceral protrusion—and followed by distinct peritonitis, are amenable to judicious treatment. They are so, because the tendency of inflammation under circumstances of moderate injury and good diathesis is not to extend, but to be restricted to the neighbourhood of the wound, and to yield to the repeated use of leeches, opium, warm water stupes, and complete repose: I have seen several cases which illustrate the truth of this observation. Three fatal cases of traumatic peritonitis* are subjoined: —

188. *General peritonitis from a penetrating wound of the liver. — Considerable effusion of serum in the head without symptoms.* — James Harrison, aged twenty-eight, born in India, tall, and of moderate strength, was admitted into the European General Hospital on the night of the 22nd October, 1838. He stated that, whilst in a state of intoxication, he had stabbed himself.* On the left side of the epigastrium there was a wound about an inch long, filled with charcoal and oil, but apparently not deeper than the muscles. It was attended with considerable tenderness of the abdomen. Twenty ounces of blood were taken from the arm, and a purgative enema was exhibited. On the morning of the 24th he still complained of general tenderness of the abdomen, attended with considerable fulness. The pulse was 120 and compressible; the tongue was covered with a thin yellow fur; there was present a short cough, from which he had suffered for some days previously; there was, however, neither vomiting nor difficulty in micturition. One hundred leeches were applied to the abdomen, and in the evening, the symptoms, having somewhat increased, twelve ounces of blood were taken from the arm, and seventy-two leeches were repeated to the abdomen; the warm bath was directed to be used, and pills of calomel and opium to be given at bed-time. On the 25th he was considerably relieved; but on the evening of the 26th the symptoms of peritonitic inflammation were again on the increase; a large blister was applied to the abdomen, and a turpentine enema exhibited. On the 27th the pulse was 120 and feeble, the countenance anxious, and there was occasional vomiting. An attempt was made to induce the action of mercury on the system by inunction, and the internal exhibition of calomel and opium. The pain was never very acute, but the symptoms progressed, and he died at 10 P.M. of the 28th.

Inspection nine hours after death. — Body stout; abdomen distended. — *Abdomen.* On tracing the wound, it was found to penetrate transversely the lower edge of the sixth rib on the left side also, the entire of the cartilage of the seventh rib, about a quarter of an inch from its junction with the other cartilages. The wound passed through the diaphragm and through the left lobe of the liver, and was about half an inch in its long diameter. The intestines adhered to the abdominal parietes, and the convolutions to each other; and among the adhesions there was much extravasation of dark bloody serum. In the pelvis, between the rectum and bladder, and in the right iliac region, there was much dark coagulated blood. All the intestines were distended with air; but, with the exception of the lymph effused on the peritoneal surface they were healthy. The liver was pale coloured. The mucous coat of the stomach was thickened, but otherwise healthy. *Chest.* — The lungs were emphysematous. In the lower lateral part of the left side of the chest there were flakes of lymph effused on the costal pleura, and blood extravasated in small quantity underneath the pleura of the diaphragm. *Head.* — There was considerable effusion of serum between the pia mater and arachnoid membrane, and at the base of the skull; also considerable venous congestion of the posterior lobes of the brain.

189. *Fracture of both thigh bones. — Abdomen bruised. — Death in fifty-four hours from peritonitis. — General redness and effusion of lymph on the peritoneal sur-*

---

* The knife was shown to me on the following morning; it was a blunt, somewhat rusty, worn, table carving knife.

faces.—*A pint of turbid serum in the cavity.*—John Birch, aged twenty-two, of the ship *Cornea* was brought to the General Hospital at 4½ P.M. of the 5th March, 1842. It was stated that he had just fallen from the yard-arm of the ship on deck; both thigh bones were fractured about the middle of the shaft; the abdomen was bruised and tender to the touch; and the breathing was oppressed and attended with sense of sinking. He passed an indifferent night, and on the morning of the 7th the tenderness and tension of abdomen had increased, and the pulse was feeble. Fomentations and enemata were used. Towards evening the tension of the abdomen had increased, and there was pain of left side complained of, with oppressed breathing. Pulse small, 120. He died at 10 P.M.

Inspection twelve hours after death.—Purple sugillations on the posterior part of the trunk. The abdomen distended. *Chest.*—The right lung adhered firmly to the costal pleura. In the left sac of the pleura about six ounces of red-coloured serum were effused. The lungs and the heart were healthy. *Abdomen.*—The intestines were distended with air. The external surface of all the intestines was of a brown red colour. The omentum was matted over the intestines, and adhered to them by bands of friable lymph, and similar adhesions existed between their convolutions. In the cavity of the abdomen there was about a pint of brown turbid serum effused. The liver and spleen were healthy. The mucous coat of the stomach was healthy.

190. *Wound of the abdomen with protrusion of intestine.*—*Vascularity of, and lymph-exudation on the peritoneum and the protruded intestine.*—A man was brought to the Native General Hospital at 9 A.M. of the 24th February, 1845, with a considerable portion of the small intestine, and a part of the attached mesentery, protruding from a wound between the umbilicus and margin of the right ribs, to the right of the mesial line. It had been inflicted by himself about three hours before. The intestine was of a bright red colour. The wound was small, and it was enlarged with the view of reducing the intestine. But, in consequence of the opposition and struggles of the individual, reduction could not be effected. The following morning, at 7 A.M., the protruded intestine, now consisting of several convolutions, was covered with a tolerably thick layer of friable red-coloured lymph, which united the protruded convolutions to each other.

Remark.—Thus, assuming the intestine to have been healthy before, we find active vascularity in the course of three hours after protrusion, followed by effusion of a layer of lymph in twenty-four hours—a process, however, which must have commenced many hours earlier. I do not find the date of death in my notes, which were made merely to record the periods of vascularity and exudation.

When attention is turned from peritonitis in individuals of good constitution, characterised by exudation of plastic lymph, to that form in which puriform or sero-puriform effusion predominates, we shall always find this difference of result attributable to conditions of diathesis.

In the first of the three cases * about to be narrated, the special character of the cachexia does not appear,—the patient is merely stated to have been long ill. The second is related to parturition; and the third is a case of circumscribed purulent effusion, probably due to cachexia from intemperance. These, however, form but a small portion of the cases of this nature which, at different times, have come under my observation. There is reason for believing that among the cachectic natives received into general hospitals

* Cases 191 to 193.

in India, death is not unfrequently hastened by the access of aplastic peritonitis, overlooked during life in consequence of the latency of the symptoms. I have more than once seen patients, under these circumstances, sink with cooling skin, collapsing features, thready pulse, and no suspicion of peritonitis; yet examination after death has proved its existence. When, in cachetic states, unexpected prostration, unexplained by discharges, comes on, we shall do well to direct our attention to the peritoneum.

191. *Peritonitis.—Purulent effusion into the cavity of the abdomen.—Lymph general on the peritoneal surfaces.*—Robert Piper, aged sixteen, seaman, ship *Oriental*, after having been unwell for a long time, chiefly with recurring constipation of the bowels, was admitted into the General Hospital on the 9th August, 1842. The abdomen was uneasy on pressure, but quite supple. Till the 16th he continued complaining of occasional pain of abdomen, and had generally an evening accession of fever. Leeches were applied two or three times; the bowels were kept open with laxatives, and an attempt was made to control the febrile accessions by the exhibition of quinine. On the 17th, the tenderness of abdomen was increased, and the pulse rose to 120, and was irritable. On the 19th, to the pain was added fulness and tenderness of abdomen, which had considerably increased by the 21st with occasional vomiting; and pyrexial symptoms were generally present. Leeches were again had recourse to, followed by blisters, and an attempt was made to induce the constitutional effect of mercury. On the 28th, wandering delirium commenced. The other symptoms persisted with increasing failure of strength, and he died on the 2nd September.

Inspection fifteen hours after death.—Body emaciated. Abdomen distended. In the abdomen there was about a pint of pus; and the interior surface of the parietes, the omentum, and the external surface of the small intestine were more or less coated with a thin layer of lymph. The body was not further examined.

192. *Peritonitis after parturition, but probably caused by blows.*—Mary Anne, a native Christian, of twenty-three years of age, was admitted into hospital, on the 26th November, 1848. She stated that she had been affected with diarrhœa for about a month. That three days before admission she had given birth to a child which had died: that two and a half hours before admission she had been kicked on the chest and abdomen. There was tenderness of the abdomen about the umbilicus, the extremities were cold, the pulse 120 and thready, the countenance collapsed. She was treated with ammoniated stimulants and opium, sinapisms and fomentations. She continued in the sunken state as on admission, with frequent vomiting and little vaginal discharge, and died on the 28th.

Inspection seventeen hours after death.—The abdomen was considerably distended; there were no marks of bruises on the external surface. There was general redness, with lymph effusion on the peritoneal surface of the small intestine, the omentum was matted to the fundus of the uterus, and there was about a pint of purulent effusion in the pelvis. The uterus, upwards of six inches long and four wide, rose like a flaccid bag above the pubes, inclined to and occupied the right iliac fossa. There was lymph on its peritoneal surface, but no redness or purulent infiltration of its structure. The inner surface as well as upper part of the vagina was lined with grey and black pultaceous adhesive matter with gangrenous fœtor, and the lining membrane when exposed by removal of the adherent exudation presented a red colour. The mucous membrane of the colon showed numerous circular ulcers.

193. *Partial peritonitis leading to formation of a large circumscribed purulent sac.*—Dewjee Gunnoo, a Hindoo horse-keeper, of twenty-five years of age, using spirits oc-

casionally, was, after two months' illness, admitted into the clinical ward, on the 18th August, 1851. He was a good deal reduced. The countenance was anxious, and the respiration thoracic. A large, prominent, distinctly circumscribed, somewhat elastic, and obscurely fluctuating swelling occupied the abdomen. It extended from the ensiform cartilage almost to the pubes. It engaged more of the right than of the left side of the abdomen. The right boundary was a vertical line dropped from the ninth rib, but the left a line passing obliquely from the seventh rib to the left of the umbilicus, and reaching the right iliac fossa. The swelling was dull throughout on percussion, it was tender on pressure, and pain was increased by decubitus on the left side. No abnormal chest signs. The pulse was small, the bowels were regular. He stated that, two months before, he had noticed a small swelling below the margin of the right ribs unattended by pain, that twenty-five days before admission this swelling, subsequent to the action of a purgative, had disappeared, but it reappeared after eight or nine days, and was situated more in the direction of the umbilicus, and since had gradually increased to its present size. He further added that he attributed his complaint to pressure made by some friends, a month before admission, for the purpose of relieving pain that existed there. He was under treatment till the 3rd September, when he died. During his stay in hospital there were irregular febrile exacerbations, with night sweats, and the swelling increased in size, and became more tense, and prominent, and painful. His friends would not permit a post mortem examination, but they did not object to the introduction of a trocar and canula, which were inserted a little above, and an inch and a half to the right of the umbilicus. On removing the trocar about half an ounce of reddish-coloured fluid escaped through the canula, and on making a good deal of pressure on the tumour, about eight ounces of flaky pus, mixed with coagula of dark-looking blood, were slowly drawn off. It was necessary, frequently, to clear out the canula, as it became stopped up with the flakes of pus. The tumour, after the removal of the pus, had not diminished much in size, but had become much softer.

Remark.—Many years ago I saw a case similar to this, both in situation and size, in an old Hindoo tailor, in company with Dr. Bird. At the urgent entreaty of the patient the fluid, of dark-red colour, was drawn off by a small trocar. The operation perhaps rather hurried the fatal issue.

Chronic Tubercular Peritonitis is an interesting and well-understood form of disease. I find among my cases four * of tubercular peritonitis. Two in Europeans, with tubercular deposit in the lungs, and two in natives without this complication. In one of the Europeans † the intestines were firmly adherent to each other, and tubercular deposit was intermixed with the organised tissue. In the second European ‡ the tubercles were miliary and semi-transparent, without adhesions, and with very little serous effusion. The appearance presented in this case by the tubercles on the diaphragmatic peritoneum of the right side was of interest; they were compressed by the liver into flattened patches, instead of standing in granular relief as elsewhere. I do not find this effect of pressure mentioned by any author, and yet some, Dr. West for example, particularly allude to the diaphragm and the surface of the liver as common seats of granular tubercular formation.

* Cases 194 to 197. † 194. ‡ 195.

In both natives there was abundant serous effusion, and the disease had been considered to be ascites. In one * the effusion disappeared consequent on an attack of cholera. In my remarks annexed to this case, attention has been called to the evidence which it affords that the peritoneum, studded with tubercles, is still fitted for absorption; and to the fact, that the supply of fluid derived from a peritonitic and pleuritic effusion delayed the fatal result.

In the other native † case there is a feature of diagnostic importance. The diagnosis of peritonitic effusion from ovarian dropsy, by percussion, is now well understood: that in the former, we generally have clearness of the uppermost surface of the swelling; in the latter, dulness all over.

Dr. Watson directs attention to two exceptional conditions which in peritoneal effusion may occasion dulness throughout as in ovarian dropsy. 1. When the distention is so great as not to admit of the floating intestines reaching the surface of the fluid. 2. When the intestines are fixed down by adhesions. Case 196 points to a third cause, viz., a contracted state of the intestinal canal in an asthenic person who, for some time previously, had used very little food. This explanation, suggested to my mind before death, was confirmed by dissection. The uniform character of the swelling and the history forbad the belief in ovarian dropsy.

194. *General peritonitis.—The lungs studded with crude tubercles.—The mesenteric glands tuberculated.—The end of the ileum, the cœcum, and colon ulcerated.—Considerable effusion in the head.*—Daniel Rumbell, aged twenty-two, of slight habit, a marine on board Her Majesty's sloop *Cruizer*, was admitted into the European General Hospital on the 19th December, 1838. During the six previous months he had suffered from frequent attacks of catarrh excited by slight exposure to cold, and latterly attended with œdematous swelling of the feet. His general health had also become much impaired. He was debilitated and emaciated, and complained of pain at the epigastrium, and across the lower part of the chest, also of dyspnœa and dry cough. The pulse was generally frequent, and there were profuse nocturnal sweats. On admission into hospital pain across the epigastrium, increased by pressure and full inspiration, was complained of; the tongue was florid but not furred; there was thirst, but no vomiting. He complained of occasional dry cough, and the pulse was 96, of good strength. During the thirteen first days of his residence in hospital, attention was chiefly directed to the abdomen, which was moderately distended and tense, with, on one or two occasions, an obscure sense of fluctuation. There was also generally tenderness on pressure, but at no time acute. The tongue was usually florid, and every evening there was a distinct febrile exacerbation. The abdomen was leeched and blistered, and on one occasion ten ounces of blood were taken from the arm. Small doses of calomel and opium were given, but the mouth did not become affected. On the 2nd of January, dyspnœa and uneasiness across the chest were complained of, and sibilous and subcrepitous rales were audible on the anterior part. The feet became œdematous, and

* Case 197. † 196.

the pulse increased in frequency and lost in strength. A blister was applied to the chest with relief; two grains of pulv. scillæ, in combination with a grain of calomel, half a grain of ipecacuanha, and a similar quantity of opium, were given thrice daily. The urine was examined, but found not coagulable. On the 4th of January there was diarrhœa for the first time during his stay in hospital, it recurred from time to time; the evening febrile exacerbations persisted; the pulse became feebler; emaciation increased, and he died on the 15th. The pectoral symptoms were not, with exception of on the 2nd of January, much complained of.

Inspection four hours after death.—Body emaciated. *Head.*—There were about three ounces of serum in the cavity of the head. *Chest.*—The liver had encroached on the cavity of the chest to the level of the third rib on both sides, and the heart was in consequence placed more transversely than is natural. The pericardium contained several ounces of serum. Both lungs adhered firmly to the costal pleuræ; and in both, there was abundant deposition of crude grey tubercles, with emphysema. *Abdomen.*—There was no distention. The peritoneal lining of the parietes, and all the viscera, with the omentum, were firmly united by adventitious adhesions. Between the layers of these adhesions there was serum in some places, and in others nodules and masses of firm, almost schirrous lymph, frequently of tubercular form. The liver was much enlarged and firm, and the cut surface presented a white mottled appearance. The spleen was also enlarged, its texture was firm, and part of the edge was matted to the left lobe of the liver by means of a thick mass of lymph. The mesentery was much thickened, and when cut showed the glands enlarged, and in many places undergoing tubercular degeneration. The mucous lining of the stomach was of a pale rosy tint, and softened. The mucous coat at the end of the ileum for the extent of several feet presented large transverse ulcerated bands. Some of which, on the separation of the peritoneal adhesions, opened into the cavity of the abdomen. The cœcum was in a similar state of ulceration, but the transverse part of the colon was undiseased. The right kidney was healthy. The left was of chocolate-red colour.

195. *Extensive ulcer on the groin.—Miliary tubercles in the lungs and underneath the peritoneum throughout its whole extent.—Follicular ulceration of the large intestine.—Three ounces of serum in the cavity of the cranium.—No head symptoms.*—Charles Sutherland, aged twenty-four, a seaman, of fair complexion and strumous habit, was first admitted into the hospital on the 16th October, 1838, affected with extensive ulceration of the left groin, and of the under and upper part of the thigh of the same side. This affection was of several months' duration, and was attributed to a venereal sore, with which he had been affected some time previously. He remained in hospital without improvement till the 17th January, when being impatient from the tedious nature of his illness, and at the want of success attending the treatment, he was discharged at his own desire. He was re-admitted on the 17th February, having been during his absence from hospital under the care of a Hakeem in the bazaar, who had used various applications, and given internal remedies, in consequence of which the mouth had become affected. At this second admission the ulcer on the groin had a more unhealthy appearance, its edges being ragged and irregular; that on the thigh had become double its former size, and had also irregular ragged edges. Sarsaparilla and hydriodate of potass were prescribed and continued for some time, and the applications to the ulcers were frequently varied. The ulcers did not improve in appearance, the general health declined, and on the 9th April he first complained of cough with scanty expectoration. The cough continued more or less troublesome, chiefly so during the three weeks immediately succeeding its first appearance. The ulcers were generally stationary, sometimes, however, for a few days assuming a more healthy appearance, and then again relapsing. The strength declined; night sweats became troublesome, the cough ceased; and on the 19th June diarrhœa commenced, and was more or less urgent, and attended with florid tongue, till the period of death on the 15th July.

Inspection six hours after death. — Body emaciated; abdomen collapsed. *Head.*— There was no turgescence of the vessels, and there were about three ounces of serum at the base of the skull. *Chest.* — There were adhesions of the upper lobe of the right lung to the anterior parietes, and opposed to these adhesions there was a crude tuberculous nodule the size of a walnut. The lowest lobe of the right lung was moderately congested with frothy serum. The upper lobe of the left lung was healthy; the lowest part of the lower lobe was in a state of red hepatisation, and at the upper part, and immediately below the pleura, there were miliary tubercles deposited. The heart was healthy. *Abdomen.* — There were about five ounces of clear serum in the cavity of the pelvis. Over the peritoneal lining of the lateral part of the abdomen, of the pelvis, and of much of the intestines, there was a blush of ramified redness, and the tunic was studded in these places with isolated miliary tubercles, transparent, none larger than a pin's head, and many smaller; in many instances they seemed to constitute the termination of a vascular ramification. Underneath the peritoneal lining of the diaphragm where opposed to the liver there was a similar tubercular deposition, but here, instead of standing in relief, it was compressed into flattened patches — a modification evidently caused by the resistance of the liver, because, on the left side of the diaphgram, where there was no resisting object, the tubercles stood out in relief as elsewhere. These appearances where much more developed on the right than on the left side of the abdomen. The mucous coat of the stomach was dotted dark red at the cardiac end, but it was healthy in texture; towards the pylorus it was mammillated and thickened. The liver was pale and mottled. The mucous coat at the end of the ileum was vascular and studded with mucous glands. The mucous coat of the colon and rectum was studded with ulcerated follicles, and in some cicatrisation had commenced. Here and there there were patches of reddish lymph, with occasionally a yellow central point like a tubercle. The mesenteric glands ranged in size from a pea to a horse bean, but they were not tuberculated. The kidneys were healthy.

196. *Chronic peritonitis.* — *Tubercular.* — *Much effusion, and complete dulness on percussion.* — Ramni Penack, aged fifty, a Hindoo female, much emaciated, was admitted on the 28th July, 1852. The abdomen was swollen, tense, fluctuating, *dull all over on percussion.* The dulness rising to the fourth rib on both sides. The feet and legs were œdematous; the rest of the chest was resonant, and vesicular respiration was distinct. The sounds of the heart were natural. There was no increased heat of skin. Pulse small, and very easily compressed. Tongue coated brown in the centre; urine scanty; bowels confined for five or six days. She stated that twenty days before admission there had been pain below the ribs, and that eight days afterwards the abdomen began to swell, and was attended by difficulty of breathing. She died at 3 P.M. of the 30th.

Inspection seventeen hours after death. — *Abdomen.*—About fourteen pints of turbid yellowish serum were found in the sac of the peritoneum. The intestines were in general much contracted, and occupied the left lumbar region, but were not fixed by adhesions. On the surface of the intestines here and there slight redness was seen. Studding the mesentery and the inner surface of the abdominal walls, chiefly at the hypogastric region, and also the pelvic viscera (bladder, rectum and ileum), were numerous miliary tubercles, ranging from the size of a mustard-seed to a small pea, and situated in the subserous tissue. Firm adhesions connected the under surface of the right lobe of the liver to the upper ends of the right kidney. The liver was smaller than natural, but did not feel indurated when incised. The gall-bladder was full of bile. The kidneys were somewhat smaller than natural, and externally mottled red and white, finely granular, and presenting numerous serous cysts. One of the cysts in the right kidney, when laid open, was found to contain puriform matter, which showed under the microscope broken-down pus corpuscles. The cortical portion of both kindeys defective. Lungs healthy; heart healthy. There was atheromatous deposit on the aortic valves.

197. *Effusion in chest and abdomen.—Access of cholera.—Disappearance of the effusions.—Bright's disease of the kidney and tubercular peritonitis.*—Mooburick Nuseeb, an African, of fifty-eight years of age, was admitted into the clinical ward on the 10th of September, 1849. He was somewhat emaciated; the abdomen was swollen, tense, and fluctuating, and somewhat tender on pressure. On the left side of the chest there was dulness below the level of the third rib, varying with change of posture, accompanied with absence of vocal thrill, and the heart's impulse was most distinctly felt to the right of the sternum. There was no febrile disturbance observed, but he complained of nausea and abdominal distention and discomfort after eating. The pulse was small, of natural frequency. The tongue not coated, but somewhat florid at the tip, and the bowels occasionally relaxed. He stated that he had been ill fifteen days, and that the uneasiness and fulness of abdomen had come on gradually during that period. On the 15th and 19th the urine was examined; its specific gravity was about 1020, and it gave no traces of albumen with heat and nitric acid. On the 20th, the occasional diarrhœa from which he had suffered since admission, passed into distinct cholera, and he died on the 26th. The rice-water-like discharges continued more or less abundant till the 23rd. The pulse became feebler, but remained distinct till shortly before death. The surface of the body was sometimes cold, at others regained its natural temperature. The urine was passed scantily on the 23rd and 25th. Drowsiness first showed itself on the evening of the 21st, and he became quite comatose before death. On the 21st the fulness and tenseness of the abdomen were much lessened; the thoracic dulness extended no higher than the fifth rib, and the heart's impulse was less to the right of the sternum. On the 25th the abdominal fulness and the thoracic dulness had almost entirely disappeared, and the heart's impulse was most distinct between the third and fourth ribs of the left side, an inch from the margin of the sternum.

Inspection twelve hours after death.—Chest.—There was not any serous effusion found in the sac of the left pleura, and the left lung was soft and crepitating. Two or three bands of firm adhesion connected the inner surface of the lung to the pericardium. The right lung was also soft and crepitating, and united by old adhesions to the costal pleura. There were no traces in the costal or pulmonary pleura of recent inflammatory action. A larger than normal portion of the heart was to the right of the mesial line. There were opaque patches here and there on the surface of the heart. A slight degree of dilatation of the left ventricle, and of thickening of the mitral valve, was observed; the right ventricle, and the aortic valves, were healthy. *Abdomen.*—The whole of the peritoneal covering of the anterior parietes was closely beset with granular deposits, each granule was about the size of a small pin's head. Similar deposit was also present on the peritoneal surface of the intestines, and the convolutions were closely and firmly adherent to one another, and, in places, here and there, to the anterior parietes chiefly below the umbilicus. The concave surface of the liver adhered to the stomach, and to the hepatic flexure of the colon, and also by old and firm adhesions to the diaphragm. There was no serous fluid in the cavity of the abdomen. The liver was harder than natural, resisting to the knife, and granular. The left kidney was considerably enlarged and flabby; and when incised the surface showed, chiefly in the body of the organ, considerable encroachment on the tubular portion by a pale buff finely granular structure. The external surface, on removal of the capsule, presented a finely mottled appearance (red and yellow). A similar state of the right kidney existed, in greater degree. The *Head* was not examined.

Remarks.—This case occurred at a time when cholera was prevalent. It presents several points of considerable interest. The abdominal effusion, co-existing with a pleuritic effusion, was due in all probability to the kidney disease, not to the pre-existing, and probably not recent, tubercular peritonitis. The incomplete collapse, and the long course of the cholera attack, are to be attributed to the replacement, from the pleuritic and abdominal effusions, of the water of the blood lost in the intestinal discharges. It shows that endosmosis and exosmosis may go on freely from a serous surface studded with grey granular deposit. It is an instance of this deposit present in the peritoneum, but absent in the lungs.

Chronic peritonitis consecutive on an acute attack, and tubercular peritonitis, chronic in its character from the commencement, are well known to pathologists. But I apprehend that idiopathic peritonitis, not tubercular, yet chronic from its outset, is not a form of disease very generally recognised.

Mr. Scott, now Inspector-General of Hospitals of the Bombay Army, at the time Surgeon of the 10th Regiment Bombay Native Infantry, called attention*, in 1842, to a very interesting form of disease which he correctly designated "Chronic Peritonitis."

The regiment was stationed at Aden at a time when, from defective arrangements, a scorbutic taint was prevalent among the native classes there, and rheumatic affections were also common.

The disease in question was most prevalent at the commencement of the cold season, and the symptoms, as observed in twenty-nine cases, were of the following nature:—There was uneasiness on pressure, or a sense of pricking or heat about the umbilicus with anorexia, distention after eating, and subsequently vomiting. The urine was scanty and high coloured, but there was no febrile heat. So little importance did the sepoys attach to these symptoms, that, in some cases, they had been present for a week or two before application was made for admission into hospital. Then signs of effusion into the abdomen succeeded at varying periods. Sometimes the men did not report themselves ill till effusion had commenced; and in others, the effusion began to appear three or four days after admission. In some there was jaundice and enlargement of the liver. A few cases, treated at the commencement, after the true nature of the disease had been determined, are believed to have recovered; but all in whom effusion had taken place, died within a month from its appearance. A post mortem examination was made in three cases. In all, the liver was hard and granular, the peritoneum was opaque; and in two there were extensive deposits of coagulable lymph among the intestines. The kidneys were healthy.

There can be no doubt that the disease was chronic peritonitis. Mr. Scott attributed it to a rheumatic diathesis which prevailed to

* "Transactions, Bombay Medical and Physical Society," No. 6, p. 153.

a considerable extent. His words are: "Perhaps what excites rheumatic pains in the muscles and joints of one man, fixes on the peritoneum in another, and creates this complaint."

When we bear in mind that Mr. Scott's report was written at a time when diathetic disease did not occupy the place in pathology which has since been accorded to it, and when little notice was taken in medical writings of rheumatic pneumonia, pleuritis, or bronchitis, it must be allowed that the words just quoted are conceived in a spirit of happy suggestion.

I would only further add that Rokitansky, and probably other pathologists also, recognise a rheumatic form of peritonitis.

On the *treatment* of peritonitis, generally, I shall be very brief.

Of the utility of general and local blood-letting, the use of opium, and gentle mercurial influence in the early stages of idiopathic peritonitis in a good constitution, there can be no question; but it must be recollected that the proportion of this form of the disease is very small. There can be no doubt that the too ready association of antiphlogistic remedies with the name peritonitis has been attended with injurious consequences in practice.

General peritonitis, secondary on other serious forms of abdominal disease, or idiopathic in cachectic constitutions, ought not to be treated by much blood-letting, or mercury. It is true that in these forms the chances of recovery are very limited; but they should not be still lessened by injudicious treatment. There ought not, in these conditions of peritonitis, associated as they generally are with marked collapse, to be any hesitation in setting antiphlogistic means altogether aside, and in trusting to opium,—after the manner recommended by Dr. Stokes,—with rubefacients, and stimulants to sustain the failing pulse.

In the chronic forms of the disease we shall have further to keep in view the character of the diathesis, and the means, gently eliminatory or other, which science may suggest for its removal or improvement. The injury often caused by active purgatives, in the treatment of peritonitis, is well enforced by Dr. Watson in his excellent lectures, and is I apprehend, now universally assented to.

SECTION II.—*Ileus and Colic.*

Setting aside cases of strangulated hernia, the instances of *ileus*, which have come before me, are few in number.

The first of the two following cases came under my observation at Kirkee, in the hospital of the 4th Dragoons, and is of the form depending upon paralysis of muscular fibre, consequent on commencing inflammation (enteritis), which Dr. Abercombie has so well illustrated in his writings. In the second, a portion of the small intestine was strangulated by old adhesions resulting from former peritonitis. To Mr. Carter I am indebted for the notes and the opportunity of inspecting the morbid appearances of a case which had come under his care. In this the obstruction was from colloid-cancerous degeneration of the sigmoid flexure. It is the only instance of malignant disease of the alimentary canal which has come under my notice.

198. *Ileus, with granular effusion on the inner surface of the ileum.—Biliary calculi.*—Mrs. Horton, aged thirty-seven, admitted into the hospital of the 4th Light Dragoons, September 6th, 1832. A few months in India. Had been for some years subject to occasional pain in the abdomen, with constipated bowels; good health in the intervals. Had an attack some months ago in Bombay, also another about ten days since, from which she recovered under the use of purgatives and leeching. In the course of the day of admission, had been affected with violent pain of abdomen; belly tender. Little vomiting. Actively treated, leeched, blistered. Some dark-coloured stools procured after the use of active purgatives and enemata. Pain undiminished, insensibility; moaning and sinking on the 7th. Died early on the 8th.

Inspection six hours after death.—Abdomen distended and tense, the integuments loaded with fat; a small quantity of serum in the cavity of the peritoneum. On the incisions being made, the intestines protruded, distended with gas and fluid. The ileum externally, principally at its most dependent parts, was dark red, and vascular, with very slight and partial exudation of flakes of lymph. There were old firm adhesions at the upper part of the ascending colon, which connected it firmly to the whole surface of the gall-bladder, and to the thin edge of the right lobe of the liver. The gall-bladder shriveled, contained no bile, but was filled with small angular earthy concretions. In portions of the descending colon and sigmoid flexure there were contractions for some extent, but no unnatural condition of the tissues. The lower end of the ileum to a considerable extent, also the cœcum, were laid open. Where the peritoneum was discoloured, there the inner surface of the ileum presented a similar discoloration, and there more especially, and elsewhere also, for the extent of about two feet, there was effusion on the inner coat of the ileum of fine granules, forming an aspect as if a moist surface had been sprinkled with fine sand: this effusion, with the thin mucous tunic, peeled easily off with the nail. The large intestine also, in part distended, contained, as well as the small, thin light-coloured feculence; no scybalous matter, no obliteration of the cells of the colon. The upper part of the descending colon was marked with red dotted softened patches of the mucous membrane; in the contracted portion no disease of the tissue. Liver somewhat dark in colour, otherwise pretty healthy. Uterus of natural size, with some vascularity of its peritoneum; but no exudation.

199. *Ileus.—Strangulation of part of the intestine by old peritonitic adhesions.*—A lady, aged twenty, of very delicate habit, the subject, it was said, of abdominal inflammatory attacks at different times in early life, had for some time been suffering from diarrhœa. On the morning of the 26th July the bowels had been relaxed, and to check this an opiate was given. About 3 P.M. was seized with excruciating pain of abdomen, with much prostration, cold skin, anxiety, and frequent vomiting. This

continued during the night, and the pain was relieved by friction and pressure. Seen by me, with Dr. Burn, on the 27th at 2 P.M. From the period of the attack no action of the bowels had taken place, though enemata had been freely used for this purpose. When seen, the abdomen tender and tense, the pain was increased by pressure and the slightest motion; pulse 120, easily compressed. Thirty-six leeches were applied, and Dover's powder, with hydrarg. cum creta, given. At 5 P.M. she had borne the leeching well; the pulse was rather more developed; tenderness and pain of abdomen continued, and just above the pubes, and inclining towards the right iliac region, there was an irregular knotty induration perceptible. The pain was constant, but it increased in paroxysms from time to time with eructations, but no return of vomiting. Five dozen leeches were applied. Seen at 9 P.M. The pain and tenderness of abdomen were very little alleviated, pulse upwards of 120, and very feeble. No discharge from the bowels, and she was anxious and exhausted. Opium one grain, calomel two grains, every third hour. 28th, 6 A.M. Had dozed much during the night. Pulse very feeble. The tenderness of abdomen and tenseness continued; no evacuation. The opium was directed to be continued without the calomel, and an enema to be exhibited in the course of the day. 5 P.M. The vomiting recurred, and was frequent. The exhaustion had been great, and the paroxysms of increased pain frequent. Some dark feculent matter was brought away with the enema. Now skin cold; pulse thready; features collapsed; breathing hurried. Stimulants were given. She died about 7 P.M. Intelligence entire to the end.

Examination fourteen hours after death.—Abdomen tense. Not much distended. The omentum vascular, adhered to the convolutions of the small intestine, dipped into the pelvis, and was adherent there. A dark reddish tint of the surface of the small intestine generally, and the stomach also at its great arch, was observed. On separating the tender adhesions of the convolutions of the intestines, and raising them from the pelvis, very dark-red effusion was found to the extent of about ten ounces, and a portion of the small intestine to the extent of about two feet was observed to be in a perfectly black state. Over this the omentum was in part matted, but the greater part of the dark-coloured portion of the intestine had sunk into the cavity of the pelvis. On examination it was found that this portion of the intestine had been strangulated. A ligamentous band passed from the free end of the appendix vermiformis to a part of the mesentery. The side of one convolution (about six inches from the ileo-cœcal valve) was united to another by a firm ligamentous band not more than quarter of an inch in length. The ring thus formed was about two inches in diameter. The strangulated portion of intestine had passed through this ring, and the size of the ring had been lessened, by part of its circumference and its diameter, having been compressed by the band connected with the appendix vermiformis. But of the exact manner of the strangulation I was not quite certain. The part strangulated was a portion of the ileum commencing a few inches above the ring which has been described.*

Ordinary *colic* from some casual error of diet is not uncommon both in Europeans and natives, and is in general readily cured by a purgative combined with an anodyne.

M. Boudin remarks † that "colique végétale" is not alluded to in the first edition of this work, and adds, that when he questioned me on the subject I seemed astonished at the name. Doubtless

* Case 86 may be referred to in connection with that now detailed.

† "Traité de Géographie et de Statistique Médicales," par J. Ch. M. Boudin. Vol. ii. p. 377. His words are,—"Nous ajouterons même, qu'ayant tout récemment interrogé M. le professeur Morehead sur la colique végétale, le seul nom de la maladie parut l'étonner beaucoup.

this impression is correct, as the name was then new to me, and I find on a careful perusal of the interesting description in M. Boudin's work, that the disease is also unknown to me.

It is said to occur in greatest degree in French ships, particularly steam vessels, in the proximity of tropical coasts. It is observed much less frequently, and in a milder form, on shore. It attacks several individuals at a time, and consists of recurring paroxysms of severe colic, succeeded by emaciation, tremors, paralysis, delirium, and convulsion. The mortality is considerable, and the occurrence of cerebral symptoms always indicates a fatal result. The water, the wine, the provisions, and the circumstances of crews thus affected, have been carefully examined, without the slightest evidence of the presence of lead. The disease has therefore been attributed to a miasmatic poison.

It is difficult to explain why this form of colic is unknown in India in English troops, or, as I believe, in the crews of English ships in tropical seas. The statement in M. Boudin's work, that English surgeons in Bombay receive a large number of patients affected with this form of colic from Scinde and the Persian Gulf, is certainly erroneous.* The European General Hospital is the only hospital in Bombay for the reception of sick sailors, and with the occurrences in this hospital I have been familiar for the last twenty years.

I quote, in connection with this subject, the only case of lead-colic which has come under my observation, and this chiefly on account of the morbid appearances found after death.

200. *Colica-Pictonum.—The colon was much distended and displaced.—Death, with head symptoms.— Only slight serous effusion at the base of the skull.* — W. Keilly, of twenty-eight years of age, a seaman in moderate condition, a painter by trade, who had at different times, after working with paint, been affected with severe colic. The last attack was about two years before he came under observation, and it continued for eight months. On the 5th of May, 1839, he came to the General Hospital in a state of intoxication. He was affected with vomiting, and complained much of pain at the epigastrium; his hands were tremulous and the bowels constipated. He had lately been engaged in painting the ship to which he belonged. The pulse was feeble, the skin damp. The pain and constipation were relieved by the warm bath and turpentine enemata, but they recurred from time to time, with vomiting, during his stay

* The words are, "Les chirurgiens Anglais de Bombay, dit M. Lemarie (thèse Montpellier, 1851), reçoivent un grand nombre des malades atteints de colique sèche des postes et des bâtiments du Sind et du Golfe Persique; ceux de Calcutta de la navigation du Gange et du Golfe de Bengale." I am not entitled to speak with the same confidence respecting Calcutta, but I have very little doubt that here also there is some misapprehension. The experience of the medical officers of the steam vessels of the Oriental and Peninsular Company would be of value on this question.

in hospital, and were attended with retraction of the wrists, and convulsive movement of the fingers. On the 8th, 9th, and 10th, he had several convulsive fits, followed by moaning, restlessness, and incoherence; accompanied with a cold, damp skin, a quick and feeble pulse. On the 11th and 12th he was delirious, and death on the latter day was preceded by drowsiness. He was treated with opiates, stimulants, blisters, and purgatives.

Inspection fifteen hours after death. — *Head.* — An ounce and a half of serum was effused in the cavity, the greater portion at the base of the skull; the substance of the brain and the membranes were in their natural state. *Chest.*—The lungs were healthy and collapsed. The heart was soft in its texture. *Abdomen.*—The whole of the large intestine was dilated and varied in calibre from about two to three inches. The transverse colon coursed along the margin of the right false ribs, concealed the liver, reached to the ensiform cartilage, thence coursed downwards at the margin of the left false ribs, thence passed directly upwards to the diaphragm, opposite to the apex of the heart, thence turned downwards and formed the descending colon; the distended sigmoid flexure occupied the hypogastric region and reached to the umbilicus; the coats were natural, perhaps thinned, and there was much thin feculence in the gut; the mucous follicles were here and there enlarged. The stomach was contracted and concealed by the colon; at its cardiac end, there were dark, extravasated patches, elsewhere the coat was mammillated, but there was no softening. The small intestine was contracted. The liver was paler than natural. The kidneys were healthy.

CHAP XVIII.

AFFECTIONS OF THE STOMACH.

SECTION I. — *Gastritis, Acute and Chronic.*

Acute Gastritis. — In my remarks on remittent fever *, it is stated that bright redness of the mucous membrane of the stomach is occasionally found after death, in the fevers of plethoric Europeans in whom irritability of the stomach had been present during life; but this condition is probably rather congestive than inflammatory.

In my notes of fatal cases of small-pox there is one in which symptoms of acute gastritis were present during life, and the characteristic morbid appearances were found after death; but with this exception, all the other cases of acute gastritis which have come under my observation have been instances of irritant poisoning.

Poisoning by arsenic, with suicidal or criminal intent, is unfortunately common in India, as is well known to medical officers connected with native general hospitals.

I have the notes of several before me, but I shall be satisfied with the narration of two, selected not only as illustrative of the symptoms and morbid appearances of acute gastritis, but also of a a remark previously made relative to the diagnosis of cholera.† In the absence of a faithful history, the following case, in a season of epidemic cholera, might very readily have been taken for one of that disease: —

201. *Poisoning by arsenic, admitted in the stage of collapse, after the active symptoms of gastritis were passed.*—Furdonjee Jewajee, a Parsee liquor seller, of thirty years of age, was brought by his friends to the hospital at 7 A.M. on the 28th February, 1851. He was said to have taken arsenic at 2 A.M., and at the same time half a bottle of brandy. He vomited frequently, and the ejected matters contained blood. He had also been frequently purged. On admission he was drowsy and restless, and the conjunctivæ were vascular, the skin cold, the pulse imperceptible, and the tongue some-

---

* Page 93. † Page 214.

what florid. He complained of pain of the loins, but not of the abdomen. He died at eleven o'clock.

Inspection four and a half hours after death.—Rigor mortis present. The heart contained liquid blood, and there was concentric hypertrophy of the left ventricle. The stomach contained about seven ounces of dark liquid blood. The mucous membrane was throughout of bright red colour, abundantly studded with dark red points of extravasated blood. There were patches of viscid mucus here and there, with white particles intermixed. Liquid blood flowed from the vessels of the dura mater, as it was divided. The pia mater was congested. The substance of the brain was redder than natural, and showed many bloody points.

Analysis.—Some of the white gritty particles from the mucous membrane of the stomach, heated with black flux in a test tube, gave a grey metallic ring. This portion of the tube, heated in a large tube, gave on its sides deposit of a white sublimate, which was dissolved in boiling distilled water; tested with the ammonio-nitrate of silver, it gave a canary-yellow precipitate, with the ammonio-sulphate of copper, a bright green precipitate, and with a stream of sulphuretted hydrogen, a yellow solution.

202. *Poisoning from arsenic in which symptoms of narcotism were prominent at the commencement.*—A Hindoo goldsmith, of about thirty years of age, was brought to the Jamsetjee Jejeebhoy Hospital on the morning of the 21st May, 1847, at 6 A.M. He had been picked up by the police on the public street. He was comatose; his pupils were dilated, the breathing was natural, the pulse frequent. There was no appearance of injury, and no emaciation or sign of long-continued sickness. As he was being lifted from the cart in which he had been conveyed to the hospital, he vomited a little bilious matter. Nothing was known of his history. Cold affusion was used to the head, and an emetic of ipecacuanha and carbonate of ammonia was given. The emetic acted readily, and he became sensible. He vomited several times during the day, and was purged two or three times, the evacuations consisting of gelatinous-looking mucus. Towards evening the pulse had become very feeble, the breathing hurried, the thirst and anxiety considerable, with occasional retching. He died about five o'clock A.M. on the 22nd instant. The only statement he made was, that he had eaten some sweetmeats the night before he was brought to the hospital. The result of the coroner's inquest was, that he had taken poison himself.

Inspection six hours after death.—The body was in good condition. *Abdomen.*—There was a general blush of redness over the peritoneal covering of the stomach and small intestine, but no effusion into the sac of the peritoneum. The stomach was opened and found to contain about six ounces of a dark watery fluid with mucous sediment, partly tinged with blood, and containing some white gritty particles. There was general redness of the mucous lining of the stomach, characterised towards the cardiac end by a dark patch-like arrangement; and towards the pyloric end there was a dark and more diffused redness leading to an almost black patch about three inches long, and two in short diameter, raised somewhat above the general level, and abraded in part of its surface. There was dark redness in patches of the mucous lining of the duodenum, and a general blush with increased secretion of mucus on that of the jejunum, and of the ileum and cœcum. The thoracic viscera were healthy, there was slight congestion of the vessels of the pia mater of the brain. For the following note of the analysis of the contents of the stomach I am indebted to Dr. Giraud:—

"About four ounces of a mucous flocculent fluid taken from the stomach, containing a few minute white brittle particles. These particles, weighing about the tenth of a grain, were sublimed in a tube into a white crystalline ring;—this, with the part of the tube on which it was deposited, being placed in a reduction tube with charcoal powder, gave a steel grey metallic ring, which, on being heated in a wide tube, was reconverted into a white crystalline sublimate. By Reinsch's process metallic deposition on copper was obtained from the above-mentioned fluid; this yielded a white crystalline sublimate, which on solution in water gave the characteristic effects of arsenious acid with ammoniaco-nitrate of silver, ammoniaco-sulphate of copper, and sulphuretted hydrogen. By the foregoing processes arsenious acid and metallic arsenic were obtained from the white particles found in the fluid of the stomach; and from the fluid itself metallic arsenic was procured, and made to pass through its various compounds of arsenious acid, arsenite of silver, arsenite of copper, and orpiment."

Remark.—The interest in this case consists in the strongly marked narcotic symptoms shown on admission into hospital. It was viewed then as a case of narcotic poisoning, and treated as such. Subsequently its nature was sufficiently evident. A circumstance, not noted in the case, attracted my attention when the narcotic symptoms were present. There was a fixed frown on the countenance, an expression of suffering not usual in simple narcotism, and to which probably more importance as a diagnostic sign should have been attached.

Chronic Gastritis. — A review of the fatal cases of disease now before me, and partly detailed in this work, show that some degree of chronic inflammation of the mucous membrane of the stomach is frequently observed in persons addicted to excesses in drinking, —indicated by streaked or dotted redness, generally at the cardiac end of the stomach, associated with softening, or a hypertrophied and mammillated state of the tissue.*

Ulceration of the gastric mucous membrane has not been frequently met with by me †; and the same remark applies to fibrous growths in the sub-mucous tissue. A small fibrous tumour is mentioned in case 50. I have also notes of the history of a soldier of the 4th Light Dragoons whom I saw in the hospital at Kirkee in 1837 in a state of great emaciation. He died shortly afterwards. The pyloric orifice of the stomach was so contracted by cartilaginous thickening as barely to permit the passage of a quill. Vomiting had only been occasionally present, and in consequence of the pale colour of the evacuations the disease had been considered hepatic, not gastric.

I have not met with a single case of malignant disease of the stomach, though the occurrence of two or three in the higher classes of Europeans, in the practice of others, has come to my knowledge. My own observation in India would lead me to infer, that malignant growths generally are of infrequent occurrence.

* Though a remark pertaining rather to the symptoms of cerebral irritation, it may be well even here to allude to the risk of mistaking the irritability of stomach sympathetic with cerebral affection, for that symptomatic of gastric inflammation. In respect to children, caution on this point is well understood, but it is also necessary in regard to adults. I have known cases of cerebral determination from undue exposure to the sun, in which the vomiting was so prominent as to tend to overshadow the uneasiness of head, the flushing of countenance, the restlessness, and tendency to mental confusion, and to divert attention from the true seat of the disease.

† Cases 89, 90.

Whether the circumstance of their having come rarely under my notice is to be attributed to absolute infrequency, or to my field of inquiry not having extended to the classes and the periods of life most susceptible of malignant disease, I am unable to determine.*

SECTION II. — *Glossitis.*

This serious disease is of very rare occurrence. I have met with only two cases. The first in a sthenic soldier of the 15th Hussars. The half of the tongue was affected; but the organ was so swollen as to fill the mouth, protrude between the lips, and cause apprehension for the result. Recovery took place under the use of general blood-letting.

The second case occurred in February 1846, in a very asthenic native child, who was brought to the dispensary of the Jamsetjee Jejeebhoy Hospital for relief. Both sides were affected, and the swollen tongue protruded from the mouth and completely prevented deglutition. Leeches and superficial scarifications were used without relief. The child was so reduced that the bleeding consequent on free incisions was dreaded, and yet the symptoms had become very urgent. I pencilled the tongue freely with nitrate of silver. On the following day the swelling was much reduced. The caustic was again used, and nothing further was necessary to perfect the cure.

I have alluded to the subject of glossitis that I might record the efficacy of the nitrate of silver in this case. It is a practical fact well worthy of being borne in recollection.

* As connected with the pathology of the stomach, I would allude to a peculiar case of injury which came under my observation in the European General Hospital in 1839. A sailor was violently squeezed between the bulwark of a steam vessel and a tense cable which passed across the epigastrium. When received into the hospital, an hour after the accident, there was an ecchymosed mark distinct on the epigastrium and opposed part of the spine. There was much collapse. He vomited some dark-coloured blood. After reaction there was much tenderness of abdomen, hurried respiration, but no return of vomiting. He died twenty-four hours after admission. After death, a pint of dark fluid blood was found in the left pleura: a large rent, through which three fingers could be passed, existed at the posterior part of the left side of the diaphragm, near to the spine. No fracture of the ribs. In the pelvis and neighbourhood of the kidney there was a pint of dark fluid blood. Transversely across the centre of the great arch of the stomach there was a strip of the mucous membrane above an inch in breadth, torn from the subjacent coat, hanging loose with lacerated edges.

SECTION III. — *Dyspepsia. — General reflections on Pathology and Principles of Treatment.*

Though "dyspepsia" occupies a prominent place in hospital returns, it is my intention to treat very briefly the train of symptoms to which this term has been applied. By dyspepsia, or indigestion, is meant more or less of such symptoms as anorexia, nausea, vomiting, epigastric distention and pain, gaseous and watery eructations. Much has been written on this affection, but the question may be suggested, whether the tendency of elaborate disquisitions on dyspepsia has not been to obstruct the progress of enlarged views in pathology and rational doctrines in therapeutics.

Indeed, I venture to predict, that the time is not very distant, when consequent on advancing generalisations in pathology, the term dyspepsia will be removed from our nosologies, just as dyspnœa has already been.

That, consequent on inflammation of the mucous membrane, or organic lesion of the stomach, the taking of food will be followed by more or less of the symptoms called dyspeptic, may be readily allowed. Gastric inflammation and organic lesion should be treated in accordance with the general principles applicable to their class, adapted to the diathesis of the individual affected.

My present remarks, however, are not intended to apply to dyspeptic symptoms thus arising, but as they occur independent of inflammation or organic disease, — the form of dyspepsia called functional.

In the first chapter of this work, and in other places also, much importance has been attached to diathesis in its bearing on etiology and therapeutics, and to no affection is this principle more justly applicable than to the so-called disease — functional dyspepsia.

In the most robust constitution, great excess in eating will be followed by imperfect digestion with its attendant phenomena, but here the pathology is clear and the indication of cure self-evident. These, however, are not the circumstances under which functional dyspepsia usually occurs. It is among the asthenic and cachectic that it is generally met with. In these states of defective assimilation of food to blood and blood to tissue, or of blood vitiated by mal-assimilation, retained excretion, or reception of external injurious agencies, the stomach partakes in the infirmity of the whole system, its functional power is enfeebled, and that quality and quantity of food which in vigorous health would be digested with ease, is followed by indigestion.

Then there are associated with these dyspeptic symptoms, phenomena which indicate derangement of other organs, as irregular action of the heart, headache, restless nights, muscular and mental languor, depressed spirits, irritable temper, morbid alvine discharges, constipated bowels, urine vitiated with urates, phosphates, or oxalates, &c. In this assemblage of deranged actions the dyspeptic symptoms are prominent, because the functions of the stomach are frequently called into exercise, the phenomena of derangement are well marked, the act of placing food into the organ is voluntary and often injudiciously performed. This prominence of the indigestion naturally tends to favour the belief that the other co-existing disorders are sequences of it. It may be admitted that as the function of the stomach is essential to recovery from asthenic and cachectic states, its frequent derangement must tend to increase these states with all their attendant evils; and thus in a limited sense the continuance of the other derangements may be said to be consequent on the persistence of the dyspepsia.

But this is not the large and practical view of the relation of all these events to each other.

The deranged digestion, circulation, assimilation, secretion, nervous and muscular functions, are conditions of the diathetic state, which, when developed, tend mutually to aggravate each other; but still they are all equally traceable to the causes which induced the asthenia or cachexia, and are only to be permanently cured by the removal of these causes and by the substitution of the causes of health.

The truly essential practical consideration in the treatment of functional dyspepsia, is to determine the causes of the asthenia or of the cachexia, to remove the individual from the sphere of their influence, and to place him in circumstances favourable to health.

The conditions of health may be summarily stated to be: relief from mental care and anxiety, a pure atmosphere, nutritious food in quantity adapted to the power of the stomach, exercise in the open air always short of fatigue, attention to the functions of the skin by ablution and suitable clothing, cheerful occupation, due amount of sleep, and avoidance of excessive evacuations. Under these influences the dyspeptic symptoms and their associated derangements will gradually disappear; but if these influences be overlooked and neglected, there cannot be restoration to health.

But this statement does not comprise all the resources of the medical art. The progress to recovery may be smoothed and hastened by various remedies, as sedatives, alkalies, tonics, alteratives, eliminants. It is not my object to enter here into the details of these means; they are well set forth in systematic works on disease and on Materia Medica, and their powers and applications should be carefully investigated by the clinical student; for, when the circumstances of the patient do not admit of change of scene and relaxation from occupation, or when the cachexia has become irremediable, these remedies, with the adjustment of diet, are unfortunately the only means by which relief may be obtained.

My present purpose has been to enforce the doctrine that these gastric and associated derangements are very generally induced by neglect of the conditions necessary to health, and are only to be permanently recovered from by a suitable adjustment of the vital stimuli, on which health depends, and without due attention to which it cannot be maintained or restored.

Articles of the Materia Medica, when the conditions of health are attended to, conduce to the cure, but in many instances are not essential to it. When the conditions of health are neglected, articles of the Materia Medica, judiciously used, may alleviate discomfort and suffering, but they are insufficient of themselves to effect recovery, and are liable, in unskilful hands, to prove injurious.*

It is from reflections such as these, that I have ventured to hint that elaborate treatises on dyspepsia tend to interfere with enlarged views in pathology and rational doctrines in therapeutics; and to predict that the term, at no remote period, will be used merely to express a symptom, not a disease.

I am very sensible that in these remarks I have laid myself open to the charge of inculcating trite and very simple principles, yet they can hardly be deemed uncalled for. It is, in fact, to the neglect of these obvious truths which lie upon the very surface of our science, that are due the exaggerated pretensions of partial systems of treatment, and the attempts to throw discredit on rational medicine.

* It would be easy to enlarge upon the evils which have resulted, and the discredit which has attached, to the profession of medicine, in consequence of the excessive and habitual use of purgative and mercurial medicines in India, as in other countries, in the treatment of the symptoms called dyspeptic. I would fain hope that the subject is now well understood.

CHAP. XIX.

ON BRIGHT'S DISEASE OF THE KIDNEY AND ALBUMINOUS URINE.

SECTION I. — *Prevalence of Bright's Disease in the hospital-frequenting classes of the natives of India.*

IN the year 1849 I first called the attention of the Medical and Physical Society of Bombay to Bright's disease of the kidney, as occurring in the hospital-frequenting classes of the native population of Bombay; and subsequent experience has confirmed my belief, that the morbid states to which the name of this eminent physician has been given, are as common in these classes of the community in India as in European countries.

I have before me the notes of fifty-eight cases which have been under my care in the clinical ward in the course of six years: thirty proved fatal, and twenty-eight were discharged, of whom nineteen were improved, and nine had received no benefit from treatment. These, however, form but a part of the admissions for this disease into the Jamsetjee Jejeebhoy Hospital during this period. Many cases have come under the observation of other medical officers in other wards of the hospital; and there is, in the following circumstance, evidence that many more must have passed through the hospital unrecorded. During these six years 782 patients have been admitted under the head "Cachexia;" and of these 493 have died. This is 12 per cent. of the total hospital deaths. The term cachexia is used in the hospital register when the imperfect history of previous illness, or the short time which has elapsed between admission and death, has prevented the discovery of the character of the cachexia, or of the existence of important organic disease. It is not to be doubted that a proportion of this class has been affected with Bright's disease. Indeed, if the relation which these structural changes of the kidney have to processes of degeneration be recollected, and, at the same time, the fact of the greater prevalence of asthenic and cachectic types of disease in warm climates be borne in mind, then, not only an equal, but a greater frequency of this affection in India, may be assumed as the fair inference from a review of all the attendant circumstances.

In respect to the occurrence of Bright's disease in Europeans in India, my dissection reports show that it was not unfrequently noticed by me in the European General Hospital. At that time, however, my attention was more given to other subjects of pathology; and I therefore believe that my observations at that period do not indicate the full proportion of this disease in the classes who resort to that hospital. Of its frequency in European regimental hospitals in India I am unable to speak; but I need hardly observe that in this, as in all other questions of pathology relating to European soldiers in India, the comparison is between them and soldiers elsewhere, and not between them and the civil population of European countries. I am also without satisfactory facts respecting this disease in officers, civil servants, and others of the higher classes of Europeans in India. Of the 311 fatal cases of officers, of which I have notes, Bright's disease is mentioned in only three, and these were subsequent to the year 1849. These data, however, as bearing on this question of pathology, may be set aside as inconclusive; for it is very evident that the attention of medical men in India has been, till very lately, imperfectly directed to its investigation.

The remarks which I am about to make have been chiefly suggested by the fifty-eight clinical cases now before me, viewed in connection with the statements and opinions advanced by European writers. They may be arranged under the heads— 1. Pathology. 2. Causes. 3. Symptoms and Treatment.

SECTION II. — *The Relation of Bright's Disease to Albuminous Urine stated. — The Morbid Anatomy and Pathology of the Fluids. — Pathology of the Secondary Affections. — The Uræmic Theory. — The Proximate Cause of Albumen in the Urine.*

Albuminous urine may occur independent of structural change of the kidney, caused by cold applied to the surface of the body, when the eliminating and sensory functions of the skin are in an abnormal condition. Under these circumstances, the urine is scanty, more or less tinged with the hæmatosin of the blood, and abounds in albumen, depending on an excessive afflux of blood to the capillaries of the kidney, with, it may be, an increase of the epithelial cells of the uriniferous tubes. But this state is transient, and may readily be removed by appropriate treatment: it has been most generally observed secondary on scarlatina.

Albuminous urine occasionally exists in connection with forms of fever, independent of renal disease. The albumen is then present in small quantity, only for a few days, and disappears with the febrile disturbance.* The history, the condition of the patient, the fact, ascertained by frequent and careful examination, of the disappearance of the albumen, will always suffice to distinguish these cases.

The various morbid states to which the term Bright's disease has been applied are characterised by urine, more or less albuminous, at some period or other of their progress. This condition of the urine is generally persistent throughout the entire course of the disease; but occasionally the albumen is absent from the urine for varying periods, and such cases may usually be distinguished from transient albuminuria, related to a febrile state, by the history, the condition of the patient, and the fact that the urine from which the albumen has disappeared is generally in abnormal quantity, and of density too low to be explained by the increase of watery constituent alone.

The prevailing opinions on the *morbid anatomy* of Bright's disease may be summarily expressed in the following terms:—

1. The kidney, when enlarged, is so: (*a*) from accumulation of epithelial cells, or of more or less degenerate lymph, in the interior of the tubuli of the cortical portion; (*b*) from exudation, external to the tubuli of the cortical portion, in the areolar matrix of the organ. The greater or less redness, and the various degrees of mottling, depend upon the proportion and situation of the blood present in the capillaries of the kidney at the period of observation.

2. When the kidney is small, granular, and indurated, it is so: (*a*) from collapse and cohesion of the sides of the tubuli of the cortical portion consequent upon the removal of pre-existing accumulations; (*b*) from atrophy of the cortical structure consequent on pressure from the contractile organisation of pre-existing cacoplastic deposit in the areolar matrix.

There has been much discussion in regard to the relative importance of deposit, external or internal to the tubes, and to the

* The presence of albumen in the urine, from the existence of blood or pus in the secretion, is apart from my present subject, and does not call for remark in this place.

nature of the deposit. Into these questions I shall not enter, but merely observe that there is one fact common to all—viz., that they tend to destruction of more or less of the secreting structure of the organ.

The following fifteen cases will illustrate the general features of the disease in the natives of India. They show the kidneys enlarged in five, of natural size in two, small in four, lobulated in six, and mottled in five. The encroachment of the cortical on the tubular portion is noted in ten, and small cysts were present in the kidney in two.

203. *A diver by occupation.—Anasarca, ascites.—Urine of low density and albuminous.—Dilatation of the right ventricle of the heart.—Hypertrophy and dilatation of the left.—Kidneys enlarged, lobulated, in a state of yellow granular degeneration.*—Suliman Seedee, a Mussulman, twenty-five years of age, an inhabitant of Zangibar, and resident in Bombay about a month. He had followed the occupations of a diver and a blacksmith, used spirits and ganja habitually, and opium occasionally. About five years before he came under observation, he was the subject of dropsical symptoms for about ten days, which made their appearance after he had been engaged in his occupation of diver. There was no recurrence of them till about five months before his admission into the clinical ward, on the 7th March, 1849. Then they had been preceded by febrile symptoms, coming on frequently with chills, not terminating by sweating, and attended with scanty urine. On admission there was general anasarca and ascites, the respiration was somewhat hurried, and dry bronchitic rales were heard in different parts of the chest; the impulse of the heart was rather increased, but the sounds were natural; uneasiness of the loins; urine copious, and passed frequently; the pulse of good strength; no febrile heat; the bowels regular, and the tongue moist and clean. He continued under treatment till the 24th April, when he died. During the first month the urine ranged in quantity from forty to eighty ounces and upwards in the twenty-four hours, was clear and pale, sometimes alkaline, at others neutral, and always gave a considerable flocculent deposit by heat and nitric acid. The dropsical symptoms were stationary; a sense of uneasiness across the chest was frequently complained of, attended with some degree of dyspnœa, cough, and crepitous rale in both dorsal regions. On the 17th April præcordial uneasiness was complained of, and there was increased dulness over the region of the heart, with accelerated action and confused sounds. The pulse was very small; and now the urine was reduced to nine ounces; the dropsical symptoms, the dyspnœa, and asthenia increased; and diarrhœa was superadded. He became somewhat drowsy, and died the 24th April. The treatment consisted of diaphoretics, diuretics, and purgatives; rubefacients, antimonials, and on two occasions leeches were used for the chest affection, and latterly stimulants were exhibited.

Inspection seven hours after death.—Chest.—The pericardium contained eight ounces of serous fluid; the cavities of the right side of the heart were dilated and filled with blood; the left ventricle was also dilated, and its walls hypertrophied; the valves were all healthy; the inner surface of the aorta near to the arch was roughened from yellow deposit. The lower lobes of both lungs adhered to the costal pleuræ firmly, posteriorly; and a considerable part (more of the right lung) of these lobes was in a state of red hepatisation. *Abdomen.*—Serous effusion, but to no great amount, was present in the cavity of the abdomen. The liver was enlarged, indurated, and its incised surface mottled. Both kidneys were slightly enlarged, and somewhat lobulated; their surface, when denuded of the capsule, was mottled dark red and yellow, and was granular. The kidneys, when vertically incised, showed much granular degeneration,—the surface being mottled red and yellow, granular, with confusion of the tubular and cortical structures. This state was most marked in the central part of the right kidney; it was more diffused in the left one. In both, in one or two places, there was tubular structure, not encroached upon; but the cortical portion external, showed commencement of yellow granular deposit.

204. *Dropsical symptoms.—Urine of low density and albuminous.—Bronchitis, diarrhœa, periostitis, erysipelas, as secondary affections.—Kidneys large, and in a state of yellow granular and fatty degeneration.—An opium eater.*—Hurrichund, a Hindoo writer, of thirty years of age, a native of Cutch, and resident in Bombay for about seven months, was the subject of primary and secondary syphilis about five years before he came under observation, but no traces of the disease were present. He admitted that he had been in the habit of eating opium to the extent of twenty-five grains daily for about four years, and that he occasionally drank spirits. About four months before his admission into hospital he had been affected with dropsical swellings, which had disappeared without any medical treatment. About a month before admission he had experienced pain in the lumbar region, and the dropsical symptoms had returned. He was admitted into the clinical ward on the 22nd April, 1849. There was œdema of the lower extremities; the abdomen was full, but without distinct fluctuation. The respiration was calm; there was no dulness on percussion of the chest. The sounds of the heart were natural, but an occasional crepitus mixed with the vesicular respiration in the dorsal regions, chiefly the left. The pulse was soft, the skin cool, the tongue moist, the bowels were reported to be regular, the urine copious, and the pain of the lumbar region, formerly complained of, had ceased. On the 24th the urine was amber-coloured, of specific gravity 1·007, and gave an abundant flocculent deposit under heat and nitric acid. During the seven months that he was under treatment the quantity of urine passed was noted daily, and there are upwards of sixty observations on the character of the secretion to be found in the diary of the case. The urine fluctuated a good deal in quantity; it was seldom less than twenty ounces in the twenty-four hours, and during the months of June and July very generally amounted to about five pints. Whether this great flow of urine was due to the diuretic remedies which he was at the time using, or to the influence on the cutaneous surface of the cold damp air of the monsoon season, is doubtful. For the most part, the specific gravity of the urine ranged from 1·003 to 1·012; and it was always very albuminous. To the low density of the urine there were several exceptions, chiefly in the month of May, when the urine was about twenty ounces in quantity: on these occasions the specific gravity ranged from 1·018 to 1·030, and then the urine was generally of a deep brown colour, and very albuminous, and sometimes febrile symptoms were present. Throughout the course of treatment the dropsical symptoms were more or less present. Bronchitic symptoms were also at times complained of, at others diarrhœa, sometimes dysenteric in character. There were also periostitis of the sternum, and erysipelas of the left thigh, in the month of October, with febrile symptoms, which tended much to increase the asthenic state. Febrile symptoms recurred about the 10th November, attended with occasional delirium; the dropsical effusions increased, and he died, with much hurry of the respiration, but without distinct coma, on the 12th November. The dropsical state was treated with diaphoretics and diuretics, and the other indications, as they arose, were attended to.

Inspection eight and a half hours after death.—The body swollen from anasarca. *Chest.*—There were about seven pints of clear serous fluid effused into the sac of the right pleura, and about one pint into that of the left. The right lung was compressed against the spinal column, did not crepitate on pressure, but was soft and tough; the left lung was crepitating. There was no redness, or other trace of inflammatory action, observed in any part of the pleura. There were about three ounces of clear serous fluid in the sac of the pericardium, but no redness of the membrane, or other trace of inflammation. The heart was of smaller size than natural, and the mitral valves were somewhat thickened. *Abdomen.*—There was about a pint of serum in the cavity of the abdomen. The liver, not enlarged, was in the first stage of hepatic congestion. The spleen was enlarged. Both kidneys were increased in size, the left one most so—it weighed eleven ounces, and the right one eight; both were somewhat lobulated, externally mottled red and yellow, but not granular. On incising the kidneys, the cortical portion of both was in increased proportion, was mottled red and yellow, and was somewhat granular and fatty in appearance; the tubular portion was encroached upon, but was quite distinct. *Head.*—The vessels of the pia mater were somewhat injected, and there was slight serous effusion into the sub-arachnoid space.

205. *Gastro-enteritis, anasarca, and ascites.—Urine of low density and albuminous.—Paracentesis.—Death from peritonitis.—Kidneys small, in a state of yellow granular degeneration.*—Imam Khan, a Mussulman Hakeem, of thirty years of age, a native of Dowlutabad, and resident in Bombay for two years and a half. He was in very indigent circumstances, and often very badly supplied with food; was in the habit of smoking ganja and tobacco, but did not use spirits. For about eleven days before his admission into hospital he suffered from fever and dysentery. He was admitted into the clinical ward on the 25th June, 1849. He was reduced in flesh; the respiration was calm; there was no dulness of the chest; and vesicular respiration was general and unmixed. The abdomen was collapsed, tender, slightly resistant, and an indurated enlargement was perceptible for two inches below the margin of the left ribs. The skin was of natural temperature, the tongue rather florid at the tip and edges, the pulse small and easily compressed; he complained of frequent calls to stool, and the evacuations, passed with griping and straining, were said to contain blood and mucus; he also suffered from occasional vomiting after eating. At first attention was directed to the removal of the dysenteric symptoms. As these improved, bronchitic symptoms appeared; and on the 11th July there was puffiness of the face and œdema of the feet. The urine was now examined, and was found to be of pale amber colour, of specific gravity 1·004, and albuminous. It was frequently examined during his illness, and varied a good deal in quantity, frequently above forty ounces in the twenty-four hours, and latterly often below twenty, the specific gravity ranging from 1·004 to 1·018, and the presence of albumen always clearly indicated. Diarrhœa succeeded an alleviation of the bronchitic symptoms, continued present for several weeks in succession, and often in an aggravated degree; the dropsical symptoms increased; there was troublesome dyspnœa; the abdomen swelled, and became tense and fluctuating. Paracentesis was had recourse to on the 9th December, and fourteen pints of clear serous fluid, of specific gravity 1·006, and giving a copious deposit under nitric acid, were drawn off. On the 11th there was general tenderness of abdomen, with a very feeble pulse. This increased, and he died on the 12th.

Inspection eleven hours after death.—Head.—There was considerable serous effusion in the cavity of the arachnoid and in the sub-arachnoid space. The vessels of the pia mater were congested; and there was about an ounce of serum in the ventricles of the brain. *Chest.*—There was about a pint of reddish serum in the sacs of the pleura. Both lungs collapsed and crepitated; the right lung was in part adherent to the costal pleura, but the left was free. The heart was contracted and smaller than natural; the valves were healthy, and there was no hypertrophy of the walls. About two ounces of serum were found in the sac of the pericardium. *Abdomen.*—About ten pints of serum in the cavity of the abdomen. The peritoneal covering of the small intestine presented in some places a dotted red appearance, and shreds of recent coagulable lymph were found upon its surface and between the convolutions of the intestine, causing tender adhesions of the convolutions to each other, and to the parietes of the abdomen. The peritoneal aspect of the trocar wound was cicatrised, and there was no greater trace of inflammatory action around it than elsewhere on the peritoneum of the anterior wall. The convex surface of the liver adhered to the diaphragm by a thin layer of lymph; the organ was smaller and harder than natural, and yet presented appearances of congestion. The kidneys were smaller than natural, and each weighed three ounces. On removing the capsule the surface appeared of a pale buff-colour, mottled red and granular. On incising the right kidney the cortical part was also of pale buff colour, with a mottling of red; it was slightly granular, and in parts encroached considerably on the tubular portion. The left kidney presented much the same appearance as the right, with this exception, that the cortical portion was pale, and the tubular less red.

206. *Anasarca and ascites.—Urine of low density and albuminous.—Was eight times tapped.—Kidneys in a state of yellow granular degeneration.*—Ahmed Senna, a Mussulman beggar, thirty years of age, a native of Scinde, and originally a cowherd. About three years before he came under observation he suffered from fever while in Scinde, and was subsequently on several occasions affected with œdematous swelling of the feet and ankles. He denied being addicted to the use of spirits, and stated that he had never taken them till two months before admission, when he was advised to do so, moderately, for the relief of the dropsical symptoms. He was in the habit of smoking tobacco, but not of eating opium. Four years before admission he had been the subject of syphilis, for which he had been salivated. He was admitted into hospital on the 28th September, 1849. There was general anasarca, and the abdomen was much swollen, tense, and fluctuating. He was under treatment in hospital till the 19th January, 1851. Throughout this period the urine was generally less than twenty ounces in the twenty-four hours, was pale, of specific gravity (varying with the quantity) from 1·007 to 1·015, and giving a flocculent deposit, more or less copious, under heat and nitric acid. From the 10th October, 1849, to the 10th November, 1850, he was eight times tapped, and about one hundred pints of fluid, in all, evacuated. After the first tapping it was discovered that the spleen was much enlarged, reaching beyond the umbilicus in the median line, and as low as the crest of the ilium; but after the latter tappings it was found to have considerably decreased in size. In the months of July and August, 1850, he suffered from diarrhœa, sometimes dysenteric in character; and during this time the fluid re-accumulated slowly in the abdomen. He died from exhaustion, and without coma. The treatment was very varied, consisting of purgatives, diuretics, with tonics and stimulants, but without any advantage. The operation of tapping was in each instance performed at the patient's urgent request, to relieve the discomfort attendant on the distention of the abdomen.

Inspection.—Abdomen.—There were about twenty-six pints of serous fluid in the sac of the peritoneum. The diaphragm was pushed up by the effusion, as high as the interspace between the third and fourth ribs. The liver was much reduced in size, and was suspended by its ligaments, separated by a considerable interspace from the concave surface of the diaphragm. Bands of old adhesions united the lower part of the right lobe of the liver to the diaphragm. After detaching the liver from its connections, it weighed twenty-eight ounces; the external surface was pale, and its peritoneal covering opaque; the surface was also granular, chiefly that of the left lobe; the tissue, when incised, appeared dense and compressed, and pale,—but had none of the lobulated appearance of cirrhosis. The body of the gall-bladder adhered to the duodenum. The spleen was of about the natural size, weighed eleven ounces, and its capsule was opaque and thickened; its texture was very indurated, and its incised surface appeared red, and abundantly studded with white spots and streaks of fibrous tissue. At the upper end the fibrous constituent was so abundant as to form a pale indurated nodule, of about the size of a pigeon's egg. The left kidney was larger than the right, and weighed about four ounces. On removing its capsule, the surface appeared somewhat lobulated, mottled red and yellow, and granular; when incised, it presented a surface also mottled red and yellow, but not granular; the tubular portion was encroached upon by the cortical, chiefly at the central parts; at the upper end there was a cyst, of about the size of a pea. The right kidney weighed three and a half ounces; the external and internal appearances were very similar to those of the left, but more marked in character. The colon was contracted, and the small intestine was gathered together in the centre of the abdominal cavity. *Chest.* —The right lung was firmly adherent to the costal pleura, but its texture was spongy and crepitating; the left lung was also healthy. The heart was of about the natural size, and weighed eight ounces; there were some opaque patches on the surface of the right ventricle; the aortic and mitral valves were healthy.

207. *Anasarca and ascites.—Urine of low density and very albuminous.—Sunk under diarrhœa.—The kidneys in a state of yellow granular degeneration.—The mucous coat of the colon and ileum with dotted red patches and granular deposit.—A spirit drinker.—Cirrhosis.*—Shaik Abdoola, a Mussulman sailor, of thirty years of age, addicted at one time to the excessive use of spirits, but not to opium or other narcotic drug, had for two months before his admission into hospital, on the 28th May, 1850, suffered from frequent vomiting, and latterly from œdema of the feet and legs. He was received into the clinical ward on the 15th June, when the abdomen was somewhat full, soft, and with an indistinct sense of fluctuation, but without any induration below the margin of either ribs. The feet and legs were also œdematous, the respiration was calm, the sounds and impulse of the heart were natural, and there was no dulness on percussion of the chest; the pulse was small and soft, the tongue moist and clean. He was the subject of a large reducible scrotal hernia of the left side, which had commenced three years previously. He continued under treatment till the 27th June, when he died. The urine in the twenty-four hours was generally above fifty ounces, was clear amber-coloured, of specific gravity from 1·007 to 1·012, and very albuminous. He became affected with diarrhœa, which increased, and caused death by asthenia. The treatment was chiefly directed against the diarrhœa.

Inspection.—The body was emaciated. *Head.*—There was some serous fluid effused in the sub-arachnoid space. *Chest.*—The lungs were collapsed and crepitating; the heart small in proportion to the body. *Abdomen.*—The large intestine generally was contracted,—its coats were thickened. The omentum was contracted, and matted over the colon. The inner surface of the large intestine was rugous and irregular, dark grey coloured, variegated of different shades, with bright red patches, and spots here and there, chiefly in the cœcum; the mucous coat had a granular appearance, and was firmly adherent to the subjacent coat. For a foot and a half the inner surface of the lower end of the ileum presented the same appearance as the large intestine; above, for about three feet, the inner surface of the ileum was rugous, of a dark red colour, with grey granular patches here and there. The portions of the ileum just described occupied the large scrotal tumour. The stomach was contracted, and the mucous coat was rugous, of dark grey colour, with some dark red patches, and covered with adhesive mucus. The liver was granular externally, and hard under the scalpel; the left lobe was very small. The left kidney was larger than the right,—its external surface was mottled red and yellow, the cortical portion buff-coloured and granular. The red colour of the tubular portion was quite distinct. The right kidney presented the same appearances as the left. The spleen was small, and denser than natural.

208. *Anasarca with ascites.—Urine of low density and generally albuminous.—Died comatose.—Kidneys small, with cysts and excess of cortical portion.—Cirrhosis.—Thrice admitted.*—Antonio de Souza, fifty-five years of age, a Portuguese inhabitant of Goa, but resident in Bombay for about eight years, and occupied as a servant in a baker's shop. For many years he had been in the habit of drinking about three ounces of spirits daily; was the subject of incomplete paralysis of the right arm from his boyhood; but, with this exception, had enjoyed good health till about three weeks before his admission into the hospital, on the 19th February, 1849, when he had become, con-

sequent on exposure to cold, he believed, the subject of intermittent fever, which after fifteen days was followed by dropsical symptoms.

State on Admission.—He was somewhat emaciated, but with general anasarca, and the abdomen full and fluctuating. The respiration was somewhat hurried, and there were dry and moist bronchitic rales general on both sides of the chest, obscuring the sounds of the heart. The pulse was feeble and somewhat frequent, the tongue slightly coated, but moist, and the skin of natural temperature. During his stay in hospital, the urine ranged in quantity from twelve to thirty ounces, was generally clear, sometimes of acid, at others of alkaline reaction, of specific gravity from 1·007 to 1·017, and very generally gave a scanty flocculent deposit with heat and nitric acid: this deposit, however, was sometimes absent. He continued in hospital till the 15th March, when he was discharged, at his own desire, with the dropsical symptoms somewhat less, and the bronchitic rales considerably decreased. He was treated with stimulant diuretics, of which squills was generally a constituent, and also at one time the ferri-potassio tartras; rubefacient applications were also used to the chest. He applied for readmission on the 27th March. The emaciation and the dropsical symptoms had much increased; the respiration was more hurried and oppressed, and the cough more urgent; the pulse was very feeble, and the urine very scanty. Under the use of eight grains of sesquicarbonate of ammonia, a drachm of spiritus ætheris nitrici, with camphor mixture every third hour, and four ounces of arrack daily, and an adequate diet, he speedily began to improve. The pulse gained somewhat in strength, the breathing became less oppressed, the urine increased to sixty ounces and upwards in the twenty-four hours, and the dropsical symptoms gradually lessened. On the 5th April the acetate of potass was substituted for the sesquicarbonate of ammonia. The urine still increased, and the dropsical symptoms had altogether disappeared by the 10th April; on the 13th, quinine and the muriated tincture of iron were substituted for the diuretic; and he was discharged on the 15th, at his earnest request. The urine was in general clear, sometimes alkaline, of specific gravity from 1·006 to 1·017, and was, except on one or two occasions, unaffected by heat or nitric acid. He was admitted again into hospital on the 23rd October, 1849. The face was puffed, the feet and legs œdematous, the abdomen swollen. He complained of cough and muco-puriform expectoration. Sounds of the heart natural, impulse feeble. He stated that since his discharge from hospital he had used spirituous liquors moderately, had been to Goa, and been exposed to the inclemencies of the weather, to which he attributed the return of the dropsical symptoms, as well as irregular febrile accessions, to which he was also subject. The pulse was very feeble; the asthenic and bronchitic symptoms increased. He became comatose on the 29th, and died on the 30th. The urine, during the time he was under treatment on this last occasion, ranged in density from 1·011 to 1·013, and was albuminous.

Inspection twenty hours after death. — *Head.* — The vessels of the pia mater were congested, and there was more than the normal quantity of serum in the sub-arachnoid space, but none in the ventricles. On incising the brain, numerous bloody points appeared, but no softening was observed. *Chest.* — The lungs adhered firmly to the costal pleura, and to the diaphragm, and when incised gave out much sero-puriform fluid on pressure. The substance was crepitating, and the mucous membrane of the bronchial tubes was of dark red colour. The heart was well covered with fat, chiefly over the left ventricle; the right ventricle was somewhat dilated; the left slightly hypertrophied; no disease of the valves, but the ascending aorta was somewhat dilated with opaque deposit, in parts ossific, on its inner surface. *Abdomen.*—There was about a pint and a half of clear serum found in the cavity. The liver was somewhat smaller than natural, with some degree of irregularity on its external surface, mottled dark red, and indurated in texture under the knife. The kidneys were smaller than natural. In the cortical portion of the left kidney there were two cysts, each of about the size of a small bean, but no distinct granular degeneration was found in any part. The cortical part of the right kidney was mottled red and buff on its surface, and it somewhat encroached on the tubular portion, but it was not granular, and there was an appearance of commencing cysts in some places.

209. *Febrile symptoms, followed by anasarca, ascites, and dysenteric symptoms.—Urine of low density and albuminous.—Death by coma.—The kidneys in a state of yellow granular degeneration.—The mucous membrane of the large intestine ulcerated, and with granular exudation.*—Elepa, a Hindoo shopkeeper, of fifty years of age, an inhabitant of Hydrabad, in the Deccan, but for twenty-five years resident in Bombay; not addicted to the use of spirituous liquors. He stated that about two months before he came under observation he left Bombay, in good health, on a pilgrimage to Nassick; that about fifteen days after his arrival there, he, consequent on exposure to wet, became affected with febrile symptoms and diarrhœa, followed by œdema of the feet and legs. He was admitted into hospital on the 29th July, 1850, feeble, and reduced in flesh; the feet and legs were œdematous; the abdomen full, and with distinct sense of fluctuation; there was no dyspnœa or sign of disease of the lungs or heart; the pulse was small and thready. The day after his admission the urine amounted to fourteen ounces, was pale, neutral, of specific gravity 1·010, and gave a copious flaky deposit under nitric acid, but less under heat; and such continued to be its character whilst he was under treatment. On the 8th August, dysenteric symptoms set in, and he died on the 17th August, having been very drowsy for twenty-four hours before death.

Inspection twelve hours after death.—Head.—There was slight turgescence of the vessels of the brain, but the substance of the organ was of natural consistence. *Chest.*—There were old adhesions on both sides, but chiefly on the right, and the base of this lung was also adherent to the diaphragm. There were about two ounces of fluid found in the cavity of the pericardium. The heart was small, but healthy in structure. *Abdomen.*—There were about two pints of clear serous fluid in the sac of the peritoneum. The liver was of natural size and consistence, but its incised surface showed the presence of congestion in the second degree; upon its external surface there were two or three opaque puckered patches of cartilaginous consistence. The spleen was smaller than natural, and its substance healthy. The left kidney was somewhat larger than the right, and on removing the capsule the external surface presented a granular appearance, and was somewhat mottled. When incised, the cortical portion was found to encroach upon the tubular, which was here and there of a dark red colour, and arranged in distinct bundles. The right kidney was smaller in size, and presented very much the same appearance as the left, with the addition of two or three small cysts, of about the size of a split pea. The apices of some of the papillæ were also somewhat indurated, and fibrous in appearance. The rectum was contracted, and its mucous membrane was thickened, and presented irregular ulcerations, the surfaces of which were covered with a deposition of granular lymph. The mucous membrane of the descending colon and sigmoid flexure was also ulcerated, but the ulcers were more follicular in character. The mucous membrane of the remaining portion of the large intestine was attenuated, and there were transverse striæ of vascularity seen, apparently an early stage of the inflammatory action, which in the rectum had passed on to ulceration and granular exudation.

210. *Vesicular emphysema of both lungs.—Displacement of the heart.—Dilatation and hypertrophy of the ventricles.—Atheromatous deposit, with ulceration, in the aorta.—Granular degeneration of the kidneys.—Urine once noted, albuminous.—Dropsy.*—Rawogee Canojee, a Mahratta gardener, of fifty years of age, resident for twelve years at Parell, was admitted into hospital on the 15th October, 1850, affected with dyspnœa and œdema of the lower extremities. He had been ill for two years, but no account is given of the nature of his illness. The chest, including the præcordial region, was preternaturally resonant; there was faint respiration, and sonorous and sibilous rales; the impulse of the heart was most distinct at the scrobiculus cordis,

and there the sounds were distinct, and no murmurs were audible. The dropsical symptoms increased, and also the dyspnœa, and he died on the 4th November. The urine passed during the night after admission was sixteen ounces, of specific gravity 1·005, and unaffected by heat and nitric acid. After the 24th it became more scanty —about ten ounces in twenty-four hours; it was of specific gravity 1·020, and gave a turbid deposit under heat and nitric acid.

Inspection sixty hours after death.—Chest.—Both lungs were emphysematous, and rose beyond the margins of the chest; they were soft and spongy. The heart was displaced downwards and towards the right side. Firm adhesions connected parts of the surface of the heart to the pericardium, and there were opaque patches on other parts of the heart's surface. The heart was enlarged from dilatation with hypertrophy of the right ventricle, and hypertrophy with dilatation of the left. There were coagula of blood in the left auricle and right ventricle. There was slight opaque deposit towards the attached margin of the mitral valve. The aortic valves were healthy; the inner coat of the aorta, from its commencement, and throughout its thoracic portion, was closely studded with variously-sized patches of atheromatous deposit. At the origin of the left carotid and subclavian arteries the deposit was ossific in character, and the inner coat was ulcerated to the extent of a quarter of a rupee piece. *Abdomen.*—The left kidney was small, the surface pale yellow, granular, in places lobulated, and the tubular portion was distinctly encroached upon by the cortical, chiefly at its central parts. The right kidney was of the natural size, but presented the same abnormal appearances as the left.

211. *Admitted in an advanced state of disease.—Hepatisation of both lungs.—Circumscribed pleuritic effusion of the right side.—Kidneys enlarged, and in a state of yellow granular degeneration.—Urine not tested.*—Balloo Ragoo, aged forty, a Maratha, a native of Poona, but resident in Bombay for ten years, was admitted into the Jamsetjee Jejeebhoy Hospital on the 1st October, 1849, affected with diarrhœa and oppressed breathing. He had been ill a month, but was unable to give any connected account of his illness. On the 5th October, Atmaram Pandurang, at the time an intelligent student of Grant College, now a graduate, made the following note of the physical signs:—"Respiration short and hurried; the whole of the posterior and lateral part of the right side of the chest is duller than natural, and here bronchial sounds, mixed with mucous rale, are heard under the stethoscope; elsewhere on this side of the chest, and in the whole of the left side, the resonance was natural, and puerile respiration mixed with mucous rale is audible. There is equal movement of the two sides of the chest, and the dulness noticed does not vary by change of position. The vocal thrill is distinct on both sides." He died on the 7th.

Inspection fifteen hours after death.—Chest.—The inner edge of the right lung adhered firmly to the pericardium, and its anterior surface from the first to the sixth rib, adhered to the costal pleura by old firm adhesions. Below the fourth rib the adhesions did not extend externally beyond the nipple, but above that rib they were general to the lateral and posterior costal parietes, as well as to the anterior. There were about thirty ounces of sero-puriform fluid in the sac of the right pleura, chiefly between the base of the lung and diaphragm, and between the costal pleura and the lung, below the level of the fourth rib. The costal and pulmonary pleuræ were there covered with flaky lymph, forming, in parts, friable bands which extended across the effused fluid. The liver was displaced by the effusion, and projected below the margins of the right ribs. The right lung was, in great part, in a state of red induration, in parts passing into grey infiltration. The left lung adhered firmly to the costal pleura; the lower lobe was in a state of red induration; the upper crepitating, but œdematous. The kidneys were both enlarged and flabby, appearing mottled externally on the removal of the capsule, and on incision considerable encroachment of the tubular portion by pale yellow, slightly granular substance was evident.

212. *The subject of intermittent fever, followed by bronchitis, and slight anasarca.—Urine of low density, and very albuminous.*—Moria Pheena, a Hindoo labourer, of fifty years of age, an inhabitant of Benares, but for four or five years employed as a labourer at Aden, which place he left about eight months before admission into hospital: he had been addicted to the use of opium—ten grains daily for about eight years; he smoked ganja occasionally, but did not take spirituous liquors. He was admitted into the clinical ward on the 20th June, 1851: he stated that he had been the subject of intermittent fever about four months before, succeeded by cough, with copious expectoration, some œdema of the arms and feet, and subsequently with swelling of the abdomen. On admission he was a good deal reduced; the abdomen was somewhat full, and obscurely fluctuating, and there was slight œdema of the legs, scrotum, and fore-arms, with puffiness of the face; the lungs and heart showed no signs of disease on percussion and auscultation; there was no induration detected in the abdomen; the pulse was small and feeble; tongue moist; the bowels rather confined; no pain of loins. He continued under treatment up to August 7th, with no change in his state. The urine ranged in quantity from thirty to seventy ounces in the twenty-four hours, in specific gravity from 1·005 to 1·015, was generally clear, of pale lemon colour, neutral, and giving a copious flocculent deposit with heat and nitric acid. The urine being free, and the dropsical symptoms slight, it was thought advisable to try whether any impression could be made on the degeneration of the kidney by cod-liver oil: he took it to the extent of an ounce, and latterly an ounce and a half daily, and at the same time quinine was used twice daily in three-grain doses; but there being no improvement in the urine, or in his general state, these remedies were omitted, and the syrup of the iodide of iron was substituted. This was not followed by any amendment, and Dover's powder and the occasional use of the warm bath were had recourse to, with lessening of the œdema of the feet. He continued under treatment till the 22nd October, when he left the hospital, having derived little or no benefit from treatment. He was again seen on the 21st December, much in the same state as on discharge. From this time he was lost sight of till the 4th April, 1853, when he was re-admitted into hospital with feeble pulse, coldish skin, puffed face, œdematous feet, full abdomen. The urine, scanty and very albuminous, became almost entirely suppressed, and he passed into a drowsy state, and died on the 17th.

Inspection sixteen hours after death.—Head.—There was much opaque granular thickening of the arachnoid membrane, at the situation of the glandulæ Pacchioni. There was increased serous effusion in the sub-arachnoid space, and there was about a drachm of fluid in each lateral ventricle. The substance of the brain was healthy. There were about three pints of reddish-coloured serum in the sac of the left pleura. The left lung was compressed against the spine, and both costal and pulmonary pleuræ were thickened by granular lymph deposit. The right lung was œdematous, but healthy in other respects. The heart did not present any abnormal appearance. The left kidney was small, lobulated, granular, and pale externally. Internally the cortical part encroached much on the tubular, particularly at the centre. The right kidney not so pale, was more granular on the surface than the left, but in other respects was in the same state. The liver was congested in the second degree.

213. *Febrile symptoms and dropsy after exposure to cold and wet.—Traces of albumen in the urine, slight throughout, finally disappeared.—Addicted to the occasional use of spirits and opium.—Finally sunk under increasing asthenia.—Granular degeneration of the kidneys.*—Shaik Isood, a Mussulman horsekeeper, of eighteen years of age, a native of Kattyawar, apparently somewhat weak in mind, and using opium and spirits occasionally, was on the voyage to Bombay, two months before he came under observation, for two days exposed to cold and wet. After this he began to suffer from irregular febrile symptoms, generally commencing with chills, and the feet and

legs became swollen. On admission into the clinical ward on the 24th August, 1851, the face was puffed, and there was some degree of œdema of the body and the extremities, but no swelling or fluctuation of abdomen. No signs or symptoms of pulmonic or cardiac disease, or of enlargement of any abdominal viscus. The pulse was small, the bowels confined, and the urine free. On the 26th the urine had been thirty ounces in the preceding twenty-four hours, was of pale amber colour, neutral, and specific gravity 1·015, and became slightly turbid, by heat and nitric acid. He was treated with Dover's powder five grains, quinine two grains, ipecacuanha half a grain, every fourth hour for four times. This was continued, with the occasional use of warm baths, and one dose of castor-oil, till the 2nd September. There was generally sweating after the bath, the febrile symptoms ceased to recur, the dropsy lessened. The urine from thirty to fifty ounces, specific gravity 1·011 to 1·015, now showed a less degree of turbidity under heat and nitric acid. The same treatment, with substitution of six grains of nitre for the quinine, was continued till the 8th, when the dropsical symptoms were gone, and the urine, unchanged in other respects, ceased to give traces of albumen. The warm bath was still occasionally used, and fifteen mimims of the tincture of the sesquichloride of iron was now substituted for the powders. He continued in the clinical ward till the 12th October, gaining strength slowly, but without return of fever or of dropsical symptoms, and with the urine free of albumen. There was occasionally turbidity by heat, but it disappeared with effervescence, on addition of nitric acid. Latterly, ten minims of the compound tincture of iodine had been added to the tincture of iron. From this date he continued in another ward of the hospital, till the 5th April, without any regular record of the symptoms. Then imbecility of mind is noted, with occurrence of febrile disturbance, painful swelling of the left lower extremity, and pain of loins. He was with difficulty persuaded to keep his urine, which on the 11th was reported to be clear and high coloured, of specific gravity 1·020 and almost unaffected by heat, but showing a dark brown colour on excess of nitric acid. On the 15th, uneasiness of the cardiac region was complained of, and the pulse was weak and irritable: no signs of cardiac disease were detected. He now became affected with diarrhœa; sank rapidly, and died on the 17th.

The inspection after death was made by Dr. Forbes Watson, the Curator of the Museum, and the following note is abridged from his description.

Inspection.—*Head.*—On removing the scalp, a small ulcerous opening was detected over the right parietal protuberance. Opposite to it the bone was absent for the space of a circle an inch in diameter. The foramen was found to be filled with dense fibrous tissue, about quarter of an inch in thickness, and adherent pretty firmly to the dura mater. At this situation the brain felt less elastic, but did not present any abnormal appearance. *Chest.*—Slight adhesions existed between the left pleural surfaces at their lower part, but otherwise no disease of the lungs. The heart was healthy. *Abdomen.*—The liver rather increased in size; the external surface rough, and the surface of an incision mottled. The mucous membrane of the large intestine, and of the ileum, about Peyer's glands, was more vascular than natural. The size of the kidneys is not noted. On removing their capsules, the surface was granular, and of brick-red colour, and the texture was friable. These appearances were more remarkable in the left kidney. A section showed encroachment of the cortical on the tubular portion, and some fat was found in the pelvis, about the mammary processes. A portion of the healthy tubular part adjoining the cortical was examined under the microscope. The tubuli were distinctly made out in several parts, but only an occasional fat molecule detected. The cortical part showed multitudes of granular cells, and an occasional fat granule.

214.—*Dropsical symptoms with diarrhœa, following exposure to cold and wet.—Urine very albuminous.—Drowsiness co-existing with sinking pulse, removed by stimulants, did not recur.—Death by exhaustion.—Kidneys large and granular.—Spirit drinking not admitted.*—Abdoolla, a Mussulman Lascar, of thirty-five years of age, and in indigent circumstances, abstaining, according to his own statement, from the use of opium and spirits. Three months before he came under treatment had suffered from œdema of the feet, removed by the remedies used, and one month before his admission on the 16th September, 1851, into the clinical ward, he, consequent on exposure to wet and cold, became affected with diarrhœa, uneasiness of the right iliac region and loins, œdema of the feet and scanty urine. On admission, he was considerably reduced. The feet and legs were œdematous. The abdomen somewhat full, but without fluctuation. No signs or symptoms of pulmonic disease. The impulse of the heart was feeble, but the sounds normal. Hepatic dulness reached half an inch below the the margin of the ribs. The pulse was small. The tongue clean but glazed. The bowels relaxed. The urine scanty, high-coloured and very albuminous. He continued under treatment till the 23rd October, when he died. Throughout the diarrhœa, with more or less abdominal uneasiness, persisted. From the 26th September, febrile symptoms began to appear, and frequently recurred. On the 22nd September the pulse became very small, and there was drowsiness, which, removed by stimulants, did not again return. The urine, examined daily, was sometimes of brownish tint, at others amber coloured. At first the quantity was below twenty ounces. After the 1st October it ranged from twenty to thirty ounces. The specific gravity was always below 1·018. The albumen was throughout very copious, often filling half the tube, and latterly there was some degree of bronchitis. He died exhausted, without coma. He was treated with quinine and opium and stimulants.

Inspection seven hours after death.—Chest.—About one pint of serum was found in the left, and half a pint in the right cavity of the pleura. The middle lobe of the right lung was somewhat emphysematous, and firmly adherent to the costal pleura by old adhesions. The rest of the lungs was healthy and crepitating, excepting the upper part of the upper lobe of the left lung, which was compressed. *Abdomen.*—About two pints of serous fluid were found in the cavity. Firm adhesions connected the convex surface of the liver to the diaphragm. The peritoneal surface presented generally an opaque appearance, and the surface of the viscus was of a yellowish (not mottled) colour. The right lobe was larger than natural. When incised the surface had also a general yellow colour, was not mottled, and had a smooth appearance. Its texture was rather soft. The mucous membrane of the ileum was healthy. No enlargement of Peyer's glands or ulceration anywhere. In the mucous membrane of the large intestine, viz., part of the transverse, and the whole of the descending, colon, the sigmoid flexure, and rectum, numerous small, circular, follicular ulcers were seen scattered here and there; some completely cicatrised and others in process of ciatrisation. No ulceration could be detected in the ascending colon or in the cœcum. The right kidney was very large; it weighed six and a half ounces. When divested of its capsule it presented a somewhat lobulated, granular surface, of a generally buff colour, with small red patches here and there. When vertically incised, the cortical portion presented also a buff mottled granular surface, encroaching upon the tubular portion, chiefly at the central parts. The tubular portion, where not destroyed, was distinct and of a reddish colour. The left kidney was similar in colour and appearance to the right, both externally and when incised, but there was more of encroachment upon the tubular portion by the buff granular cortical part. It weighed seven ounces. Under the microscope a small portion scraped from the yellow granular substance showed an amorphous granular appearance. No oil globules.

215. *Syphilis, primary and secondary. — Mercurial influence. — Slight dropsy. — Albuminous urine, pain of loins, dysentery. — Fatal. — Bright's disease. — Ulceration and granular exudation on intestinal mucous membrane.—Cirrhosis.—A cretified guinea-worm encysted between the right lung and the pericardium.* — Shaik-Hussain-Adam, a Mussulman drummer, a native of Madras, of thirty-five years of age, and using spirits habitually to the extent of two ounces daily, suffered from primary syphilis, for

which he was salivated five years before he came under observation. From this time, however, till six months ago, his health had been good; then he experienced irregular febrile accessions, with much pain of the limbs, particularly of the tibiæ. For these symptoms he was received into the hospital; and while under treatment, orchitis came on, the 21st June, 1853, relieved by leeches, succeeded on the 25th by pain of loins and scanty urine, which on examination was found to be albuminous. He was transferred to the clinical ward on the 28th. Reduced in flesh, with œdema of the face and feet, pulse of moderate volume and jerking; no signs of cardiac disease, but bronchitic rales were audible in different parts of the chest. The liver was felt below the ribs, and the spleen was enlarged. The pain of loins, testes, and joints continued. There was slight heat of skin, with venous murmurs above the middle of the clavicles. The appetite was impaired, and he vomited occasionally. On the 1st July the urine was fourteen ounces, of light amber colour, and gave a deposit with heat and nitric acid. Under the occasional use of the warm bath, infusion of chiretta and diluted nitric acid, or the tincture of the sesquichloride of iron, there was lessening of the dropsical symptoms and some degree of general improvement up to the 15th, when dysenteric symptoms began to show themselves, and an abscess to form in the left natis, associated with frequent febrile accessions. Under these complications he sank without drowsiness, and died on the 27th July. The vomiting had been troublesome throughout. The urine had ranged from sixteen to thirty-eight ounces, specific gravity, 1·007 to 1·012, and was always albuminous.

Inspection nineteen hours after death. — There was not any effusion into the sac of the peritoneum. The kidneys weighed about four ounces each. The external surface was mottled red and white. The cortical portion encroached upon the tubular, and the latter was in some places indistinct, and in others spread out and expanded. The liver weighed 2 lb. 6 oz. There was much atrophy of the left lobe, and the external surface had an irregular puckered aspect. The mucous membrane of the end of the ileum ascending, transverse, descending colon and rectum presented a mottled brown and red granular appearance. There was extensive sloughy ulceration of the mucous membrane of the cæcum, and the tissue around was dark red, almost black in colour. Peyer's glands were not enlarged. The pleural and pericardial sacs were free of effusion. The lungs were crepitating but did not collapse. Between the inner surface of the middle lobe of the right lung and the pericardium, and connected to both by areolar tissue, there was an indurated tubular-looking body about three inches long, and much convoluted at one end. It resembled a guinea-worm. The large bronchial tubes contained frothy mucus, and their lining membrane was vascular. There was congestion of the left lung. The heart was abnormally small—concentric hypertrophy of the left ventricle—no disease of the valves.

Remark. —The cretified guinea-worm, situated between the lung and pericardium, is of interest. It is not unusual to find them in this state in subcutaneous areolar tissue in the dissecting-room of Grant Medical College.

216. *Dysentery, dropsy.—Albuminous urine, with fat globules, in an old spirit drinker and opium eater.—Fatal.—Ulcerated intestines.—Kidneys enlarged.—Fatty degeneration.*—Baldeen Pectum, aged sixty, a Hindoo barber, a native of Lucknow, and residing for the last twenty years in Bombay, drinking spirits freely in his early youth, and using opium occasionally in more advanced age, became affected with diarrhœa six months, followed by scanty urine and dropsical symptoms one month, before admission into hospital, on the 27th September, 1853. He was emaciated. The countenance was anxious and puffed. The upper and lower extremities were œdematous. The abdomen resistant, and uneasy on pressure in the course of the colon. The diarrhœa persisted. Had cough, but no signs of cardiac disease. The pulse was hardly perceptible and the skin coldish. On the 2nd eight ounces of urine of light amber colour, and specific gravity 1·010, gave a copious white precipitate by heat and

nitric acid. He continued to sink under the diarrhœa, and died on the 8th October without coma. The urine continued albuminous and scanty, and showed epithelial cells and abundant fat globules under the microscope.

Post mortem examination three hours after death.—Body emaciated. *Chest.*—There were firm old adhesions of the lungs on both sides all around. The right lung was very œdematous, in parts hepatised, and broke down under the fingers. The left lung was spongy and crepitating. There was about an ounce of fluid in the cavity of the pericardium. Heart diminished in size. The cavities were contracted and the valves healthy. On the anterior surface of the right ventricle there was an opaque, white, membranous patch the size of quarter of a rupee. *Abdomen.*—There were about eight ounces of turbid serum in the cavity of the abdomen. The intestines collapsed. The peritoneal surface of the intestines had an opalescent appearance; but no trace of inflammation was observed on the peritoneal surface of the anterior wall of the abdomen. There were large ulcerated patches here and there on the mucous membrane of the large intestine, evidently consequent on the separation of sloughs. About a foot of the mucous membrane of the ascending portion, and the commencement of the transverse colon, was in a dark grey and sloughy state. Similar disease was observed in the cœcum and also at the end of the rectum. There was redness of the mucous membrane of the ileum, as well as other parts of the small intestine; but no softening or ulceration observed. The stomach was distended, reached across the abdomen into the right hypochondriac region, and occupied half the space between the margins of the right false ribs and the right crest of the ileum. The mucous membrane of the stomach was healthy. The liver was not enlarged. It was of a dark brown colour both externally and internally. The right kidney weighed eleven ounces; externally it was of a pale yellow colour and lobulated; when incised, the surface presented, for the most part, a pale yellow granular appearance; the tubular portion had disappeared, except at the ends of the kidney, where there remained two or three bundles of bright red colour. The left kidney weighed nine ounces, and the morbid appearance was the same as that of the right kidney, with the exception of the tubular portion, which was more abundant and still present in the body of the organ. The scrapings of the surface, placed under the microscope, showed epithelial cells abounding with fat globules, similar to those observed two days before death in the urine. The spleen was somewhat increased in size, and the structure was found to be firm and hard on incising it.

217. *Dropsy.—Albuminous urine.—Death from dysenteric symptoms.—Kidneys enlarged, with fatty degeneration.—Redness in patches of the intestinal mucous lining.—Habits not known.*—Chimajee, a Hindoo horsekeeper, of thirty years of age, and of whose habits there is no note, after two months' illness, was admitted into hospital on the 4th June, 1852. The face was puffed, the feet and legs œdematous, and the abdomen tumid and fluctuating. He also suffered from febrile symptoms. The urine was scanty, of specific gravity 1·017, and gave a copious flocculent deposit with heat and nitric acid. It was tested several times and always found to be albuminous. He became affected with diarrhœa, lost strength rapidly, and died on the 17th June, without head symptoms.

Inspection thirteen hours after death by Mr. Carvalho.—Chest.—Both lungs were collapsed. The whole of the middle lobe of the right lung and the posterior part of the first and third lobes were in a state of red hepatisation and easily lacerable. There was congestion of the posterior parts of the left lung, but no hepatisation. The heart was normal in size and structure. *Abdomen.*—The liver was about the natural size and of normal structure. The mucous membrane of the lower end of the ileum, and of the whole of the colon, was of dark grey colour, with streaked patches of redness here and there, chiefly at the end of the ileum and rectum. No ulceration, thickening, or enlargement of the follicles. Both kidneys were considerably enlarged. The right weighed eleven and a half ounces, the left eleven, when denuded of their capsules. Both, when incised, presented a similar appearance. The cortical substance was found considerably augmented, pale yellow, fatty-looking, and encroaching much on the tubular structure which was of reddish colour. Under a cursory examination with the microscope numerous fat globules were apparent. The spleen was somewhat enlarged in size.

Under the continuance of Bright's disease, the quality of the *blood* is changed. The albumen and the red corpuscles decrease, the water increases, and an excess of urea is present. The *urine* may be defective, normal, or increased in quantity; and may contain varying proportions of albumen, be deficient in urea, and of diminished density.

Dropsy is of frequent occurrence. Some degree of anasarca and ascites was present in forty-six of my cases. The effusion may take place under two sets of circumstances. 1. In the early stages of the disease, while yet there is no deficiency of blood in the system, from the decided application of cold to the surface of the body. 2. In advanced stages, when cachexia is apparent, the blood watery, and all the actions of the system manifestly enfeebled. The occurrence of dropsy in these latter conditions is also very generally favoured by abstraction of heat from the surface of the body. My cases chiefly, though not exclusively, illustrate this second form.

In estimating the relation of dropsy to Bright's disease, we must not lose sight of the fact, that the structural changes throughout a considerable part of their progress are unattended by this symptom. Cases observed by me in the European General Hospital and reported in the chapters on Fever, Dysentery, and Hepatitis, confirm this truth.

The relation of Bright's disease to *head symptoms*—drowsiness, coma, convulsion—has been much dwelt upon by all observers in European countries, and is supposed to substantiate a pathological theory.

Head symptoms—drowsiness, or coma—were present in eight of my cases. In four * there was general exhaustion sufficient to explain these symptoms. In one (214) the drowsiness was not at the close of the disease, but some days previously, associated with failing pulse, and removed by stimulants. In two there were febrile symptoms of that kind, which not unfrequently lead to drowsiness and coma, irrespective of kidney disease. In one (203) there was complication of heart disease to which the head symptoms were as fairly chargeable as to the affection of the kidney.

* Of these, three, 208, 209, 212, are detailed.

Nor do my cases confirm the opinion, that when head symptoms take place, they may be explained by the existence of intercranial serous effusion. I have already shown* that increased serous effusion in the cranium, without head symptoms, is a common occurrence in India; and of my twenty post-mortem examinations of Bright's disease, there are three (204, 205, 207) in which increased intercranial effusion existed without head symptoms.

The relation of Bright's disease to *structural change of the heart*, has also been much insisted on. Not only has valvular disease been observed, but hypertrophy of the left ventricle†, without affection of the valves or of the aorta, has also been noticed, and regarded in the theoretic pathology of this disease. Complication of cardiac disease existed in six of my cases, and in one the aorta alone was affected. In two‡ of the six cases there was aortic disease, but the subject of one had followed the occupation of a diver, and the heart affection, more particularly the dilatation of the right ventricle, was probably as much due to this as to the aortic lesion. In one (210) of the six cases, there were old pericardial adhesions, and considerable emphysema of the lungs. In three there was disease of the mitral valve, and the subjects of two had formerly suffered from rheumatism. I have not met with a single instance of simple hypertrophy of the left ventricle. My observations, then, do not show a very frequent or evident relation between cardiac and renal disease; and a similar inference may be drawn from the facts stated by me in a subsequent chapter on pericarditis and organic affections of the heart. As bearing on this question, I would refer to two of my cases, in which an anæmic cardiac murmur was present. That this symptom should occasionally occur in a disease characterised by deteriorated blood is very probable, and the fact suggests a caution lest anæmic be mistaken for organic murmur; an error the more likely to arise when the mind of the observer is fully preoccupied with the idea, that disease of the heart is a very frequent sequence of Bright's disease of the kidney.

Various other secondary affections have been observed in the course of this disease—as pleuritis §, pericarditis, bronchitis,

* Chapter on Remittent Fever, p. 90.

† Dr. Bright, in the First Volume of Guy's Hospital Reports, records this state of 22 cases in 100.

‡ Cases 203, 208.

§ The relation of puriform pleuritis and peritonitis, secondary on hepatic abscess, to the cachexia of Bright's disease, has been already suggested in the chapter on Hepatitis, p. 369.

pneumonia, peritonitis, cirrhosis, diarrhœa, and dyspeptic symptoms. Of all these, occasional instances have come under my notice.

The morbid actions in the kidney which lead to disorganisation by deposits internal or external to the tubuli, and their ulterior changes, may be fairly attributed to a degenerate state of the processes by which constituents of the blood, in the renal capillaries, are assimilated to tissue, or appropriated to secretion. This abnormal action may be dependent on a pre-existing altered condition of the blood, the precise nature of which is unknown, but which forms part of those states of the system to which the terms "asthenic" and "cachectic" are applied. The morbid changes in the kidney will doubtless be favoured by the capillary circulation becoming the seat of inflammation. It is very probable that, when the structural lesion has taken place apart from *well-marked* cachexia, inflammatory action has been an operative condition.

The opinion that the organic change of the kidney is the result of a blood-poison seeking for local elimination, is altogether hypothetical, and hardly accordant with the fact of relation to various and different cachectic conditions which even a toxœmic theory of disease must attribute to separate poisons.

That the dropsical, cerebral, cardiac, and other secondary affections are dependent upon *uræmia*, is another favourite pathological theory. It is sufficiently plausible, and may ultimately prove correct; but I cannot avoid the conclusion, that it has been inferred from very insufficient premises, and too hastily and generally adopted. It may be admitted that when a part of the secreting structure of the kidney has become unfit, excess of urea in the blood, and defect in the urine, are probable sequences; but at the same time it should be borne in mind, that when an important organ becomes gradually unfit for function, then all the other actions of the system gradually harmonise with this defect. The lungs slowly unfitted by tubercular deposit, or the liver by cirrhosis, does not lead to excess of carbonic acid, or of bile in the blood, but to an anæmic state of the general system. The blood is by degrees reduced to the quantity which these imperfect organs are capable of depurating. For a similar reason, when the kidney becomes gradually disabled, it follows that there will be defect of urea in the urine, but by no means, necessarily, excess of this excretion in the blood. On the contrary, the inference from analogy is, not that there will be excess of urea in the blood, but that the blood will be brought down to that quantity which the kidney is competent to purify.

But chemistry has detected urea in excess in the blood in Bright's disease. On this point the questions may be put: (*a*) what proportion do the cases, in which the blood has been analysed by competent inquirers, bear to the total number of cases of Bright's disease which have been clinically studied? (*b*) Has care been taken, in selecting cases for analysis, to discriminate the recent from the advanced, the rapidly from the slowly-occurring structural lesions? (*c*) There are cachectic states from malaria, scurvy, mercury, syphilis, insufficient food, &c., in which the secondary affections, noted in Bright's disease, also occur. What amount of information do we possess in respect to the proportion of urea in the blood and in the urine, in these varied and frequently-occurring conditions? (*d*) Moreover, the cerebral and dropsical symptoms do not usually take place in chronic cases till the advanced stages of the renal affection have arrived. When dropsy occurs earlier, it, as well as many of the other secondary phenomena, may be removed by treatment and remain absent for months or years. Yet all this time the urine is albuminous, and in theory there is uræmia, but why is the poison quiescent?

Frerichs, appreciating this latter difficulty in regard to the secondary nervous affections, has propounded the theory that urea does not, while in that state, exercise a poisonous influence, but only after decomposition and formation into carbonate of ammonia. This theory, to be good for anything, will require to be extended in its application to all the other secondary affections which pathologists have, equally with the head symptoms, attributed to uræmia.

It is consequent on reflections such as these that I have ventured to suggest that the uræmic theory of the secondary affections of Bright's disease has been too hastily adopted, and on data altogether insufficient for the logical affirmation of an important pathological doctrine.

The facts as they now stand relative to the kidney-degeneration itself, and the secondary affections which attend on it, seem to me merely to afford another illustration of that general law on which I have already so frequently insisted, viz., that structures in cachectic states are apt to be injured and unfitted for function by degenerate processes of assimilation; and that, when this occurs in an important organ, the effect must be to aggravate the cachexia by reducing the blood and the actions dependent on it to a degree proportionate to the impairment of the organ. Further, that in cachectic states, various secondary affections are apt to arise, under the influence of slight, sometimes even without appreciable, exciting causes.*

That special structural changes may, at some future time, be proved to be related to special cachexiæ is very probable; but this advance in science can only be achieved by time and a far more extended range of investigation than has as yet been applied to these subjects. The hasty generalisations, too characteristic of pathological inquiry of late years, serve to retard sure and steady progress, and to detract from the philosophy of medical research.

Having in view, in the remarks which have just been concluded, the uræmic doctrines which have been applied to the pathology of the secondary affections of Bright's disease, I have confined my observations to the supposed alteration of the blood in respect to the proportion of urea; but the blood is also said to be defective in its proportion of albumen, in the ratio of the excess of the albumen in the urine. (*a*) It may perhaps be inquired whether, in thus relating the loss of albumen in the blood to the gain of albumen in the urine, sufficient attention has been given, in the cases submitted to analysis, to the fact of presence or absence of dropsical effusion; for surely when dropsy is present, deficiency of albumen in the blood may more fairly be attributed to its presence in the effusion than to its transudation into the urine. (*b*) Again, is it not likely that deficiency of albumen in the blood will be found equally characteristic of other dropsies as of renal dropsy? (*c*) Further, is it not probable that much of the deficiency of albumen in the blood may be attributable to the coexisting anæmic state? (*d*) In a word, pathologists in explaining a defect of albumen in the blood in Bright's disease, seem to lay

* That when an important organ is structurally unfit, the co-existing cachexia may favour one secondary affection rather than another, is very true and very intelligible. In malarious and scorbutic cachexiæ, secondary dysentery or dropsy are sufficiently common, but when certain structural changes of the liver co-exist, there is still greater liability to secondary dysentery and ascites, in consequence of the obstruction to the portal circulation. When heart disease co-exists with cachexia, general dropsical effusions more certainly take place. When we recollect the function of the kidney in regulating the proportion of water in the blood, there need be no difficulty in understanding why a cachexia, attended with certain structural changes of this organ, should have more of secondary dropsical affections than cachexiæ unassociated with this structural change; but I am unable to appreciate the necessity of calling in the aid of a special toxœmia, in explanation of the dropsy of Bright's disease, more than in that of the many other pathological states with which this symptom is also often associated. I shall have to return to the subject of dropsy in a subsequent chapter, which may be considered in reference to my observations now made.

chief weight upon one event—albumen in the urine—to the exclusion of other co-efficient events—dropsical effusion, and general anæmia.

The supposed accordance of the latest theory of urinary secretion, and albumen in the urine in Bright's disease, is certainly not exempt from difficulty and doubt. In regard to normal secretion it is assumed that the peculiar arrangement of the capillaries of the Malpighian bodies leads to an abrupt retardation in the velocity of the current of the blood passing through them; by which, and by the aid of cilia, facility is given to the escape, by transudation, of the water of the blood from the Malpighian capillaries. It escapes without albumen. In regard to the presence of albumen in Bright's disease, it is argued that defect of the processes between the blood external to, and the epithelial cells internal to, the cortical tubuli, leads to retardation of the blood in the Malpighian bodies behind; hence transudation of the serum of the blood takes place, just as obtains in a dropsical effusion from venous obstruction. We are further told that after a time under this deranged action the walls of the Malpighian capillaries become thickened.* In the early stages of the disease when the urine is scanty, and the Malpighian capillaries, we may assume, as yet unthickened, this explanation of the proximate cause of albumen in the urine is perhaps satisfactory. But when we refer to the advanced stages, when the urine is more than normal in quantity, and the walls of the Malpighian capillaries are said to be thickened, the explanation fails to convince, for it is not in accordance with the theory of normal secretion. In Bright's disease with excess of urine there must be a continuous current through the capillaries as in the healthy state; but in the latter we have a condition of the capillary walls more favourable to transudation, yet the albumen is retained, and only transudes when the condition of the capillary walls is, from hypertrophy, less favourable for the process. It seems to me, however, that this difficulty rather invalidates Mr. Bowman's theory of the function of the Malpighian bodies than the explanation of the albuminous urine; for in order to complete the theory of urinary secretion, advanced by this distinguished physiologist, is it not necessary to show some reason why, under circumstances described as so favourable to transudation, the albumen is retained during the process which is supposed to take place normally in the Malpighian capillaries? Is there

* "On the Diseases of the Kidney:" London, 1852. By George Johnson, M.D., p. 240.

any other instance of free transudation, through thin capillary walls, in which the water of the blood is not accompanied by a portion of the albumen?

SECTION III.—*Etiology.—Scarlatina not influential in India.—Relation to Caste, Age, Occupation, Habits, Season.—Cold an exciting cause sometimes of the Kidney Disease, generally of the Secondary Affections.*

The frequent occurrence of dropsy, with albuminous urine, during convalescence from scarlatina, and the history of occasional cases of Bright's disease in European countries, have suggested the idea that scarlatina may be related, as a cause, to Bright's disease. This may be true of these countries, but it cannot be of India; for I have elsewhere * stated that there, scarlatina, if not altogether unknown, is undoubtedly very rare.

The native population of Bombay is very varied and fluctuating, and includes all castes, and the inhabitants of different and widely separated countries. This is well shown in the following classification of my fifty-eight cases of Bright's disease.

Hindoos, 19—natives of the following districts:—

Bombay	4	Mooltan	1
Concan	2	Benares	1
Deccan	2	Lucknow	1
Cutch	1	Country not stated	7
Jeypoor	1		

Mussulmans, 22—from

Bombay	2	Scinde	2
Concan	1	Mooltan	1
Deccan	2	Khorassan	1
Cutch	1	Lucknow	1
Kattywar	1	Cabool	1
Guzerat	1	Arabia	1
Bengal	2	Africa	1
Madras	1	Not stated	3

Parsees, 8—from Bombay and Surat.

Christians, 9—chiefly Portuguese, from Goa.

From this statement it is evident, that the frequency of Bright's disease in Bombay is not attributable to the influence on the native resident population, of the example of the lower classes of Europeans who frequent the port. It rather justifies the belief that further inquiry will show that this disease prevails in certain classes of the varied tribes and natives of Asia and Africa, as well as of Europe.

* Chapter on Eruptive Fevers, p. 199.

The ratio per cent. of these fifty-eight cases in the different castes stands thus:—

Mussulmans	36·9 per cent.
Hindoos	32·7 "
Christians	15·5 "
Parsees	13·2 "

But in order to determine whether these data suggest the probability of a greater prevalence in one caste than another, it is necessary to show the ratio of the hospital admissions of these castes. It is as follows:—

Hindoos	33·9 per cent.
Mussulmans	28·9 "
Christians	16·2 "
Parsees	6·8 "

On comparing these two ratios we find that they show the greatest proclivity to Bright's disease in Parsees and Mussulmans. In the ratio of castes to the hospital admissions, females are not included; but the women of all castes are 14 per cent.; and of the fifty-eight cases of Bright's disease, two were females, which is 3·4 per cent. But these data do not justify any inference relative to *sex*, because my clinical researches were pursued chiefly in the male wards of the hospital.

In classifying my cases with reference to age, occupations, habits, and season, the following results appear:—

AGES.

From 15 to 20	3
" 21 " 30	27
" 31 " 40	16
" 41 " 50	8
" 51 " 60	2
Not stated	2
	58

OCCUPATIONS.

Baker	1	Pilgrims	3
Barbers	2	Sailors	6
Beggars	3	Servants	2
Cooks	8	Sepoys	2
Coachmen	8	Shopkeepers	2
Diver	1	Weavers	2
Hakeems	2	Writers	2
House painter	1	Women	2
Labourers	7	Not stated	2
Liquor sellers	2		
			58

HABITS.

Spirit drinkers	20	Spirits, opium, and ganja	1
Opium eaters	4	Not stated	11
Ganja smokers	4	Denied use of spirits or narcotics	9
Spirit drinkers and opium eaters	7		
Spirit drinkers and ganja smokers	2		58

MONTHS OF ADMISSION.

January	6	August	5
February	2	September	16
March	2	October	11
April	2	November	4
May	2	December	3
June	4		
July	1		58

The bearing of these facts on the etiology of Bright's disease may be thus stated:—

1. The great number, forty-three, between the ages of twenty-one and forty, is consistent with the opinion, that intemperate habits are influential. 2. Seventeen occupations are named, but twenty-nine of the cases are comprised under four, viz.: cooks, coachmen, labourers, and sailors, all of which, more or less, involve exposure to alternations of heat, cold, and wet, and imply habits usually more or less intemperate. 3. The habits of only thirty-eight are stated, but in these, the use of spirits, opium, or ganja, singly or combined, is acknowledged. 4. Twenty-seven were admitted in September and October, months in which neither cold nor wet are influential as exciting causes of disease. But considering that a very large proportion were not residents of Bombay, and that all were admitted in advanced stages of the disease, the period of admission into hospital has no bearing on the etiology. September and October, the months immediately succeeding the rainy season, are those in which the influx of strangers is great, and to this circumstance the large number of admissions in these months is doubtless attributable.

The inference from my cases is, that there exists a relation between structural degeneration of the kidney, and the cachectic states induced by the habitual use of spirits and narcotics.

They however afford no evidence of the influence of syphilis in causing Bright's disease, because though a syphilitic taint is recorded of eleven cases, they all, with two exceptions, are also included in the list of spirit drinkers, opium eaters, or smokers of ganja.

Malaria is a fertile source of cachexia in India, and conduces, as we have already found, to degeneration of structure in the liver and spleen. It is interesting to inquire whether this influence is also exercised on the kidney. It is difficult to separate the effects of malaria from the other causes already named, for they are often combined together. It is, therefore, sufficient to note, that, in nineteen of the fifty-eight cases, the influence of malaria on the system is clearly recorded.

That inflammation, though by no means essential, is often operative in producing the structural lesions of this disease, is probably true. If so, we may expect occasional evidence of the ordinary exciting causes of inflammation acting as the exciting causes of Bright's disease. Therefore, we can be at no loss in understanding how this disease may, in some instances, be clearly traceable to the influence of external cold. Indeed, the functional relation of the skin and the kidney might lead us to anticipate that interruption of the actions of the former (more particularly if previously disordered), by reduction of its temperature, may be followed by inflammation or other derangement of the latter.

So much, then, in regard to the causes of the renal disease. We have next to inquire into those of the secondary affections. I shall not again advert to the question of uræmia; for I have already expressed my opinion that it ought to be regarded as still *sub judice;* the more so, as the phenomena of the disease are, for practical purposes, sufficiently explainable on certain general well-understood pathological principles. That a more intimate knowledge of deranged actions ought to be earnestly sought for, is not denied; but a practical art, such as medicine, is as likely to be damaged, as advanced, by uncertain science; and it is therefore well not to set aside useful and safe, though incomplete principles, for others which, though full of promise, are still hypothetical, and may lead us into errors of practice.

In the cachectic state, associated with Bright's disease, there is ample explanation of the predisposition which exists in the system to become affected with inflammatory and other forms of disease. In *this* cachectic state, as in others, of which I have previously treated, the deranged actions are very generally excited by the application of external cold to the surface of the body. In regarding cold as an exciting cause of the secondary affections of Bright's disease, we must remember the lessened capacity for the generation of animal heat in cachectic states; and when our inquiry has reference to tropical countries, we have also to recollect the relation of heat-generating power to climatic temperature. Further, in respect to the class of individuals from which my experience in Bright's disease has been chiefly derived, there is, in inadequate clothing and insufficient habitations, another circumstance favourable to the abstraction of heat from the surface of the body. On referring to my cases for confirmation of the influence of cold as an exciting cause, I find that the dropsy has been attributed to cold or wet by the patients themselves in seven instances, and that it occurred in sixteen others at times when the heat-abstracting conditions of the cold or rainy season were operative.

SECTION IV. — *Symptoms.* — *Referable to the Kidney.* — *Condition of the Urine.* — *Treatment.* — *Of the Kidney Disease.* — *Of the Secondary Affections, chiefly the Dropsical Effusions.*

Symptoms. — In cases in which the scanty, high-coloured, and very albuminous character of the urine rendered probable the existence of preternatural, inflammatory, or other afflux of blood to the kidneys, this inference has been further confirmed by the presence of more or less uneasiness in the lumbar region, with sometimes nausea and vomiting. But in the large proportion of my own observations this has not been the character of the urine, and pain of loins has not been a common symptom.

The disease has generally been indicated in my cases by the occurrence of dropsy in cachectic individuals, suggesting inquiry into the state of the urine. In order to the detection of this disease, the safe practical rule is, that in all asthenic or cachectic states — whether simple or complicated — we ought to search for Bright's disease of the kidney by examining the urine, just as in all cases of rheumatism and of idiopathic fever we search for pericarditis and pneumonia by percussion and auscultation. Indeed, I have previously remarked that in asthenic and cachectic states the clinical rule should be invariably observed of determining, by the application of all the diagnostic means at our command, the presence or absence of local disease; for, without this preliminary step, the prognosis will be needlessly uncertain, and the treatment vacillating and unsafe. My present remark, in reference to Bright's disease, is merely an application of this general rule.

In all the cases in which the *urine* was carefully examined, its albuminous character and low density have been well marked. It has been, for the most part, of pale amber or lemon colour, clear and neutral, varying in specific gravity from 1·003 to 1·018.* In quantity it has generally ranged from twenty to forty ounces in the twenty-four hours; and in cases beyond these limits it has more frequently exceeded forty ounces than fallen short of twenty. My earlier cases occurred before much attention had been given to the microscopic character of the urine; but in the later ones the characteristic tube casts, epithelial debris, and oil globules, were frequently observed.

Treatment. — The treatment resolves itself into that which is appropriate for the *disease of the kidney*, and that which conduces best to the removal of the several secondary affections.

When uneasiness of the loins, scanty, very albuminous, and high-coloured urine, indicate excess of blood in the kidney, then local depletion from the loins by cupping or leeches, the use of the warm water, vapour, or hot air bath, the removal of constipation, and confinement to bed, are appropriate and efficacious means of cure. When the state of constitution is such as to contra-indicate loss of blood, much diaphoresis, or other evacuation, then dry cupping, a moderated use of baths, and a greater attention to warm clothing, is the modification of treatment required. By these means the lumbar uneasiness will disappear, and the urine will gradually become more copious and of lighter colour. The persistence or not of albumen will depend upon whether the excess of blood has been in a kidney previously healthy, or affected with structural degeneration.

In cases in which freedom from lumbar pain, and a flow of pale urine, of normal or increased quantity, point to the absence of excess of blood in the kidneys; but in which the presence of albumen and a low specific gravity of the urine, generally with a co-existing cachectic state, prove the existence of structural degeneration, the indication of cure as respects the kidney, is to promote, moderately, the function of the skin by great attention to clothing, and to endeavour to lessen the general cachexia by well-adjusted tonic regimen and remedies. The cases observed by me have been chiefly of this nature, and the remedies which have seemed to me most efficacious, have been *preparations of iron*, combined with *quinine*, in instances in which the influence of malaria was suspected.

* The specific gravities are noted as observed with a urinometer, graduated for a temperature of 60°. These observations have been made at a mean temperature of about 80°; and may be sufficiently corrected by an addition of 2° to each specific gravity.

Though by this course of treatment we can hardly hope to remove the structural degeneration when fairly established, yet we may expect to check its progress, and lessen the predisposition to attacks of the secondary affections. Moreover, though we may not be sanguine enough to anticipate the restoration of structures already degenerate and changed; still there is surely no more likely method of effecting an object so desirable, than by that regimen and those remedies which tend best to re-induce normal assimilation to blood and to tissue.

In noticing the treatment of the secondary affections, I shall consider first the *dropsical effusions*, as being the most frequent, and perhaps the most important, of them. When dropsy comes on early in the disease, it is generally accompanied with the symptoms which indicate excess of blood in the kidney, and will be best removed by the means already recommended as most appropriate for this state, viz., local blood-letting, the warm or vapour bath, attention to the bowels, and confinement to bed. When dropsy, as is most frequently the case, occurs in the more advanced stages of the disease associated with a cachectic state, and not characterised by scanty urine and lumbar uneasiness, then the following rules of practice may be observed:—

1. Attention to the functions of the skin by warm clothing, and the occasional use of the warm bath, is a ruling indication in the management of all the forms of dropsy.

2. When the effusions, from situation or degree, are not of a nature to interfere much with the functions of important organs — as the lungs, the heart, or the kidneys themselves — the treatment of the dropsy simply resolves itself into that adjustment of regimen and tonic remedies, which is most likely to ameliorate the nutritive condition of the blood. With improvement in the general system, the dropsical effusion will disappear.

3. When the dropsy, from situation or extent, interferes with the functions of important organs, the reduction of the effused fluid by evacuation from the blood becomes an important indication in the treatment. The channel of elimination must be selected according to the circumstances of individual cases.

4. When there is no evidence of gastro-intestinal irritation, evacuation by *purgatives* holds out the greatest prospect of speedy relief — bitartrate of potass combined with jalap or gamboge, and elaterium, are the most useful remedies of this class. In asthenic states, complicated with dropsy, purgatives may probably be given to a degree which would be unsafe in similar states of constitution

unattended by dropsy, because the effusion is a ready source of supply to the blood of that fluid which has been eliminated from the intestinal surface.* But risk from the use of purgatives in the dropsy of Bright's disease rests on the fact of the proclivity which obtains in this, as in all other cachectic states, to muco-enteritis, from the application of irritants to the mucous surface. This difficulty is very likely to arise in tropical countries, and in my own practice it has proved very generally obstructive to the use of this class of remedies.

5. When purgatives are contra-indicated, then we may select between evacuation by diaphoresis or diuresis. If there be no congestion of the kidney to remove, I doubt whether much will be gained by evacuation by the skin. Indeed, in those cases of dropsy with renal congestion, in which determination to the skin in general acts so beneficially, the good effected is not by diaphoresis, but by the restoration of improved circulation and secretion in the kidney itself. The frequent use of the warm bath must tend to increase the cachexia; therefore, in the kind of cases of which I now treat, diaphoresis, beyond that which is involved in my first rule, is inexpedient.

6. When there are no symptoms of excess of blood in the kidneys, when purgatives are contra-indicated, when the dropsical symptoms are such as to call for speedy removal, — then we must use combinations of *diuretics*, as the acetate of potass, with tincture of squills and of digitalis, and spiritus ætheris nitrici. The addition of the potassio-tartrate, or other salt of iron, or of quinine, is often very useful. When the state of the constitution suggests the use of stimulants, the sesquicarbonate of ammonia may with advantage be substituted for the acetate of potass.

7. I have already said that, when the dropsy is not present to that extent which interferes with important functions, evacuation from the blood is not required; for the effusions will disappear under attention to the state of the skin, and improvement in the condition of the general system. And it may now be added, that when, under these circumstances, the intestinal discharges and the quantity of urine are adequate, we are likely to do harm by the use of evacuant remedies, for they tend to increase the asthenia.

* In the chapter on Peritonitis I have narrated a case (197) in which cholera came on in the course of Bright's disease, with dropsy, and in which I attributed the slow course of the cholera to the fact that the loss to the blood by intestinal discharges was supplied from the fluid of the dropsical effusions.

8. While appropriate evacuants are being used in those cases in which the degree of the dropsy calls for reduction by evacuation, great attention must, at the same time, be given to the regimen, and to the tonic or stimulant remedies, which may be indicated for the correction of the diathesis. Success in the treatment of such cases will be commensurate with the skill and steadiness with which these two indications are simultaneously carried out.

It is unnecessary to explain the details of treatment of the *secondary inflammations* in Bright's disease. They must be conducted with reference to the state of the constitution, the improvement of which must also be kept in view as a leading indication in the management of the case. Hence the great importance of ascertaining, in respect to all asthenic inflammations, whether they are co-existent or not with structural degeneration of the kidney. The only secondary inflammation which I shall notice, in consequence of the frequency of its occurrence in India, is dysentery. The treatment must be conducted in accordance with those principles which I have already elsewhere so fully explained, combined with much attention to warmth of the surface of the body.

To conclude. In Bright's disease, as in other structural degenerations, for the restoration of which the powers of the animal system are inadequate, we have impressed upon us the importance of careful inquiry into the causes, with the view of preventing their action. It is thus, in respect to these forms of disease, that we shall best apply the resources of medical science in prolonging life.

It may seem that by making no reference in my remarks on treatment to the uræmic theory, and the therapeutic principles which it naturally suggests, the value of medical art has not been fully appreciated. I would, therefore, on this question of practice, express my belief that, in the present state of the science, the only conditions which justify the use of eliminant remedies are excess of vascular action, adequate amount of blood and diminished excretion; and that the eliminant should be selected with reference to the excretion which is most markedly defective.

Some degree of asthenia or cachexia is always present in the chronic forms of disease supposed to be dependent on an abnormal materies in the blood; and attention to the amount and variety of elimination which is involved in a well-adjusted tonic regimen, holds out, it seems to me, a better and a safer prospect of benefit from the therapeutic principle in question, than the empiric use of special eliminant medicines. A well-adjusted tonic regimen implies a just attention to pulmonary, cutaneous, alvine, and urinary excretion. It aims, also, at bringing about increased activity of those actions by which food is assimilated to blood and blood to tissue; and every step of success towards this end must improve the structural fitness and other functional conditions of excreting organs, and lead to augmented excretion. Increased excretion is a necessary sequence of increased assimilation. That these are sound principles of practice, in the present uncertain state of the pathology of blood diseases, cannot, I think, be questioned; but I venture to go further than this, and to predict, that even with that greater knowledge of blood poisons and of excretions which chemical science has yet to confer on pathology, these principles will still prove applicable and essential.

CHAP. XX.

ON ABNORMAL STATES OF THE URINE.

SECTION I. — *Preliminary Pathological Remark. — A want of Information in respect to the Normal Condition of the Urine in India.*

ALBUMINURIA has, in the last chapter, been related to transient congestion, or to structural degeneration, of the kidney: the proximate cause is therefore supposed to exist in the secreting organ itself. But there are other abnormal conditions of the urine occurring without structural change of the kidney, whose proximate cause is believed to reside in derangements of primary or secondary assimilation: the precise nature, however, of these derangements is unknown. But before noticing these abnormal states of the urine, a preliminary question suggests itself for consideration, — In what respect does the normal condition of the urine in warm climates differ from that in cold?

In the months of July, August, October, and November 1852, and in February and March 1853, Mr. Sebastian Carvalho, an intelligent graduate of Grant College, while officiating as one of the medical officers of the Jamsetjee Jejeebhoy Hospital, conducted a series of observations on the urine of five healthy Hindoo Ward boys, with the view of determining the normal quantity and specific gravity of the secretion. The average quantity amounted to about forty-two ounces in the twenty-four hours, and the specific gravity was found to range from 1·007 to 1·016.* But on other questions

* In my remarks on the urine in Bright's disease of the kidney, I stated the specific gravity observed in my cases to range from 1·003 to 1·018; or, when corrected for temperature, from 1·005 to 1·020. The normal specific gravity, as deduced from Mr. Carvalho's observations, does not accord with this. The inference I believe to be simply this — that further and more extended investigation is necessary, in order to establish a trustworthy standard of the normal state of the urine both in Europeans and natives in India.

relative to the quality of the urine, no light has been thrown by these observations. They were submitted by Mr. Carvalho to the Grant College Medical Society, and a summary statement of them has been published.* I have already † expressed my belief that all the solid excreta are considerably less in India than in colder climates; and the investigations just referred to, so far as they go, tend to strengthen this opinion in regard to the urine.

SECTION II. — *Chylo-serous Urine.—Short Notice of its Pathology and Treatment.*

This term has been applied to urine of a milky, opaque appearance, coagulating on the application of heat or addition of nitric acid, and sometimes spontaneously. The opacity depends upon fatty matter, the coagulability by heat on albumen, and that which occurs spontaneously on the presence of fibrine. This abnormal state of the urine has been generally noticed in association with more or less asthenia or cachexia, and has been attributed to faulty assimilation, and not to disease of the kidney; because, in the few instances of which post mortem appearances are recorded, this organ has been found healthy; and, on the other hand, restoration to health, with coincident normal urine, has not been infrequent. Prout‡ had met with thirteen cases of this disease; and as seven of them occurred in residents of hot climates, it was inferred that the affection was probably more common in tropical than in temperate countries. Still it cannot be viewed as of frequent occurrence in India. There is the case of a female reported § by Dr. H. H. Goodeve; also one ‖ of a female observed by Dr. Pearse, with a careful chemical analysis by Professor Mayer. These are the only recorded Indian cases with which I am acquainted. My personal knowledge of the disease is limited to eight cases. The first, made known to me at Belgaum in 1830, occurred in an European officer's wife. The urine coagulated spontaneously into a white gelatinous mass: with the termination of this case I am not acquainted. The second was observed by me about 1839, in the European General Hospital at Bombay. The

* "Transactions, Medical and Physical Society of Bombay," new series, No. 2.

† Page 4.

‡ "Nature and Treatment of Stomach and Renal Diseases," 4th edition.

§ "Transactions, Medical and Physical Society of Calcutta," vol. viii.

‖ "Transactions, Royal Medical and Chirurgical Society," vol. xxxiv.

subject was a young female born in India, of European parents, and the wife of a warrant officer of the garrison. She was pale and feeble, the urine was white and spontaneously coagulated into a jelly-like mass. Much variety of treatment was adopted without benefit. This patient left the hospital, and was lost sight of for about two years, when I accidentally met her in the ward visiting a friend. She had lost her pallid appearance, and was in good condition. I inquired into her state of health; but so completely had the former abnormal condition of the urine passed from her mind, that the object of my questions was not at first readily understood. It appeared that after leaving the hospital she had gone to Scinde to join her husband, who was on duty there. Her general health improved, and the urine became normal without the use of medicines of any kind.

The remaining six cases are annexed in detail to these remarks; three of them occurred in Parsees, one in the clinical ward, and two communicated to me by Mr. Dossabhoy Bazunjee, a zealous graduate of Grant College. The fourth was observed in a Hindoo by Mr. Carvalho. The fifth is extracted from Mr. Balchrishna Chintoba's report of the Poona Charitable Dispensary for 1858. The sixth occurred in a Portuguese servant, under my own observation.

I shall not speculate on the nature of the faulty assimilation by which fatty and proteine principles, instead of being normally appropriated, are excreted with the urine. Albuminous and chylo-serous urine would seem to differ simply in this, that in the former, albumen is the only proximate principle present, whereas in the latter, albumen, in greater quantity, is associated with fat and frequently with fibrine. There is in the chylo-serous urine a more complete transudation of organic constituents of the blood on the *free* surface of the uriniferous tubes. Though it may probably be added that urea is deficient in albuminous, but not in chylo-serous urine; yet it may be doubted whether investigation has been sufficiently extensive in both affections to justify an assertion so positive.

There is good reason for relating both derangements to cachectic states, that is, to mal-assimilation. In Bright's disease, degenerate proteine and fatty principles are deposited *in* the structures of the kidney, and albumen transudes with the urine. In chylo-serous urine the proteine and fatty principles are separated from the blood at the kidney, *with* the urine, and no part is left behind to clog and destroy the structure of the organ. In both affections proximate principles unsuited, from some cause or other, for their normal purposes, are carried to the kidney. In the one they are partly deposited in the organ to the injury of its structure, and are partly removed with the urine. In the other all are removed with the urine, none are deposited in the kidney. Such, I think, is the view which, in the present state of pathology, we are justified in taking of the points of resemblance and difference between these two diseases. Why, in the one, the same principles are all excreted, and in the other partly deposited in the kidney, is one of the many questions which pathology has yet to determine. I would further remark, that the doubts which I ventured to express, relative to the generally received explanation of the proximate cause of albuminous urine in Bright's disease, are increased by the fact of the greater albuminous transudation which takes place in chylo-serous urine.

On *treatment* a very few remarks will suffice. The indication is to remove the cachectic state, in other words, to correct the error of assimilation; and six of my cases distinctly show, that all means having this object in view failed till suitable change of air was enforced. The balsams, lytta, diosma, gallic acid, preparations of iron and other remedies supposed to have special influence on the urinary organs, have signally failed—a further proof that the proximate cause of the disease is not to be sought for there.

218. *Urine thick, white, opaque, coagulating with heat and nitric acid.—No improvement under the use of varied remedies.—Recovery by attention to the general health, chiefly to change of air.*—A Parsee, of twenty-one years of age, following the occupation of English clerk, of temperate habits, never the subject of syphilis, but of weak constitution, consulted Mr. Dossabhoy Bazunjee on the 13th October, 1851. There was no indication of pulmonary or cardiac disease, but the pulse was feeble, the appetite impaired, and he attributed his feeble health to close application to study. He was also the subject of reducible femoral hernia of the left side. He stated that for six or seven days he had been voiding thick, white opaque urine, without, however, frequent calls to micturate. This state of the urine had been attended with pain of the loins and limbs, but no distinct fever. He had never suffered thus before. The urine, on being examined, was found to be white, thick, and opaque, of specific gravity 1·040, and gave a copious white flocculent deposit under heat, and on the addition of nitric acid. He was treated with creosote and tincture of the sesquichloride of iron, and plain nourishing food; a rubefacient liniment of turpentine oil, liquor ammoniæ, and olive oil was applied to the loins. This treatment was followed till the 29th October, by which time he had gained in flesh, the pulse had improved in strength, the uneasiness of loins was less; the urine, for the most part unchanged in character, was, however, occasionally clear, of amber colour, slightly acid, and unaffected by heat and nitric acid. The same treatment was continued, with exception of the liniment to the loins; and on the 1st November he went to the seaside at Breach Candy, and resided four days with a friend. There he improved in general health, the urine also became clear, and remained so for four days after his return home to the Fort of Bombay. On the fifth day the urine was clear in the morning, but in the middle of the day had become white and opaque as before. Mr. D. Bazunjee recommended a longer resi-

dence at Breach Candy, but another practitioner undertook to cure him by other means. The infusion of diosma, balsam of copaiva and aperients, with restricted diet, were freely tried. He became emaciated and feeble, and the urine remained unchanged. About the 15th December he again became a patient of Mr. D. Bazunjee, and I was asked to see him in consultation. The tincture of the sesquichloride of iron, with tincture of lytta, was prescribed. He improved in flesh and strength, but the urine continued white, thick, and opaque. And on the 14th March he again went to Breach Candy, and remained there for two and a half months. In ten days the urine became clear. He returned home on the 1st June in good health, and afterwards continued so. While at Breach Candy he took no medicine, and lived on good food without any particular restriction.

219. *Urine thick, white, opaque, coagulating with heat and nitric acid.—No improvement from medical treatment.—Recovery from change of air.*—On the 1st May, 1852, a Parsee, of forty-five years of age, of stout frame and temperate habits, never the subject of syphilis, nor under the influence of mercury, but generally in the enjoyment of good health, consulted Mr. Dossabhoy Bazunjee. No visceral disease could be detected; but he complained that his urine was white, thick, and opaque, and that the calls to micturate were generally six times in the night and four in the course of the day. He had suffered thus for five months, and had been treated with balsam of copaiva and various other remedies, with some relief. The urine, when examined, was found to be of high density, and to give a copious flocculent deposit under heat and nitric acid. Mr. D. Bazunjee prescribed creosote, without benefit; then tincture of the sesquichloride of iron, with tincture of iodine, tincture of lytta, gallic acid, and sulphuric ether were in succession tried, with as little success. On the 15th July medicine was omitted, and change of air recommended. This advice he could not follow for twenty days, during which time the urine continued unchanged. About the middle of August he went to reside at Negaon. He remained there for a month, became quite well in fifteen days, and has continued in good health since his return home.

220. *Urine opaque and white, occasionally coagulating spontaneously.— Recovery from change of air.*—A Hindoo clerk, of twenty-three years of age, attended the Jamsetjee Jejeebhoy Hospital, as an out-patient, from the 21st May to the 1st July, 1851. He was under the care of Mr. Sebastian Carvalho, to whom I am indebted for the following information. Five years before he had been affected with white opaque urine, which continued for two months,—then ceased, he thought, not from the remedies used, but gradually and spontaneously. He remained well till eight months and a half before he came under observation at the hospital, when the urine suddenly became opaque and milky, but without pain of loins or fever. On admission the urine was milk-like, of specific gravity 1·012, and gave a copious coagulum by heat and nitric acid; and the rest of the urine was left clear. Blood and mucus were also present, and subsided to the bottom of the vessel. Latterly the urine spontaneously separated into a coagulum and a pretty clear fluid; it was frequently passed with pain, and obstructed by coagula in the urethra. His only other complaint was of weakness. He was treated with tonics without benefit. He ceased attendance that he might avail himself of change of air, from which he is reported to have soon recovered, and after his return to have continued in good health.

221. *Urine milky, coagulating by heat and nitric acid, becoming clear by addition of sulphuric ether.— No improvement from treatment.— Change of air recommended.— Result not known.*—Coverjee Maneckjee, a Parsee schoolboy, of sixteen years of age, and temperate habits, but in feeble health, was admitted into the clinical ward on the 12th December, 1852. With exception of slight bronchitis, he was free from thoracic or abdominal visceral disease. He stated that, six months before admission, his urine had begun to be scanty, and that two months ago it had assumed a milky appearance. There was also pain of loins. The urine was passed without pain, except occasionally

from urethral obstruction by coagula. He continued under observation till the 2nd January. The urine was of milky appearance, coagulated with heat and nitric acid, lost its turbidity by addition of sulphuric ether, ranged in quantity from twenty-five to forty ounces, and was of specific gravity from 1·022 to 1·030. He was treated with gallic acid, phosphate of soda, and creosote, without the least benefit, and was discharged with a recommendation to proceed to Surat for change of air. The result is unknown.

222. *Chylo-serous urine removed by change of air.*—Junardhun Kesho, a Hindoo clerk, of twenty-one years of age, applied at the Poona Dispensary. He was in reduced health, and on the 17th September, 1858, passed a pint of curdy urine, of specific gravity 1·012, giving a cloudy deposit with heat and nitric acid. There was no fever nor syphilitic taint. He was treated with gallic acid, then with the tincture of the sesquichloride of iron; but the urine continued opaque, with a brick-red tint. He went for change of air on the 22nd, and on the following January was reported well, and the urine natural.

223. *Chylo-serous urine removed twice by change of air.*—Antone ——, a Portuguese butler, about forty-five years of age, left Bombay for Goa in May 1854, after having been for some months the subject of chylo-serous urine, with occasional fever and generally impaired health. During the voyage the urine began to clear, became normal, continued so at Goa, and he returned to Bombay in perfect health in about a year and a half. After about a year's residence in Bombay, the chylo-serous urine, impaired health, and occasional fever returned; and he went again to Goa in May 1857. The urine became clear on the voyage, and continued so when I last saw him, on the 3rd November, 1857, five days after his second return to Bombay.

SECTION III.—*Saccharine Diabetes.—Infrequent in India.—Diuresis.*

In this abnormal state of the urine we have another illustration of disease depending on faulty, primary, or secondary assimilation; differing, however, from that which has just been considered, in that the defect is in the processes by which the *non-azotised* principles of food are converted to their purposes of usefulness in the system. The result is, that sugar exists in excess in the blood, and is excreted with the urine; hence the great abundance of this secretion, its saccharine quality, and its high specific gravity.

For details on these points, and on the cachectic phenomena which are associated with saccharine diabetes, I must refer to the many excellent treatises which have been written on this disease.

Prout, during the period in which he had seen only thirteen cases of chylo-serous urine, witnessed 500 of diabetes. From this fact some idea may be formed of the comparative frequency of the two affections in European countries. The number of cases of diabetes in India, of which I have had personal knowledge, amounts to six. The first occurred about the year 1836, in the Hindoo Jemadar of the Governor's escort at Dharpooree, in the

Deccan. This officer died two or three months afterwards. Another, in the person of a Mahomedan gentleman of advanced age, about whom I was consulted in 1854, by Mr. Atmaram Pandurang. The remaining four cases are narrated in this section: three, two males and one female, were Parsees; the fourth was a native of Goa. I have no reason for supposing that in the experience of others, diabetes has been found a more common disease than it has proved to be in my own. Prout was disposed to relate diabetes to malarious influence. The infrequency of the disease in India is not in conformity with this opinion; nor does it countenance the idea that abuse of mercury, or syphilitic taint, have much to do with the etiology of diabetes. When we recollect that numerous classes subsist chiefly on cereals and other vegetable food, we, in theory, might anticipate that diabetes would be a more common disease in India than in those countries in which animal food is more generally consumed. This, however, does not seem to be the case. Such facts tend to show that much of the pathology of saccharine diabetes is still unknown.

224. *Diabetes.—Symptoms improved somewhat under the use of creosote and muriate of morphia.*—Muncherjee Ruttonjee, a Parsee cook, of twenty-eight years of age, whilst on his return from China, about twenty-three months before he came under observation, landed at Singapore, and there, without appreciable cause, for the first time experienced extreme thirst and frequent desire to micturate. Since that time both these symptoms have continued and increased. After his return from China, he resided for three months in Bombay; then proceeded to his native town, Surat; and, after a residence there of about eight months, he again set off for China, unrelieved of his complaint. Twenty days before admission into the clinical ward, on the 9th March, 1850, he had returned from China to Bombay. He was a good deal emaciated, was affected with urgent thirst and dryness of the fauces, and micturated frequently and copiously. The gums were swollen and the teeth loose, the appetite was keen, the tongue dryish and slightly florid at the tip, and the bowels rather slow. The skin was of natural temperature, and dry; the pulse 100, of tolerable volume, and soft. There were no signs of pulmonary or cardiac disease. The abdomen was full, but soft, without uneasiness or abnormal dulness. He complained of a general sense of weakness, slept badly, from uneasiness in the course of the tibiæ, burning in the soles of the feet, and frequent calls to pass his urine. He stated that the urine increased in quantity after oleaginous articles of food and vegetables, and that when voided on the same place for two or three successive days, the spot appeared as if whitewashed. He was unable to assign any particular cause of the complaint; but a sister had died, after two years' illness, with similar symptoms. No other member of his family, however, had been thus affected. Much variety of medicine had been used, and he had been salivated about a year before admission. He continued under observation till the 4th April. The urine was generally of amber colour, and of specific gravity from 1·035 to 1·040. On admission twenty-four pints were passed during the night; but it gradually decreased, and after the 14th March ranged from seven to three pints in the night. The thirst lessened, and he improved somewhat in appearance. He was treated chiefly with creosote in two-minim doses thrice daily, a draught with the solution of the muriate of morphia at bed-time, and the occasional use of the hot-air bath. The diet consisted of milk, eggs, mutton, with succulent vegetables.

225.—*Diabetes.—No improvement from preparations of iron, permanganate of potass, and opium.*—Ruttonjee Dhunjeebhoy, a Parsee sweet-meat seller, of twenty-five years of age, and using spirits to the extent of two ounces daily, was admitted into the clinical ward on the 10th October, 1853. He was much reduced and complained of pain of loins, weakness of the lower extremities, and frequent micturition. The countenance was anxious, the pulse small, and slightly jerking; the skin of natural temperature, and dry; the tongue thinly coated, and somewhat florid at the tip; the gums slightly swollen, and tender; and the bowels confined. With exception of an occasional bronchitic râle, there was no sign of pulmonary or cardiac disease. The abdomen was retracted and free of induration or dulness. He rested badly at nights. He stated that he had suffered from dysenteric symptoms for about two years, for which much variety of treatment had been unsuccessfully followed till three months ago, when he was treated in the hospital with opiates and stimulants, and the dysenteric symptoms were removed. Then, for the first time, he observed an increase in the urine, and attributed it to the remedies which had been used. These, he said, had caused thirst, and led him to drink much water. On the 12th eight pints of urine had been passed during the night; it was clear, of pale amber colour, neutral, of specific gravity 1·033, and on addition of sulphate of copper, liquor potassæ, and application of heat, a yellowish brown precipitate was thrown down. He continued under treatment till the 7th November. The urine ranged from three to eight pints in the night, and continued of high specific gravity. The asthenia increased. He was discharged at his own earnest desire. He was treated first with preparations of iron and opium, and then the permanganate of potass was substituted for the iron, and a diet of eggs, mutton, and a limited portion of bread, and two ounces of arrack daily was given.

226. *Diabetes.—Not improved by treatment.*—Sorabye, a Parsee female, of twenty-six years of age, much emaciated, and affected with boils, was, after a year's illness, admitted into hospital on the 20th May, 1850. The tongue was florid. The pulse feeble and quick. The urine ranged from six to twelve pints, and was of specific gravity from 1·030 to 1·036, and yielded sugar on evaporation. The thirst was urgent, and the appetite voracious. Opium, quinine, creosote, and Dover's powder were used, and a diet of milk, eggs, chicken, and little bread was given. She gained somewhat in flesh, and the tongue was less florid, but in other respects was at the time of her discharge, on the 29th July, in the same state as on admission. I saw her again in the month of October, when the symptoms remained unchanged.

227.—*Diabetes.—No improvement from permanganate of potass, or from creosote alone, but marked benefit from addition of opium.*—Cosmo de Souza, a native Christian, of forty-five years of age, an inhabitant of Goa, a cook by occupation, and habitually using spirits, was admitted into the clinical ward on the 10th November, 1852. He was reduced in strength, the pulse was small and jerking. He complained of dimness of vision, sleepless nights, frequent and copious micturition. The tongue was moist and clean, the bowels slow, the appetite keen, and the thirst urgent. No signs of thoracic or abdominal disease. He stated that these symptoms had first made their appearance at Belgaum five years before, and had persisted with little intermission. The urine on the 12th was five pints, of specific gravity 1·033, and gave a scanty brown precipitate with sulphate of copper and liquor potassæ. The patient seemed to have discovered, and alluded to, the sweet taste of his urine. He continued under treatment till the 21st December, when he was discharged at his own request; the urine having decreased to about fifty ounces, and specific gravity to 1·022; his general state had also improved. He was again seen on the 28th December, and the urine was examined. It was of specific gravity 1·025, and gave merely a trace of sugar with Trommer's test. He was afterwards seen on the 24th January, when the specific gravity of the urine was 1·028, and a considerable brown precipitate was thrown down with the sulphate of copper and liquor potassæ. During his stay in hospital he was treated first with permanganate of potass without improvement, then with creosote, also without any change in the urine; but on the addition of a grain of opium at bed-time, the urine decreased from 100 to 60 ounces, and during the twenty days that he subsequently continued in hospital ranged from forty to eighty ounces. He had full diet, but without any special arrangement.

Diuresis.—Cases of abundant limpid urine, of low specific gravity, are occasionally, though rarely, observed in India. I recollect two well-marked instances of this affection. The first, a European, employed in the government remount stables, who, about the year 1837, consulted me for this affection, and for partial amaurosis of one of his eyes. The urine was very copious and limpid, and was about 1·005 or lower in specific gravity. The abnormal state of the urine, unaffected by medical treatment, after a time reverted to its normal standard, and some improvement took place in the amaurosis. This individual is still (1860) in Bombay, and for many years subsequent to the period adverted to has enjoyed good health.

The second case was of an Indo-Briton, who applied at the Jamsetjee Jejeebhoy Hospital, towards the end of 1853. The urine was very copious, of low specific gravity, and gave no traces of sugar. He was much emaciated and out of health. I have no notes of the particulars of this case, or of its further course.

Section IV. — *Uric, Oxalic, and Phosphatic Diathesis.*

The presence of insoluble urates, oxalates, and phosphates in the urine, is also a consequence of faulty primary or secondary assimilation, sometimes due to error in the quantity or quality of the food, at others to defect in the processes themselves. The subject has of late years received much attention, and the risk is, that too much importance may be attached to the ascertained facts, both in reference to pathology and therapeutics. The probability is, that further investigation of the morbid states of the urine in India will lead to results similar in kind to those which have already been obtained in European countries.

These abnormal conditions of the urine may be practically considered from two points of view.

1. As leading to the formation of urinary calculi, and all their attendant evils. The opinion at one time entertained that these were of rare occurrence in India, has been long since disproved in Bengal, by the experience of Burnard, Brett, Twining, Darby,

Cole, and many skilful lithotomists, graduates * of the Bengal Medical College; in the Nizam's territories, by Dr. W. C. Maclean; and in Bombay, by Peet, Ballingall, Ritchie, and Bhawoo Dajee.†

* Of the many skilful lithotomists trained in the Bengal Medical College, I would name Ram Narain Doss, the present teacher of surgery in the military class of the college, as the most conspicuous. He has performed the operation above two hundred times with good success. Also Mr. C. E. Raddock, who has communicated an interesting report of his cases of lithotomy in the 4th number of the "Indian Annals of Medical Science."

† On this subject I quote the following extract from my retrospective address to Grant College Medical Society for the year 1857:—

"Mr. Bhawoo Dajee, in continuation of a former paper published in the 2nd number of the 2nd Series of the 'Transactions of the Medical and Physical Society,' communicated five additional cases of lithotomy. In four the operation was performed by the author; in one by Mr. Narrayen Dajee. Two were of Mahomedans, three of Hindoos. The ages of three ranged from 7 to 10; of the remaining two the ages were 55 and 60. In all, the symptoms of calculus had been present from 3 to 6 years; in all the operation was successful. The calculi extracted weighed from 3 to 4½ drachms. But neither in the six cases previously reported, nor in those now under notice, is there any account given of the chemical composition of the calculi.

"Mr. Sadashew Hemraj contributed three cases of lithotomy successfully performed at Bhooj. Two in children 4 years of age; one of 12. The composition of the calculi is not stated. The same defective information exists relative to 41 of the 50 calculi now in the Grant College Museum.

"The etiology of urinary calculus is imperfectly understood. It is, therefore, very important that, in the investigation of this form of disease, information should be carefully sought in regard to all points which may serve to elucidate the causes which produce it. It is very desirable that the place of birth and of residence, varieties in modes of life from habits of caste or difference of circumstances, and the chemical composition of the calculi, should be inquired into and recorded. Mr. Bransby Cooper, in the year 1851, in a paper published in the 7th volume of the 2nd series of Guy's Hospital Reports, relative to the cases of lithotomy performed by Mr. Coles of the Bengal army in the Punjaub, remarks on the importance of determining whether a relation existed between the climate and peculiar systems of diet and the composition of urinary calculi; and he throws out the suggestion, that in theory it may be expected that in India, where vegetable food is more exclusively used by large numbers of the people, a greater proportion of oxalate of lime calculi would be found to exist. With the view of setting before you the results which may be deduced from existing records of Indian calculous disease, I have referred to the several sources of information within my reach. There are cases recorded, with chemical analysis, in the 'Transactions of the Medical and Physical Society of Calcutta,' by Burnard, Spry, Twining, Brett, and Darby; in Guy's Hospital Reports by Coles; and in the catalogue of the Grant College Museum there is an analysis by Dr. Watson of nine calculi extracted by Dr. Ritchie at Mooltan. The cases adverted to amount to 77. Eleven consisted of uric acid, or urate of ammonia; 48 of uric acid associated with oxalate of lime or phosphates; 7 of oxalate of lime alone; 7 of oxalate of lime and phosphates; one of phosphates alone.

"Dr. Simpson, of Tirrhoot, in the 3rd number of the 'Indian Annals of Medicine,' gives the analysis of 186 cases, with a mortality of 4·8 per cent. He makes no allusion to mixed calculi, but classes them all under the heads of urates, phosphates, oxalates. Of the first 76; of the second 68; of the third 42; which gives a per-centage of 40·8 urates; 36·6 phosphates; 22·6 oxalates.

2. As indications of mal-assimilation, the urates being often related to excess of food and sthenic states, the oxalates and phosphates to asthenic and cachectic states. They are signs of deranged actions, very useful to note in practice, but often serving merely to confirm an inference already sufficiently evident from other symptoms. They indicate the propriety of the regimen and remedies which are calculated on general principles to remove the deranged constitutional states on which they depend. They do not indicate the use of chemical remedies with the view of altering the state of the urine, unless the formation of urinary calculus be apprehended; and, then even, such remedies are not entitled to rank higher than temporary palliatives.

The presence of blood, pus, and mucus in this secretion, in their relation to disease of the urinary organs, and the decomposition of urea, is well understood and need not be described in this work.

"Mr Ruddock, Sub-Assistant Surgeon of the Bengal Service, in the 4th number of the 'Indian Annals of Medicine,' reports 77 cases of lithotomy, with a mortality of 6·7 per cent.; but he is silent on the chemical composition of the calculi.

"These data show that uric acid entered into the composition of 135 out of 263 calculi; but this is, doubtless, far short of the truth, for it is very improbable that Dr. Simpson's 68 phosphates and 42 oxalates were, all of them, free of uric acid.

"In Dr. Golding Bird's work there is an analysis of 374 calculi in Guy's Hospital Museum. Uric acid entered into the composition of 269. So far, then, as inquiry has as yet gone, there are no grounds for believing that oxalate of lime calculi occur in greater proportion in the natives of India than in those of England, yet the question cannot be viewed as settled without more extended and more careful investigation."

Since these remarks were written, Mr. H. Vandyke Carter, Professor of Anatomy and Physiology, Grant Medical College, has carefully analysed the urinary calculi in the Museum and arrived at the following conclusions:—

"1. That in the Bombay Presidency the proportion of calculi having oxalate of lime for their nucleus, or wholly composed of it, is about twice as great as in England, taking for comparison certain standard collections there. 2. That the proportion of calculi having uric acid, or a urate for their nucleus or entire substance, is considerably less in India than in England; in the former, urate of ammonia calculi are somewhat more frequent than uric acid calculi: the opposite is the case in England. 3. That the number of calculi wholly composed of earthy phosphates, or having them for a nucleus, is proportionately much fewer in India than in England: the difference being chiefly owing to the rarity of mixed phosphates in the former." *

* "Transactions, Medical and Physical Society of Bombay," No. 5, New Series, p. 147.

CHAP. XXI.

ON PNEUMONIA.

SECTION I. — *Pneumonia. — Rare in Europeans in Bombay. — Asthenic Form common in Natives.*

PNEUMONIA is a rare disease in Europeans in Bombay. I am unable for the six years of my own service in the European General Hospital to separate the admissions of pneumonia from those of bronchitis and pleuritis: they have all been recorded in the hospital returns under the head "Thoracic Inflammations." The register of admissions might supply the means of subdivision, but it is not at present within my reach. On referring to my "Cases* illustrative of the Pathology of the Diseases of Bombay," chiefly observed in the European General Hospital, I find only eight of pneumonia, and five of them were consecutive on measles. Of the three other cases, one occurred in a dissipated clerk serving in a public office, and the attack came on obscurely during a series of successive days of intemperance; the second in a seaman suffering from delirium tremens; the third in a warrant officer of the garrison, terminated in red and grey induration, with several gangrenous excavations. In the returns of the European General Hospital for the succeeding ten years, from 1844 to 1853, kindly supplied to me by Dr. Stovell, twenty-two admissions of pneumonia are recorded: of these, two died. On examining my notes of cases of sick officers, it appears that of 1,699 cases which passed under my review, only five of pneumonia are noted: four of these proved fatal; in one there was a gangrenous excavation, and in the remaining three the disease had passed on to induration or hepatisation.

In respect to the natives of India, however, the results are very different. In them pneumonia, of asthenic type, is sufficiently

* "Transactions, Medical and Physical Society of Bombay," 1st Series, Nos. 2, 6, 7.

common. Mr. Allen Webb has published* an account of this disease, as observed in 1845, at the dispensary of Cawnpore, in the upper provinces of Hindostan, by Dr. Edward Goodeve; and in the jail at Midnapore, in Bengal, by Mr. Green, in the same year. Mr. Webb had also himself frequently observed pneumonia in natives in the lower belt of the Himalayan range. During the six years, from 1848 to 1853, 313 admissions of pneumonia took place in the Jamsetjee Jejeebhoy Hospital. Of these 103 were under my immediate care in the clinical ward; and the following remarks will chiefly relate to the pathological and therapeutic deductions which these cases have suggested.

Seventy-six of the cases were of primary pneumonia, and twenty-seven † were of pneumonia complicating intermittent or remittent fever.

In the chapter on Remittent Fever it was stated that primary pneumonia, and that which complicates malarious fever, would be considered together. When this arrangement was originally adopted, it seemed to me that questions relative to the pathology, symptoms, and treatment of inflammation of the lungs might arise, in the consideration of which a comparison of the two forms might be found useful. In the observations which I am about to make I shall use the term *primary pneumonia* in its generally received sense; while for convenience sake, I shall designate by the term *febrile*, the pneumonia which complicates intermittent and remittent fever. In this restricted sense, then, the word febrile, when applied to pneumonia, has been used in this chapter.

My comments on these clinical cases have been arranged under the heads—1. Etiology. 2. Pathology. 3. Symptoms. 4. Treatment.

SECTION II.—*Etiology.—Relation to Sex, Age, Caste, Habits Constitution, and Season.*

Sex.—The question of the influence of difference of sex in predisposing to pneumonia is not affected by these cases—they were all of males.

Age.—The greater or less prevalence and mortality of this disease at different periods of life is a subject of interesting inquiry;

* "Pathologia Indica," by Allan Webb, B. M. S., 2nd edition: Calcutta, 1848.

† Of these, twenty-three complicated remittent fever, and four intermittent fever.

but the class of inmates of the Jamsetjee Jejeebhoy Hospital is not calculated to advance it. They are chiefly adults, and consist for the most part of day-labourers, peons, cart-drivers, domestic servants, and sailors. Many of them are natives of other parts of the country, resorting to Bombay, for a season, in pursuit of the means of subsistence. They are generally individuals in the vigour of life. Of the subjects of the present cases, fifty-seven were between the ages of twenty-one and thirty; twenty-two between thirty-one and forty; eleven between ten and twenty; and nine above forty.

Caste.—The castes from which these patients were selected have been, with one exception, Hindoo, Mussulman, and native Christian: there were forty-nine Hindoos, forty Mussulmans, and thirteen native Christians. This is about the ratio of the total hospital admissions of these several castes. In this statement, then, there is no evidence of liability to pneumonia being caused by peculiarities in the customs of these different classes. Yet there is an interesting fact observable in these cases, which is probably related to caste-customs. The mortality among the Hindoos and Mussulmans has been about one in three; that of the native Christians not quite one in six. On referring to the duration of the disease before admission, I find that of the seventy-one recovered cases, only twenty were admitted within five days of the commencement of the attack: of these, nine were native Christians. From this statement it is a fair inference, that though pneumonia has been as prevalent among native Christians as the other two castes, yet it has been much more successfully treated, in consequence of their earlier application for relief.*

Habits and state of constitution.—The state of constitution and the habits of these patients, have in all probability assisted in causing the disease. Of one hundred and one individuals whose state of constitution on admission is noted, sixty-three were asthenic, and the condition of thirty-eight is stated to have been good or tolerable. Of the asthenic patients, about one in three died; of the others about one in four.

The habits of seventy-seven are stated: of these, forty-six admitted that they were in the practice of using spirituous liquors; thirty-one denied it.

Seasons.—On referring to the total hospital admissions of pri-

* That the difference of the rate of mortality from pneumonia in Christians extends to all forms of disease is shown by the fact—that the general hospital mortality is, in Hindoos, 19·48, in Mussulmans, 15·56, and in Christians, 9·93.

mary pneumonia during the six years to which these remarks relate, it is found that in the year 1849 the number was one-third more than the average of the other years. On comparing the monthly admissions for the whole period, it appears that in the six months from December to May, the admissions were 182; but in the six months from June to November, they were 131—a difference of fifty-one in favour of the winter and spring. These results are deduced from the consideration of 313 cases.

In M. Grisolle's elaborate work on pneumonia, there is a table which exhibits the months of admission in Paris of 296 cases. It will be useful to compare these two statements *, with the view of determining to what extent there is correspondence or difference in the seasons of greatest prevalence of pneumonia in the climates of Paris and Bombay. In both we find the disease more common in the six months from December to May than in those from June to November. But the difference is more marked in one climate than in the other: in Paris it is 190, in Bombay fifty-one. When the month of November is excluded, and the admissions in the two places from June to October are compared, it appears that in Bombay they amount to one hundred, in Paris to thirty-one.

There is, then, in Bombay, a greater proportion of admissions in summer and the first half of autumn than in Paris. The reason is evident. June, July, August, and September are the monsoon months in Bombay—the season of the periodical rains. We have at this time wet, a moist atmosphere, and high winds, as causes of reduction of the temperature of the surface of the body.

These remarks have had reference to *primary* pneumonia. But when we regard the periods of admission of the twenty-seven cases of *febrile* pneumonia, we find that the greatest monthly number

* The statements in detail are subjoined:—

	Bombay.	Paris.
January	30	20
February	39	40
March	32	47
April	21	62
May	27	40
June	23	8
July	9	13
August	18	3
September	21	5
October	29	2
November	31	22
December	33	34
	313	296

was in July. When we compare the six months from June to November with those from December to May, we find that the admissions in the former amounted to twenty-two, in the latter only to five. The difference between the seasons of greatest prevalence of primary and febrile pneumonia in Bombay would seem to be well marked. The explanation is clear. Primary pneumonia is most common in the cold months of the year; but febrile pneumonia, on the other hand, is necessarily most common in the months in which malarious fevers chiefly prevail. This fact is important, as it tends to facilitate the diagnosis of the two forms, and affects the principles of treatment.

Causes assigned.—The patients generally have not attributed the attack to any particular cause. Nine traced it to cold or wet, eight to fatigue and exposure, and ten to blows more or less recently received. When we consider the season of greatest prevalence of the primary form, the occupations of the inmates of the hospital, their exposure to vicissitudes of weather, their scanty clothing, and defective habitations, we are justified in regarding reduction of the temperature of the surface of the body as the common exciting cause of pneumonia in India, as elsewhere.

SECTION III.—*Pathology.—Preliminary Question relative to the affected Capillaries.—Rate of Mortality.—Duration of Illness before Admission.—Stage of the Disease.—Which Lung most frequently affected.—Period of Residence in Hospital.—State of the Lung on Discharge.—Morbid Anatomy.*

Preliminary Remarks.—The first question which naturally arises, relative to the pathology of pneumonia, is the determination of the precise seat of the inflammation. I do not mean, whether the walls of the pulmonary air cells or their connecting areolar tissue are the structures affected: this, though much discussed by pathologists, has never appeared to me a very important or difficult point to establish. If in inflammation of mucous and serous membranes we generally find that the deranged action tends to extend to and cause exudation in the areolar tissue subjacent to them, it is improbable that inflammation of the pulmonary cell-wall can exist without tending to extend and to cause exudation in the areolar tissue which connects the cells together, as well as into the cells themselves. The question to which I allude is, whether the capillaries of the *bronchial* arteries, or those of the *pulmonary* artery, are the seat of inflammation. The answer appears to me simple and evident. If we adopt the opinion, at present generally received, that inflammation is an altered state of the nutritive processes of the affected part, depending upon something faulty in one or other of the conditions of normal nutrition, then the capillaries concerned in inflammation must necessarily be only those which circulate, in their normal state, arterial blood for purposes of nutrition. The capillaries of the bronchial arteries are the nutrient vessels of the visceral pleura, of the mucous lining and other structures of the bronchial tubes, and of the connecting areolar tissue of the constituent parts of the lung; and we can hardly avoid the conclusion that they are also the nutrient vessels of the pulmonary cell-walls. These capillaries are unquestionably those involved in visceral pleuritis, and in bronchitis; and when we regard the frequent relation of these affections to pneumonia, it is reasonable to conclude that the same kind of capillaries are concerned when the inflammation is of the pulmonary cell-walls, and of the areolar tissue which connects the cells to each other.*

The capillaries of the pulmonary artery, on the other hand, convey venous blood to the air cells, for distribution on their walls, in order that the physical process of endosmosis and exosmosis may take place between the gases of the blood and the atmospheric air. It does not seem probable that the blood in these capillaries takes any part in the nutrition of the cell-walls. It is, therefore, a just conclusion that these capillaries and their blood cannot be agents in the altered state of nutrition of the pulmonary cell-walls, and their connecting areolar tissue, which we designate by the term pneumonia. Though the capillaries of the pulmonary artery are not the capillaries directly engaged in inflammation, yet their deranged action has much to do with the pathology of pneumonia.

The phenomena which attend on the first inspiration after birth, on asphyxia, vesicular emphysema, and other pathological states of the lungs, teach us the following facts:—

1. That the pulmonary capillary circulation is contingent on

* I am, of course, aware that some physiologists hold that the blood in the pulmonary capillaries, passing into the arterial state, becomes nutrient of the cell-walls. The subject is not susceptible of demonstrative proof; but surely the argument from analogy supports the opinion that the bronchial are the nutrient capillaries. It seems to me quite as reasonable to suppose that the blood flowing in the channel of the aorta is nutrient of its walls, as that the arterialised blood of the pulmonary capillaries is nutrient of the tissues around it. Both bloods are flowing in their respective channels with objects in view, special, and not related to the nutrition of the tissues immediately adjoining to them.

the processes between the blood in the pulmonary capillaries and the air in the pulmonary air cells being in action.

2. If this aëration of the blood is impeded from want of sufficient air or from thickening of the cell-walls, or the cells becoming filled with liquid or solid deposits, the pulmonary capillary circulation on such cell-walls becomes languid, and soon stops:—the blood distends the vessels, and stagnates in them. Now, additional blood is no longer sent into the branches of the pulmonary artery which conduct to these defective cells; but it passes in excessive quantity into adjoining branches, to be conveyed to the capillaries of adjoining healthy cells, in order that it may be aërated there. If, however, the blood thus sent in excessive quantity to these adjacent healthy cells be greater than their extent of surface can readily aërate, dyspnœa is caused. Short and hurried respirations merely express the fact that all the cells of the lungs are not admitting air, and that the diminished extent of surface thus arising is being compensated for by the greater frequency of the respiratory acts. Difficulty of breathing is only experienced when there is want of harmony between the quantity of blood in the vascular system and the extent of the effective pulmonary surface.

Let us now endeavour to apply these principles to the pathology of the disease before us.

When the pulmonary cell-walls become somewhat thickened from the turgescent state of the bronchial capillaries, and when secretions are present in the cells, in the degree which interferes with, but does not altogether prevent, the admission of air, then we may believe that some degree of aëration is still carried on, that the pulmonary capillaries become somewhat distended, and that the circulation of the blood is impeded in them, but as yet is not altogether obstructed. Such I believe to be the condition of the lung in the first stage of pneumonia. The inflammation continues, the thickening of the cell-walls increases, the inflammatory deposits take place in greater abundance into the cells, and now the aëration of the blood at these cells is physically impracticable: the pulmonary capillaries become turgid with stagnated blood, and the circulation in them becomes altogether obstructed. Such I believe to be the state of the lung in the second stage of pneumonia: its spongy structure has become solid; the solidification depending, in part, it may be assumed, on inflammatory exudation into the cells, in part also, however, on the stagnated blood in the close-set meshes of the pulmonary capillaries. This latter condition of consolidation is not stated with sufficient prominence by pathological writers on this disease. It explains well how the consolidation of the lung sometimes takes place rapidly, and how it sometimes is very speedily removed. It is evident that if part of the consolidated condition has depended on pulmonary capillaries turgid with blood stagnated, but not coagulated, and aëration becomes re-established in the affected cells by reduction of the inflammation, then this stagnating blood will at once be set in motion, and the consolidation that depended upon it be speedily removed.

My belief, then, is, that the capillaries of the pulmonary artery are not the inflamed capillaries of pneumonia; but that consequent on inflammation of the pulmonary cell-walls, the action of the pulmonary capillaries becomes deranged in the manner explained. This derangement constitutes the danger of pneumonia, as of all other forms of pulmonary disease. Moreover, the deranged action of the pulmonary capillaries takes a part in producing the striking morbid appearance of the lung in pneumonia —I mean its hepatisation.

In this view of the pathology of pneumonia, we have also a satisfactory explanation of the relation between hypostatic consolidation of the lung, and the hepatisation of pneumonia. In hepatisation, there is in the pulmonary capillary turgescence which is present, the condition of hypostatic consolidation; but there are also, in addition, the consolidating conditions derived from the direct products of inflammation.

These are not mere idle speculations, for, as we shall presently find, they have an important reference to symptoms, as well as to questions of treatment. The subject is analogous to that which has been previously discussed, relative to the capillaries engaged in hepatitis.*

Rate of Mortality.—There were 76 cases of *primary* pneumonia. Of these 24 died—a mortality of nearly 29 per cent.,† if two cases fatal from cholera be excluded.‡

* Page 325.

† In my subsequent statements regarding the rates of mortality, I shall not exclude these cholera cases.

‡ It will be observed, that the tabular statement at the end of this chapter gives for the total hospital admissions of pneumonia a mortality of 38·6 per cent. This is in part explained by the supposition that there may have been cases admitted in such an advanced and hopeless state of disease as to be unsuited for clinical instruction,

There were twenty-seven cases of *febrile* pneumonia: of these eight died; in two the fatal result was caused more from co-existing meningitis than pneumonia; yet, in estimating the rate of mortality of this form, we may not exclude any of the usual contingencies of malarious fever. The rate of mortality of the febrile cases was not quite 30 per cent.

The rate of mortality of primary pneumonia has been nearly as high as that of the febrile form: hence we are probably justified in assuming that this inflammation, complicating malarious fever, is not so severe as when it occurs in its primary form. Were it otherwise, the mortality of the febrile form would be higher, for in it we must always attribute death, in part, to other conditions of idiopathic fever as well as to the pneumonia.

But 29 per cent. seems a large mortality from primary pneumonia. We have already found in the diatheses of a large proportion of the patients one condition favourable to high mortality from disease. Still it is very necessary, with the view of satisfactorily testing the success or failure of treatment, to inquire into the following points:—

1. The duration of illness before admission.
2. The stage of the disease on admission.
3. The extent and part of the lung affected.
4. The length of time under treatment before recovery or death.
5. The state of the lung on discharge, in the cases discharged from hospital.

Duration of illness before admission.—The following tabular

and therefore to have been excluded from my selection for the clinical ward. Allowance must also be made for errors of diagnosis, liable to occur in large hospitals served by different medical men often overtasked with duty. This latter observation, probably more or less true of all countries, is correct of civil and military hospitals in India—more especially in seasons of unusual sickness, or amid the distractions and labours of active service. It is also particularly applicable to those forms of disease—of the chest for example—in which much care, time, and patience are required to establish the diagnosis with that precision and accuracy of which the present state of the science is capable.

I am most desirous of impressing on the Indian practitioner the injury which is likely to result to pathology and therapeutics, by applying to their elucidation data which are unsuited for the purpose. The least reflection must convince any one that there is little in common between the figured statements of disease in hospitals, as usually compiled, and the results of the scrutiny of a series of attentively considered and carefully recorded clinical cases. Most certainly nothing in common, but the use of figures, between pathological and therapeutic deductions, from military and naval hospital statistics, and the inferences from the numerical method as practised by Louis and those who are *truly* his followers.

statement exhibits the duration of illness of the patients before admission.

Duration of Illness of Patients before Admission.

	Recovered.		Died.		Total.
	Primary	Febrile.	Primary.	Febrile.	
1 to 5 days	17	3	1	1	22
6 to 10 „	18	8	8	—	34
11 to 15 „	6	6	4	2	11
16 to 20 „	5	—	1	3	9
21 to 30 „	2	2	2	2	8
31 and upwards	4	—	8	—	12
				Total .	103

The mortality of the *primary* form, admitted within five days from the commencement of illness, was 5·5 per cent. The single fatal case occurred in a Parsee of intemperate habits; was in the second stage, and complicated with pleuritic effusion and albuminuria.

The mortality of the *febrile* form, admitted within five days from the commencement of illness, was 25 per cent. The single fatal case occurred in an individual affected with fever and bronchitis: pneumonia came on subsequently, and proved fatal seventeen days after admission.

The mortality of *primary* pneumonia, admitted between six and ten days from the commencement of illness, was 30 per cent. In seven of the eight fatal cases the disease was in the second stage on admission. In four the pneumonia was double, and in three of them the disease was in the second stage, in one in the first.

Of the eight cases of *febrile* pneumonia, admitted between six and ten days from the commencement of illness, none proved fatal.

The mortality of both forms, admitted above ten days from the commencement of illness, was nearly 47 per cent.

When we regard all the admissions of *primary* pneumonia, within ten days from the commencement of illness, the rate of mortality is found to be 20 per cent. But when we consider the *febrile* cases from the same point of view, the mortality falls to 8 per cent. Yet for the periods above ten days, the mortality of both forms is the same,—47 per cent. The lower mortality of febrile pneumonia, within ten days from the commencement of illness, is of interest: it seems to show that the pneumonia does not come on till some time after the commencement of the fever. It is, therefore, probable, that in all the cases of febrile pneumonia admitted within ten days from the commencement of illness, the pneumonia has generally been either in the first stage, or only passing into the second.

Stage of the Disease.—Of the *primary* form eight were in the first stage. Of these two died; in one the pneumonia was double, in the other it was complicated with much bronchitis in a man of sixty years of age.

Sixty-four cases of primary pneumonia were admitted in the second stage. Of these twenty-seven were double, thirty-four were single, and confined to part of a lung, and three were of one entire lung. If we class together the cases of double pneumonia and those of one entire lung in the second stage, we find that the mortality was 36·6 per cent.; but the mortality of single pneumonia in the second stage, involving only part of a lung, has been 17·6 per cent. The mortality of the aggregate admissions of primary pneumonia in the second stage, has been 26·5 per cent.

Four admissions of primary pneumonia took place in the third stage: all were fatal.

Of the *febrile* form, five cases were admitted in the first stage: one proved fatal, admitted after twenty days from the commencement of the fever, complicated with muttering delirium and drowsiness.

Twenty-two of this form were admitted in the second stage. Of these, fourteen were double, eight single. The mortality of the former was 35 per cent., of the latter 25 per cent.

Lung affected.—In comparing the frequency of pneumonia in the lung of the different sides, and in the different parts of the lung, I shall class the primary and febrile forms together. Of both lungs (double pneumonia) there were forty-six cases, with a mortality of 32·6 per cent. Of the right lung there were thirty-nine cases, with a mortality of 33·3 per cent. Of the left lung there were eighteen cases, with a mortality of 22·2 per cent. Of the cases in which the right lung was affected, the entire organ was involved in three: this did not occur in any of the instances in which the disease was confined to the left side, therefore, when these three cases are deducted, the mortality for the right side is reduced to 25·3.

In regarding these rates of mortality, we must always bear in mind that they relate to a series of cases of which the admissions in the first stage were only about 13 per cent.

In this statement the proportion of double pneumonia appears much greater than has usually been observed. This is, in part, owing to the two forms having been classed together. Of the twenty-seven cases of febrile pneumonia, we had the disease double in seventeen. When we consider the primary form alone, we find of double pneumonia twenty-nine; of the right lung thirty-three; of the left lung fourteen. This is still an unusual proportion of double pneumonia.

When we direct our attention to the part of the lung affected in these cases, it appears that in seventy-nine the lower or middle parts, or both, were engaged, and of these the mortality was 26 per cent. In fifteen cases the upper lobe was affected, and of these the mortality was 26 per cent. In nine the entire lung, double or single, was affected, and the rate of mortality was 77 per cent.

The greater liability of the lower part of the lung to become affected with pneumonia is well shown in these cases. The great mortality of the disease when an entire lung is involved also appears; but the opinion that pneumonia of the upper part of the lung is more fatal than that of the lower, is not confirmed by these cases. It was believed by Louis, that individuals above the age of fifty were more liable to pneumonia of the upper lobe than those of earlier periods of life; but eleven of my fifteen cases were under the age of thirty-one.*

* Subsequent observation in India has tended to confirm my opinion that pneumonia of the upper lobe is more frequent than is generally supposed, is not more dangerous, and is not most common in individuals above the age of fifty. It also shows that, in India at least, there is a greater liability to error of diagnosis between pneumonia and phthisis in their second stages, than would exist under the generally received opinion that pneumonia is seldom exclusively in the upper lobes. I am satisfied that a too ready belief in the common opinion has led me, on more than one occasion, to diagnose phthisis in the second stage instead of pneumonia in the second stage.

The subject is so important, that I do not hesitate to submit a short summary of the additional cases which have come under my notice since the remarks in the text were written; the aggregate thus amounts to twenty-one cases.

1. Bapoo Rawa, a Maratha, twenty-five years of age, admitted with remittent fever attended with delirium, on the 5th December, 1856. There was cough. Dulness and coarse crepitus were detected in the right infra-clavicular region on the 11th, and phthisis was diagnosed. The fever ceased. The dulness lessened, and he was discharged on the 16th December without any trace of disease in the right infra-clavicular region.

2. Chota Padren, aged twelve, was, after three days' illness, admitted on the 5th January, 1857. He was out of condition, there was much fever with pain of limbs. The dorsal regions were examined, and no pulmonary disease detected. Continuance of febrile exacerbation with cough led to a more thorough examination, and on the 7th there was found dulness of the left infra-clavicular, mammary and axillary regions with bronchial respiration. Acetate of ammonia and nitre were given, and water compresses applied to the affected regions. The febrile symptoms lessened, crepitus appeared in the dull regions, and on the 22nd the state of the upper part of the left lung was normal and he was discharged well on the 31st.

Residence in hospital.—In considering the duration of residence in hospital, let us separate the recovered from the fatal cases.

Of recovered cases, twelve primary and two febrile were discharged within ten days; twelve primary and eleven febrile between eleven and twenty days; thirteen primary and three febrile between twenty-one and thirty days; fifteen primary and three febrile above thirty-one days.

There were fifty-seven cases discharged at different periods above ten days; eighteen of them, indeed, above thirty-one days. From this statement we may infer, that though pneumonia in the second stage is frequently recovered from, yet a considerable time is generally required to ensure the restoration of the lung to a healthy or useful state.

Of the fatal cases, fourteen primary and five febrile died within ten days from admission, three primary and two febrile between eleven and twenty days, two primary and one febrile between twenty-one and thirty days, and five primary upwards of thirty-one days. The fact of nineteen of the thirty-two fatal cases having proved fatal within ten days of admission shows the advanced stage at which a great portion of them must have come

3. Rama Itoo, a Hindoo, aged thirty, after six days' illness, was admitted on the 4th January, 1858, with dulness, bronchial respiration, and crepitus of the left infra-clavicular, mammary and scapular regions. There was also crepitus in the right infrascapular region. Under the use of quinine, stimulants, nourishment, and a water compress to the chest, the cough and fever lessened, the dulness and bronchial respiration decreased, and he left the hospital contrary to advice on the 12th, at which time there was no fever nor cough, but the defective resonance and the bronchial respiration on the left side were not altogether gone.

4. Pestonjee Dorabjee, a Parsee, aged forty, had been in hospital two or three times with fever and suspected tubercles in the upper right lung, but after discharge he had gained so much in flesh as to remove the suspicion of phthisis. He was re-admitted on the 4th February, 1857, with remittent fever. The tongue was florid at the edges, and there was occasional vomiting and cough. On the 7th there was dulness and imperfect respiration in the right infra-clavicular region, with bronchial respiration and crepitus in the scapular region. On the ninth the physical signs were the same, and the sputa had a faint rusty tinge. The fever continued for two days with some delirium and slight jaundice, then lessening of the fever and cough, and on the 12th there was coarse general crepitus in the right infra-clavicular region. On the 14th the dulness was less and the crepitus was being replaced by vesicular respiration. The fever no longer recurred. He gradually improved and was discharged on the 23rd March in good flesh, without cough, and with normal resonance and breath sounds in the right infra-clavicular region.

5. Mahadoo Sawnut, a Mahratta sepoy of the 6th Regiment, Bombay Infantry, aged twenty-two, was admitted into hospital at Poona, on the 15th April, 1859. He had fever with marked remissions and exacerbations. The chest was examined on the 17th, but nothing abnormal was detected. On the 19th the fever continued, the respiration was hurried, and wandering delirium was present. I saw this patient for the

under treatment. It confirms the direct statement made on this point in a former part of these remarks.

State of lung on discharge.—Seventy-one cases were discharged from hospital. Of fifty-one cases of *primary* pneumonia the lung was quite* restored in thirty-three, improved in thirteen, not improved in five, and in one not recorded. Of nineteen *febrile* cases the lung was restored in sixteen, improved in two, and in one not recorded.

When we class the two forms together, we find that sixty-two were admitted in the second stage, and only nine in the first stage. It has appeared that in forty-nine of the discharged cases the lung was restored. If we deduct from these the nine cases admitted in the first stage, we have of sixty-two cases of pneumonia in the second stage forty recoveries. Of the remaining twenty-two the lung was improved in fifteen, not improved in five, and not recorded in two.

Morbid anatomy.—There was a post-mortem examination made in fifteen of the twenty-four fatal cases of primary pneumonia, and in seven of the eight fatal cases of febrile pneumonia.

In eleven of the cases the solidified lung was in a state of

first time on the morning of the 20th, on the occasion of my weekly visit to the hospital, and was struck with the hurried breathing and defective movement of the left side. The subclavian, mammary and scapular regions of that side were dull, and bronchial respiration was present. I called the attention of the medical officer to the pneumonia in the second stage, complicating fever, which he had overlooked. A few leeches were applied, and quinine, with one grain of calomel and antimonial powder, was given every second hour, and sesquicarbonate of ammonia in the intervals. On the 21st the sputa, previously tenacious, had become less so, the respiration less hurried, but the delirium still occasional. On the 23rd, the respiratory murmur began to return; and on the 28th, when I again saw him, the dulness was gone and the respiration quite restored. He was discharged on the 1st May. This case shows very forcibly the importance of frequent systematic auscultation and percussion in remittent fever in natives of India. The medical officer in this instance was a gentleman of much intelligence, and in general quite alive to the importance of these methods of investigation, but in this case he had been satisfied with one cursory examination on the second day after admission.

6. John Dias, aged thirty, a cook, after five days' illness, was admitted, on the 18th December, 1857, with fever, slight jaundice, delirium, adhesive yellow-tinged sputa, and solidification of the left lung, chiefly noted in the axillary and scapular regions. He died on the 14th, and on inspection the whole of the left upper lobe was in a state of grey hepatisation, with friable lymph on its pleural surface. The upper part of the lower lobe from above downwards passed from grey into red hepatisation, and the thin part of the base of the lung was spongy and crepitating. The right lung was healthy. There was commencing Bright's disease. This was a case of pneumonia commencing in the upper lobe, and passing downwards.

* By this I mean that the removal of the dulness on percussion, and return of the vesicular respiration, indicated that the lung had become permeable and fit for function.

induration, either red or grey. This condition, compared with readily lacerable hepatisation, occurs in this hospital in a greater proportion even than this series shows: it is related to asthenic states, to a protracted course, and not unfrequently to advanced period of life. True hepatisation, on the other hand, usually occurs in better states of the constitution, and after a more rapid course: in the febrile form it has existed in greater proportion than induration. Of the seven cases of febrile pneumonia there was hepatisation in five, and induration in two; whereas in the fifteen cases of primary pneumonia there was induration in nine, and hepatisation in six. Whether the grey induration is to be regarded as an advanced stage of the red or brown, or a distinct variety from the commencement, has been a question: these cases rather countenance the former view. Tubercular deposit was observed in only one case, a febrile one: it was in small quantity in the upper lobe of the left lung.

In three of the cases—two primary, and one febrile—the hepatisation, in places, occurred in nodules: the pneumonia had been in part lobular; but in all there were also hepatised portions of considerable extent. There was no reason for supposing that these instances of lobular pneumonia were dependent on pyæmia: they were more probably cases in which bronchitis had passed into pneumonia, for in all of them increased redness of the bronchial mucous lining was well marked.

Though there are no cases of pyæmic pulmonary abscesses in this series, yet several have been observed in the hospital. Pyæmia will be considered in a subsequent chapter.

Pleural adhesions have generally proved the co-existence of pleuritis, more or less recent. The absence of pleuritis occurs, more frequently in febrile than in primary pneumonia: of the seven fatal cases of the former, examined after death, it is distinctly stated that in two of them there were no traces of pleuritis, and yet in both there was much red hepatisation of the lung.

Thick cacoplastic membranous, almost cartilaginous, deposits were found in one or two cases, connecting the surfaces of the pleura together. One case seemed to show that the deposit takes place in the first instance on the surface of the pulmonary pleura, and advances to some degree of thickness, before it forms adhesion with the opposed costal pleura. In the case referred to, the anterior part of the upper lobe of the right lung adhered to the costal surface by a thick membranous, almost cartilaginous, layer; while on the same part of the left lung there was an opaque membranous deposit, but no adhesion.

Bronchitis, to greater or less extent, has also been noticed as a frequent complication: it occurred in greater proportion in the febrile form.

Cavities were found in the lungs in five* cases. They ranged in size from a small orange to a split pea. In all there were several cavities: they existed both in the upper and lower lobes, and had formed in the midst of grey induration. In case 228 the different stages of the process were well shown; in it, scattered in the grey induration, were dark-red points, from the size of a pin's head to that of a hemp seed; and there were also cavities from the size of a split pea to that of a pigeon's egg, with an inner surface, moist, and of dark-red colour. In the grey indurated part, inflammatory stasis of blood had probably taken place, here and there followed by molecular loss of vitality, hence softening, liquefaction, and the formation of cavities at these points: this seemed to me to be the process by which in two of these cases the cavities had been formed. In the three others the appearance of the cavities, the fœtor of their contents, or of the sputa during life, indicated that the loss of vitality had not been molecular merely, but of portions of tissue more or less extensive: that the cavities had been formed by a process of gangrene.†

* There was a sixth case, in which cavernous respiration was present; but the body was not examined after death.

† The occurrence of gangrene of the lung, unpreceded by inflammation, is not common. There are two cases in my notes which seem to me to have been of this nature.

The first was a marine of Her Majesty's ship *Endymion*, of twenty years of age. He had suffered from adynamic remittent fever, and was under treatment for consecutive dysentery. *Chest.*—The lungs did not collapse, the anterior parts were inflated, the posterior œdematous. On the posterior part of both lungs there was a green discoloured portion, which broke down readily under the knife, and gave out much greenish frothy serum. The cellular tissue was plainly disorganised, and the serum seemed to have been contained in a small cyst, rather than in the natural tissue of the lung (gangrene with serous effusion into the cellular tissue of the lung, not preceded by condensation of that portion of the lung). No hepatisation of any part of the lungs. Heart healthy. *Abdomen.*—The stomach, much distended, occupied the entire space between the ensiform cartilage and umbilicus; its mucous coat was lined with adhesive mucus, and presented throughout a dusky rosy tint, without softening. The liver was rather enlarged, olive-green in colour, and mottled; no abscess. The transverse portion of the colon was opened; the mucous coat presented numerous ulcers in different stages, many of them cicatrising. Spleen natural; kidneys healthy.

The second occurred in a destitute Mahomedan pilgrim, of fifty years of age, with puffed face, œdematous feet, short and hurried respiration, puriform sputa, some degree

In none of the five cases in which cavities existed was tubercular deposit observed in the lungs: three of them are here detailed:—

228. *Pneumonia, extensive of right lung.—Grey induration with cavities formed in the upper lobe by molecular gangrene.*—Pandoo Gunnoo, a Hindoo, of thirty-five years of age, a native of Carlee, following the occupation of a peon, and not addicted to the use of spirits, was, after fifteen days' illness with fever, cough, pain of back and loins, admitted into the clinical ward on the 5th September, 1849. He was emaciated. The respiration was hurried. There was dulness of the subclavian and lateral regions, and of the whole posterior part of the right side of chest, greatest in degree in the supraspinous and dorsal regions. In all these situations occasional subcrepitus was heard, with blowing respiration under the clavicle and under the spine of the scapula. In the left side of chest no abnormal sign was detected; but the respiration was puerile in parts. The sounds and impulse of the heart were natural. There was elastic and uneasy fulness of the abdomen, above the umbilicus. The feet were œdematous. The skin was above the natural temperature. The pulse was small and somewhat frequent. The tongue was slightly florid at the tip and coated posteriorly. The voice was hoarse, and the breath very fetid. On the 8th the chest was again carefully examined: under the acromial end of the right clavicle and in the axilla, the respiration was cavernous, sometimes almost amphoric, and pectoriloquy was distinct. In the right lateral and dorsal regions the respiration was bronchial, with occasional crepitus and subcrepitus in the former. He continued under treatment till the 21st, when he died. There was hectic fever, frequent hard cough, with grey puriform sputa. Diarrhœa supervened on the 16th, and hastened the fatal issue. He was treated with anodynes chiefly till the diarrhœa came on, when acetate of lead with opium was given.

Inspection six hours after death.—The larynx and trachea were healthy. *Chest.*—The left lung was crepitating and inflated: there were old adhesions between the inferior lobe and the costal pleura and diaphragm. The right lung adhered firmly on all sides to the parietes of the chest: the upper lobe was in a state of grey induration with many irregular excavations; the largest was situated near the apex, of the size of a small egg, and another, somewhat smaller, existed at the lower and outer part; the excavations in process of formation were surrounded by a dark-red layer, and the contents of all consisted of dark grey, sero-puriform, very fetid fluid; the lower lobe was in a state of grey hepatisation, with the exception of its inner and lower half, which was healthy and crepitating. *Abdomen.*—On opening the abdomen some fetid gas escaped. Firm adhesions connected the anterior parietes to the omentum and colon, which passed horizontally across the abdomen from one side to the other, just above the umbilicus. The liver had contracted firm adhesions with the stomach, diaphragm, and anterior parietes of the abdomen; and its outer covering appeared to be denser than natural. The structure was healthy. Besides the adhesion with the liver, the stomach was also adherent to the spleen; its mucous surface was not examined. The spleen was not enlarged; it adhered on all sides to the diaphragm, abdominal parietes, and the stomach. The left kidney was larger than the right; both were flabby, but of healthy structure. Other parts not examined.

---

of dulness of the right dorsal lateral and scapular regions, with occasional subcrepitus. No albumen in the urine. *Inspection.*—Old adhesions united the posterior part of the right lung to the walls of the chest. The posterior part of this lung, for about four inches in length and three in width, was in a state of gangrene—reduced to a dark-grey fetid pulpy state. The surrounding pulmonary tissue was in part healthy, in part œdematous; but without trace of sanguineous engorgement or hepatisation. The heart was healthy. Two pints of serous fluid were effused in the cavity of the abdomen.

229. *Grey, almost cartilaginous, induration of the lower part of the right lung, with several excavations by process of gangrenous molecular softening.—The several stages of the process well shown.—Bright's disease of the kidney.*—Pandoo, a Hindoo labourer, a native of Coorla, of thirty years age, was, after three months' illness, admitted into the clinical ward on the 11th September, 1848. He was much reduced, affected with cough, puriform expectoration, and daily febrile accessions coming on at irregular times. He had suffered thus for two months. He pointed to the right false ribs as the seat of pain when he coughed, and this he believed to have been caused by a fall from a horse some years before; but he was wanting in intelligence, and not distinct in his statements. The breathing was rather hurried, and the pulse feeble. In consequence of disturbance from the cough, it was some days before a satisfactory examination of the chest could be made. On the 17th, there was large mucous rale in the right axilla. On the 27th, cavernous respiration in the right axilla, dulness of the right scapula and dorsal regions, with occasional crepitus in the latter, were noted; also vesicular respiration general on the left side, with occasional crepitus in the dorsal region. On the third October, cavernous respiration, and pectoriloquy, were reported in the right axilla, and at the inside of the inferior angle of the right scapula. Vesicular respiration was absent in the right lateral region, and bronchial sounds were heard there. On the 8th, the right dorsal and lateral regions were completely dull, and the signs of a cavity continued. There was very troublesome cough with copious puriform expectoration and frequent hectic fever. On the 13th October, the urine gave a flaky deposit with heat and nitric acid, and on several subsequent occasions also evinced traces of albumen. The feet became œdematous, and he died on the 24th October. Small blisters were applied to the right side of the chest. He was treated with anodynes, expectorants, and tonics.

Inspection four hours after death.—Chest.—The left lung adhered firmly to the costal pleura; its upper lobe was emphysematous, but elsewhere it crepitated, was nowhere consolidated, and did not give out much fluid of any kind when incised. The right lung adhered very firmly to the costal pleura at the lateral and dorsal parts; also to the diaphragm. The upper lobe was crepitating, with, at its very apex, an emphysematous bulla, the size of a walnut. The third lobe was consolidated throughout, and covered by a membranous layer of lymph, at least quarter of an inch thick at the base of the lung, where opposed to the diaphragm. This lobe was in a state of grey induration, almost cartilaginous when incised, but branches of the pulmonary artery and veins and bronchial tubes could be traced ramifying through the indurated substance. At the very edge and back part of this lobe there was about an inch square of crepitating tissue, and at the upper part were several irregular excavations, the largest the size of a pigeon's egg, with moist dark red walls, and membranous investing tissue. They had the character of gangrenous excavations, but wanted the gangrenous fœtor. On making a vertical incision in the indurated lobe, below and somewhat posterior to these excavations, there was found at the upper part another cavity, the size of a small bean, with dark red sides; and a little lower down, one the size of a split pea. Still lower in the lobe there existed dark red spots distinct, isolated with considerable interspaces, from the size of a hemp-seed to a pin's head, evidently the first stage of what would have formed excavations. The heart was healthy. *Abdomen.*—The liver, enlarged, was not particularly examined. Both kidneys were somewhat enlarged, the left most so, somewhat lobulated and mottled externally. When incised, the surface of the cortical part presented a granular appearance, very streaked and mottled red and buff, and some of the bundles of the tubular part were surrounded by a distinct buff-coloured band. When examined through a lens, the surface of the incision had a glistening fatty look.

230. *Grey and red induration of the upper lobe of the right lung with gangrenous excavation.*—Dulla, a Hindoo servant, a native of Sawunt Waree, using spirits habit-

ually, was admitted into the clinical ward on the 27th February, 1849. He stated that, three years before, he had been struck with the stock of a musket at the lower part of the sternum, and that immediately afterwards he vomited blood. He soon recovered from the effects of the injury, and did not then suffer from cough. On admission he was a good deal emaciated, had frequent cough, with copious muco-puriform sputa in roundish masses. The voice was hoarse, and the breath very fetid; decubitus was dorsal, and attempts to lie on the left side excited cough. He suffered from hectic fever and diarrhœa. He had been affected with these symptoms for six weeks, and he stated that his father, at an advanced age, had died of pulmonic disease. The respiration was somewhat hurried and oppressed. There was dulness on percussion of the right subclavian, mammary, and lateral regions, decreasing from above downwards. The respiration was bronchial in these dull regions, and the resonance of voice was very distinct below the right clavicle and a little below and internal to the nipple. The respiration was puerile on the left side, but there was no dulness of that side, nor any rales. He sank rapidly under the diarrhœa, and died on the 8th March.

Inspection five hours after death.—The left lung, with exception of a few hepatised nodules the size of a horse-bean in the upper lobe, was soft and crepitated under pressure. The upper lobe of the right lung was in a state partly of grey and partly of red induration, and there was a gangrenous excavation at the apex the size of a large orange. In the indurated parts adjoining the cavity, there were a few dark grey portions the size of a bean (commencing gangrene). The two lower lobes were in a state of red induration, with exception of the posterior thin edge of the third lobe, which was soft and crepitating. The heart was healthy. The kidneys were normal. The end of the ileum and the large intestine, as far as the ascending colon, were opened: the mucous membrane was not ulcerated.

In many of these cases, as may generally be noted when there is solidification of a considerable part of a lung, a more or less emphysematous or inflated state of the permeable parts of the lung was observed.

Bright's disease of the kidney was present in only three of the twenty-two cases examined after death: in two of them there was red hepatisation, lobular in character in one, in the third case there was grey induration, with cavities. On referring to my cases of Bright's disease, it appears that pneumonia was present as a secondary affection in five of twenty fatal cases. Of these, two were in a state of induration, and three of hepatisation. Thus, then, the observations made in this hospital tend to show a relation between pneumonia and Bright's disease.

My investigations have not as yet confirmed the supposed frequent relation between heart disease and pneumonia. Disease of the heart was not present in any of the cases in this series, but pneumonia was found in two of the seventeen fatal cases of cardiac disease examined after death, and included in my remarks in a subsequent chapter on disease of the heart.

In one case there had been circumscribed empyema of the right side, and perforation of the under part of the middle lobe of the lung at its fissure with the third lobe had taken place: this part of the middle lobe had formed the vault of the sac. The purulent effusion had also opened into the pericardium, and excited pericarditis. In the left lung there was grey induration, and cavities by softening.

The complication of pleuritic effusion, serous or puriform, was observed in only two of the fatal cases of this series. One, just adverted to, was circumscribed empyema and primary pneumonia. The other was febrile: the effusion was of red-tinged serum. These results, however, by no means express the frequency of this complication. It was present in five of the recovered cases, four primary, and one febrile; and I have met with it in several other cases at different times. Defective vocal thrill, the appearance of a friction murmur as the dulness lessened, the presence of crepitus at some period or other, and of sputa more or less copious, have been the signs on which the diagnosis of this complication has been determined. On the whole, my experience tends to confirm the generally received opinion relative to the combination of pneumonia, and some degree of pleuritic effusion, — that the prognosis is more favourable in the combined than in the separate affections. We may believe that both commence simultaneously, and may suppose that they mutually influence each other: the solidification of the lung may limit the amount of the pleuritic effusion; the pleuritic effusion may limit the degree of the solidification of the lung. The advance of the morbid change in both is thus checked, and a greater tendency to restoration results.

SECTION IV. — *Symptoms.—Fever, Pain, Dyspnœa, Cough, Delirium, Character of the Sputa.—Physical Signs.*

Fever, not hectic in character, was observed in ninety-two cases, viz., in all of the febrile form, and sixty-five of the primary.

The remittent * character of the fever was well marked in all the cases of the febrile form. It was also distinctly observed in a considerable proportion of the cases of primary pneumonia. The remittent character of symptomatic fever is of frequent occurrence, both in the medical and surgical practice of this hospital, and may be regarded as a feature of symptomatic febrile disturbance in the natives of India generally, more particularly in the asthenic. It is of practical importance to watch for the remission, for reasons to be explained when the treatment of pneumonia comes under

* I do not think it necessary to separate the four cases in which the fever was intermittent in type.

consideration. This remittent type of symptomatic fever probably depends on the influence of malaria pre-existing in the constitution, and is excited by local inflammation, just as intermittent fever may be excited by exposure to cold in the same state of the system. The inflammation is the exciting cause of the fever. The state of constitution, previously engendered by the influence of malaria, determines the type which that fever assumes. These views we shall find are confirmed by the results of treatment. But whatever the true explanation may be, the fact is undoubted that symptomatic fever in asthenic natives affected with pneumonia in Bombay is in many instances markedly remittent in type.* So much so, indeed, that it is frequently a difficult question of diagnosis to decide whether the particular instance ought to be classed as primary or febrile pneumonia.

In determining this diagnosis, the following considerations have chiefly influenced me, in respect to the febrile form:—

1. The distinctness of the exacerbation and remission.

2. The history showing clearly that the febrile phenomena had taken precedence by some days of the symptoms of pneumonia.

3. The state of the tongue, as regards fur, floridity, dryness.

4. The presence of much restlessness at night, with some degree of delirium when the pneumonia was not far advanced.

5. The fever presenting adynamic phenomena. This was, however, an occurrence only of the advanced stages: it was observed in five of the cases of this series.

Attention to these circumstances will in general suffice to establish this diagnosis. Still, with patients admitted in the advanced stages of disease, with imperfect histories of their previous illness, difficulty will be occasionally experienced.

When the pneumonia has existed for some time in the second stage, very generally, the cessation of the febrile disturbance takes precedence for a time — longer or shorter, according to the previous duration of the disease — of the restoration of the lung to its healthy state. The discontinuance of the fever, when not replaced by that of hectic type, is usually attended by improvement of the other symptoms, as by lessening of the cough and dyspnœa. It is, however, to the *physical signs* that we must turn for information regarding the real condition of the lung. In many cases— nearly all of the febrile form, and in a considerable proportion of the primary form — it will be found that the cessation of the fever,

* Remarks of a similar tenor have already been made at p. 74. I now apply them to a particular disease, as previously done in respect to hepatitis, p. 374.

and the lessening of the cough and dyspnœa, are attended by a corresponding improvement in the physical signs. The dulness becomes less, the bronchial respiration is gradually replaced by vesicular murmur, the crepitus redux is sometimes heard, and after a period more or less long the signs of complete recovery reappear. In other cases, however, of the primary form, in which the lung has been for a longer time consolidated, we find that days may pass before improvement in the general symptoms is followed by signs of decrease of the consolidation: then these signs begin to return, and by a slow process the lung is more or less completely restored. It is reasonable to assume, that though in these latter cases the process of recovery is so slow as to require some time before, by a lessening of the signs of consolidation, it gives evidence of its being in progress, yet its commencement, or its tendency to commence, is coincident with the termination of the fever and the improvement in the other symptoms. These facts have an important bearing on treatment as I shall presently endeavour to show.

Hectic fever was noted in eight cases. They were all of the primary form; five of them were cases in which cavities existed, and which proved fatal. Three of them were discharged cases, two with the lung somewhat improved, and one with no change.

Pain.—When we inquire into the frequency with which pain in some part of the chest has been complained of, we find that it was present in only forty: thirty-four of these were primary, which is rather more than half of this form; five were febrile, which is a little less than a sixth of this form.

The less complaint of pain in the febrile form accords with the results noted under the head Morbid Anatomy. There, it is stated that pleuritis was more frequently absent in the febrile than in the primary form.

Pain below the margin of the right false ribs was noticed in thirteen cases: they were all of the primary form. In three there was pain also at the margin of the left ribs. In six in which there was pain below the margin of the right ribs, there was also some degree of abnormal dulness on percussion in the same situation.

In only one of these thirteen cases (a fatal one) was there reason for connecting the pain with the existence of hepatic inflammation. In this single instance abscess was found in the liver after death. In my remarks on disease of the heart in a subsequent chapter (page 592), it will appear that in six of thirteen cases of that affection there existed pain and some degree of abnormal dulness at the margin of the right ribs. This was attributed to congestion of the liver, consequent on obstructed passage of the blood through the heart. That congestion of the liver is also apt to occur consequent on obstruction to the passage of the blood through the lungs in extensive pneumonia, is an old observation of pathologists. That it is correct, I believe, from having witnessed a congested state of the liver after death in several cases of pneumonia.

When pain below the margin of the right ribs is present in pneumonia, associated with abnormal dulness, we shall generally be right in relating it to hepatic congestion. The pneumonia may be either of the right or the left side, but the hepatic congestion probably indicates that it is extensive.

There are, however, other cases in which pain is experienced at the margin of the right ribs, but which are unattended with abnormal dulness. In these the pain is probably sympathetic, like that not unfrequently observed at the margin of the left ribs in pericarditis. When the pneumonia is of the right lung, we shall have this kind of pain, if present, at the margin of the right ribs; if the pneumonia, on the other hand, be of the left lung, the pain will be at the margin of the left ribs. But we may expect to find this symptom more frequently on the right side, because pneumonia of the right lung is more common than that of the left. This sympathetic pain was noticed in seven cases of the present series: but my remarks are not grounded on these cases alone, for the symptom has been noticed by myself and others in other cases in the general wards of the hospital.

The occurrence of hepatitis secondary on pneumonia doubtless occasionally takes place; therefore, when pain is felt at the margin of the right ribs, this fact should be borne in mind. Still, these cases observed in India would seem to justify the opinion that the co-existence * of these diseases is not common. It was noticed in one only of 103 cases of pneumonia, and that in an instance in which the event was unlikely to occur, for the pneumonia was of the upper part of the left lung. But pain at the margin of the right ribs, unconnected with hepatitis, has been observed in twelve of the 103 cases.

* It must be understood that I speak of hepatitis secondary on pneumonia: pneumonia secondary on hepatitis is more common. I do not now allude to the co-existence of these diseases taking place in this latter order, but only in the former.

I have called attention to this symptom *, — and I shall follow the same course in connection with heart disease, — in order that an error in diagnosis may not be committed, and pneumonia be mistaken for hepatitis. This I have known to occur; therefore I am satisfied that the caution is not uncalled for.

Dyspnœa. — Some degree of shortness and hurry of the respiratory acts was noticed in ninety-one cases: of these sixty-seven were primary, and twenty-four were febrile. Thus there remain nine of the first form, and three of the second in which this symptom was not noted.

Though some degree of dyspnœa has been observed in so many instances, yet in the great proportion of them it was by no means urgent, and in many might have been overlooked, had not the cases, from the circumstance of being collected together for purposes of clinical instruction, been submitted to careful investigation and record. The reason why the dyspnœa was slight, and might readily have escaped notice in many of these cases, is sufficiently explained by the asthenic state of so many of the affected.

The degree of dyspnœa in this disease is always an expression of the degree in which there is disproportion between the amount of blood to be aërated, and the extent of the pulmonary surface.

In an individual of sthenic constitution, in whom the blood is abundant and the full extent of the pulmonary surface is required for aëration, pneumonia of a small extent of lung will be attended with marked dyspnœa. But when the quantity of blood has been for some time reduced, as always happens in asthenic states, then the full extent of the pulmonary surface is in excess of what is necessary: part of it may become unfitted for function by pneumonia, and yet dyspnœa be hardly noticeable. In these statements we have the explanation of the latency or obscurity of the symptoms of impaired function of the lungs in asthenic pneumonia.

When the treatment of the sthenic forms of the disease comes under consideration, we shall find that it is of importance to remember that dyspnœa indicates a want of proportion between the quantity of the blood and the extent of the aërating surface; and that it may be lessened, or removed, in one or two ways — either

* It is hardly necessary to caution against the error of mistaking uneasiness at the margin of the right ribs, with dulness, consequent on displacement of the liver from pleuritic effusion, for the conditions to which reference has been made in these remarks.

by restoring the pulmonary surface to its structural fitness, or by reducing the blood till it has become in proportion to the diminished extent of that surface.*

Cough was present in ninety-eight cases,—seventy-two primary, and twenty-six febrile.

The little urgency of the cough in pneumonia has been very generally remarked by writers on this disease. The opinions which I have ventured to express on the general pathology of pneumonia seem to me to afford a ready explanation of this peculiarity. Cough merely expresses the fact that there exists in the bronchial tubes some obstacle to the free transmission of air to the cells beyond: it is a forcible expiratory act, called into exercise to remove the cause of the obstruction. It is reasonable to suppose that if the air cells beyond become unfit for aëration, and the venous blood is no

* In some cursory notes on the thoracic inflammations in the European General Hospital, presented by me to the Medical and Physical Society in May 1845, and published in No. 6 of the "Transactions," the following remarks are made:—"Pneumonia is certainly a disease of infrequent occurrence in Bombay; but it may not be altogether misplaced to remark here, that partial and circumscribed pneumonia is by no means a rare complication of the fevers to which natives are liable in the cold season in the Deccan, and I believe in Guzerat. If the febrile symptoms persist without intermission for two or three days, if the skin be dry, the tongue not furred to the extent that might be expected, where the digestive organs are much deranged; then a careful stethoscopic examination will probably detect the existence of crepitous rale in some part or other of the chest — most frequently in the neighbourhood of the mammary region; and this may be when there has been no complaint of pain, no cough, and attention has not been called to any difficulty of respiration. In these cases, attentive observation will detect an altered expression of countenance, not amounting to anxiety, but which probably marks the implication of some important organ. The person feels ill, but seems unable to explain to another the nature of his feelings; the body is inclined forwards, the lips are dry and parted, the respiration is somewhat hurried, but often not more so than a general and uncomplicated febrile condition might explain. The stethoscope will resolve the doubt, and the free use of tartar emetic, combined with blood-letting, general or local, and blisters, according to circumstances, will, if the disease has not been allowed to go too far, effect a cure, and prove the accuracy of the diagnosis." These remarks were grounded on what I had seen of the diseases of natives in former periods of my service in the Deccan, and on the Mahabuleshwur Hills. My experience since in the Jamsetjee Jejeebhoy Hospital has corrected my error in regard to the infrequency of pneumonia in Bombay. But my chief object in reverting now to what I had previously written is, that I may have the opportunity of observing, that though there is nothing in my experience since at variance with the tenor of these remarks on the obscurity and importance of febrile pneumonia, yet we ought not to lay much stress on general symptoms such as those I have detailed. In treating the malarious fevers of the natives of India, percussion and auscultation of the chest should be invariably practised with daily regularity. It is a practical rule quite as important in the management of this class of disease, as the search for the signs of pericarditis and endocarditis is in the course of acute rheumatism. He is a careless observer of disease who finds himself taken by surprise by the discovery of pneumonia in remittent fever, or pericarditis in acute rheumatism.

longer sent to them, but, instead, to the healthy adjacent cells,—then any obstruction existing in the tubes leading to the impervious cells is no longer the same evil as when the cells were efficient and blood was sent to them for aëration: hence there is no longer the same demand for cough to clear them. The solidified lung in pneumonia is in the state just described, and such seems to me the best explanation of the little urgency of the cough in this disease.

Delirium was observed in eleven cases. This symptom, when present in primary pneumonia, occurs in the advanced stages: it is of very unfavourable import. It was observed in three cases of the primary form: they were all fatal, one with pneumonia of the upper part of the left lung in the third stage with cavities, the other two were double pneumonia in the second stage.

The remaining eight cases in which delirium, generally associated with some degree of drowsiness, was noted, were of the febrile form: in four there was recovery, and in four death. Therefore this symptom, more particularly when occurring early in the disease, and when not attended with adynamic phenomena, is not of the same unfavourable import in febrile as in primary pneumonia.

The character of the sputa.—The rusty adhesive sputa characteristic of pneumonia were noted in only seventeen cases,—twelve primary, and five febrile; of these fourteen were recoveries, and three proved fatal. In the other cases the sputa were untinged, mucous, and more or less adhesive; in a few cases none are recorded.

In seven cases red muco-puriform sputa are stated to have been present: they were all of the primary form. Four proved fatal, and in all of them there existed cavities in the lungs; in two, verified by post-mortem examination, but in two not examined after death, cavities were believed to have been present, in consequence of cavernous respiration having been recognised during life. In three the patients were discharged: they were cases in which hectic had been present; in one there was no improvement of the lung, but in two some degree of improvement had taken place. In none of the three were cavities suspected to exist. From these cases, then, and from another to which I shall presently advert, the appearance of this character of sputa does not necessarily indicate the existence of cavities in the lungs.*

* This is the red-tinged muco-puriform sputa, to which I have already alluded in my remarks on hepatic abscess, as occurring in states of asthenic pneumonia, and

Physical signs.—It is unnecessary that I should enlarge on a subject now so well understood as the physical signs of pneumonia. The accuracy of the statement relative to the stage of the disease on admission, and the state of the lung on discharge, depends on these signs. On this point I would merely observe, that abnormal dulness on percussion, bronchial respiration, with some degree of crepitus in the adjacent parts, and presence of vocal thrill, were the signs held to indicate the existence of the second stage; while disappearance of the abnormal dulness, and replacement of bronchial by vesicular respiration (even though the latter continued somewhat feebler than on the sound side) have been held to signify that the lung had become restored to functional fitness.

There is one caution which it may be useful to make. The frequency with which enlargement of the spleen is met with in India, makes it necessary that we should be careful not to mistake abnormal dulness of the left dorsal region, caused by it, for dulness from hepatisation of the lung.

SECTION V.—*Treatment.*—*General and Local Blood-letting, Tartar Emetic, Mercury, Blisters, Quinine, Liquor Potassæ, Stimulants.*—*Concluding Remarks.*

General blood-letting was held to be expedient in only three of the 103 cases of pneumonia which form the subject of my present remarks, and even in these it was adopted to a very limited extent. This fact shows clearly the general character of the constitution of the persons affected, and the stage of the disease at which they usually came under treatment. It is not to be explained on the supposition that I entertain peculiar views in regard to the unsuitableness of general blood-letting in the treatment of inflammatory disease. On the contrary I entirely agree with those who think that a pulse above the natural frequency, full and firm, associated with increased heat of skin, and co-existing with inflammation of an important organ, indicates the propriety of general blood-letting. But we, at the same time, cannot impress too firmly on our minds, that these are conditions of the pulse which co-exist only with the *early* stages of inflammation in individuals of *sthenic* constitution. Whilst thus, then, expressing my belief in the efficacy of general blood-letting in appropriate

which is not to be distinguished, I believe, from that which I formerly considered to be pathognomonic of hepatic abscess having opened into the lung. I would refer the reader to those observations (p. 383).

circumstances, in the treatment of inflammatory disease, I am unable to concur in those views which regard it as a remedy *peculiarly* appropriate in pneumonia. The opinion that blood-letting may be carried to a greater extent in pneumonia than in other inflammations, rests, it may be supposed, on the observation of the great relief to the dyspnœa which generally follows the loss of blood; and on the inference that this relief may be received as proof that there has been a corresponding improvement in the inflamed lung. Such an inference, however, may surely be erroneous. Dyspnœa, as already explained, depends on a want of just proportion between the quantity of blood in the vascular system, and the extent of the pulmonary aërating surface. In pneumonia the extent of that surface is lessened; more blood is sent to the healthy part of the lung, and dyspnœa results. By reducing, by venesection or other means, the amount of blood circulating in the system, we necessarily relieve the dyspnœa. But this may have been effected without any improvement in the state of the inflamed part. Indeed, it is distinctly stated by Dr. Alison *, as a result of his clinical observation, that auscultation may indicate a continuance and even an extension of the disease for a considerable time after the breathing has been effectually relieved by blood-letting. Let us admit, then, that blood-letting in pneumonia may afford relief on two distinct principles: one common to it with other inflammations, the other peculiar to itself, and related to the function of the organ. But it by no means follows on this account that the rules for its use should in any respect differ from those which obtain in inflammation generally. Blood-letting, within certain limits, is a valuable therapeutic means in certain states and stages of inflammation. Carry it beyond these limits, use it in other states and stages of inflammation, and it becomes injurious. This principle is equally true of pneumonia as of other inflammations. When the circumstances, as indicated by the pulse and skin and stage of disease, are inappropriate, we may not use blood-letting in pneumonia merely to relieve dyspnœa: this would be the mere palliation of a symptom, purchased by increasing the tendency to death by syncope. It would be as if in idiopathic fever complicated with diarrhœa and stupor, we were to give full opiates and check the former, with the certainty of increasing the tendency to death by coma.

The statement made, with the view of inculcating free blood-

* "Outlines of Pathology," p. 281.

letting, by Andral *, and repeated by Dr. Watson †, that it is useful in pneumonia on the principle applicable to all inflammations, and also on the principle in accordance with which the exclusion of light is useful in ophthalmia, and rest in an inflamed joint, is, I apprehend, in its latter part, of very doubtful accuracy. If the opinions which I have ventured to express in a former part of this chapter be correct, viz., that after the affected pulmonary cells have, for a time, been the seat of inflammation, they become unfit for function and no longer exercise it; then blood-letting can do no good to them, by relieving them from function, as the exclusion of light and attention to rest do to the inflamed eye and joint. It does good to the *healthy* cells by relieving them of part of that excess of function which they had been required to assume. But the only way in which the loss of blood can be of use to the *affected* cells is by lessening the inflammation, in the way in which other inflammations are lessened by the same means. The benefit thus gained is augmented, not by the *repose* of these cells, but by the *resumption of function* on their part setting the blood in their pulmonary capillaries again in motion.

Local blood-letting. — Though there has been more scope for the use of local than general blood-letting in these cases, still the application of this means has also been limited in degree: not so much as regards the proportion of instances as the extent to which it was considered expedient to carry it.

In twenty-one of the cases cupping was used; in thirty-six, leeches were applied. We have, then, an aggregate of fifty-seven cases in which local blood-letting was practised: of these forty-six recovered.

The total admissions within the fifth day from the commencement of illness were twenty-two. Of these twenty recovered; and in all of them local blood-letting formed part of the treatment.

Between the sixth and tenth days there were thirty-four admissions. Of these, twenty-six recovered: local blood-letting was used in eighteen of them.

But if we confine our attention to primary pneumonia, this latter statement gives too favourable an estimate of the success of treatment. Of the twenty-six recoveries between the six and tenth days, eight were of febrile pneumonia; and I have already observed, that though the fever had been of that duration on admission, the pneumonia was probably of more recent origin.

* "Clinique Médicale," vol. ii. p. 378.

† "Lectures on the Principles and Practice of Physic," vol. ii. p. 91, 3rd edition.

From these data, then, we are justified in concluding that when pneumonia is seen within five days, or a little over it, even in the classes to which the inmates of this hospital belong, local blood-letting to some extent is an appropriate and efficacious remedy.

Of the forty-six recovered cases in which local blood-letting was used, there remain eight admitted above the tenth day of illness.

Of the eleven fatal cases in which there had been local blood-letting, three were admitted between the sixth and tenth day, and eight above the tenth day, dating from the commencement of illness.

It appears, that of forty-seven cases of pneumonia admitted after the tenth day, local blood-letting was had recourse to in sixteen. Of these forty-seven cases, twenty-five recovered, and local blood-letting had been used in eight of them. We find, then, that for pneumonia admitted after the tenth day, the scope for local blood-letting is very limited; for even in those for whom at the time it seemed admissible, there were as many deaths as recoveries.

The principles which have been observed in directing local blood-letting have been the symptoms and signs of pneumonia existing with that condition of pulse and skin which, on general therapeutic principles, justifies the use of this means.

To those, who, by clinical experience, have yet to become familiar with the varying conditions of the pulse and their indications, it may be said that in the natives of India, generally, we are not likely to meet with the state of pulse and skin which indicates local blood-letting, co-existing with a primary pneumonia of upwards of ten days' duration.

Tartar emetic. — We have found that in these cases there was little opportunity of practising general blood-letting. There has been also, and for the same reasons, little opportunity of giving tartar emetic in free doses. I am, however, from former experience, perfectly sensible of its efficacy in suitable cases.

This remedy, however, has been used to some extent * in sixty-six of the cases: of these, forty-nine were recoveries, and seventeen proved fatal.

Thirty-three of the recoveries were admitted under ten days' illness, and in twenty-four of them local blood-letting had also been used. Sixteen were admitted above ten days' illness: in five of

* From a sixth to half a grain every second, third, or fourth hour.

these tartar emetic was given alone, and in eleven it was combined with quinine.

It may be inferred then, from these statements, that in many of the recovered cases for which local blood-letting was considered appropriate, the moderate use of tartar emetic was also held to be indicated, and that it assisted the cure. That in some, in which local blood-letting was had recourse to, tartar emetic was omitted, either in consequence of co-existing gastro-enteric irritation, or from the treatment with mercury having been preferred. Further, that in some cases, for which local blood-letting was not considered appropriate, tartar emetic was used, generally in combination with quinine, on a principle to be subsequently explained.

The principles which have been stated relative to local blood-letting, may be also applied to this moderate use of tartar emetic, viz., that those states of pulse and skin and symptoms, which indicate the propriety of local blood-letting, justify the use of tartar emetic, provided it be not contra-indicated by the presence of an irritable state of the gastro-intestinal lining. But we may probably go further than this, and say that, if we are careful to guard against the tartar emetic causing increased evacuation from the bowels, we may use it in instances of pneumonia with febrile disturbance, in which the small volume and compressibility of the pulse are such as to contra-indicate local blood-letting or other evacuation. We may act thus because, by this cautious use of tartar emetic, we are not adding directly to the asthenia; and if by its use we can reduce the degree of febrile disturbance, we thereby certainly lessen an influence which tends rapidly to induce asthenia.

Mercury. — Calomel and opium were given with the view of inducing mercurial influence, in twenty-one cases. Of these, twenty were of the primary form, and the following remarks have exclusive reference to them.

Fourteen were recoveries, six proved fatal. The constitutional effect of mercury was produced in eleven of the recovered cases, and in two of the fatal ones. In the remaining seven it was necessary to omit the remedy, from some cause or other adverse to its continuance. The cases in which mercury was used were in the second stage of the disease. In the fourteen recovered cases, seven were admitted within five days from the commencement of illness, five between the sixth and tenth day, and two after the tenth day.

Of the eleven recovered cases in which mercurial influence was induced, there was complete restoration of the lung in seven; but in four only improvement. Of the seven restored cases, four were admitted within five days, and three between the sixth and tenth day. Of the four improved cases, two were admitted within five days, and two above that period.

Let us now take eight of the cases in which mercury was used, and regard them from another point of view. In three the commencement of improvement in the lung was coincident with the tenderness and swelling of the gums. In three the improvement of the lung distinctly took precedence of the usual indications of mercurial action. In two there was no improvement.

Let us now follow the six fatal cases in which mercury was given. The two, in which mercurial influence was induced, had been ill for upwards of twenty days before admission: in one of them dysenteric symptoms with hectic fever came on, and in the other, hepatitis ending in abscess. Of the four other fatal cases in which it was necessary to discontinue the mercury, three were admitted between the sixth and tenth day, and one within five days.

Let us now address ourselves to the question, whether this series of cases affords evidence favourable to the mercurial treatment of pneumonia.

Of the seventy-one cases discharged from hospital, the lung was restored in forty-nine, and improved in fifteen. Of the restored cases seven had been brought under the influence of mercury, and forty-two had been cured without it; and of these latter cases thirty-seven had been admitted in the second stage. Of the improved cases, in eleven the improvement was effected without mercury; they were all in the second stage.

It may, however, be objected to this statement that the febrile cases have been included, while, with one exception, mercury was only used in the primary form.

Let us exclude, therefore, from the discharged cases admitted in the second stage those that were of the febrile form, and there will remain twenty-five cases of restored primary pneumonia, with eighteen of them cured without mercury; and of improved cases thirteen, with nine of them without mercury. Further, let us recollect that, of the seven cured cases in which mercurial influence had been induced, in three the improvement in the lung commenced before the usual evidence of the action of mercury had appeared; it may, therefore, be argued that the improvement was independent of this remedy.*

From a careful consideration of these facts, it must be acknowledged that in these cases there is little evidence of the therapeutic value of mercury in the treatment of pneumonia. But because we have found little proof, in a particular field of practice, of the advantage of this agent, it by no means follows that it may not be expedient and useful under some circumstances of the disease. These cases have borne no testimony to the efficacy of general blood-letting, or the free use of tartar emetic, but the utility of these means in suitable instances has not on this account been called in question. Nor may we doubt the advantages to be derived from mercury when the conditions are appropriate for its use. It is most important that we should endeavour to determine the states of pneumonia in which mercury is likely to be beneficial, in order that we may have recourse to it only in these, and abstain from it in those for which it is unsuitable and injurious.

For the treatment of *sthenic* pneumonia in its first stage, or as it begins to pass into the second, general blood-letting and the free use of tartar emetic are, I apprehend, the appropriate remedies, because we are almost certain, under such circumstances, of finding the full and firm pulse, and the increased heat of skin, which indicate the propriety of these measures. But when the disease has gone on, and passed into the second stage, or has come under treatment at this period, then, in addition to the degree of local blood-letting and of tartar emetic indicated by the state of the pulse and skin, we should give calomel and opium in such manner as shall most safely effect a gentle mercurial influence. But when the failing volume and strength of pulse, and reduction of the temperature of the skin, indicate a deficiency of blood, and a feebly acting heart, then, whether this state be consequent on long duration of the disease, or on too antiphlogistic treatment in a constitution originally sthenic, or co-exist with the earlier stages of the disease in a constitution originally asthenic, we must abstain from the use of mercury, because in this condition of the blood, and of the heart, it will increase the exhaustion: instead of favouring the removal of lymph-

* This argument has been generally used, but its force may be doubted. There is nothing unreasonable in assuming that the mercury may have influence on the blood and the diseased action which it is intended to remedy before it has been carried to the degree of causing tender and swollen gums.

deposits, mercury will favour their degeneration into pus or sero-pus.

If I were asked to state a rule on this point of practice which might be applied to clinical purposes, I should be disposed to say that calomel and opium should only be given in the second stage of pneumonia, *in addition to* tartar emetic; but that when the pulse and skin contra-indicate the use of tartar emetic, mercury is also contra-indicated. In sthenic pneumonia it will be found, that after the tenth or twelfth day this remedy will no longer be appropriate; while, for the asthenic form, it is altogether unsuitable. It not only increases the asthenia, and favours softening or gangrene of the indurated lung, but the calomel and opium are very apt to cause irritation of the intestinal mucous lining, and lead to dysentery or diarrhœa: this is a most unfortunate complication of asthenic pneumonia, and ought most carefully to be guarded against. The result in several of the fatal cases of this series was hastened by exhausting diarrhœa.

For the treatment of the second stage of the *febrile* form, mercurial action is most inexpedient. We have, as I shall presently show, a more powerful agent in the sulphate of quinine.

Blisters.—Blisters have been used in eighty-two cases; of these fifty-two recovered. It appears, then, that this remedy has been had recourse to in a greater number of cases than any other of the means which have been noticed. This has occurred, because blisters are applicable to a greater variety of circumstances,—to the more advanced stages of those cases in which local blood-letting and antimony have been used, as well as to those for which these means have been considered inappropriate.

This greater experience of the use of blisters might seem to justify a positive opinion on their therapeutic value; but such is not the case. It is difficult to come to a satisfactory conclusion on this point of practice. They are used in those more advanced stages of disease in which we cannot look for marked and speedy improvement from any remedies, and in which we must be satisfied with steady, progressive, though slow amendment. When the stage of pneumonia suitable for local blood-letting has passed, blisters may be had recourse to with some prospect of advantage. If applied too early in the disease, they are apt to re-excite febrile disturbance and to be injurious. If used in very asthenic states, they are sometimes followed by troublesome ulceration, and the continued irritation thus arising does harm, by increasing the asthenia. For these reasons, then, we must be cautious. The blisters in these cases have never been larger than four inches square. The liquor lyttæ has been the preparation generally selected.*

Quinine.—The sulphate of quinine has been given in fifty-six cases: of these thirty-seven were primary and nineteen febrile; of the former twenty-seven were recoveries, of the latter fifteen.

In the treatment of *febrile* pneumonia, in addition to the local blood-letting, tartar emetic and blisters, which the symptoms may justify, quinine should be given in adequate doses *during the remission.* It may be combined with tartar emetic. From five to eight grains of quinine, with from one-sixth to one-fourth of a grain of tartar emetic, given at intervals of two or three hours for five or six doses, will, in general, suffice to check and then stop the febrile recurrences. When this effect on the febrile symptoms has been produced, it will generally be found that improvement in the pneumonia will at once commence; and in a large majority of cases, if the recurrence of the febrile state be prevented for some days, the inflammation of the lung will be speedily removed. That this is a therapeutic fact I am satisfied from the observation of many cases. Indeed, I am not acquainted with anything more striking and satisfactory in the whole range of rational therapeutics than the progressive but speedy restoration of a hepatised lung, co-existing with fever of remittent type, *when the exacerbations have been controlled by the adequate use of quinine.* It is true that small local detractions of blood, the application of small blisters, and the use of quarter-grain doses of tartar emetic, have been generally used at the same time; but it is quite impossible for any one familiar with disease, and the action of these means in these degrees, to attribute the benefit chiefly to them, and not to the prevention of the febrile exacerbation by the quinine. But this is merely another illustration of a therapeutic principle already explained, and inculcated in the chapters on intermittent and remittent fever.

The same principle of treatment has been also applied to many of the cases of *primary* pneumonia in asthenic subjects.

In my remarks on "Symptoms," I stated that the symptomatic fever of primary pneumonia in asthenic natives is not unfrequently

* Though confining my observations to blisters, I by no means undervalue other derivants, as turpentine, sinapisms, dry cupping, and water compresses. The last application may be used with advantage in all stages.

distinctly remittent in type, and it seemed to me reasonable to assume that it became so in consequence of the operative influence of malaria. Actuated by these views I have latterly, in all cases in which the remission was well marked, given quinine in combination with antimony, in the same manner as in the febrile cases, and very frequently with the same good effect; though I think that the improvement in the lung has taken place more slowly. It is nevertheless true, that in some of the cases in which even the remission has been well marked, we have met with disappointment; the quinine failed to control the exacerbation. When this occurs the remedy must be omitted, and the other usual means appropriate for the case be trusted to.

Liquor potassæ.—Some years since my attention was called to the use of liquor potassæ as a deobstruent remedy in the second stage of pneumonia.* It has been used by me in many cases for which mercury was considered unsuitable. It was given in doses of from half a drachm to one drachm and a half every third or fourth hour in ten of the recovered cases of this series, and was in general continued for several days. In some the proportion of liquor potassæ was diminished, and from six to ten grains of sesquicarbonate of ammonia were added, when the state of the pulse indicated the propriety of a stimulant. The general impression left on my mind was favourable to the use of liquor potassæ; but this impression has not been confirmed by a careful consideration, not only of this series of cases but also of all other hospital cases in which it had been used. I can only find two, and they are not satisfactory, in which quinine on the principle just explained was not at the same time given. Being already satisfied of the therapeutic value of quinine in appropriate cases, I cannot feel sure of that of the liquor potassæ, when the two remedies have been given at the same time. Further careful clinical observation is therefore necessary to satisfy me of the deobstruent efficacy of liquor potassæ in the second stage of pneumonia. The same remark may be made of the internal use of iodide of potassium, and the external application of the compound iodine ointment. I have had recourse to both on several occasions, but am unable as yet to offer any opinion on their utility.

Stimulants.—There often comes a period in the treatment of pneumonia, and it may arrive very early in the asthenic form,

* I much regret that I am unable to refer to the publication in which the liquor potassæ was recommended. I omitted to make a note at the time, and I have been unsuccessful in my search for it. It was in one of the periodicals.

when the failing pulse, the lowered temperature of the skin, and the feeble expectorating efforts indicate the necessity for stimulants. The earliest tendency to this must be watched for, and stimulants be freely and assiduously given. The sesquicarbonate of ammonia with tincture of squills, wine, and arrack, are the most useful. At the same time chicken broth or beef tea must be frequently administered; and sinapisms or warm turpentine applied to the chest. By these means, if adopted in good time, cases which appeared hopeless have been occasionally saved, more especially in youthful subjects.

Concluding Remarks.—In the review of these cases it has been found that a large proportion of them came under treatment in the second stage of pneumonia, and that when the disease was confined to part of one lung, the rate of mortality was 17 per cent. I am not acquainted with other recorded data exactly similar with which to compare these results. But the impression on my mind previous to my service in the Jamsetjee Jejeebhoy Hospital had always been that pneumonia in the second stage was a more fatal disease.

If, on the whole, success has attended the management of these cases, it is very expedient to endeavour to explain all the principles in accordance with which it has been directed. In a previous part of these remarks I have stated, that in many of the cases a considerable time was required for the restoration of the lung; and that in many the cessation of the febrile symptoms and the relief of cough and dyspnœa, were not at once followed by lessening of the signs of consolidation of the lung, but that several days elapsed before this began to appear. The efficacy of local blood-letting, of tartar emetic, of occasional mercurial influence, of blisters, and of quinine, has been acknowledged, and an endeavour has been made to explain the principles on which these remedies have been respectively used. But we do not find in these principles anything that provides for the management of that period in the course of the disease when there is persisting consolidation of the lung, with little or no febrile disturbance, and little or no cough or dyspnœa, yet I am satisfied that it has been on the proper treatment of this condition of the disease that the successful issue of many of these cases has depended. If so, then, it is necessary that I should explain what the nature of this treatment has been, and the principles on which it has been conducted. In this state of the disease, the pulse will be found to be of small volume, and easily compressed

This character of the pulse, with absence of febrile * disturbance, at once indicates the appropriate method of cure. Antiphlogistics of every kind, especially mercury, should be abstained from; and the tonic regimen and remedies best fitted gradually to increase the quantity of blood, improve its condition, and strengthen the action of the heart should be used. A light nutritious diet with suitable stimulants, pure air, nitric acid, quinine, and preparations of iron, are the means most suitable.

That at different periods in the history of medicine there have been great errors in practice, is a truth which, with a view to future improvement, we are bound to keep steadily before us; and perhaps no better illustration can be found than the wavering principles which have characterised the practice of medicine during the last twenty years and more. Those of us who were familiar with practice at the commencement of this period must have witnessed the destructive freedom with which antiphlogistic remedies were not unfrequently applied; and must be sensible that there then was a very general disregard of tonic means.

When, on the other hand, we turn our attention to the present state of practical medicine, we may discern a tendency to commit the opposite error — to neglect antiphlogistic remedies and to misapply tonics and stimulants; to lose sight of great leading principles, and to act too much under the guidance of a fragmentary, and as yet very imperfect, knowledge of animal chemistry.

If this be true, it is peculiarly the province of those who have practised during this period of vacillation and uncertainty, — who have witnessed the advantages of the judicious use, and the evils of the abuse, of antiphlogistics and tonics, — to endeavour to hold the balance true between these two leading therapeutic principles, by stating the impressions which these varied opportunities may have left upon the mind.

Considerations of this nature induce me to explain, more fully than may seem necessary, my reasons for attaching so much importance, in certain states of pneumonia, to the decided intermission of antiphlogistic, and the substitution of tonic treatment. The principles which I am about to state are applicable, more or less, to all inflammations.

It may be confidently affirmed, that when a tissue is inflamed, a

* I have not thought it necessary to notice those cases in which, with continuance of consolidated lung, we have hectic fever coming on, not cessation of the febrile disturbance. Such cases must be managed on the ordinary principles observed in the treatment of structural disease and co-existing hectic fever.

leading aim in its cure is the maintenance of a normal state of the capillary circulation in the structures around. It matters not whether the restoration is to consist merely in stagnating blood being again set in motion, or in serous or lymph effusions being absorbed, or in the organisation of lymph, or in the change of lymph into pus with organisation of a bounding sac and processes for the evacuation of the pus and the after reparation of the abscess, or in the granulation and cicatrisation of ulcers. Whichever of these actions must be gone through before the inflamed structure can resume its state of integrity, it should be a main object in the management of all to bring about and maintain a normal quantity, quality, and rate of movement of the blood in the capillaries around and in the general vascular system. If there be symptomatic fever, with a pulse full, firm, and frequent,—the quantity, quality, and rate of movement, of the blood in the capillary system are abnormal, and our means of correcting this derangement are blood-letting and other antiphlogistic remedies. But when the pulse becomes soft and of moderate volume, improvement in the inflammation by general antiphlogistic treatment will cease, for under its use the pulse will become small and compressible, indicating a quantity, quality, and rate of movement of the blood in the capillaries around the inflamed part and in the system generally, as adverse to restoration, by whatever processes it is to be effected, as the opposite conditions of sthenic symptomatic fever: under these circumstances of inflammation we cannot hope to do good, unless our regimen and remedies be decidedly tonic.

These may seem very narrow principles, yet they are very useful in practice. They may seem trite and simple, yet they are often lost sight of under the seductive influence of transcendental theories, inapplicable in the present state of the science. But, after all, they reach further than at first may appear.

In the state of pneumonia to which reference is now being made, mercury is an injurious deobstruent, for it spoils the quality and lessens the quantity of the blood. But it is probable enough that a deobstruent may yet be discovered free from this defect, and therefore applicable to the treatment of this kind of consolidation of the lung; still a tonic influence on the blood, and on the heart, must be a leading indication of cure, for unless there be an adequate capillary circulation immediately around the deposits, there can be no absorption from the influence of any deobstruent. Again, the idea that many inflammations are dependent on a *materies morbi* in the blood is gaining ground as a pathological theory—very probably a true one; if so, its elimination by the excreting organs may become a chief object in the treatment. Still the maintenance of a normal state of the capillary circulation by antiphlogistics or tonics, as the case may be, must always be a leading aim, for without it we can have no adequate action of the excreting organs, and consequently no sufficient elimination from the blood. It would be easy to multiply illustrations in proof, that whatever *special* therapeutic indications may in after times arise in the treatment of particular forms of disease, based on physiological or chemical facts as yet undiscovered, there must always be the *over-ruling* principle of maintaining, as far as practicable, a normal condition of the blood and a sufficient capillary circulation general and local. This we must endeavour to effect, in some forms of disease by antiphlogistics, in others by tonics; the state of the pulse, and of the general system, determine the question.

SECTION VI.—*Statistics of Pneumonia.*

TABLE XXXV.—*Admissions and Deaths, with Per-centage, from Pneumonia, in the Jamsetjee Jejeebhoy Hospital at Bombay, for the Six Years from* 1848 *to* 1853.

	1848 to 1853.		Monthly Average.		
	Admissions.	Deaths.	Deaths on Admissions.	Admissions on total Admissions.	Deaths on total Deaths.
January . .	30	12	40·0	1·4	2·7
February . .	39	10	25·6	2·1	3·1
March . . .	32	17	53·1	1·5	4·4
April . . .	21	8	38·1	0·9	2·4
May . . .	27	14	51·9	1·2	4·8
June . . .	23	6	26·1	1·1	1·9
July . . .	9	5	55·5	0·4	1·6
August . . .	18	7	38·9	0·9	2·1
September . .	21	8	38·1	1·01	2·5
October . .	29	15	51·8	1·3	4·4
November . .	31	4	12·8	1·4	1·2
December . .	33	15	45·5	1·4	3·8
Total . .	313	121	38·6	1·2	2·9

CHAP. XXII.

ON PLEURITIS, BRONCHITIS, AND ASTHMA.

SECTION I. *Pleuritis.—Symptoms, Causes, Pathology, Treatment.*

INFLAMMATION of the pleura is more common than that of the substance of the lung, because pneumonia seldom occurs without co-existing pleuritis, and simple pleuritis is not an unfrequent disease.

The admissions of pleuritis in the European General Hospital for the ten years, from 1844 to 1853, amounted to sixty-eight, with one death, whereas those of pneumonia did not exceed twenty-two, with two deaths. The admissions of pleuritis into the Jamsetjee Jejeebhoy Hospital during the six years, from 1848 to 1853, were sixty-one, with nineteen deaths, a mortality of 31·2 per cent. The cases treated by me in the clinical ward during the same period, numbered twenty-five, and the deaths seven. The admissions of pneumonia into the hospital and the clinical ward, during the same period, were respectively 313 and 103. These data would suggest that, in Europeans in India, pleuritis is more common than pleuro-pneumonia, but that in natives the converse obtains: they are, however, too limited to justify a general inference of this kind.

The following brief observations have reference to the twenty-five cases which formed a subject of study in the clinical ward. They are arranged under the heads, Symptoms, Causes, Pathology, and Treatment.

Symptoms.—In cases admitted after the occurrence of pleuritic effusion *pain* was not usually complained of; but inquiry into the history generally led to the conclusion that this symptom had been present at the commencement of the attack. Impaired respiratory movement of the affected side was noticed in all.

A distinct *friction murmur* was observed in ten cases. Its most common situation was about the inferior angle of the scapula, or in the lateral region. In eight the murmur was primary: I do not mean that it occurred in that early stage which precedes effusion, but that from the period of the disease and the degree of co-existing dulness, it was judged not to be a redux friction murmur. The redux murmur was noted in three cases: in two it had not been present on admission, but had appeared as the lessening dulness indicated absorption of the liquid effusion; in the third, the murmur was primary on admission, disappeared with increasing effusion, but again reappeared in association with increasing absorption. *Œgophony* was recorded in only one case of pleuritis consequent on fracture of a rib. *Bronchial respiration* was noticed in relation to the degree of effusion. *Dulness on percussion* — more or less extensive, more or less complete — was observed in every case. In some the shifting character was present, in others it was absent. Defective vocal thrill generally co-existed with the dulness.

In cases in which the effusion was considerable, the size of the affected side was notably increased. In two of this class the absorption of the fluid was followed by distinct contraction. In the cases in which the effusion was in the left side — displacement of the heart, in those of the right side — displacement of the liver was noticed.

Causes. — Cold was doubtless the ordinary exciting cause. In some, however, the affection was attributed to blows received in squabbles, and in two to a strain while working. In two the inflammation had probably depended on peculiarity of diathesis; in one who had suffered from syphilitic rheumatism, all the characteristic physical signs were present, and recovery took place; in the other, cachectic from intermittent fever and long the subject of diarrhœa, the bowel complaint was checked, pleuritis of the left side with effusion, dulness, absence of vocal thrill, and displacement of the heart, took place, and was removed on recurrence of the diarrhœa, but death resulted from exhaustion.

Pathology. — These cases show that when the constitution is good, and the management careful, recovery may be expected even though the physical signs have proved the existence, for several successive days, of considerable effusion. The left side was affected in fourteen cases, and the right in eleven. In none was it distinctly double. The seven fatal cases, with one exception already noticed, occurred in asthenic individuals, admitted in advanced stages of effusion. In four a communication existed between the effusion and the lung, as was proved in three by examination after death; in one by several small openings, in another by a large opening into a gangrenous excavation, and in the third by direct communication with the left bronchus. In this last case there was also perforation by ulceration of the second, fourth, and sixth intercostal spaces, with a fluctuating swelling in these situations, and partial absorption of the costal cartilages. In that case, which communicated with the gangrenous excavation, there was a second collection, the size of a cocoa-nut, circumscribed between the base of the left lung and the diaphragm. In the fourth case there was no inspection after death; but the character of the sputa, the tympanitic resonance on percussion, and the amphoric respiration, had left no doubt that communication existed between the lung and the pleural sac.

I have seen two cases of recovery by discharge of the contents of a circumscribed pleuritic effusion through the lung. One, a Hindoo lad, in whom, while under treatment for adynamic remittent fever, pneumonia of the lower part of the left lung, as indicated by crepitus and bronchial respiration, took place. This was followed by circumscribed effusi o of the upper part of the left side, proved by great dulness and absence of breath-sounds, then, by perforation of the lung, shown by the sputa, the tympanitic resonance in the previously dull regions, and the presence of amphoric respiration. There was gradual and slow restoration to health, with permanent dulness of the upper part of the left side, very imperfect breath-sounds there, but no cognisable difference in the appearance of the two sides. The second case was of a young European female, of tubercular diathesis, who, after obscure pectoral symptoms, suddenly expectorated a large quantity of fetid pus. At this stage of the affection I saw this patient. There were no signs of consolidation, or cavities, of the upper part of either lung. About the inferior angle of the left scapula, passing into the lateral region, there was defective sound on percussion for a limited space, and no breath-sounds. I concluded, not that tubercular excavations existed in the lungs, but that a circumscribed pleuritic effusion had opened into the lung. The opinion given, that gradual restoration to tolerable health would take place, was verified. The expectoration gradually ceased; and when next I saw this patient, several years afterwards, there had been absence of pulmonic disturbance for a long period.

The few cases which have formed the subject of these remarks, suffice to prove that pleuritic effusion is not unfrequently circumscribed, and that a considerable extent of pulmonary surface — generally its anterior part — may become adherent to the costal pleura. The facts are important because they serve to qualify the import, in diagnosis, of the situation and shifting nature of the dulness, and the character of the breath-sounds.

Further, there are two cases before me in which the circumscribed effusion existed between the anterior wall of the chest and the anterior surface of the lung, and extended into the infra-clavicular region, causing dulness and leading to the erroneous diagnosis of tubercular phthisis.

Treatment.—The principles of treatment in pneumonia are also applicable to pleuritis. Local blood-letting, small blisters, and tartar emetic were the antiphlogistic remedies used in those cases. Mercurial influence was induced in only one, but without benefit, for the dulness continued when the patient was discharged. In cases in which, from the state of constitution and the duration of disease, it is reasonable to conclude that the existing effusion is serous and removable, it must always be remembered that absorption is improbable before time has been allowed for the circulation in the capillaries of the pleura to return to a normal state, and for the exudations to become organised into areolar tissue. Whilst waiting with this view, small blisters or other mild derivants may be applied to the affected side. The further general treatment, whether antiphlogistic, expectant, or tonic, will depend upon the state of constitution, as explained in my remarks on the treatment of pneumonia. But at this stage diuretic remedies also may be used with advantage. In several of the cases now under review, the decrease of the effusion, consecutive on an increased flow of urine by diuretics, was well marked. Acetate of potass, nitrous ether, and tincture of squills, were the remedies used. In cases in which, from diathesis, duration of the disease, extent of effusion, and hectic symptoms, empyema has become probable, the general treatment must be regulated in accordance with the principles applicable to a similar condition of the system, however induced.

A special practical question arises in the treatment of pleuritis, viz., whether the effused fluid should be removed by paracentesis or not. On this point I am without experience. Dr. Barlow, in his instructive "Manual of the Practice of Medicine," thus remarks on this question of practice: — "In short, the objections to the operation may be thus summed up: where it is safe and likely to be successful, it is unnecessary, but where it seems to be called for by the permanence of the effusion, it is more dangerous and generally unsuccessful." In estimating this opinion, it should be borne in mind that it is grounded on experience in a field— Guy's Hospital,—in which this operation has been practised on an extensive scale. Dr. Barlow is careful to enjoin, that when the operation is considered expedient, it should be performed in the manner recommended by Dr. Hughes and Mr. Edward Cock, and to which I have already referred in my remarks on the puncture of hepatic abscess.*

SECTION II. — *Bronchitis.* — *Asthma.*

Bronchitis.—The admissions from bronchitis into the European General Hospital at Bombay during the ten years, from 1844 to 1853, have amounted to 223, and the deaths to fourteen, which gives a mortality of 6·2 per cent. on the admissions, and shows that the proportion of cases of this disease to the total sick treated in the hospital has been, for this period, 1·77 per cent.

The number of sick from bronchitis in the Jamsetjee Jejeebhoy Hospital for the six years, from 1848 to 1853, has been more than double that from pneumonia. The admissions amounted to 707, and the deaths to 57, a mortality of 8·07 per cent. The ratio of cases of bronchitis to total hospital sick, has been 2·7 per cent.

On instituting, in respect to bronchitis, the comparison, previously made regarding pneumonia, of the relative portion of admissions at different periods of the year, it will be found that there has been a great uniformity throughout the year. For example: the admissions, from December to May, were 366, and the deaths 29; those from June to November, were 341 and 28. The probable inference from this statement is, that the rainy season, included in the second half year, is as efficient an exciting cause of bronchitis as the cold months of the first half year.†

* Page 410.

† For seventeen years, from 1837 to 1853, the "thoracic inflammations," doubtless chiefly bronchitis, in the Byculla Schools, amounted to 518 with two deaths. For the half year from December to May, the admissions were 227; from June to November, 291; but the greatest number in one month was in May, 85,—whereas, the number in January was 21. I am unable to offer any explanation of the excess in May. It has, however, not been uniform, because 48 of the 85, were in the Mays of 1840, 1844 and 1853, and none in 1841, 1847 and 1852.

It is unnecessary to enter into questions of practical detail relative to a disease so well understood. It is sufficient that the practitioner applies to bronchitis in India the lessons of watchfulness and care, more especially in regard to young children, which have been inculcated by European writers.

Asthma.—The term asthma has been used in its common acceptation, to signify that pathological state compounded of varying proportions of bronchitis, emphysema, and bronchial spasm. It is sufficiently common in natives of India, more particularly in the cold and wet seasons of the year. I have already * expressed my belief that this disease is occasionally related to malaria as a cause, and is then most successfully treated with quinine and preparations of iron; and above all by a prolonged residence in a non-malarious climate of suitable temperature.

Vesicular emphysema of the lungs is often present in great degree, and is indicated by the well-known physical signs, of altered form of the chest, increased resonance on percussion, faint vesicular respiration with rhonchi, prolonged expiratory acts, displacement of the heart and liver, accompanied with general anæmia.

Section III.—*Statistics of Bronchitis.*

Table XXXVI.—*Admissions and Deaths, with Per-centage, from Bronchitis, in the Jamsetjee Jejeebhoy Hospital at Bombay, for the Six Years from* 1848 *to* 1853.

	1848 to 1853.		Monthly Average.		
	Admissions.	Deaths.	Deaths on Admissions.	Admissions on total Admissions.	Death on total Deaths.
January	66	5	7·6	3·1	1·1
February	55	3	5·4	2·9	0·9
March	68	5	7·4	3·1	1·3
April	55	5	9·1	2·6	1·4
May	69	6	8·7	3·1	2·1
June	49	5	10·2	2·3	1·6
July	51	4	7·9	2·5	1·3
August	43	2	4·6	2·2	0·6
September	66	4	6·1	3·2	1·3
October	60	4	6·6	2·6	1·2
November	72	9	12·5	3·3	2·7
December	53	5	0·9	2·3	1·3
Total	707	57	8·07	2·7	1·4

* Page 55.

CHAP. XXIII.

ON PHTHISIS PULMONALIS.

SECTION I.—*Causes, Symptoms, Pathology, and Treatment.*

IN stating the result of my investigations, I shall keep in view the researches of Louis, and other European writers on this disease.

During fifteen years, from 1838 to 1853, the admissions of phthisis into the European General Hospital at Bombay, amounted to 184, and the deaths to 79, a ratio of 0·93 per cent. on the total hospital admissions, and 6·1 per cent. on the aggregate deaths.

The admissions of natives with phthisis into the Jamsetjee Jejeebhoy Hospital, during the six years from 1848 to 1853, have amounted to 445, and the deaths to 268, a ratio of 1·7 per cent. on the total hospital admissions, and 6·5 per cent. on the total deaths. But this statement does not fully represent the proportion of phthisical disease in the inmates of this hospital. The remark made at page 465, relative to the admissions registered under the title "Cachexia" is applicable to phthisis pulmonalis, equally as to Bright's disease. Seventy-nine cases of phthisis have been treated in the clinical ward during these six years. Of these forty-two proved fatal, and inspection after death was made in thirty-one.

I have also before me the reports of seventeen fatal cases, noted during my service in the European General Hospital, and already published.* In my notes of 311 fatal cases of European officers in the Bombay Presidency, phthisis was the cause of death in eight.

I shall arrange the brief observations which these data suggest under the heads: — 1. Causes. 2. Symptoms. 3. Pathology. 4. Treatment.

Causes.—The erroneous opinion, at one time, entertained of the rarity of phthisis pulmonalis in tropical countries, has been long

* "Transactions, Medical and Physical Society of Bombay," Nos. 2 and 6.

since corrected by the medical statistical reports of the British army, and information from other sources. I have witnessed the disease in Europeans, Indo-Britons, and in many of the Asiatic races. Whether the access of phthisis is usually postponed to a later period of life in warm climates, is a question which existing data are insufficient to solve. Of nine European seamen who died in the European General Hospital, seven were upwards of thirty years of age, and one of them had attained the age of fifty-two. Two European pensioners also died at the ages of fifty-three and forty-nine. In respect to the eight fatal cases of officers; in three the age was above thirty, in one it was twenty-three, in another seventeen, and in three it is not recorded. The ages of seventy-eight of the clinical cases of natives have been given; four were below twenty years of age, fifty-eight between twenty and forty, fifteen between forty and sixty, and one upwards of sixty.

These facts probably tend to indicate a later development of the disease in India than in European countries; but they are too limited to suggest more than the expediency of further inquiry.

The admissions of phthisis into both hospitals have been pretty equally distributed throughout the different months of the year, with, however, a slight excess in favour of the half year from June to November. For example, the admissions into the European General Hospital and the Jamsetjee Jejeebhoy Hospital, for the half year from December to May, were respectively 82 and 218; whereas, for the half year from June to November, they were 102 and 227. The inference that the rainy season is unfavourable to the course of phthisis, which may be drawn from this statement, is confirmed by a remark made by Dr. R. H. Hunter relative to the effect, on the health of Her Majesty's 2nd Regiment, of change from Poona to Bombay, at the commencement of the monsoon of 1836. Dr. Hunter says "all the phthisical cases began rapidly to decline as the moist weather set in, and all proved fatal in the course of the monsoon." *

Whether malarious cachexia favours the development of tubercular disease, is a question of interest; and tropical countries necessarily afford the best field for its investigation. In seven of the seventy-nine clinical cases, attacks of intermittent fever were reported to have preceded the pulmonary symptoms, and in four others the febrile disturbance which co-existed with the phthisical symptoms was rather malarious than hectic in character. Still

* "Transactions of the Medical and Physical Society of Bombay," No. 1, p. 23.

these facts do not justify the supposition of a predisposition to tubercular disease from malarious influence: for in the classes who resort to hospitals in India, it is very likely that the admissions of any other form of disease would evince evidence of the taint. in a proportion quite as great. Nor does my experience in India afford any support to the opinion of Lancisi and others, that malaria is preventive of pulmonary phthisis.

The data before me relate exclusively to males, and, therefore do not show whether the greater prevalence of phthisis in females than in males, established in respect to European countries, obtains in India or not.

Symptoms.—The general symptoms and physical signs of phthisis in India do not present any peculiarities.* Hæmoptysis had been present before admission in seventeen of the clinical cases, and it was observed in three during the time they were under treatment. In one of them the hæmorrhage was considerable in quantity, and took place very shortly before death. A cavity with red-tinged walls was found at the apex of the right lung, and another the size of a walnut, filled with blood, existed at the upper part of the left lung. Hoarseness of voice was present in eighteen of the cases.

Pathology.—It has been supposed that phthisis runs a more rapid course in warm than in cold climates, after it has fairly commenced. My cases are not of a nature to throw any light on this question, for the record of the previous history is, in general, not sufficiently precise, and probably unworthy of being fully depended upon. Yet the general opinion may be safely hazarded, that in all diseases which include destructive degeneration of structure and co-existing hectic fever, the rapidity of the course will bear relation to the number and degree of the debilitating influences to which the individual is exposed. As in warm climates elevated temperature and malaria are causes of debility, additional to those existing in cold climates, it is a reasonable inference that, after tubercular softening has fairly commenced, a fatal issue is likely to follow sooner in a tropical than in a temperate climate. Moreover, as re-

* It has seemed to me that that the accuracy of diagnosis in cases, in which the ordinary symptoms of cough, expectoration and dyspnœa are not well marked, is sometimes prevented:—1. By an emphysematous state of the adjoining pulmonary tissues preventing dulness. 2. Many cavities, none sufficiently large or empty to give a tympanitic sound on percussion, may lessen dulness. 3. In cases of general anæmia, in which pulmonary expansion is diminished, there may be slight infra-clavicular dulness from defective expansion: this may suggest the suspicion of commencing tubercular deposit, but it will disappear with the removal of the anæmia.

spects phthisis pulmonalis, it should be remembered that the course of the disease is always very dependent on the early access and the extent of intestinal ulceration, and that this is a morbid state to which the residents in warm climates are particularly prone. On the other hand, however, it may be argued, that inasmuch as the rate of progress of tubercular phthisis may depend on intercurrent pneumonia or bronchitis excited by cold, the resident in warm climates has in this respect an advantage over the inhabitant of colder climates. This may be true of the well-clothed and cared-for European, but the argument has no application to the hospital-frequenting classes of the native community; they, from constitution, from insufficient clothing and habitations, are as much exposed to the injurious effects of cold and wet as the dwellers in more northern latitudes.

In fifty-two of the clinical cases, at the time of admission, the disease had passed on to the stage of softening; in twenty-four the tubercles were still in their solid state, and in three there was doubt.

With one exception, both lungs were affected in all; and of fifty-five of these, we have information as to the side in which the disease had made most progress. It was furthest advanced on the left side in thirty-six; on the right side in nineteen. The observation universally made by European writers, that the tubercular deposit commences in the upper lobes and travels downwards, is equally true of the disease in India. I would remark, however, that I have witnessed cases of transition, as it were, between tubercular deposit and grey induration, in which there seemed to be a blending of the position-character of pneumonia and phthisis: the acme of the disease was neither in the upper nor the lower part of the lung, but rather midway between. This observation is not unimportant as regards diagnosis, for we certainly meet in practice with cases in which the signs of excavation are distinct at the inferior angle of the scapula, without signs of consolidation in the upper part of the lung. Such are, probably, of the pathological character just adverted to.

In twenty-nine cases examined after death, in which the tubercles had softened, a single cavity was found only in two; in all the others the cavities were numerous, and in different stages.

The deposits of tubercle usually take place at many points; these increase in size by accretion, and aggregate into nodules. The same order of progress occurs in the process of softening:

commencing at points, increasing in size, and coalescing into excavations of various forms and dimensions. It is important to keep this fact before the mind, because it gives a significance to the early and undoubted signs of tubercular softening—I mean the variously sized but sharply defined moist ronchi. My cases exhibit that constant co-existence of pleuritic adhesion with fatal tubercular pulmonary disease, which has generally been noted by other observers. The adhesions have a distinct relation to the stage of the disease. They are not unfrequently absent in the miliary stage, but are invariably present when excavations have formed. They take place in accordance with that protective law, which has in view the prevention of the effusion of abnormal fluid collections into serous sacs. Pleuritic adhesions were observed in all my inspections after death.

The morbid appearances of pneumonia have been less frequently present. There was hepatisation in twelve cases, and sanguineous engorgement in six. The frequent absence of the signs of inflammation of the pulmonary tissue, affords conclusive evidence that the deposition of tubercular matter is not necessarily a result of inflammatory action. But, on the other hand, the not unfrequent occurrence of intercurrent pneumonia requires to be carefully borne in mind and regarded in treatment.

Louis found the larynx diseased in one fourth of his cases, and the epiglottis in one sixth. My observations in India show fully an equal proportion of this complication. In eighteen of seventy-nine there was hoarseness of voice. In thirty-one cases inspected after death, the larynx was ulcerated or abraded in nine, the epiglottis in six, and the trachea in 7.*

In fifteen cases, a turgid or ulcerated state of Peyer's glands, and in sixteen, circular ulcers in the large intestine, were found after death. In only one case was there reason for attributing the intestinal ulceration to tubercular deposit and softening. My researches, as already previously stated†, have not suggested to me that there is any difference between the morbid process which leads to the formation of circular ulcers in the large intestine in phthisis, and that which causes the same form of ulcer in dysentery, consecutive on hepatic abscess, or simple and primary.

Diarrhœa was absent in only five of the seventy-nine cases. Of these five, only one proved fatal; the tubercles were in a miliary

* I need hardly remark, that the morbid state of the different parts of the air tubes was not unfrequently noticed in the same case; and that these numbers (nine, seven, six) do not represent twenty-two instances of phthisis.

† Page 369 (foot note.)

state, and there was no intestinal ulceration; death had been caused by co-existing hepatisation of the lung and pleuritic effusion. The mesenteric glands were noted as tubercular in seven cases, but this probably does not represent the full proportion, because in many there is no record of the state of these structures, which gives rise to the impression, that they had occasionally been overlooked.

In two, miliary tubercles existed in the subperitoneal tissue. Case 195 is an additional instance of this morbid condition.

In one case perforation of the intestine took place. In two, the liver was found in a state of cirrhosis.

Fatty liver was observed by Louis in one third of his cases, but much more frequently in females than in males. This morbid state has not been found to co-exist with phthisis in the same proportion in England. It was noticed in only one of my thirty-one fatal clinical cases, but they were all males, and probably my attention has not been sufficiently fixed on this question of pathology. I attach no weight, then, to my observations on this point.

Bright's disease of the kidney has been noted in only one of the cases.

Treatment. — On this subject it is needless to enlarge. The principle now generally admitted,—that the indication for the prevention, cure, and stay of this disease, is the application of a well-arranged system of tonic regimen and remedies — must command the assent of every practical physician. Cod-liver oil has of late years been extensively used in phthisis in India as in other countries, and though the cases, which have formed the principal subject of my present remarks, were generally either admitted in a stage too advanced, or were too short a time under observation, to afford evidence of the efficacy of this remedy, still proof has not been wanting to me in other fields of practice. Though I am fully persuaded that the diathetic treatment of phthisis, as now generally pursued, is correct, still it is necessary to be careful, and to guard against its tendency to withdraw the attention from the occasional occurrence of intercurrent pneumonia, and the modification in treatment which this contingency necessarily enjoins.

Section II.—*Statistics of Phthisis Pulmonalis.*

Table XXXVII.—*Admissions and Deaths, with Per-centage, from Phthisis Pulmonalis, in the Jamsetjee Jejeebhoy Hospital at Bombay, for the Six Years from* 1848 *to* 1853.

	1848 to 1853.		Monthly Average.		
	Admissions.	Deaths.	Deaths on Admissions.	Admissions on total Admissions.	Deaths on total Deaths.
January . .	34	23	67·7	1·6	5·1
February . .	34	18	52·9	1·8	5·6
March . . .	41	18	43·9	1·9	4·7
April . . .	40	21	52·5	1·9	6·6
May . . .	36	23	63·9	1·6	8·0
June . . .	32	22	68·7	1·5	7·2
July . . .	39	26	66·6	1·9	8·5
August . . .	29	29	100·0	1·5	8·8
September . .	53	19	35·9	2·5	6·1
October . .	33	31	93·7	1·1	9·1
November . .	41	18	43·9	1·4	5·4
December . .	33	20	60·6	1·4	5·0
Total . .	445	268	60·1	1·7	6·5

CHAP. XXIV.

ON PERICARDITIS AND ENDOCARDITIS.

SECTION I.—*Introductory Remarks.*

IN this and the following chapter I shall describe affections of the heart and aorta, as observed by me in natives of India, and shortly allude to these diseases in Europeans.

Fifty-six cases have been received into the clinical ward of the Jamsetjee Jejeebhoy Hospital, during the six years from 1848 to 1853. I shall consider them under two heads. 1. Twenty-five cases of pericarditis and endocarditis, in the present chapter. 2. Thirty-one cases of structural disease of the heart and aorta, in the chapter which follows.

This inquiry will tend to correct the erroneous impression which has existed, that acute rheumatism in India is rarely associated with pericarditis or endocarditis. The relation of cardiac disease to previously existing rheumatism is apparent in twenty-nine of the fifty-six cases; and in all probability it would have been evident in a still greater number, had the record of all been equally complete.

When we compare the admissions under the head "Rheumatism" into our Indian hospitals with those which take place into hospitals in Europe, we may expect to find in the former a smaller proportion of affections of the heart. The explanation, however, is sufficiently simple. In the greater number of cases of rheumatism treated in hospitals in India, the disease is chronic; it is unattended with swelling of the joints or febrile disturbance, and occurs for the most part in persons cachectic from malaria, syphilis, scurvy, mercury, imperfect means of subsistence, &c. It is not, I need hardly observe, in association with *this* form of disease that pericarditis and endocarditis have been so frequently noticed in European countries.

It may be that *acute* articular rheumatism is not so common in

India * as in colder climates, yet it is by no means rare; and a complicating pericarditis or endocarditis is, I believe, as frequent an occurrence in the one country as in the other.

Of no rule in practice am I more thoroughly convinced than that it is as incumbent on the practitioner in India as in Europe, carefully to watch and search for the physical signs of pericarditis and endocarditis in every case of acute rheumatism. If this rule be neglected, the co-existence of these diseases in India will necessarily continue to be considered an unusual event.†

Section II.—*Causes, Symptoms, and Treatment.*

The important practical facts deducible from the twenty-five cases of pericarditis and endocarditis are arranged under the following heads:—

* This statement, written some years since in India, has been fully confirmed by recent opportunities of observing the great frequency of acute articular rheumatism in hospitals in London.

† In No. 11 of the "Indian Annals of Medical Science," for January 1859, there is a very interesting communication from Dr. Gordon, Surgeon of the 10th Regiment, on "Rheumatism and allied diseases." The author concurs with me in opinion that acute rheumatism is not so common in India as in colder climates, but dissents from my statement that pericarditis and endocarditis are as frequent a complication of acute rheumatism in the one country as the other. He justly explains the discrepancy between us, by observing, that my results had reference to the inmates of civil or general hospitals,—his, to regimental hospitals; for it is a great error to compare the statistics of communities so different as the inmates of civil, and military regimental hospitals. The greater proportion of men invalided for heart disease in the United Kingdom than in India, seems to me to prove, as is explained in the text, the comparative rarity of acute rheumatism in India, rather than the infrequency of pericarditis, as a complication, as Dr. Gordon supposes.

The subject of cardiac disease in Europeans will come under consideration in the concluding section of the next chapter, and I would only now remark that my opportunities of judging of its frequency in regimental hospitals, at different periods of my service, have not been few, and that many cases have come under my observation. Indeed the only case of acute endocarditis unconnected with rheumatism which I have ever witnessed, was in the hospital of the 12th Lancers, at Kirkee, in June 1857. The patient was admitted on the 16th with palpitation and uneasiness of the cardiac region, but no abnormal sounds were detected; and it so chanced that the day on which I examined him, towards the end of the month, was the first on which a mitral murmur was discovered. This patient was left behind when the regiment went on service, and I had the opportunity of watching him in the depôt hospital. The murmur persisted, and on the 21st August, increased præcordial dulness, not present at first, indicated commencing hypertrophy and dilatation. There is no *à priori* reason why acute articular rheumatism should be less accompanied with percarditis in soldiers in India than in Europe. The kind of data necessary to prove the contrary must be limited, and while the question is still *sub judice*, I would again urge that a careful search for the physical signs of pericarditis and endocarditis should be the rule of practice in every case of acute rheumatism in India, both in civil and military hospitals.

I. The proportion of cases of pericarditis and endocarditis, and of both combined.
II. The result of the cases.
III. Relation to difference of sex.
IV. The proportion of cases in different castes.
V. Classification, with reference to Age.
VI. The different occupations of those affected.
VII. Relation to habits of life.
VIII. The months of the year in which most prevalent.
IX. Relation of the disease to rheumatism, cachexia, and pulmonary inflammation.
X. The leading symptoms and signs treated of under the following subdivisions:—
   1. Pain at margin of the left ribs.
   2. Pain at the præcordial region.
   3. Increased action of the heart.
   4. The state of the pulse.
   5. The absence or presence of fever.
   6. Difficulty of breathing.
   7. Anxiety of countenance.
   8. Occurrence of delirium.
   9. Increased præcordial dulness.
   10. Purring tremor.
   11. Præcordial fulness.
   12. Friction murmur.
   13. Jogging movement of the heart.
XI. On the treatment of the disease:—
   1. Blood-letting, general and local.
   2. The application of blisters.
   3. Mercurial influence.

I. *The proportion of cases of Pericarditis and Endocarditis, and of both combined.*—Thirteen would seem to have been of pericarditis alone. But in regard to six, the details are not sufficiently stated to justify the exclusion of co-existing endocarditis; they must, therefore, be regarded as doubtful, though the probability is in favour of pericarditis alone.

There are four cases of endocarditis alone: of these, the mitral valve was affected in three, and the tricuspid valve was believed to be so in one.

There are eight of pericarditis and endocarditis combined: in three the aortic valves, in four the mitral valve, and in one both aortic and mitral valves were engaged. In seven, the pericarditis took precedence of the endocarditis, and in the remaining case the endocarditis was first observed.

II. *The result of the cases.*—Nine of the twenty-five cases proved fatal. Of these eight are in the list of pericarditis, but five of them are classed with those in which the co-existence of endocarditis was not disproved. One is in the list of pericarditis and endocarditis combined. Two of the fatal cases occurred in association with rheumatism, two were present in individuals of very cachectic habit, and four were instances of pericarditis secondary on pneumonia, pleuritis, or phthisis pulmonalis.

Of these last four fatal cases, in two death took place from pulmonic disease. In the first the pericardial inflammation had terminated in adhesions, in the second in opaque patches on the surface of the heart, and the endocarditis in valvular disease.

It will subsequently appear, that of the twenty-five cases, seventeen were associated with rheumatism, two with cachexia; four were secondary on pulmonic disease, and two primary or idiopathic. It has just been stated, that of the rheumatic cases two were fatal, of the cachectic all, of the pulmonic two*, and of the primary one. The deduction from these cases is therefore comfirmatory of the usual observation, that in pericarditis associated with rheumatism, the prognosis is much more favourable than under the other circumstances in which the disease arises.

Of the sixteen discharged cases, in five no signs of cardiac disease were left behind, and recovery was regarded as complete. They were, with one exception, cases of pericarditis; in the exceptional case endocarditis was also present. In three the signs of valvular disease were so slight, that it is very probable they also should be included in the list of perfect cures.

Of the eight cases in which complete restoration did not take place, in one valvular disease was left, in six valvular disease and pericardial adhesions, and in one pericardial adhesions alone. The adhesions were in six inferred to exist from the severity of the symptoms, and the distinctness and duration of the physical signs, but in one there was greater certainty, in consequence of a well-marked and persistent jogging motion of the heart.

III. *Relation to difference of sex.*—Of the cases under examination, four were females, but only three of these were hospital patients. Of the four, two were Hindoos and two Parsees. These data are much too limited to justify any attempt at precise comparison of the frequency of the disease in the two sexes. So far as they go, they show as great a prevalence in females as in males. The proportion of total female admissions into hospital during the period to which these cases refer was about one to seven males, and there is nearly the same proportion in the admissions from pericarditis and endocarditis. Moreover, as the clinical ward was for males only, I am satisfied, that in regard to the female inmates of the hospital, there has not been the same care in looking for the disease.

IV. *The proportion of cases in the different castes.*—The caste of twenty-three of the cases only is stated, but from these I shall exclude the females, so as to admit of a more accurate comparison between the affected and the total hospital admissions of the different castes. The classification of the females according to caste

* Two in which death took place from pulmonic disease long after the pericarditis are excluded.

has not been attended to in the hospital returns of disease. There are, therefore, nineteen cases to be considered under this head: of these nine, nearly one half, are Hindoos. The proportion which the Hindoo male hospital* admissions bear to the total male admissions is not quite one half. There are four cases of Parsees, nearly one fifth of the affected, but the proportion of the total male Parsee hospital admissions is about one twelfth. There are four cases classed under the head Christians in the hospital returns, viz. three Portuguese and one European. The proportion of total hospital Christian admissions is about one fifth. There are two cases of Mussulmans, being one ninth and a half of the affected, whereas the proportion of Mussulman hospital admissions is rather more than one third.

From these data, then, it would seem that there is about an equal liability to pericarditis and endocarditis in the Hindoo and native Christian classes, but that compared with them, these affections are more than twice as common among Parsees, and not one fourth so frequent among Mussulmans. It will not fail to be observed that of the four female cases, two were also Parsees, making six Parsees affected out of a total of twenty-three. Under a subsequent head it will appear that all the cases which occurred in Parsees were in association with acute articular rheumatism. These facts confirm the general impression on my mind, that acute articular rheumatism, with pericarditis and endocarditis, is more common among Parsees than any of the other classes of the native community of Bombay. Of the comparative exemption of the Mussulman population, as shown by these statements, I am unable to suggest any explanation; and it would be waste of time, and might lead to error, were I to speculate on deductions from data so limited.

* *Total number of Hospital Admissions from* 1848 *to April* 1852.

	Males.	Females.	Total.	Hindoos.	Mussulmans.	Christians.	Parsees.	Females.	Total.
1848-49.	3,045	487	3,532	1,154	1,064	482	145	487	3,532
1849-50.	3,653	589	4,242	1,335	1,377	681	260	589	4,242
1850-51.	4,133	713	4,846	1,712	1,347	715	359	713	4,846
1851-52.	3,543	583	4,126	1,486	1,064	629	364	583	4,126
Total.	14,374	2,372	16,746	5,687	4,852	2,707	1,128	2,372	16,746

V. *Classification with reference to age.* — The ages of only twenty-three of the cases are recorded: —

From 10 to 20	7
„ 21 „ 30	10
„ 31 „ 40	4
„ 41 „ 50	2
	23

The lowest age is seventeen, and the highest fifty. Seventeen cases were between the ages of seventeen and thirty, four between thirty-one and forty, and two between forty-one and fifty. Of those between seventeen and thirty, fourteen occurred in connection with rheumatism, — a fact which goes to support the common statement that rheumatism, with pericarditis and endocarditis, is a disease rather of the earlier than the advanced periods of life.

VI. *The different occupations of those affected.* — Of five cases, including three females, the nature of the occupation is not stated. That of the remaining twenty was as follows: —

2 Sailors	1 Labourer.
3 Servants	1 Carpenter
3 Fruit, vegetable and fish hawkers	1 Grain seller
	1 Schoolmaster
2 Beggars	1 Oil seller
2 Sepoys	1 Dyer.
1 Baker	1 Cook.

On examining this statement, it appears that of the twenty persons, sixteen followed occupations which, more or less, lead to exposure to wet or vicissitudes of temperature: this is the case of sailors, hawkers, beggars, sepoys, bakers, cooks, dyers, and labourers.

VII. *Relation to habits of life.* — It is stated of only five of the twenty-five cases, that there was addiction to the use of spirituous liquors; of these two were Parsees, two Hindoos, and one a Portuguese; one patient was habituated to opium smoking.

In regard to the remaining nineteen cases, it may be inferred of the greater number that they were not of intemperate habits.

VIII. *The months of the year in which most prevalent.* — The admissions occurred in the following months: —

3 in January	3 in July
2 „ February	3 „ August
0 „ March	1 „ September
1 „ April	4 „ October
0 „ May	2 „ November
4 „ June	2 „ December

The relation of the disease to cold and wet is also very well shown in this statement. There are nine cases in the cold months of November, December, January, and February. Those of February were admitted in its first half — one had been ill fifteen days, the other eight days, they are therefore justly classed with the occurrences of the cold season. There are fifteen in the rainy season, in the months of June, July, August, September, and October. Of the four which occurred in June, three were admitted after the 20th, and are consequently correctly classed as admissions of the rainy season; and of two the relation to wet as a cause is distinctly recorded. Of the four cases in October, three are correctly classed as admissions of the rainy season: they were received into hospital before the 12th of the month, and two of them had been ill fifteen and ten days respectively. The fourth admission in October was of a very susceptible individual, who had on a former occasion suffered from rheumatism. The single case which occurred in the hot season, in the month of April, was a Parsee female in good circumstances, who on previous occasions had suffered from rheumatism.

IX. *Relation of the disease to Rheumatism, Cachexia, and Pulmonic Inflammation.* — In seventeen cases the disease was associated with acute articular rheumatism. In sixteen the rheumatism was present at the period when the cardiac symptoms appeared, and afterwards co-existed with them. In one case the rheumatic symptoms were not present with the cardiac symptoms, which occurred in an individual who had some years previously suffered from an attack of acute rheumatism, and in whom the diathesis, at the period of the attack of pericarditis, may be assumed to have been still present. Of these seventeen cases, eight were Hindoos, six Parsees, two Christians, and one a Mussulman: six were of pericarditis alone, four of endocarditis, and seven of pericarditis and endocarditis combined.

Of the remaining eight cases, in which rheumatism was absent, two occurred in very cachectic states of the system; in one the cachexia was distinctly syphilitic, and in both, pericarditis alone was present. Four were extension of inflammation from the lungs or pleura, and were with one exception cases of pericarditis: in the exceptional one endocarditis also existed. Two must be looked upon as instances of primary pericarditis.

Of the total cases of pericarditis and endocarditis there was only one in which, so far as the record shows, Bright's disease of the kidney existed.

We notice distinctly in these cases the greater relation that subsists between endocarditis and acute articular rheumatism, than between pericarditis alone and rheumatism. All the cases of endocarditis, single or combined, were, with one exception, associated with rheumatism; whereas of the thirteen cases of pericarditis, seven were unconnected with rheumatism; and of the six cases in the list of uncombined pericarditis noted as occurring in association with rheumatism, it is not improbable that in two of them endocarditis was also present. Of the two cases of apparent primary pericarditis, one is peculiar in its nature, and will presently be made the subject of comment.

X. *The leading symptoms and signs observed.*—In analysing the symptoms, attention must be confined to twenty-two cases; for of three the record is so incomplete as to render their exclusion necessary.

Pain at the margin of the left ribs was present in seven cases, in some extending to the præcordial region, and in two or three to the epigastrium and abdomen generally.

Præcordial pain, either alone, or associated with pain at the margin of the left ribs, existed in eight.

To consider this symptom from another point of view, pain (præcordial and hypochondriac) was observed in ten cases; in two it was confined to the margin of the left false ribs, in three to the præcordial region, and in five it was common to both situations. Of these ten, six were of pericarditis alone, thus leaving four of this form in which pain was not observed; two were of endocarditis, leaving two of this form in which pain was not present; and two were of pericarditis and endocarditis combined, leaving six of this form not characterised by pain.

From these statements, then, it appears that we are justified in referring the symptom pain more to pericarditis than to endocarditis; for of the eighteen cases of pericarditis, simple and combined, pain was present in eight; but of the twelve of endocarditis, simple or combined, pain was characteristic of only four. These cases also confirm the now generally admitted fact, that in a considerable proportion of instances of pericarditis and endocarditis pain is not complained of. Of the twenty-two cases now under review, pain was present in ten, but absent in twelve.

Increased action of the heart is noted as having existed in eight cases. In five, pericarditis and endocarditis were combined; in two, endocarditis, and in one pericarditis existed alone: thus there would seem to be a more frequent relation between increased action of the heart and endocarditis than between it and pericarditis. Of the twelve cases in which endocarditis, simple and combined, was present, palpitation existed in five; but of the ten cases in which there was pericarditis alone, palpitation is noted of only one. It is further evident from this statement, that in a large proportion of cases of pericarditis and endocarditis, the action of the heart is not notably increased. Of the twenty-two cases under review, of eight only is increased action recorded as a symptom.

Impulse remote. — In one case the impulse of the heart is stated to have seemed distant and obscure.

The state of the pulse. — In sixteen cases the character of the pulse differed markedly from the healthy standard. In four it was *jerking*; of these, three were of pericarditis and endocarditis combined, and one of pericarditis alone. As the jerking pulse is not noted of any case of simple endocarditis, it may probably be inferred that this character of pulse is more related to pericarditis than endocarditis. It occurred only in simple or combined pericarditis.

In eleven cases the pulse is described as *small*, and in some it was also sharpish; six were of pericarditis, three of endocarditis, and two of pericarditis and endocarditis combined. It may, therefore, be inferred, that smallness of the pulse is as frequently referable to endocarditis as to pericarditis.

In only one case is the pulse stated to have *intermitted*, and this feature was not observed till long after the acute symptoms of pericarditis had ceased, and the disease was believed to have terminated in adhesions.

From a consideration of these cases, then, we may infer that an abnormal pulse is more frequently observed in pericarditis and endocarditis than pain or palpitation; that its most common quality is smallness associated with occasional sharpness, then a jerking character; but that an intermitting pulse, formerly looked upon as symptomatic of pericarditis, is of infrequent occurrence, and that we shall err, if we allow it weight in determining the diagnosis.

Febrile symptoms were observed in fifteen cases: of these five were of pericarditis alone, three of endocarditis, and seven of pericarditis and endocarditis combined. Fever, then, would seem to be as frequently related to endocarditis as to pericarditis. A reference to the remaining eight cases, of which febrile disturbance is not recorded, will show that in some of them fever had been present in the earlier stages of the illness, though it was not noticed when the patients were under observation in the hospital. In others, in which the disease was consecutive on pulmonary inflammation, it was impossible to relate the febrile symptoms to the pericarditis, rather than to the previously existing pulmonary disease.

The review of these cases, in reference to the presence or absence of fever, goes to show that pericarditis and endocarditis rarely exist without some degree of pyrexia. This was particularly true of those associated with acute articular rheumatism, and in them, no doubt, the fever was as much due to the affection of the joints as to pericarditis and endocarditis. But there is more than this; for I am satisfied that a close observation of cases of acute articular rheumatism will very generally show, that coincident with the commencement of pericarditis or endocarditis, there is a marked exacerbation of the febrile disturbance. The increase of fever in more than one case of acute rheumatism (for some days under treatment, and in which the state of the heart had been regularly inquired into), has led me to suspect the occurrence of pericarditis or endocarditis; and on careful examination the physical signs have, in each instance, confirmed the suspicion.

It is not improbable, that in acute rheumatism, in the sthenic constitutions of the inhabitants of European countries, with fever greater in degree and more continued, febrile exacerbations may not be so significant as I believe them to be in acute rheumatism in the asthenic constitutions of the natives of India, with fever, less in degree, and remittent in type. It is when the exacerbation becomes longer in duration, occurs at irregular periods, or is of increased severity, that it becomes indicative of the access of cardiac inflammation.

Some degree of hurry and shortness of breath were present in eight of nineteen cases; for under this head I have also excluded those instances of pericarditis associated with pulmonic disease. Of the eight cases, four were of pericarditis alone, two of endocarditis, and two of pericarditis and endocarditis combined. In none did the difficulty of breathing amount to orthopnœa.

The expression of countenance was observed to be anxious in five cases; two were of pericarditis, one of endocarditis, and two of pericarditis and endocarditis combined.

The occurrence of delirium was noted only in one case. The occasional presence of nervous symptoms in acute rheumatism and pericarditis, independent of direct affection of the brain, first pointed out by Dr. Watson, though not illustrated by these cases, is practically very important. I can call to mind more than one case of head symptoms misunderstood at the time, but which were afterwards suspected to be of this nature.

The review which has just been made of the general and local symptoms of pericarditis and endocarditis, goes to confirm the now well-established fact that it is to physical signs we must trust for the means of forming a precise diagnosis of these diseases; that without these signs many cases will escape detection, and very few will be recognised with certainty.

PHYSICAL SIGNS.—*Increased præcordial dulness* was present in nine cases: of these four were pericarditis alone, and five pericarditis and endocarditis combined—in all, the dulness probably depended on effusion into the pericardium. In two, the pyramidal form of the dull region was well marked; in two, effusion was found after death, and in a third, also fatal, no post mortem examination was made. In three of the six in which recovery took place, the dulness disappeared by absorption of the effusion: this was verified some time afterwards in one case by dissection. In the three remaining recovered cases, there was persistence of some degree of dulness, dependent, it was believed, on hypertrophy and dilatation of the left ventricle of the heart: these were instances in which considerable valvular disease existed.

Purring tremor was present in only three, and was accompanied with friction sound. The tremor, then, in these cases, was probably consequent on pericarditis, and not on mitral valvular disease.

Præcordial fulness was observed in only two, and was, apparently, caused by effusion into the pericardium.

Friction murmur.—The number of cases of pericarditis alone, and combined with endocarditis, amount to twenty-one; but from these, four must be excluded, in which no examination of the region of the heart had been made. Of the seventeen cases which remain, friction sound was heard in fifteen: it was absent in two—in one, consequent on the considerable effusion as indicated by the extent of the dulness, but in the other it is not noted, because I could not satisfy myself of its presence, though others at the time thought that it existed.

The duration of the friction sound is stated in nine cases: in two it was present upwards of thirty days, and the result was in all probability adhesion of the surfaces; in two the friction murmur was heard for twenty and twenty-one days—in one adhesion was suspected, in the other * it was proved to exist by subsequent dissection; in two the sound was present for fourteen days with in one probably opaque patches, and in the other adhesions; in one case the murmur existed for seven days, and adhesions in all likelihood resulted; in one the sound was heard for four days, and probably some degree of opacity of the surface was left behind; in one the murmur was audible for three days only, and in this case, on dissection many months after complete recovery, opaque patches were found here and there on the surface of the heart, but no adhesion.

In five of the cases in which friction murmur had been present, there was the opportunity of examining the body after death. In three a considerable time had elapsed between the period at which the sound had been audible, and death; in two † patches of organised lymph existed on the surface of the heart, but there was no adhesion of the surfaces; in one firm adhesions united the heart to the pericardium. In two cases death occurred at the time when the friction sound existed; in one ‡ there were eight ounces of reddish serum in the sac of the pericardium, and flakes and shreds of lymph were deposited on the surfaces; in the other § twelve ounces of clear fluid were found in the sac of the pericardium, three hours after death,—this fluid spontaneously coagulated into a gelatinous mass when removed from the body, but there were no flakes of lymph deposited on the surfaces, and no vascularity of the serous covering of the heart, or lining of the pericardium.

Four of the fatal cases confirm the generally received, and no doubt correct, opinion, that the friction murmur is for the most part dependent on the roughening of the surfaces from lymph-deposits; but case 235, if correctly observed, would seem to show that effusion of the liquor sanguinis (the fibrine being as yet undeposited in the solid form) is adequate to cause a friction sound. The case was for a very short time under observation, and that immediately before death. Moreover, the abnormal sound may possibly have proceeded from the great vessels compressed at their origin by the fluid — a cause which has been suggested ‖ as adequate to produce abnormal sound in pericardial effusion. For these reasons, I am unwilling to attach undue importance to this case; yet it seems to me to justify inquiry on the following points: —

1. Is it not probable that in exudations of liquor sanguinis from the inflamed capillaries of serous linings of closed sacs, the

* Case 232. † Cases 231, 233. ‡ Case 234. § Case 235.

‖ "Walshe on Diseases of the Lungs and Heart," p. 216, 1st edition.

deposition of the fibrine, in the solid form, does not take place so soon as is generally supposed?

2. Whether the movement of the liquor sanguinis (the fibrine as yet in the liquid form) between the serous surfaces is inadequate to produce a friction murmur; and whether, in considering this question, we ought not to bear in mind those cases of pericarditis in which this sound is present from the commencement, and to account for which has always been a difficulty, — explained by some on the supposition that the surfaces are roughened from the turgid state of the capillaries which precedes effusion, by others, as Dr. Hope *, on the improbable idea that lymph may be effused in the dry state, as first suggested by Laennec?

In two† of the fatal cases in which the friction sound was distinct, death took place several months afterwards — in one from cholera, in the other from pulmonary disease. In both, opaque patches were found on the surface of the heart, but no adhesion between it and the pericardium. In case 233 there was also valvular disease, and it may be argued that an endocardial murmur may have been mistaken for a friction sound. But this objection cannot be urged against case 231: in this, the friction murmur had been undoubted, and the valves and heart were quite healthy, with the exception of a few opaque patches on the surface of the right ventricle. This case establishes the fact, that there may be friction sound, then disappearance of it, and no greater structural change than a few opaque patches on the surface of the heart. Though this fact may now be admitted, still the statement made relative to the duration of the friction murmur, as observed in these cases, leaves little room for doubt, that when this sign ceases, after having been present for fourteen days and upwards, adhesion between the heart and pericardium has probably taken place.

The following are the five fatal cases in which friction murmur was observed: —

231. *Pericarditis.—Friction murmur distinct, and then altogether disappearing.—He was cured.—Eight months afterwards, death from cholera.—Opaque patches on the surface of the heart.—No pericardial adhesions.*—Tayjah Dongur Sing, a Hindoo fruit-seller, twenty-eight years of age, in tolerable condition, for six years addicted to opium-smoking, was admitted into the clinical ward on the 28th June, 1850, having been ill only since the day preceding. The countenance was somewhat anxious, the respiration short and hurried (sixty-eight in a minute), and almost entirely abdominal; the skin was of natural temperature; the pulse seventy-six, rather small, but

* Hope's Treatise on Disease of the Heart, 4th edit., p. 144.

† Cases 231, 233.

sharpish; and the tongue was a good deal furred. On percussion of the anterior part of the chest no defective resonance was detected, and vesicular respiration was distinct and unmixed. In the præcordial region, over a spot about an inch and a half in diameter, just internal to the nipple, there was heard a murmur, partly of a rubbing, partly of a creaking character. In this situation there was tenderness on pressure. The sounds of the heart were distinctly audible, and the impulse was not much increased. He pointed to the præcordial region, and to the margin of the left false ribs, as the seats of pain, felt since the day preceding his admission. The pain did not extend to the back or left shoulder. He was quite free of all pain of the limbs; but he stated that he had suffered eight years previously from a severe attack of swelling and pain of the joints, chiefly the knees and ankles; and the marks of scarifications were still visible on the knees. For this affection of the joints, he had also undergone two long courses of mercury, and continued ill for seven months. Subsequently, however, he had enjoyed good health. The only circumstance to which he could attribute his present illness was exposure to wet, to which he had been subjected ten days previously. Forty-eight leeches were applied to the præcordial region, followed by a blister; three grain and then two-grain doses of calomel with one eighth of a grain of tartar emetic, and one fourth of a grain of opium, were given every fourth hour. On the 30th June the gums were tender, and the calomel was omitted; on the 1st July the mercurial influence was still more developed. On the 29th June the friction murmur was still distinct; on the 30th it had disappeared, and was not again heard. He was discharged well from the ward on the 10th July. This patient again presented himself at the hospital on the 21st August, having experienced some uneasy sensations in the præcordial region, but the sounds and impulse of the heart were natural; and after the action of some aperient medicine he was quite relieved, and left the hospital on the 22nd August. He was not again seen till the 7th of March, 1851, when he was admitted in the collapsed state of cholera, that disease being at the time prevalent: re-action did not take place, and he died on the evening of the 10th.

Inspection.—Chest.—There was no increased quantity of fluid found in the pericardium, and there were no adhesions between the pericardium and the heart. The inner surface of the pericardium was pale, and without deposit of any kind. The heart was rather small; there was no dilatation of any of its cavities. Over the centre of the anterior wall of the right ventricle there was an opaque patch, about half an inch long and quarter of an inch in breadth, which, with moderate traction with the forceps, could be separated from the pericardial covering of the heart in the form of a thin firm layer of areolar tissue. The free surface of the patch was quite smooth. At the upper part of the left ventricle there was a smaller and a thinner patch. Elsewhere, here and there on the surface of the heart, other opaque spots were noticed. The endocardium was healthy, and so were also the valves. There were two or three small spots of commencing deposit on the inner surface of the ascending aorta.

Remarks.—This case has been already published by me in the *London Medical Gazette*, of the 16th May, 1851. It was so because at the time Dr. W. S. Kirkes had called in question the commonly received opinion, which maintains that when there has been acute pericarditis, with friction murmur, followed by disappearance of the murmur and restoration to tolerable health, this result has been effected by pericardial adhesion. This case confirms Dr. Kirkes' opinion; and, I think, definitely proves that we may have friction murmur and recovery, without any other structural change than the opaque white patches so frequently observed on parts of the surface of the heart.

232. *Phthisis pulmonalis.—Secondary pericarditis.—Friction murmur, distinct for twenty days.—Death eighteen months afterwards.—Firm pericardial adhesions —Bright's disease of the kidney.*—Kannyah, a Hindoo baker, thirty-two years of age, a native of Bangalore, and lately arrived in Bombay from Poona, was admitted, after

eleven days' illness, into the clinical ward, on the 27th September, 1849. He was reduced in flesh, and the respiration was short and hurried. The whole of the right side of the chest was dull on percussion, the dulness increasing from above downwards. In places there was crepitus rale, in others bronchial respiration. He continued under treatment till the 11th December. There were febrile symptoms, with evening exacerbations. The sputa, at first in part rusty and adhesive, frothy and clear, subsequently became opaque, and were expectorated in detached masses. The dulness on the right side and bronchial respiration continued for some time unchanged, but at the period of his discharge had considerably lessened. During his stay crepitus was heard in the left dorsal region.

He was re-admitted on the 14th June, 1850. He had improved in health after leaving the hospital, till five days before his re-admission, when, consequent on exposure to cold, he had a return of febrile symptoms, cough, and dyspnœa. There was dulness, with large crepitus, and bronchial respiration in the left mammary, lateral, dorsal, and scapular regions. On the right side crepitus was also audible; but nothing is noted regarding the resonance on percussion. The sounds and rhythm of the heart were natural. He continued suffering from febrile and pulmonic symptoms till the 23rd June, when a distinct friction murmur, synchronous with the heart's action, and obscuring the sounds, was heard between the left nipple and the sternum. The pulse was frequent and jerking. The murmur continued distinct till the 13th July, when it ceased; and there was left some degree of roughness and shortness of the first sound. On the 3rd August, and for some time afterwards, the impulse of the heart was distinct between the third and fourth left costal cartilages, but it was not perceptible below the nipple. The febrile and pulmonic symptoms continued, but became less in severity; the dulness and bronchial respiration of the left side lessened in degree, and he was discharged in improved health on the 20th September. He continued in tolerable health for about a year, when he began again to suffer from cough and febrile symptoms, and was re-admitted into the clinical ward on the 6th January, 1852. He was a good deal emaciated. The respiration was short and hurried; there was dulness on percussion of the right scapular and dorsal regions, but undue resonance of the subclavian region. In all these regions there was blowing respiration and increased resonance of voice. The left subclavian and axillary regions were somewhat dull on percussion, and there was bronchial respiration mixing with occasional subcrepitous rale. There was no increased præcordial dulness, and nothing abnormal was detected in the sounds and impulse of the heart. There was dulness on percussion for an inch and a half below the margin of the right false ribs, and some uneasiness on pressure there. He complained of frequent cough. The sputa were copious, puriform, and in detached masses. The pulse was small and frequent. There was no diarrhœa. He died on the 10th January. During his second admission the urine gave no trace of albumen on the one occasion on which it was examined. During his last admission it was examined on the 9th January, when it was stated to be twenty ounces in quantity, of brown colour, specific gravity 1·035, giving a deposit under heat and nitric acid, which became of a brown colour.

Inspection fourteen hours after death.—Head.—The vessels of the pia mater were congested, and about two ounces of serous fluid were found at the base of the skull. *Chest.*—The mucous membrane of the trachea presented here and there a blush of redness: there were also small red points on that of the larynx. The lobes of the right lung were firmly adherent to each other. The two upper ones were completely solidified by aggregation of crude tubercles. About an inch and a half below the apex of the upper lobe, and near to its posterior surface, there was a cavity the size of a pigeon's egg, lined by a smooth membrane. The inferior lobe, also, had scattered crude tubercles, with intercurrent sanguineous engorgement. Both lobes of the left lung were more or less solidified, but the upper one more so, from tubercular deposit; there was no cavity. The internal surface of the pericardium was firmly, closely, and generally adherent to the outer surface of the heart. The left ventricle of the heart was slightly dilated, but there was no hypertrophy of its walls. The valves of both sides were healthy. *Abdomen.*—The external appearance and size of the liver were natural. When incised, it was found to be congested in the second degree. The spleen was healthy. Both kidneys were slightly enlarged, somewhat lobulated, mottled red and pale yellow, and finely granular externally; their incised surfaces were in general pale: the cortical portion of both was somewhat enlarged and encroached upon the tubular. These changes were most marked in the left kidney. The stomach and intestines were not examined.

233. *Asthenic pneumonia, leading to red induration of the upper lobes.—In its course, pericarditis and endocarditis of the left ventricle and auricle, causing structural disease of the mitral valve.—Not traced to rheumatism.—Dilatation of all the cavities of the heart.*—Sebastian Fernandez, a native of Goa, thirty-one years of age, following the occupation of a servant, and using spirituous liquors, was admitted into the clinical ward on the 15th July, 1850. He was a good deal reduced, had been under treatment in the hospital a month before for cough, from which on previous occasions he had also suffered. Subsequent to his discharge from hospital, and about fifteen days before his second admission, the cough had become more troublesome, and for the last eight days had been attended with febrile symptoms, coming on with chills at irregular times, and terminating with sweating; and the sputa had been tinged with blood. The respiration on admission was observed to be slightly hurried; there was some degree of dulness on percussion of the left subclavian region, and the general character of the respiration there, as well as in the left scapular region, was more bronchial than normal. The sounds and impulse of the heart were natural. He continued suffering from cough—the physical signs unchanged—occasional accessions of fever, and slight dysenteric symptoms, with a pulse decreasing in strength, till the 31st July, when, for the first time, some degree of preternatural præcordial dulness was observed. The dulness extended from the third to the fifth rib, and from the left margin of the sternum to the nipple. At the fourth costal cartilage, internal to the nipple, both sounds of the heart were distinct, and continued so in a direction upwards. About an inch below and external to the nipple there was a rough murmur, obscuring the first sound, but the second was tolerably clear. On moving the stethoscope downwards and outwards, about an inch and a half below and external to the nipple, the murmur became louder, and obscured both sounds of the heart. The features were contracted, and the pulse was scarcely perceptible. The bowels were relaxed, and he had vomited frequently. He continued under treatment till the 29th September, when he was transferred to another ward. During this period occasional febrile symptoms were present. The pulse was in general small, sometimes irritable. The action of the heart was increased; the præcordial dulness somewhat extended. The cardiac murmur continued as described, but latterly it was less rough, and somewhat fainter, and did not obscure both sounds. The pulmonic symptoms and signs continued, and there was more or less gastro-enteric irritation present. The urine showed no trace of albumen. He was treated with stimulants, tonics, and anodynes, and small blisters were applied to the præcordial region. Shortly afterwards he left the hospital, and was not again heard of till the 24th February, 1851, when he applied for re-admission, and was received into the clinical ward. He complained chiefly of discomfort and distention of the abdomen after eating, and the breathing was hurried. Dulness on percussion of the right subclavian and axillary regions was noted, with a bronchial character of the respiration there, as well as in the left subclavian and scapular regions. The præcordial dulness extended from the third rib to the margin of the left false ribs, and transversely from the right margin of the sternum to half an inch external to the nipple. The action of the heart was increased. A little internal to the nipple there was a blowing systolic murmur, which became more audible in a direction downwards, but gradually disappeared in a direction upwards; the second

sound of the heart was distinct. The pulse was small and feeble, the dyspnœa increased, and he died on the 5th March.

Inspection twelve hours after death.—Chest.—The lungs did not collapse. The left lung adhered firmly to the costal pleura throughout its entire extent; the greater part of the upper lobe was in a state of red induration, the lower lobe was somewhat condensed, and a good deal of frothy serum oozed out when it was cut; there was no pleuritic effusion. The right lung was unconnected by abnormal adhesion to the costal pleura; the upper lobe was in a state of red induration similar to that of the left side, but rather less in degree; the posterior part of the third lobe was also condensed, and the anterior crepitated feebly; the bronchial tubes were filled with frothy serum, and the mucous membrane was red; there was no pleuritic effusion. The heart extended from the third to the seventh left rib. There was no fluid in the sac of the pericardium. Opaque thickened patches existed on the surface of the heart, chiefly that of the right ventricle. The cavity of the left ventricle was dilated, but the walls were of natural thickness; the mitral valve was considerably thickened, and the auriculo-ventricular opening was so contracted as not to allow the point of the little finger to pass through. The free margins of the aortic semi-lunar valves were thickened. The left auricle was also dilated, and its lining membrane presented an opaque thickened appearance throughout, with granular effusion here and there, in patches. There was considerable dilatation of the right auricle and ventricle, and both contained firm fibrinous coagula. *Abdomen.*—The liver was rather smaller than natural, but healthy in structure. The kidneys were healthy.

234. *Empyema of the right side of the chest.—Secondary pericarditis.—Friction Murmur.—Lymph effusions found after death.*—Miguel Rozario, aged thirty-five, a native of Goa, a cook by occupation, had been in bad health for some time before his admission into the Jamsetjee Jejeebhoy Hospital, on the 23rd July, 1852. He was affected with cough, and with dyspnœa, and the indurated edge of the liver projected for two or three inches below the margin of the right ribs. The dyspnœa increased and there were occasional febrile symptoms, and on the 13th August a distinct friction murmur was perceived in the præcordial region, best heard at the apex. There was slight increase of præcordial dulness. The face became puffed, the feet and hands œdematous, and he died on the 19th.

Inspection thirteen hours after death.—Chest.—The right sac of the pleura contained several pints of purulent fluid; the lung was compressed, and the liver was displaced downwards. The surfaces of the pleura were covered with flaky lymph. The left lung was healthy. The pericardium contained about eight ounces of blood-tinged serum, and flakes and shreds of lymph adhered generally to its inner surface. The heart was of natural size, and there was no disease of the valves.

Remarks.—For this case I am indebted to Dr. Haines, under whose care the patient was. I had not an opportunity of seeing the patient during life, nor the morbid appearances after death.

235. *Acute arachnitis and pericarditis, leading to considerable effusions, coagulating into a jelly-like mass when removed from the body.—Friction murmur.—In a pregnant female.*—Joomkee, a Hindoo female, a beggar, thirty years of age, was brought to the Jamsetjee Jejeebhoy Hospital on the evening of the 9th August, 1852. She had been found alone in a house by the police, and was believed to have been ill for several days. She was quite comatose, and the pupils were dilated; the skin was somewhat above the natural temperature: the breathing was hurried: the pulse was small and frequent. The upper limit of the præcordial dulness was the lower border of the second left rib, the lower limit was the upper border of the sixth rib; the inner the middle of the sternum, and the outer a vertical line drawn along the external margin of the nipple. The impulse of the heart was increased, and a thrilling sensation was communicated to the hand when placed on the præcordial region. The action of the

heart was tumultuous, and the sounds confused. There was distinct induration below the left false ribs. She was in about the sixth month of pregnancy, and the fœtal pulsations were audible to the left of the fundus of the uterus. During the 10th the coma continued; the pulse became feebler; the breathing more hurried, and at the evening visit a friction murmur was heard at the second left costal cartilage, but not at the apex—here the sounds were still confused. She died early on the morning of the 11th.

Inspection three hours after death.—*Head.*—About eight* ounces of fluid flowed from the cavity of the arachnoid and base of the skull, and speedily coagulated into a jelly-like mass. It was of red colour, but this was probably due to some admixture of blood which had escaped from the sinuses, wounded in removing the dura mater. There was no increased vascularity of the membranes, or redness of the substance of the brain. The ventricles were empty. *Chest.*—The diaphragm rose high in the chest. The lungs showed no traces of disease. The pericardium was distended, and occupied a space extending from the first to the fifth left rib, reached to the right border of the sternum, and on the left side half an inch beyond the nipple. It contained about twelve ounces of clear greenish fluid, which speedily coagulated into a tremulous jelly-like mass. There was no vascularity of any part of the inner surface of the pericardium or outer surface of the heart, and no trace of lymph deposit. The endocardium, the valves, and muscular tissue of the heart, presented no appearance of disease, unless a greater degree than usual of redness of the muscular structure may be so considered. There was no dilatation of any of the cavities, and they contained little blood, and no fibrinous coagula. The spleen was considerably enlarged. The liver was of natural size, and healthy. Both kidneys were somewhat larger than natural, but their structure was healthy. The gravid uterus extended as high as the umbilicus, and contained twins between the fifth and sixth month.

Jogging movement of the heart was noticed only in one case, and in this the history pointed to pericardial adhesions as the probable result: it may, therefore, be looked upon as tending to confirm the opinion entertained by Dr. Hope relative to the import of this sign.

XI. *On the treatment of the disease.*—The following observations have reference to seventeen cases:—

In none was *general blood-letting* required; the constitutions of the patients admitted into the Jamsetjee Hospital are for the most part too asthenic to justify the use of this antiphlogistic means.

In eleven, local blood-letting by leeches was had recourse to. The stage of the disease, and the state of the pulse and skin, were the guides to the adoption and degree of this measure. Of its efficacy, when the circumstances are appropriate, there can be no doubt.

In fourteen cases, one or more *blisters*, from three to four inches square, were applied to the præcordial region. The liquor lyttæ was the preparation generally selected, and it was usually applied after suitable local depletion, or in cases for which the latter mea-

* The character of the cerebral effusion is the only fact in this case not witnessed by myself. I am indebted to Mr. Sebastian Carvalho for the statement. The heart and pericardial effusion were seen by me.

sure was considered inappropriate. Blisters were not used more frequently, when liquid effusions were believed to be present, than when they were supposed to be absent. Looking upon the derivant action of a counter-irritant as a means which tends to favour the restoration of normal circulation in the inflamed capillaries, and believing that this is necessary to ensure the absorption of liquid effusions, or the organisation of lymph-deposits, it seems to me, as regards the application of blisters, an immaterial question which of these processes must be brought into action before recovery can take place: in both, a more or less complete return to normal capillary circulation in the structures adjoining the deposits, is essential.

Mercurial influence was induced in ten cases. In all, with one exception, local blood-letting had also been used, and in all blisters applied. Of these ten cases, three were of pericarditis alone, one of endocarditis, and six of pericarditis and endocarditis combined. Five of the ten cases in which mercury was used, recovered; but in the other five, though life was saved, structural change remained behind. Of the eight cases classed under a former head as recoveries (p. 564), mercurial influence was induced in five; but in three it formed no part of the treatment, which in one consisted of local blood-letting and blisters, in another of blisters, in a third of Dover's powder and nitre alone. The mercury was given every third, fourth, or sixth hour, in the form of calomel, in two or three-grain doses, combined with a quarter or half a grain of opium; and in cases in which there was much febrile disturbance, from a quarter to a third of a grain of tartar emetic was added. The calomel was used with caution, so as not to cause a greater effect than slight swelling of the gums, and gentle ptyalism; and this state was maintained for several days. The mercurial treatment was never had recourse to without a strict inquiry into the state of the patient's constitution, with the view of ascertaining the likelihood of a scorbutic or other cachexia. This care is essential in the treatment of the class of patients who resort to this hospital, and indeed, I might add, of natives of India generally.

We find, then, that of ten cases brought under the influence of mercury, five recovered,—but in these local blood-letting and blisters had also been used; and that of eight cases in which recovery took place, mercurial action, preceded by blisters and leeches, had been induced in five, but in three mercury had not been given. In this statement, then, we have no striking proof of the efficacy of the mercurial treatment of pericarditis and endocarditis: yet my impression is in favour of its cautious adoption in suitable states of the constitution, and stages of the disease.

The present state of therapeutic science teaches us that mercury, under some circumstances, favours the absorption of lymph-deposits; and so long as this doctrine remains unrefuted, it is the course of prudence to yield to it some measure of our faith, and to act in some degree under its guidance. At the same time, however, we must never forget, that if mercury may influence for useful ends states of the blood well constituted as regards fibrine and red corpuscles, it can hardly fail to cause harm in opposite conditions. But these principles have been already fully explained and enforced in various parts of this work.

In one case in which the use of mercury was contra-indicated, *liquor potassæ* was substituted, because in similar asthenic states many good recoveries of pneumonia in the second stage seemed to have been brought about by this remedy.

CHAP. XXV.

ON ORGANIC DISEASE OF THE HEART AND AORTA.

SECTION I. — *In Natives of India.*

THIS section records the clinical history of twenty-eight cases of structural disease of the heart, and three of aneurism of the aorta. The important facts may be arranged under the following heads:—

I. The nature and situation of the structural change.
II. Relation to difference of sex.
III. The proportion of cases in the different castes.
IV. Classification with reference to age.
V. The different occupations of those affected.
VI. Relation to habits of life.
VII. Relation to the months of the year.
VIII. Relation of the structural changes to pericarditis, endocarditis, and rheumatism.
IX. Relation to Bright's disease of the kidney.
X. The leading symptoms and signs, treated of under the following heads:—
1. Dyspnœa.
2. Dropsy.
3. Præcordial pain.
4. Pain below the margin of the right ribs.
5. Scapular pain.
6. Character of the pulse.
7. Præcordial fulness.
8. Increased impulse of the heart.
9. Præcordial dulness.
10. Dulness below the margin of the right ribs.
11. Character of the murmurs.
12. Præcordial thrill.

XI. On medical treatment.

I. *The nature and situation of the structural changes.*—Of the thirty-one cases, eighteen proved fatal in hospital, and two in all probability, shortly after discharge. Of the eighteen fatal cases an examination of the body after death was made in seventeen. Let us first notice the structural changes which existed in them.

In eleven there was *dilatation of both ventricles of the heart;* in six, associated with disease of both aortic and mitral valves; in four with disease of the mitral valve, and in one with disease of the aortic valves alone.

In ten there was *dilatation and hypertrophy of the left ventricle.* In these, with two exceptions, there was dilatation of the right ventricle also; in five there was disease of both the aortic and mitral valves, in three of the mitral valve, and in two of the aortic valves only.

In one case there was *hypertrophy of the right ventricle*, associated with obstructive disease of the pulmonary semi-lunar valves. It is here narrated:—

236. *Contraction of the orifice of the pulmonary artery, probably congenital.—Much hypertrophy, without dilatation of the right ventricle of the heart.—No disease of the left side.*—Mahadoo Babajee, a Hindoo beggar, fifteen years of age, of short stature, and disproportionately large head, a native of Alibag, in Angria's Colaba, and resident in Bombay from his childhood, was admitted into the clinical ward on the 22nd September, 1850. He stated that from childhood he had suffered from dyspnœa, occasional cough, and pain of the præcordial region; that he was liable to febrile attacks; that on one occasion his abdomen had become very tumid; that for four months before admission he had experienced pain, without swelling, of the large joints, and to these symptoms occasional headache had been added. On admission, the respiration was observed to be slightly hurried; the skin was cool; the pulse small and easily compressed; the abdomen somewhat full, but supple; the tongue coated with a white fur; the bowels regular, and the urine free. The chest sounded well on percussion, with exception of slight increase of the præcordial dulness, which extended vertically from the fourth to the sixth rib, and transversely from the middle of the sternum to the left nipple. The respiratory murmur was somewhat puerile in character, and without rales. The action of the heart was somewhat increased, and its apex beat in the intercostal space between the fifth and sixth rib, at the left border of the sternum. There was a systolic murmur, best heard a little below and internal to the nipple, continuing distinct upwards and to the right side, and fading in the opposite direction. The second sound was normal. No thrilling sensation was experienced on placing the hand on the præcordial region. He remained under treatment till the 26th November, when he was discharged, little relieved. During his stay, the physical signs of heart disease continued as on admission. He complained of dyspnœa, of cough, occasional pain of the joints, of headache, and febrile disturbance from time to time. The pulse was always small, and easily compressed; the urine free, specific gravity from 1·012 to 1·020, and without trace of albumen. This patient was re-admitted into the hospital on the 19th March 1851, affected with febrile symptoms. The systolic murmur was still present; also dry bronchitic rales. He was attacked with symptoms of cholera on the 23rd, and died on the 24th.

Inspection twenty-four hours after death.—Head.—The calvarium, chiefly the occipital and frontal portions, was very thick, being more than quarter of an inch, but without any increase of the density of the diploe. The furrows of the middle meningeal artery were deeply grooved. The membranes of the brain were very much congested. The substance of the brain was firm, showed more bloody points than usual, and the cortical portion was of darker tint than natural. *Chest.*—The heart weighed seven ounces and a half. With exception of the right auricle there was no dilatation of the cavities. The walls of the left ventricle were of natural thickness; those of the right ventricle were thicker than those of the left—they were rather more than half an inch thick. The orifice of the pulmonary artery was of size only sufficient to permit the passage of half the length of an ordinary dissecting case blow-pipe, and the surface towards the cavity of the artery, and immediately surrounding the opening, had a rough and papillated appearance, as of firm granular-lymph deposit. The orifice seemed to be constructed by adhesion of the free edges of the semi-lunar valves, with exception of their central part. The valves, however, were very little thickened, and a probe passed readily into the little pouch between them and the internal surface of the artery. The trunk of the pulmonary artery was of diminished capacity, and the walls were thinner than natural. The aorta and its valves were healthy. The lungs were not congested with blood; in parts they were dry and woolly, and the surface somewhat irregular, from slight emphysema.

Remarks.—Presuming on the rarity of disease of the valves of the right side of the heart, it was supposed that the aortic valves were the seat of disease in this case; but my belief is that a more careful inquiry into the situation at which the murmur was best heard would during life have led to a correct diagnosis. The stunted growth, the absence of dilatation of the cavities of the heart, the freedom from dropsical symptoms or other signs of congestion, and the small pulse, all show that the blood was maintained in very reduced quantity; indeed, it was only by an adaptation of the quantity to the very contracted pulmonary orifice that the circulation of the blood could have been carried on. The complete absence of congestion of the lungs, so different from what obtains in most forms of heart disease, was interesting, but of easy explanation.

In the four following cases there was *aneurism of the left ventricle.* In all, the opaque state of the endocardium showed that endocarditis had at a former period been present, and was probably the cause of the atrophy and impaired irritability of the muscular fibre which had led to the formation of the aneurismal pouches. In three of the cases there was disease of the mitral valve, and in one, of the aortic valves.

237. *Dilatation of both ventricles.—Hypertrophy of the left.—Disease of aortic valves and the well-marked results of pericarditis and endocarditis, consecutive on rheumatism, related to syphilis.*—Ahmeenah, a Hindoo female, thirty-nine years of age, had, about a year before she came under observation, been the subject of syphilis, followed by pain and swelling of almost all the joints, and latterly by dyspnœa, and fulness of the epigastrium. She was admitted into the hospital on the 14th December, 1848, affected with general anasarcous swellings, dyspnœa, and cough. There was præcordial dulness from the third to the seventh rib, and from the middle of the sternum to an inch external to the left nipple. The impulse of the heart was increased, and a sawing murmur took the place of both sounds, and was loudest between the third and fourth rib, about half an inch to the left of the sternum, continuing audible as the stethoscope was moved towards the clavicle, but lessening in the direction of the apex. There was occasional sibilus mixing with the respiration. The pulse was feeble. There was fulness and uneasiness at the epigastrium, and hepatic dulness extended to within an inch of the umbilicus. The urine was not albuminous. The dropsical symptoms and the dyspnœa increased; and she died on the 25th December.

Inspection.—On examining the body after death, the pericardium was found to extend from the second to the seventh rib, and its cavity contained about four ounces of serum. It was connected to the surface of the heart, chiefly over the left ventricle, by firm adhesions. The serous covering of the heart was for the most part thickened and opaque. The heart was much enlarged—there was dilatation of both ventricles, with hypertrophy of the left; the tricuspid and mitral valves were healthy. The lining membrane of the left ventricle, towards the aortic orifice, was for a considerable extent opaque, and much thickened. There existed at the upper part of the septum a thimble-like depression about an inch in diameter, lined by thickened endocardium, roughened by granules of lymph. The ring of the aortic valves felt cartilaginous and firm, but there was no dilatation of the aorta.

238. *Aneurism of the left ventricle of the heart, consequent on endocarditis and pericarditis.*—Mahomed Allee, aged forty, a Mussulman, a native of Bengal, resi-

dent for fourteen years in Bombay, following the occupation of a sailor, and not intemperate in his habits, was admitted into the clinical ward on the 6th November, 1849, and died on the 12th of the same month. He was a good deal reduced; the countenance was anxious; the respiration hurried; the pulse feeble and intermitting. He was easiest when on the right side, or in the sitting posture. Decubitus on the back or the left side led to much aggravation of the dyspnœa, and anxiety; and in consequence of the suffering which they occasioned, minute and repeated examinations of the chest were impracticable. The præcordial dulness extended from the fourth costal cartilage to the seventh, and transversely from the middle of the sternum to just external to the left nipple. The impulse of the heart was somewhat increased. There was a systolic murmur audible at the fourth costal cartilage, increasing in the direction of the apex, decreasing above the base. The second sound was natural. He complained of constant pain about the left scapula, but none of the præcordial region. The pain at the left scapular region had existed for about three months, but the dyspnœa came on only nine days before his admission into the hospital. About two inches below and external to the left nipple there was a depressed cicatrix—the mark, he said, of a gun-shot wound received during the late war in Scinde. Was never affected with rheumatism, or pain of the præcordial region.

Inspection.—Chest.—The lungs collapsed on opening the chest, and there was about a pint of serous effusion in the sacs of the pleura. The upper lobes of both lungs, more especially at their apices, contained many scattered miliary tubercles, with some induration of the intervening pulmonary tissue; the rest of the lung healthy and crepitating, but somewhat congested. The pericardium contained about two ounces of serum. The heart was much enlarged; it occupied vertically a space between the lower margin of the second rib and the level of the seventh, and transversely from the sternal junction of the second right rib to the left nipple. There were firm close adhesions between the pericardium and the posterior and upper part of the left ventricle; also general thickening and opacity of the serous covering of the heart. The left ventricle was very much dilated. At its apex, and posteriorly below the mitral valve, it was dilated into two distinct pouches. The latter pouch was large enough to hold a small orange, its walls were membranous and opaque, and it contained fibrinous coagula. The rest of the walls of the ventricle was of natural thickness. There was slight thickening of the mitral valve; the orifice of the aorta was dilated. The right ventricle was also dilated; the semi-lunar valves were healthy. There was no morbid appearance found in the interior of the chest corresponding with the cicatrix on its exterior. *Abdomen.*—There was about a pint of serum in the cavity of the peritoneum. The free lower margin of the liver was about three inches below the ensiform cartilage, and about an inch below the margin of the right ribs, and the organ was somewhat congested. The kidneys were healthy.

239. *Rheumatism, followed by pericarditis and endocarditis.—Disease of the mitral valve.—Dilatation of the right side of the heart.—Dilatation and hypertrophy, with circumscribed aneurism of the left ventricle.—Death expedited by acute general peritonitis.*—Abdool Rahman, a Mussulman horsekeeper, fifty years of age, an inhabitant of Hydrabad, in the Deccan, and a resident in Bombay for about six years, was admitted into the Jamsetjee Jejeebhoy Hospital on the 13th December, 1849. He had been addicted to the use of spirituous liquors for several years, smoked ganja and tobacco, and latterly also took opium. About three years before admission he had suffered for a month from pain of the large joints, unattended with swelling he said; but that since then there had been no recurrence. For a year and a half he had experienced more or less dyspnœa, easily increased by exertion, but unattended with cough, till about eight days before admission, when cough began to be troublesome, and the dyspnœa to be more urgent, followed in two or three days by puffiness of the face and œdema of the feet and legs; and in this state he was admitted into hospital.

The respirations were twenty-six, and chiefly abdominal. With exception of increased præcordial dulness, the chest sounded well on percussion; but sibilous and subcrepitous rales were present more or less in all parts of the lungs. The præcordial dulness extended vertically from the third costal cartilage to the margin of the left false ribs, and tranversely from the middle of the sternum to about three inches external to the nipple. The impulse was forcible, extensive, and heaving, and the apex beat between the sixth and seventh ribs, an inch external to the nipple. There was a systolic bellows murmur very distinct below the nipple, and in the direction of the apex, but becoming faint above the base. The second sound was distinct, but wanting in sharpness. The skin was cool; the pulse 96 to 100, small, easily compressed, and slightly jerking He complained of cough and dyspnœa, — both increased at night, the latter becoming very urgent on slight exertion. The abdomen full and supple, without any sense of fluctuation; and there was dulness below the right false ribs for about two and a half inches, and extending upwards as high as the level of the sixth right rib. The bowels were slow, and the urine reported free. He continued under treatment till the 4th March; the dropsical symptoms disappeared, and the dyspnœa and cough were much alleviated. The general character of the pulse was small, irregular and unequal, and varying in frequency. The rhythm of the heart's action was often observed to be irregular, two pulsations being succeeded by a period of considerable repose, and a distinct thrill was in general perceptible on placing the hand on the præcordial region. The dulness of the præcordial region, and the character of the murmur and of the second sound, continued unchanged. The urine was free, of varying density, and never albuminous. He was treated chiefly with combinations of camphor mixture, sesquicarbonate of ammonia, spiritus ætheris nitrici, tincture of hyosciamus, and preparations of squills. After his discharge from the hospital, he from time to time presented himself at the morning visit, and the physical signs of heart disease were found to continue without change. At length he was re-admitted into the clinical ward on the 21st August, 1850. The abdomen was tense, tender, and fluctuating; the pulse frequent, and almost imperceptible; dyspnœa urgent. He died about twelve hours after admission.

Inspection nine hours after death. — *Chest.* — On opening the cavity of the chest, the lungs collapsed, and were found crepitating. There were old adhesions of the costal and pulmonary pleuræ of the right side. The pericardium was in relation with the anterior wall of the chest from the first to the sixth rib, and tranversely beyond the right margin of the sternum to the right, and beyond the nipple to the left. There was no adhesion of the pericardium to the heart, but the surface of the heart, more particularly of the left ventricle, was covered with opaque patches. The right auricle was very much distended. There was also much dilatation of the right as well as of the left ventricle, and in both were found coagula of blood. The walls of the left ventricle were for the most part of natural thickness, with the exception of one place in the internal wall, midway between the apex and the mitral valve, where the coats were much thinned, the muscular tissue being almost removed, so as to form a pouch the size of a walnut. The endocardium surrounding the margin of the pouch for about half an inch was opaque and thick. The mitral valve was thickened, so as to permit regurgitation into the auricle. The aortic valve and the aorta were healthy. *Abdomen.* — About two pints of turbid serous fluid were found in the cavity of the peritoneum, and an abundant effusion of coagulable lymph over the surface of the intestines formed tender bands of adhesion between them and the parietes, and between the convolutions. In several places the adhesions circumscribed collections of serum. The liver was rather smaller than natural, and its substance felt hard under the knife; its external surface was granular, but there was no very distinct appearance of cirrhosis of its incised surfaces; the external surface was covered with patches of coagulable lymph; its anterior margin was firmly adherent to the ascending colon as well as to the diaphragm. In the mucous membrane of the cœcum there was an ulcer about the size of a rupee; and in that of the ascending colon there were three or four smaller ulcers, with patches of redness here and there. The other parts of the intestinal canal were healthy. Both kidneys were somewhat lobulated externally, and, when incised, the cortical portion presented a slightly granular appearance; the apices of some of the pyramids seemed somewhat indurated and fibrous. The spleen and stomach were healthy.

240. *The former subject of rheumatism. — Dilatation of the left ventricle. — Disease of the mitral valve. — Much thickening of the endocardium. — An aneurismal sac at the apex.—Also the marks of former pericarditis.*—Shamoo, a female, forty years of age, a Hindoo milk-seller, a native of Aurungabad, and resident a month in Bombay, was admitted into the Jamsetjee Jejeebhoy Hospital on the 7th August, 1852. The face was puffed; the feet and legs œdematous; the respiration short and hurried; the skin coldish; and the pulse small, and easily compressed. The præcordial dulness extended vertically from the second intercostal space to the margin of the left false ribs, and transversely from the right border of the sternum to beyond the left nipple. The impulse of the heart was feeble. There was a faint systolic murmur, most distinct at the apex. At the base the sounds were confused, but the murmur was hardly audible. The abdomen was rather full, and was dull on percussion for about three inches below the right false ribs and the sternum, where there was uneasiness on pressure. She stated that three years before she had suffered from rheumatism, and that fifteen days before admission there had been a severe febrile accession, preceded by chills, which continued for three days, and was followed by œdema of the legs, and uneasiness of the abdomen. She continued with little change in the symptoms, and died on the morning of the 11th August.

Inspection three hours after death.—Chest.—Eight ounces of reddish serum were found in the pericardium. The heart was considerably enlarged. There were opaque patches on the anterior surface of the right ventricle, and at the apex of the heart there was a patch the size of a dollar, of thick organised areolar tissue, somewhat reddened, adherent firmly to the surface of the heart, but forming no adhesion with the inner surface of the pericardium. The left ventricle was much dilated, and the walls were in places somewhat thickened. The endocardium of the posterior surface of the left ventricle was converted into an opaque thick membranous layer, with here and there cacoplastic yellow deposit, about two lines in thickness. There were also opaque thickened patches of the endocardium of the anterior surface. At the apex there was a pouch in the thickened endocardium, large enough to hold a walnut, corresponding to the patch of adventitious tissue on the external surface; the muscular covering of the pouch was much thinned. The mitral valve was opaque and thickened, not ossified. The aorta and valves were healthy. There was no dilatation of the right ventricle, and the valves were healthy. The lungs were healthy and crepitating. The body was not further examined.

In six there was both *aortic* and *mitral valvular disease*, in six disease of the *mitral valve* only, in two of the *aortic valves* alone, and in one * of the *pulmonary semi-lunar valves.*

The co-existence of dilatation of both or one of the ventricles of the heart, with various stages of valvular disease has been shown.

In nine cases the existence of former pericarditis was proved by the presence of *opaque patches on the surface of the heart;* and in two of these adhesion between the pericardium and the surface of the heart also existed.

* Case 236.

In six there was in the *opaque condition of the endocardium* of the left ventricle evidence of previous endocarditis.

Both the pericardium and endocardium had been affected in five cases.

In five there was *effusion of serum* exceeding two ounces, in the sac of the pericardium.

In the following case *rupture of the left ventricle of the heart* had taken place: the muscular fibre had probably undergone *fatty degeneration.*

241. *Rupture of the heart from fatty degeneration.* — John Amarago, a sailor, fifty-five years of age, was admitted into the Jamsetjee Jejeebhoy Hospital on the 6th March, 1852, with bronchitic symptoms. The pulse was soft, and rather full, and there was some heat of skin. He died suddenly and unexpectedly the day after admission, no information having been obtained in regard to his previous history.

Inspection. — The pericardium was distended with bloody serum, mixed with clots. The left ventricle was ruptured longitudinally in two places, about an inch apart from each other, in the upper and outer part of the ventricle. The fissures were one an inch, the other half an inch in length; one extended through the substance of the wall of the ventricle, and opened into the cavity obliquely; the other was a rupture of the external fibres only. The walls of the ventricle were somewhat thickened, but there was not any dilatation of the cavity. Over the right ventricle there was more than the usual amount of adipose tissue, and in two situations in the substance of the left ventricle were two distinct, defined, light yellow, granular-looking patches, occupying half the thickness of the wall, The aortic valves were healthy. There were points of deposit on the inner surface of the ascending aorta.

Remarks. — Though unfortunately a microscopic examination was neglected, there can be no doubt that the heart in this case was affected with fatty degeneration.

In three cases there was *dilatation* of the ascending portion of the aorta, and in one the aorta was *contracted.* In three there were thickened patches *of athermatous deposit* on the inner surface of the aorta.

In two cases there was *aneurism* of the thoracic, and in one of the abdominal aorta. One of the former and the latter are here detailed.*

* I find in my notes the following two additional cases of aneurism of the aorta, observed subsequent to my return to India; also one of perforation of the aorta and death by hæmorrhage.

1. A Hindoo admitted in November 1856. There was much dyspnœa; considerable tumefaction with dulness at the epigastrium. The dulness extended above the ensiform cartilage. There was dulness of the right dorsal region; clearness but absence of breath sounds in the right lateral and mammary regions. Dulness on percussion at the sternal end of the right subclavian region, with pulsation there greater than at the heart, with single murmur at times, but disappearing when the pulse at the wrist was faint. No abnormal cardiac sounds detected, but the heart action was feeble. No difference of pulse. He died thirty-six hours after admission.

Inspection.—The upper lobe of the right lung was displaced by a large aneurismal dilatation, the size of the fist, involving the whole of the ascending aorta, stopping at the arch and not affecting the vessels given off from it. The aortic orifice was

242. *Great dilatation of the ascending aorta and the arch. — An aneurismal tumour at the commencement of the descending aorta. — There was no external swelling, but the other signs of the disease were well marked.* — Sungoor Seedee, a Mussulman sailor, an inhabitant of Bahrein, and of African extraction, forty-one years of age, was admitted into the clinical ward on the 9th January, 1849. He was somewhat reduced in strength, and the respiration was rather short and hurried, and easiest in the sitting posture. There was no marked dulness of the chest. He had occasional cough, with scanty muco-puriform expectoration. Sonorous rale was audible in the left scapular region, but elsewhere the vesicular respiration was good. There was no increased impulse of the heart at the præcordial region, and the two sounds were distinct, but from the third rib upwards in the line of the sternum, inclining to the right towards the sternal junction of the right clavicle, there was a heaving impulse, very evident under the stethoscope, indistinctly so to the hand, attended with a single sound, but no murmur. When in the recumbent posture, there was occasional wheezing observable in the respiration. The pulse at the left wrist was 104 in the sitting posture, and of good strength; the pulse at the right wrist, and in the right carotid artery, was imperceptible. The abdomen was soft; the tongue was moist and clean; no difficulty

---

enlarged; the valves slightly thickened. There was inadequacy of the valves, from increased size of the orifice. Hypertrophy with dilatation of the left ventricle—dilatation of the right. Congestion of posterior parts of the lungs. Much congestion of the liver, which explained the epigastric fulness.

2. Balloo Krishna, a Hindoo labourer, twenty-eight years of age, was under treatment for supposed pleuritis in the early part of November 1856. He was discharged, and some days afterwards when sleeping exposed, he became affected with great dyspnœa, and was again admitted on the 28th November. There was urgent orthopnœa, with the face and trunk bent forwards. The dyspnœa, always great in degree, increased in paroxysms, and was attended with muco-puriform expectoration. The voice was feeble, and there was some difficulty of deglutition. The pulse feeble; the skin coldish. No disease of the heart or aorta detected, though carefully sought for. He experienced slight relief from the cautious inhalation of chloroform in small quantities. He died on the 7th December.

Inspection.—An aneurismal tumour, the size of a hen's egg, communicating by an opening, the size of a rupee, with the posterior wall of the aorta at the commencement of the arch, was found crossed obliquely by the innominate artery, and also by the left carotid and subclavian, both displaced somewhat to the left. The sac was filled with a coagulum, from which a fibrinous band extended down the ascending aorta into the left ventricle. The inner surface of the ascending aorta was roughened and thickened from atheromatous deposit. Some dilatation of the left ventricle. No other cardiac disease. There was congestion of the liver, and the thin edges of the lungs were solidified from collapse.

A curious case of perforation of the aorta was kindly communicated to me by Dr. Crawford, who also allowed me to examine the morbid structures:—

3. A soldier of the 18th Royal Irish swallowed a piece of chicken bone—came to hospital—pain at lower part of sternum, and symptoms of gastric irritation; very little difficulty of swallowing. On the sixth day profuse hæmatemesis and death.

Inspection.—A narrow (two lines broad) piece of bone, one and a half inch long, very pointed and sharp, lay in a sloughy depression, two inches long, three quarters wide, of the lower and back part of the œsophagus; it had penetrated the aorta. The sloughy state extended to the tissues between the œsophagus and aorta, but had not reached to those of the aorta. Under an effort of vomiting, the sharp point impacted vertically in the mucous membrane, had penetrated the aorta, then a process of ulceration and sloughing, by which the bone was loosened, and hæmorrhage the consequence.

in deglutition. When sitting he experienced uneasiness at the epigastrium; when recumbent the uneasiness extended over the chest and shoulders. He had first observed these symptoms two months before he came under observation, and they had gradually increased. He attributed his illness to his having often been obliged to lift heavy weights on board ship. During his stay in hospital, his nights were restless; he had occasional cough, and uneasiness about the sternum. On the 13th there was a slight murmur audible at the top of the sternum, but it was not again heard. Decubitus was easiest on the right side. He complained of difficulty of swallowing on the 25th, and there was some degree of febrile excitement. The breathing became disturbed, and the pulse feeble. He gradually sank and died, without any marked change in the symptoms, on the 30th January.

Inspection twenty-five hours after death.—*Chest.*—Just above the semi-lunar valves the aorta became dilated to about four times its natural calibre. The dilatation involved the ascending aorta, the arch, and commencement of the descending aorta; it included all the coats of the artery, with probably an exception at the commencement of the descending aorta, where there seemed to be a separate pouch, closely adherent to the bodies of the fourth, fifth, and sixth dorsal vertebræ, and filled by firm and fibrinous coagula. In the ascending portion of the aorta there was a loose coagulum, and at the commencement of the arteria innominata there was thickening, with irregularity of the surface of the lining membrane. The dilated arch of the aorta pressed upon the trachea just above its bifurcation. The dilated pouch at the commencement of the descending aorta made pressure on the œsophagus. The lower lobe of the left lung adhered by recent adhesions to the costal pleura, and hepatised nodules were felt on pressing it. The heart was healthy.

243. *Aneurism of the abdominal aorta.*—*Death by rupture.*—Soorga Chunderbund, a Mahratta washerman, forty years of age, in the habit of smoking tobacco and drinking moderately, was admitted into the clinical ward on the 21st March, 1848. He was considerably reduced in flesh; the countenance was anxious; and he moved about with a stooping gait. In the epigastric region, chiefly, but not altogether, to the left of the median line, reaching to the umbilicus, and extending below the arch of the left false ribs, from the ensiform cartilage downwards, there was a round indistinctly circumscribed swelling, becoming more prominent on decubitus on the right side. The swelling was strongly pulsating anteriorly and laterally, but there was no bruit audible under the stethoscope. In the rest of the abdomen, along the margin of the right ribs and the ensiform cartilage, and in the left hypochondrium above the upper margin of the tumour, the sound was tympanitic on percussion. The action and sounds of the heart were natural. He complained of pain of the loins, of impaired appetite, and uneasiness after food. The pulse was somewhat full, and the bowels slow. He stated that about a year previously, whilst engaged in ironing clothes, he felt a slight pain, first at the epigastrium, and that six months after he perceived a small pulsating swelling, which gradually attained the size which it presented on his admission. He died suddenly the day after admission.

Inspection eight hours after death.—There was a large quantity of blood (several pints) between the layers and at the root of the mesentery. Just below the superior mesenteric artery, and extending below the giving off of the renal arteries, there arose from the anterior surface of the aorta a tumour larger than a goose's egg, filled with coagula, and ruptured at its apex, which extended between the folds of the mesentery. The vena cava was pushed before the tumour, and was apparently compressed.

Of the seventeen cases examined after death, the state of the *lungs* is not mentioned in the report of two. In six there was *congestion* of part of the lungs: five of these were cases in which there was dilatation of both ventricles, and one dilatation with hypertrophy of the left ventricle. In five there was *œdema* of the lungs, and in all of them dilatation of both ventricles was present. In four there was more or less serous effusion into the sacs of the pleura, and in these there was also dilatation of both ventricles; in three the pleural effusion was associated with œdema of the lungs. In five, old pleural adhesions existed. In two there were *hepatised nodules* here and there in the substance of the lungs. In one *tubercles* existed; in one *emphysema*. In one the lungs were reported to be healthy. In these statements we find the relation between congestion of the lungs, serous effusion into the sacs of the pleura, or into the pulmonary air cells, and heart disease, well illustrated.

Cases not fatal in hospital. — There were thirteen of this class: two, as already stated, were believed to prove fatal shortly after the patients were discharged.

Of these thirteen cases, in eight there was hypertrophy and dilatation of the left ventricle.

In seven there was mitral valvular disease, in one aortic valvular disease, in one disease of the tricuspid valve, and in one aneurism of the arch of the aorta.

II. *Relation to difference of sex.* — Of the twenty-four cases, there are only three females. The observations made under this head, in reference to pericarditis and endocarditis, are equally applicable to the present division of the subject (p. 564).

III. *Proportion of cases in the different castes.* — Of the thirty-one persons, fifteen were Hindoos, nine Mussulmans, six Christians, and one a Parsee. On comparing this statement with the corresponding one in the preceding chapter* it will be observed that the proportions of Hindoos and Christians are very similar, but those of Mussulmans and Parsees are altogether opposed. This result makes it evident that the data have been too limited to justify any general conclusion on this point.

IV. *Classification with reference to age.* — The ages were as follows: —

From 10 to 20	3
„ 21 „ 30	10
„ 31 „ 40	11
„ 41 „ 50	5
„ 51 „ 60	1
„ 61 „ 70	1
	31

* Page 564.

The lowest age was fourteen, and the highest sixty-five. Between the ages of fourteen and thirty there were thirteen cases, and of these, five were in individuals who were reported to have suffered from rheumatism. Between the ages of thirty-one and forty there were eleven cases, and of these, four had been affected with rheumatism. Between the ages of forty-one and fifty there were five cases, and of these, two had suffered from rheumatism. Of the two cases between fifty-one and sixty-five, one had also been affected with rheumatism.

When we compare this statement with that under the same head relative to pericarditis and endocarditis *, we find that in the present, the range is considerably more extensive — it is between the ages of fourteen and sixty-five instead of seventeen and fifty. We observe, also, that the cases below twenty are considerably fewer — less than one half; that between twenty-one and thirty they are also less numerous, but between thirty-one and forty the proportion is more than double.

Of the thirty-one cases, twenty-one occurred between the ages of twenty-one and forty, and of these, nine had suffered from rheumatism; of the remaining ten cases, three had suffered from rheumatism.

V. *The different occupations of the affected.* — Excluding the three females, and four whose occupations are not mentioned, the remaining may be classed in the following manner: —

Sailors.	9	Servants	4
Labourers	4	Beggar	1
Horsekeepers	2	Plasterer	1
Washermen	2	Tailor	1
	17		7=24

There may be observed in this statement the same relation between probable exposure to cold and wet and heart affections, as was noted relative to these influences, and pericarditis and endocarditis: the reason is evident. But there is another point of interest in the etiology of heart disease, which is also illustrated — the frequency of the affection in individuals whose occupations require active muscular exertion. Of the twenty-four cases, the seventeen in the first column were thus circumstanced, and it is worthy of note that of the three cases of aortic aneurism, two occurred in washermen †, the third in a sailor.

* Page 566.

† It is unnecessary to state for the information of the Indian reader, but it may be for that of the European, that the method of clothes-washing in India necessitates considerable, violent muscular exertion of the arms and upper parts of the body.

VI. *Relation to habits of life.*—The habits of only twelve are mentioned: of these four were not addicted to the use of spirits, but eight were; four of them were Hindoos, two Mussulmans, one Parsee, one native Christian.

VII. *Relation to the months of the year.*—The admissions occurred in the following months:—

2 in January	4 in July
2 „ February	4 „ August
3 „ March	5 „ September
1 „ April	0 „ October
0 „ May	4 „ November
2 „ June	4 „ December.

As regards structural disease of the heart *itself*, it is not probable that we shall find any connection between admission into hospital and the season of the year. But when we recollect that admission is generally sought for relief from the secondary affections—dropsical effusions, and bronchitic attacks—we may be prepared to find the same relation between cold and wet and admission for heart disease, that we found to obtain between these states of the weather and pericarditis and endocarditis.* This statement confirms such expectation; eleven cases were admitted in the cold months of November, December, January, and February, and fifteen in the wet months of July, August, and September; in the hot months of April, May, and October only one case was admitted.

VIII. *Relation of the structural changes to Pericarditis, Endocarditis and Rheumatism.*— Excluding the three cases of aortic aneurism, and confining my observations to the twenty-eight cases of heart-disease, it appears that the existence or not of previous rheumatism has been stated of twenty cases; of these twelve had experienced, but eight never, an attack of this disease.

IX. *Relation to Bright's disease of the kidney.*—There are seventeen cases in which examination of the body after death was made: in seven of them the condition of the kidneys is not mentioned; of the ten remaining cases, in six the kidneys were healthy; in four there was some degree of Bright's disease, but in none had it proceeded to any great extent. This statement, so far as it goes, shows a more frequent association of structural disease of the heart and Bright's disease, than the corresponding one in the preceding chapter† did between this affection of the kidney and pericarditis and endocarditis. In my notice of Bright's disease‡, it appeared that cardiac disease had been noted in six

* Page 566. † Page 567. ‡ Page 482.

cases. Thus, we have an aggregate of ten cases in which these two affections were combined. But in four, the cardiac disease was fairly traceable to rheumatism; and in the remaining six, though rheumatism was not mentioned in the history, yet the evidences of pericarditis and endocarditis were found after death, and the kidney-disease was apparently of later date than the heart-disease. Therefore my cases do not tend to confirm the relation of antecedence and sequence between Bright's disease and disease of the heart.

X. *The leading symptoms and signs.*—*Dyspnœa.*—The breathing was somewhat short and hurried in twenty cases. Of these, thirteen were fatal: in eleven there was dilatation of both ventricles, in one dilatation and hypertrophy of the left ventricle, and in one hypertrophy of the right ventricle. In three of the fatal cases the lungs were found more or less congested after death, in five there was œdema, in one pleural effusion, in one emphysema, in one old pleuritic adhesions, in one the lungs were reported to be healthy, and in one there was no note of the appearances. Thus in eight of the twelve cases the dyspnœa was accounted for by the presence of pulmonary congestion or œdema.

Of the ten cases not fatal, there was in seven, it was believed, dilatation with hypertrophy of the left ventricle and disease of the mitral valve, in two there was disease of the aortic valves, and in the third of the tricuspid valve.

From these data, it would appear that dyspnœa has been generally associated with dilatation of the ventricles, and consequent congestion and œdema of the lungs.

Dropsical symptoms were more or less present in sixteen cases: of these ten were fatal; in nine of them dilatation of both ventricles, in one dilatation and hypertrophy of the left ventricle were found after death. In the six not fatal there was dilatation and hypertrophy of the left ventricle, and disease of the mitral valve.

We find, in this statement, a close relation between dropsical symptoms and conditions of the heart which must involve more or less systemic venous obstruction.

Præcordial pain was not noted in any case.

Pain below the margin of the right ribs was present in six, and was attended with dulness on percussion in the same situation. In four there was dilatation of both ventricles, and in two dilatation and hypertrophy of the left ventricle. The pain and abnormal dulness were undoubtedly due to congestion of the liver. These symptoms are practically important from the risk of mistaking them for indications of hepatic inflammation. This error was committed in one instance, and I am satisfied that the caution now given is not uncalled for. (See p. 529.)

Scapular pain was present in one case, in which aneurism of the left ventricle was found after death.

Character of the pulse.—The state of the pulse is distinctly noted in eighteen cases. In fourteen it was *small:* of these, there was disease of the mitral valve alone in nine, of both aortic and mitral valves in three, of the aortic valves alone in one, and of the pulmonary semi-lunar valves in one. The pulse was reported to be *irritable* in two cases: in one there was disease of both mitral and aortic valves—in the other of the mitral valve alone, and in this case the pulse was also sometimes characterised as small. It was *jerking* in nine cases; of these, four were fatal, and in all there had been diastolic murmur during life, and aortic valvular disease was found after death; of the five not fatal, there was diastolic murmur in three. In the remaining two the jerking pulse was noted only at the left wrist—it was small at the right; in one dilatation of the aorta was suspected, in the other this character might have been due to the anæmic condition of the patient, for it had ceased before he left the hospital. The pulse was *intermitting* in one case, and in this there was disease of the mitral valve, dilated aortic orifice, and ventricular aneurism. In two cases the pulse was *irregular:* in one there was aortic and mitral valvular disease, and in the other mitral disease alone.

From this statement it appears that smallness is the character of pulse generally met with in cardiac valvular lesion, and that it may be held to indicate mitral regurgitation, or obstructive aortic disease. In four of the cases in which the pulse was jerking, the existence of aortic regurgitation was not only made clear, by the discovery of aortic valvular affection after death, but also by the presence of aortic diastolic murmur during life. In three of the cases not fatal, diastolic murmur was present, and hence aortic valvular regurgitation was diagnosed.

In my observations on the pulse in the preceding chapter*, I have pointed to the rarity of an intermitting pulse in pericarditis and endocarditis; and now in the cases of structural disease, we find this character of pulse present only in one. The pulse, then, has been observed to intermit in only two of fifty-six cases of varied affections of the heart. It is therefore evident, that intermittence

* Page 569.

of the pulse is a symptom of little value in the diagnosis of cardiac disease.

Præcordial fulness was noted in only one case, in which there was dilatation of both ventricles, hypertrophy of the left, and disease of the aortic and mitral valves.

There was *increased impulse* of the heart in thirteen cases—of these eight were fatal: in six of them there was dilatation of both ventricles, and hypertrophy of the left, in one dilatation of both ventricles, with aneurism of the left, and in one hypertrophy of the right ventricle. In the five not fatal, there was probably—judging from the præcordial dulness—dilatation and hypertrophy of the left ventricle.

There was abnormal *præcordial dulness* noted in twenty-two cases: of these twelve proved fatal, and in nine of them there was dilatation of both ventricles, in two dilatation and hypertrophy of the left ventricle, and in one hypertrophy of the right ventricle.

Of the ten cases not fatal, there was in eight believed to be dilatation and hypertrophy of the left ventricle, in one dilatation of the right ventricle, and in one aortic valvular disease, with, probably, some degree of dilatation of the left ventricle.

In twelve there was *increased dulness below the margin of the right ribs.* Of these, seven were fatal: in five there was dilatation of both ventricles, and in two dilatation and hypertrophy of the left ventricle alone. In three of these cases the condition of the liver after death is not mentioned, in two it was increased in size and the substance mottled red and white from congestion, in one there was mottling but no increase of size, and in one there was no increase of size noted but tendency to cirrhosis. Of the five cases of hepatic dulness, not fatal, in four there was dilatation and hypertrophy of the left ventricle, and in the other dilatation of the right ventricle. Under this head might also have been included a case in which there was dulness below the margin of the right ribs, from displacement of the liver downwards by pleuritic effusion.

*Character of the murmur.**—There was *a mitral systolic mur-*

* It is very necessary, more particularly in native hospitals, to remember the fact of anæmic cardiac murmurs, so as to avoid errors in diagnosis. The state of constitution, the basic systolic character of the murmur, the absence of præcordial dulness, the occasional presence of venous hum, and the disappearance of the sound with improvement in the general system, ought in general to suffice. I do not allude to this subject without good reason. About three years ago, cardiac disease was reported to be very common among the native workmen at Aden. Then followed a period of wonder and

mur alone observed in ten cases, and of these the termination was fatal in five. There was found after death in one slight thickening of the mitral valve and aneurismal dilatation close to it, in one the mitral valve was thickened, and permitted regurgitation and an aneurismal pouch existed between this valve and the apex of the heart, in one there was no thickening of the mitral valve but the auriculo-ventricular opening was of greater than natural diameter and must have permitted regurgitation, in one the mitral valve was opaque and thickened with an aneurismal pouch at the apex of the heart, and in one there was general thickening of the mitral valve with ossific deposit chiefly at the free margin. In all these cases the aortic valves were healthy.

There was in three cases a *mitral systolic and a diastolic murmur:* the result was fatal in one, and much thickening of the mitral valve was found after death. In this case there was also an aortic systolic murmur, and disease of the aortic valves.

There was a *mitral systolic and diastolic murmur, with both sounds of the heart audible at the base,* observed in three cases: one, narrated below, proved fatal, and much ossific thickening of the mitral valve and some degree of thickening of the aortic valves were found after death.

244.—*Acute rheumatism.—Pericarditis, and endocarditis.—Dilatation of the right side of the heart.—Dilatation and hypertrophy of the left ventricle.—Ossific state of the mitral valve.—Hepatic congestion.*—Mahadoo Ruggoo, aged twenty-four, a Hindoo labourer, of originally robust frame, a native of Sattara, but resident in Bombay for a period of three years, following the occupation of a boatman, addicted to the use of spirits for a year, was admitted into the clinical ward on the 10th August, 1849. About twelve months before, consequent on exposure to wet and cold, he became affected with febrile symptoms, pain and swelling of the large joints, succeeded by uneasiness of the chest, dyspnœa, and cough. The pectoral symptoms and the affection of the joints had continued more or less. On admission, the breathing was short and hurried; the pulse irregular and feeble; the skin of natural temperature; the bowels reported to be regular. The only abnormal dulness of the chest was of the præcordial region—it reached from the third to the seventh rib, vertically, and transversely from the left border of the sternum external to the nipple. The impulse of the heart was feeble; the sounds were distinct, but distant, and there was no murmur. Dry bronchitic rales, with occasional crepitus, were heard here and there throughout both lungs. The abdomen was full, but not resistant. There was dulness on percussion two inches below the margin of the right ribs, and midway between the ensiform cartilage and the umbilicus, and uneasiness was complained of on pressure of the dull parts. With little alteration in these symptoms, he continued till the 2nd of September, when the impulse of the heart was observed to be somewhat increased,

---

correspondence and the final solution, that anæmic had been mistaken for organic murmur. The mistake was the less excusable, because the tendency to a scorbutic taint had always existed more or less in the Indian native troops and workmen at Aden.

and a distinct rough murmur was audible just below the nipple, external to it, and obscuring both the sounds of the heart; but the sounds of the heart were both heard at the third costal cartilage and upwards. The cough, the dyspnœa, pain of joints from time to time, the heart signs last noted, the bronchitic rales, and occasional crepitus, the hepatic dulness and tenderness, with occasionally pale intestinal evacuations, continued with little change, and on the 20th September there were added puffiness of the face, œdema of the feet and ankles, and some degree of drowsiness. At this time cholera was prevalent in Bombay, and this patient became affected for several days with vomiting and watery purging, and considerable collapse, during which the dropsical symptoms much decreased. They recurred on cessation of the purging; the dyspnœa continued; he became delirious and drowsy, and died comatose on the 5th October. The cardiac murmur was last heard on the 1st October. The urine was frequently tested; at first it was free and of low density; latterly it was scanty; it never showed any trace of albumen. Leeches were on one or two occasions applied to the epigastrium, and blisters to the præcordial region. An attempt was made to induce the constitutional effect of mercury, but it was necessary to desist, in consequence of the irritable state of the bowels. The rest of the treatment consisted of diuretics, or stimulants, or depressants, according to the indications.

Inspection nine hours after death. — *Head.* — The inner surface of the scalp was slightly tinged yellow. The brain and the membranes were not congested with blood, and were in every respect healthy. There was about one ounce and a half of serous fluid at the base of the brain. *Chest.*—The lungs did not collapse very freely. In places there were a few bands of recent adhesion between the costal and pulmonary pleuræ, and there was very little serous effusion in the sacs of the pleura. The situation of the heart corresponded to the dull space noted on admission. The pericardium contained about five ounces of serum, but there was no perceptible alteration in the appearance of its serous surface. The heart was larger than natural; its serous covering to a considerable extent, particularly over the right ventricle, presented an opaque appearance, but nowhere were there traces of recent lymph; a considerable quantity of dark coloured liquid blood flowed from the divided vessels of the right side; the right ventricle was considerably dilated; the tricuspid and pulmonary valves were healthy; the left ventricle was dilated, and its walls, perhaps, of little more than natural thickness, the mitral valve was converted into a thick ossific irregular mass, and the aortic valves were somewhat thickened but not by earthy deposit. The ascending aorta and the arch were narrower, and their coats somewhat more attenuated than natural. The left auricle was considerably dilated, and yellow opaque patches, somewhat raised above the surface, were seen on its serous covering. The posterior part of the left lung was very much congested, and somewhat indurated, but not distinctly hepatised. There were several red indurated nodules, the largest the size of an egg, in different parts of the right lung, especially in the upper lobe. *Abdomen.*—About a pint of dark-coloured serous fluid was found in the peritoneal cavity. The liver was almost of natural size; when incised, it presented a mottled red and buff-coloured appearance, and was somewhat indurated. The kidneys were healthy.

Remarks.—This case is of interest in many points of view. The heart-disease was clearly related to an attack of acute rheumatism. On admission, a faulty diagnosis was formed from the presence, but faintness, of the sounds of the heart, and the absence of all murmur. The dulness of the præcordial region, and the feeble pulse, were attributed to pericardial effusion. Increased bulk of the heart and disease of the valves were not suspected. Again, when increased impulse of the heart, with a rough murmur at the nipple, obscuring both sounds of the heart, were noted, a fresh accession of pericarditis, with lymph effusion, was suspected — for I was not then aware of what this case and subsequent ones have since taught me, that a mitral murmur may obscure both sounds at the apex, but leave them distinct at the base.

There was *aortic systolic murmur alone* in one case; also *diastolic* murmur in one. Neither were fatal.

Aortic systolic and diastolic murmur was present in four cases, and in all the result was fatal: in one the aortic valves were diseased, and the mitral healthy; in one the aortic valves were much thickened, the mitral valve also, and in this, as already mentioned, a mitral systolic and a diastolic murmur were also present; in one there were warty-like deposits of lymph on the aortic valves, with disease of the mitral valve, but no mitral murmur had been recognised during life; in one the aortic valves were thickened, and the orifice patulous, and there was very slight disease of the mitral valve. In three of these cases the pulse was jerking; in one it was small.

The sounds of the heart were confused, without distinct murmur, in three cases, both fatal: in one there was hypertrophy and dilatation of the left ventricle, with disease of the mitral and aortic valves,—but the murmurs were not heard, on account of the disturbed and laboured action of the heart. In the other there was considerable dilatation of the cavities of both sides, and some thickening of the aortic and mitral valves.

These statements support the opinions generally entertained in regard to cardiac murmurs. They show the relation between murmurs best heard at the base, and aortic valvular disease, and that of murmurs best heard at the apex, and mitral valvular disease. The fact that a mitral murmur obscuring both sounds at the apex may co-exist with audible first and second sounds at the base was first taught me by case 244. I am not acquainted with any writer on the physical signs of heart-disease who states this fact, with the exception of Dr. Walshe.* The case to which I have just referred occurred to me some time before the publication of this excellent work. The fact that a mitral murmur may co-exist with audible first and second sounds at the base is not only of diagnostic value, but seems to me to favour those views of the sources of the sounds of the heart which do not attribute much of the first sound to tension of the mitral valve. The sounds of the heart being confused, and murmur being absent, though valvular disease is present, is practically important as regards the diagnosis of cases first submitted to observation in very advanced stages, when the feebly acting heart is oppressed and transmits imperfectly the blood through the orifices.†

* Walshe on the Diseases of the Lungs and Heart, pp. 223—226.

† Dr. Stokes, in his Treatise on Diseases of the Heart and Aorta, has some excel-

Præcordial thrill was observed in only two cases: one proved fatal; and there was hypertrophy and dilatation of the left ventricle with aneurism, and mitral valvular disease. The other was not fatal, and mitral valvular disease was believed to be present.

XI. *Medical treatment.*—Dilatation of the cavities, hypertrophy of the muscular fibre of the heart, associated with structural change of the valves, is an incurable form of disease. All that we can attempt is to regulate the bodily and mental states in such manner as shall maintain the actions of the heart as unembarrassed as possible; and to remove, by appropriate means, the secondary dropsical and bronchitic affections when they occur. The only practical points to which I shall advert are,—1. The signal benefit frequently derived, under failing action of the heart in valvular disease, from preparations of iron, and the free assiduous use of ammonia and other stimulants. I have witnessed several cases in which imminent peril was averted, and life prolonged, by these means. On the other hand, I have never met with a case of confirmed valvular disease in which *digitalis* or other sedatives were not distinctly contra-indicated; and I look upon the association which used to exist in the minds of practical men between digitalis and heart-disease as a very serious, and, I believe, now generally admitted, error in therapeutics.* 2. A comparison of the dropsical effusions from cardiac-disease, and those from Bright's disease, shows the greater scope for the exhibition of hydragogue cathartics and diuretics in the former. The following case is a good illustration of the efficacy of elaterium in this form of disease:—

245. *Aortic and mitral valvular disease. — Hypertrophy, with dilatation of the left ventricle.— General dropsy.—Rapid relief from elaterium.—Discharged.*—Moorbaruck Seedee, an African sailor, of twenty-five years of age, and large frame, but reduced by

lent observations on an error of another kind—that of mistaking the murmur of old-standing valvular disease for that depending on recent endocarditis. This involves a question of diagnosis, which should never be absent from the mind in the investigation of cardiac disease.

* The contents of this chapter were presented very much in their present form to the Medical and Physical Society of Bombay in 1852, and published in the first number of the second series of the Society's "Transactions." Since then, Dr. Stokes's work on the Diseases of the Heart has been published. The perusal of this admirable treatise has not suggested to me the expediency of, in any respect, modifying this analysis of my own clinical experience. In regard to the observation to which this note is referred—on the value of stimulants and the danger of depressants of the muscular fibre of the heart—I would direct the attention of the clinical student to the valuable practical principle on which Dr. Stokes insists in various passages of his work—that the important question in organic valvular disease is the quality of the action of the muscular fibre, *not* the mere condition of the valves.

sickness, was received, on the 3rd September, 1852, into the clinical ward. The face was puffed, and the breathing was short, hurried, and oppressed. There was general anasarca, a swollen and fluctuating abdomen, and shifting dulness on both sides of the chest to above the lower limit of the subclavian regions. The pulse was of moderate volume, of natural frequency, with a peculiar thrill. The præcordial dulness could not be distinguished from the general dulness. The impulse of the heart, though extended, was very feeble, and the apex beat two inches directly below the left nipple. Both sounds of the heart were obscured by murmurs; one, blowing, best heard at the base and in the line of the aorta; the other, musical, best heard at the apex and to its left. The only history he gave was, that ten months before, while on the voyage from Muscat to Aden, the dropsical symptoms came on and had persisted. He was treated for three days with elaterium, which acted well, and rapidly reduced the dropsical effusions. A diuretic of acetate of potass, spiritus ætheris nitrici, and tincture of squills, was then used. The urine increased to upwards of fifty ounces daily, and gave no trace of albumen. The dropsy was altogether removed, and he was discharged on the 18th September. The pulse had lost its thrilling feel, was of moderate volume, and compressible. The breathing was easy. The præcordial dulness extended from the lower margin of the third costal cartilage to the seventh rib, and from the median line to one vertical from the nipple. The two murmurs continued distinct, and possessed the same characters as on admission. The hepatic dulness reached upwards to the fifth rib, and inferiorly to a line extended from the tenth right to the seventh left rib.

He was re-admitted on the 16th November. The dropsical symptoms had returned, but not to the same degree. The cardiac signs were unchanged, but the pulse was feebler and again jerking, and bronchitic dry rhonchi were present. A similar course of treatment was followed again, with removal of the dropsy, and he was discharged on the 1st December. The pulse, however, had not resumed its former volume, and continued jerking. The mitral murmur had lost its musical character and become rough.

Remarks.—An African sailor, sailing along the coast of Arabia, becomes affected with general dropsy and marked symptoms of hydrothorax. This case a few years ago would have been called, in the language of Indian nosology, beriberi, and an air of mystery have been thus thrown over one of the simplest events in pathology.

SECTION II.—*In Europeans in India.*

Disease of the heart and aorta is not uncommon in Europeans in India. Many years ago Dr. R. H. Hunter*, in a series of interesting reports, addressed to the Medical and Physical Society of Bombay, directed the attention of the profession in India to the frequency of cardiac-disease in Her Majesty's 2nd or Queen's Royal Regiment, and suggested the probability that it was owing to undue parading in the tight thick dress of the European soldier, so unsuitable for the climate of India. At the period now referred to, I enjoyed the privilege of frequent communication with Dr. Hunter, and on many occasions had the opportunity of witnessing his cases, and appreciating the accuracy and care with

* "Transactions, Medical and Physical Society of Bombay," No. 1, p. 239; No. 2, p. 222; No. 5, p. 47.

which he diagnosed cardiac and pulmonary disease, at a time when the physical signs of these affections were not so well understood, or so generally studied, as at present.

In the European General Hospital also many instances of cardiac and aortic disease in sailors and others came under my observation. Seven of the former and two of the latter have been elsewhere detailed by me.*

The subject, however, requires further careful clinical and statistical investigation, for the following reasons:—

1. Dr. Gordon † is of opinion that disease of the heart bears an inconsiderable ratio to the admissions of acute ‡ rheumatism; but the exact ratio is not stated. He further thinks that the number of men invalided in consequence of disease of the heart in India, is not a tithe so large as in the United Kingdom. No precise data are given, but my own experience, as stated above, as well as subsequently, convinces me that the disease is not very unfrequent.

2. Facts for determining the ratio of heart-disease to acute rheumatism, and of invaliding from heart-disease in India, do not, I believe, as yet exist — not only from a want of clinical information on the disease itself, but also because cases are not unfrequently returned "Carditis," in which the derangement of the heart's action is merely functional. I make this latter statement with much confidence; not only of Europeans in the Indian army, but in the British army also. In respect to the former, I some years since satisfied myself by carefully examining the invalids sent to Bombay with "disease of the heart;" in several it did not exist: in respect to the latter — in 1857, 1858, and 1859 — when, as superintending surgeon at Poona, I weekly visited all the European hospitals at the station.

3. Palpitation, increased at night and by mental and physical excitement, without cardiac pain, dulness, or murmur, generally in pale young soldiers, is surely not unusual in hospitals in India, and is not unfrequently erroneously returned "carditis." It may often be traced to drinking or smoking in excess, to exposure to the sun, and to the debilitating effects of elevated temperature and frequent recurrences of fever or other forms of disease augmented by medical treatment unduly depressing. It is also sometimes

* "Transactions, Medical and Physical Society of Bombay," No. 6.

† "Indian Annals of Medical Science," No. 11, p. 7.

‡ The word "acute" does not occur in the passage adverted to, but it is evidently implied by the context; in fact, the question entirely rests upon it.

feigned. If these be the causes it necessarily follows, that the affection will vary much in different regiments: I am acquainted with some in which it was hardly known, and others in which it was very common.

Dr. Gordon remarks*: "As far as my experience goes, there is, as already stated, no want of care among medical officers in making minute examination of the cases under their care." To this statement a large part of my experience leads me cordially to assent; but there remains behind a portion which tells me that it is not invariably applicable.

It is on these grounds that I conclude, that, cardiac disease in Europeans in India has still to be clinically and statistically investigated.

* "Indian Annals of Medical Science," No. 11, p. 16.

CHAP. XXVI.

ON SUN-STROKE.*

THE influence of high atmospheric temperature in exciting or modifying febrile and other forms of disease, has been elsewhere explained in this work.† In the present chapter I propose to describe effects of direct or indirect solar heat—more immediate, often very urgent—which have less of the character of unmixed fever, and evince earlier and greater disturbance of the brain, the heart, and the lungs.

But as in inflammatory remittent, ardent continued fever, and the type compounded of these, there is often disturbance of the brain, heart, and lungs; and, as in sun-stroke, there is the heat of skin, the frequency of pulse and defective secretions, characteristic of fever,—difficulty has been sometimes experienced in drawing the line between fever and sun-stroke, and in keeping distinct the pathology, etiology, and therapeutics of these two forms of disease. In the first edition of this work sun-stroke was treated very briefly‡,

* Of the many names applied to this affection—insolation, coup de soleil, ictus solis, heat apoplexy, heat asphyxia, sun fever, calenture, erethismus tropicus—I have, after much consideration, selected the simplest, because it involves no pathological theory, and expresses merely, what all admit, that the chief exciting cause is great solar heat, direct or indirect, and that the attack is often sudden and dangerous.

† Pages 8, 57, 61, 81, 162, 164, 363, 437, 642, 650.

‡ Not only very briefly, but I fear, also, very unintelligibly, if I may judge from the manner in which my opinions have been misunderstood and misrepresented.

Mr. Scriven in a paper on "Sun Fever," in the 4th volume of the "Indian Annals of Medical Science," at pages 502 and 503, notices my remarks on the effects of elevated temperature, and misstates my opinions in the following instances:—

1. By combining statements in the 3rd chapter of the 1st volume on ardent continued fever with others in the 19th chapter of the 2nd volume on sun-stroke, he represents me to say, that, the blood is unduly heated in ardent fever, and that undue heating produces no chemical change of the blood. Whereas there is no allusion to a heated state of the blood in my chapter on ardent fever; and the manner in which "materies" is used, in contrasting the causes of remittent fever, and of ardent fever, must satisfy the most casual reader that a "materies" introduced from

because, though occasional cases occurring in my hospital practice had made me sufficiently familiar with the general clinical characters

without was referred to. The words are "in the former (ardent fever*) there is no 'materies' in the blood, as in the latter (remittent fever), exercising a sedative influence on vital actions and requiring time for elimination" (vol. i. p. 264). The only observation on undue heating of the blood, is in the following words at page 585 of the 2nd volume. "From a review of all the attendant circumstances, it seems to me not an unreasonable suggestion to offer that the temperature of the blood may become much increased, and that to this altered condition of the blood the deranged actions may in part be due."

2. Mr. Scriven writes: "Dr. Morehead I see still looks upon it (sun-stroke) as an inflammatory disease, and recommends early bleeding, tartar emetic, &c., and this too, under the head of diseases 'to the extreme degree' of which 'the terms coup de soleil, &c., have been given;' and amongst which he considers encephalitis and phrenitis may be included. On the post-mortem appearances, however, of those extreme cases in which the brain is found healthy, he does not touch, and, seems not to entertain the idea of such patients dying from cerebral syncope."

Whereas (*a*) the word "inflammation" is not once used in my remarks on sun-stroke. It was purposely avoided, because I do not consider the disease to be an inflammation. (*b*) The early bleeding and tartar emetic are recommended by me in ardent fever. The only allusion made to them in connection with sun-stroke, is in the following words. "In the commencement of the second degree" (that is the stage of cases of sun-stroke in which the pulse is frequent, full, and firm), "the same means are still indicated." (*c*) Blood-letting &c., are not recommended by me in the extreme degree of sun-stroke; on the contrary, my words are "but in the advanced stages of this degree (second), and in the third degree from its commencement when coma co-exists with a rapid feeble pulse, blood-letting, and free purging, if had recourse to, will necessarily expedite the fatal issue;" and again, "cold effusion frequently applied, and the exhibition when practicable of ammoniated stimulants, from time to time, are the means which hold out the fairest prospect of good." (*d*) The object of my incidental allusion to encephalitis or phrenitis is to express my belief, that, if there is such a disease as the phrenitis of Cullen in tropical climates, it is those occasional cases of sun-stroke in which the delirium is violent. The logical inference from my remarks is, not that sun-stroke is an inflammation but that the phrenitis of Cullen is not an inflammation. (*e*) The term cerebral syncope is not used by me, because I think it objectionable; but if it be implied that the depression of the action of the heart, and the tendency to death by syncope in extreme cases, are not recognised by me, I can only remark, that in the description of symptoms and treatment much prominence is given to them; indeed, in the latter, it is twice emphasised by italics. The words are, "as soon as the *impairment* of the cerebral functions sets in, the pulse begins to fail in strength, and when coma is fairly established it becomes small and rapid. In the most aggravated form, that in which there is coma at the outset, the pulse is small and rapid from the beginning. It appears then that co-existent with the *oppression* of the brain, there is always a marked sedative influence operating on the action of the heart."

To a medical writer, whose sole object ought to be to elicit truth, the free and fair criticism of others must always be very acceptable. But when he finds his opinions on important questions of pathology and treatment perverted by garbled references and inaccurate statements, it is a duty which he owes to himself and to the character of medical literature to enter his protest against the proceeding.

* This and other parenthetical passages in this note are not in the original text, but their introduction is necessary, to render the quotations intelligible when separated from the context.

of the disease, still it seemed to me inexpedient to enlarge upon my own limited experience, in a work professing to be chiefly the record of personal research. The late contingencies of public service in India have, however, enhanced the importance of sun-stroke as a disease of our armies; and my altered official position on my return to that country has afforded me the opportunity of collecting information, and thus in a measure participating in the experience of others. The following clinical history is drawn from these and other sources*, as well as from my own previous practical knowledge of the disease.

* The papers before me, to which chief attention has been given, are:—

1. A short sketch of the medical topography of the fortress of Bukkur, and the cantonment of Sukkur, &c., in 1839, by I. Don, M.D., staff surgeon. "Transactions, Medical and Physical Society of Bombay," No. 3.

2. Some remarks upon the climate of Sukkur in Upper Scinde, during the months of April, May, June, and July 1846, with an account of the fever prevailing there during these months, by N. Hefferman, M.B., H.M's 60th Rifles. "Transactions, Medical and Physical Society," No. 10.

3. Manuscript notes, by Dr. Crawford, 18th Royal Irish, on coup de soleil, as observed by him in H.M's 51st Regt., in operations at Rangoon, in April 1852, kindly lent for perusal.

4. Report of a board of medical officers, assembled by order of Major-General Sir Hugh Rose, K.C.B., commanding Central India Field Force, dated 18th May, 1858, to investigate circumstances connected with the death of several men of H.M's. 71st Highlanders, before Koonch, on the 7th May, 1858, as well as other points referred to in a letter from the superintending surgeon of the force No. 65 of 1858, dated 8th May, 1858, to the chief of the Staff. President: Surgeon A. Stewart, 14th Light Dragoons. Members: Surgeon W. Simpson, 7th Regt.; Assist. Surgeon O'Brien, 3rd Bombay European Regt.

5. Reports on coup de soleil in H.M's 71st Regt. (right wing) in Central India, 1858, by W. Simpson, M.D., Surgeon, H.M's. 71st Regt.

6. Cases of coup de soleil, in the 3rd European Regt., Central India Field Force, by T. W. W. Ward, Esq.

7. Cases of coup de soleil, at Shikarpoor, by Assistant Surgeon, A. K. Simpson, M.D.

8. Cases of coup de soleil, in the 3rd troop H. A., by Assistant Surgeon J. H. Wilmot, M.D. The last five papers are in the "Transactions, Medical and Physical Society, Bombay," No. 4, new series.

9. Major-General Sir Hugh Rose's despatch on the operations attending the capture of Calpee, dated Gwalior, 22nd June, 1858.

10. The summaries of twenty-seven cases fatal in Rajpootana and Central India kindly shown to the author by C. White, Esq., Deputy Inspector-General of hospitals in Bombay.

11. Manuscript report by Assistant Surgeon Lofthouse, 14th Light Dragoons, lent for the author's perusal, by the Deputy Inspector-General.

12. Queries issued to medical officers of the Central India Field Force, by Superintending Surgeon Arnott, with replies thereto from Assistant Surgeon Naylor, Field Hospital, Jhansi; Assistant Surgeon Lofthouse, 14th Light Dragoons; Surgeon Ward, B. European Regiment; Surgeon Ewing, 95th Regiment, and Assistant Surgeon Sylvester, forwarded by Dr. Arnott, for the author's perusal.

13. Manuscript report of the 25th Regiment, N.I. for the year 1858-9, while in Central India, by Dr. W. Stuart, Surgeon of the Regiment.

14. Manuscript case of an engineer at Kotra, in Scinde, by Assistant Surgeon Niven.

I shall class my remarks under the heads:—1. Symptoms. 2. Pathology. 3. Etiology. 4. Treatment.

SYMPTOMS. — When the various descriptions of sun-stroke are carefully considered, a want of uniformity in the symptoms is apparent; and when the investigation is still further pursued, it is evident that the discrepancy depends upon the circumstance that in sun-stroke the tendency to death is by three different ways: (1) by coma; (2) by syncope; (3) by coma and syncope combined. I shall succeed best in rendering the symptoms intelligible by describing those which, though not all present in every instance, may be regarded as typical of these three varieties, and then remarking more particularly on the phenomena which have chiefly attracted the attention of observers as characteristic of the disease.

With the view of rendering my own remarks more easily understood, and of obviating the necessity of frequent circumlocution, I shall designate the first variety—that in which there is death, or tendency to death, by coma—the *cerebro-spinal;* the second—that in which there is death, or tendency to death, by syncope—the *cardiac;* and the third—in which there is death, or tendency to death, by coma and syncope combined—the *mixed.*

1. *The cerebro-spinal variety.*—In this the premonitory symptoms are headache, more or less severe, delirium, tendency to drowsi-

15. Private notes on this and allied subjects, from Deputy Inspector-General W. M. Muir, M.D.

16. Remarks on the disease termed insolatio or heat apoplexy, with observations on its pathology by Marcus G. Hill, Officiating Assistant Garrison Surgeon, Calcutta. "Indian Annals of Medical Science," vol. iii. p. 188.

17. On Sun Fever, by J. B. Scriven, Esq. "Indian Annals of Medical Science," vol. iv. p. 496.

18. On erethismus tropicus, by J. R. Taylor, Esq., Deputy Inspector of Hospitals. "Lancet," 21st and 28th August, 1858.

19. Coup de soleil in India, by R. H. A. Hunter, Esq., 1st Class Staff Surgeon. "Medical Times and Gazette," December 18th, 1858.

20. On heat apoplexy, coup de soleil, or sun fever, by James Ranald Martin, Esq., F.R.S. "Lancet," 1st, 8th, and 15th January, 1859.

21. Heat apoplexy, summary of a report of sixteen cases in H.M's. Regiment, Barrackpore, by Thomas Longmore, Esq., Surgeon, 19th Regiment. "Lancet," March 26th, 1859.

22. On insolatio, sun-stroke, or coup de soleil, by W. Pirrie, M.D., Assistant Surgeon, H.M.'s 71st Regiment. "Lancet," May 20, 1859.

23. Brief notice of a paper on coup de soleil by Dr. Peet, Professor of Medicine, Grant Medical College. "Transactions, Medical and Physical Society of Bombay," No. 4, new series, Appendix, p. xxix.

24. Manuscript report on sun-stroke, occurring in K Battery, Royal Artillery, at Baroda, in May 1859.

Numbers 13 and 24 have since been published. "Transactions Medical and Physical Society," No. 5, new series.

ness, flushing of the face, increased vascularity of the conjunctivæ, and a dry hot skin. The pulse is accelerated, full, occasionally jerking, but generally easily compressed; there is much thirst, and the urine is scanty and high coloured, with sometimes a frequent desire to micturate. More or less of such symptoms as these may continue for some hours, and then, without further aggravation, may be gradually removed by appropriate treatment, or, after varying periods, sometimes, indeed, so transient as to escape notice, they assume the following characters:—The drowsiness increases, the pupils contract, convulsive twitching of the muscles is observed, the respiration becomes somewhat hurried and oppressed, the action of the heart is tumultuous, the pulse still frequent becomes smaller and more compressible, and the heat of skin increases in pungency. Now succeed coma and dilated pupils, sometimes preceded by convulsion; the respiration becomes more oppressed and slower, and often stertorous, the countenance swollen and livid, the action of the heart still tumultuous, but feebler, and the pulse rapidly sinks. Death may thus take place in from two to nine hours from the commencement of the attack, and the skin continues pungently hot to the close, and even for some time after death.

2. *Cardiac variety.*—Sometimes without premonitory warning, generally consequent on direct exposure to the sun, the individual falls down insensible, makes a few hurried gasping respirations, and instantly expires.* This is death by syncope. Or a sense of faintness and prostration is experienced, with vertigo, dimness of vision, dilated pupils, drowsiness, from which the patient may be roused by pinching, loud speaking, or sprinkling the face with water. There is constriction of the chest, with sighing respiration, a sense of weight or sinking at the epigastrium, with nausea and sometimes vomiting. The face and lips are pale, the skin is generally cold and clammy, with exception of the head, which is somewhat hot. The pulse is feeble, and generally slow. In a large proportion recovery will take place from these symptoms under judicious management; on the other hand the pulse may sink, the respiration become more sighing and irregular, and death result, sometimes preceded by convulsion.

3. *The mixed variety.*—The premonitory symptoms—of longer or shorter duration—are headache, delirium, drowsiness, vertigo, prostration with tendency to weep or to laugh on being questioned †; a sense of constriction of the chest, nausea, vomiting, palpitation, the pulse frequent, soft, small, and compressible; the countenance

* Dr. Pirrie. † Dr. Simpson.

is pale, the skin sometimes hot, at others rather cold. Such symptoms may be gradually recovered from, or aggravation may take place, characterised by convulsion, coma, oppressed breathing, lividity of lips and nails, failing pulse, a skin sometimes hot but moist, at others cold and clammy, with death, partly by coma, partly by syncope.

Remarks on some of the principal symptoms.—*Delirium* is sometimes present in the premonitory stage of the *cerebro-spinal* and *mixed* forms. It is occasionally though rarely violent, and when so, is generally of short duration; for, unless subdued, it speedily terminates in convulsion and coma.

Convulsion is liable to occur in all the forms, preceding the coma in the first and third, and occurring very shortly before death in the second.

Coma.—The insensibility of syncope, which attends more or less the *cardiac* variety, is pathologically distinct from the coma of the other two. It ceases with the reviving action of the heart, and does not return unless on a recurrence of the syncope. Recovery from incomplete coma, in the first and third forms, is not unfrequent; but such cases require to be watched with great care, for the tendency to relapse is great. The patient may have seemed alert in the comparative coolness of the morning, but as the day advances, the drowsiness may recur and pass into complete coma sometimes preceded by convulsion. Dr. Simpson truly observes,—"No patient can be considered out of danger till the skin becomes cool and moist." Recovery from complete coma would seem to be occasional, but rare. Dr. Taylor expresses himself with more confidence on this point than any other writer. In the cases which he witnessed at Ghazeepore in 1843, recovery from deep coma was rare; but in his subsequent experience at Rangoon in 1852, he found that in cases of insensibility, sometimes lasting from one to three hours, and in some instances attended with one or more epileptic fits or convulsions, cold affusion in the shade was successful—not one case terminated fatally. The difference he attributed to the treatment. At Ghazeepore there was copious abstraction of blood in all the cases;—at Rangoon blood-letting was abstained from, and cold affusion used.

The *pupils* are generally contracted when the drowsiness of the first and third forms is passing into coma, or when convulsion impends; but they become dilated when the coma is complete. There is also some degree of dilatation with the insensibility of the second form.

The *respiration* in the *cardiac* and *mixed* varieties has the irregular, gasping character of syncope, with a sense of constriction of the chest. Coincident with the coma of the first and third forms, the breathing becomes laboured and slow, and in cases in which the access of coma is speedy and complete, it is a striking symptom from the outset of the attack.

The *tumultuous action* of the heart—greatest in degree in the cerebro-spinal variety—is also present in the mixed, and is most marked in the stage of coma; but it is not then regarded merely as a consequence of the impeded pulmonary function, but as due to a more direct influence on the heart itself. This view is probably correct, because cardiac disturbance of this kind is not unfrequently observed as a single derangement, after undue exposure to solar heat: it very likely precedes in many cases the attack of the cardiac form.

The *pulse* is frequently full, sometimes firm, at the commencement of the first form, when the premonitory symptoms have been of considerable duration; but as the drowsiness advances it becomes compressible, and sinks as the coma increases. In the third variety, the pulse is wanting in volume and power from the very commencement; and in the second it is always small and often slow.

The peculiar, dry, pungent *heat* of skin is observed chiefly in the coma and premonitory stage of the cerebro-spinal and mixed forms; and is always in greatest degree in sthenic Europeans recently arrived from colder latitudes.

A cold clammy skin, usually, though I believe *not* invariably, attends the syncope of the cardiac form: it is also noticed sometimes in the mixed form, and in this too the skin is occasionally hot and moist. It is not improbable that in this latter form the skin will be hot and dry in Europeans recently arrived, as was the case in the 71st Regiment; but occasionally cold and clammy in natives, and asthenic Europeans long resident, as happened in the 14th Light Dragoons. Both these regiments suffered in Central India in the same field: the first had been only three months in India, having reached it by the overland route; the second had served about twenty years.

Colour of the skin.—During the premonitory stage of the first variety, the face is flushed and the general surface redder than natural, but when coma and oppressed breathing supervene, it becomes swollen, more or less purplish and finally livid. In the second variety, the face and general surface are pale. This is also often the case at the commencement of the third form, but in this, towards the close, when coma and dyspnœa are established, the lips and nails become purplish and livid.

Nausea and vomiting, preceded by giddiness and dimness of vision, are most common in the cardiac and mixed forms, and are related to the syncopal condition.

But as is well known, nausea and vomiting are also not unfrequently indications of cerebral disturbance. It is important to remember that in occasional cases of the cerebro-spinal form, the premonitory symptoms may be uneasiness of head, slight suffusion of the eyes, listlessness and fretfulness of manner, with irritability of stomach so great as almost exclusively to engage the attention of the observer. These are often perplexing. The vomiting is symptomatic of cerebral disturbance, and if it be rightly understood, and the appropriate remedies used, the result will be satisfactory; but a grave error will be committed if the principal derangement is overlooked, and the treatment directed to the secondary and sympathetic disorder.

The *bowels* are not affected with any characteristic derangement; they are often natural, sometimes constipated, at others relaxed. This last condition when present will in general, probably, be found to have preceded the attack of the second variety.

The *urine* is high coloured and scanty, in association with the increased heat and cerebral disturbance of the first and third forms. A frequent desire to micturate is sometimes a premonitory symptom, to which Mr. Longmore has specially called attention: in referring to it he very justly observes, "If this symptom should prove to be a general precursor of the attack it might be rendered valuable as an indication of the approaching danger, which, by early and proper care, might then probably be averted; and its presence at a time when heat apoplexy was prevalent would make the surgeon alert to obviate the more serious symptoms which might be expected to follow."

Convalescence.—In the milder attacks of the *cardiac* form, recovery, when no abiding state of debility is present, is often rapid. During the operations of the Central India Field Force in May and June 1858, it was not unusual for officers and men struck down to be recovered by cold affusion on the field and to return to duty.

The premonitory symptoms of the other two varieties, when slight and brought under treatment at the commencement, may be recovered from by two or three days of careful management. But when these symptoms have been greater in degree, or of longer duration, or have partially merged into those of the more advanced stages, then recovery may be characterised by prostration of strength, partial paralysis, blunted sensation, imperfect respiration, and deranged secretions.

PATHOLOGY.—The post-mortem appearances in the cerebro-spinal and mixed forms are varying degrees of congestion of the cerebral vessels and of serous effusion in the sub-arachnoid space and ventricles, varying degrees of engorgement of the lungs, of the right side of the heart, and of the general venous system, with more or less congestion of the abdominal viscera. The blood is always fluid. The post-mortem appearances referable to the cardiac form have not yet been carefully studied, but doubtless they are those which follow death by syncope, from paralysis of the fibre of the heart, when the cavities of both sides are filled with blood; or from spasm of the heart, when the so-called concentric hypertrophy is found.

I concur with those who think that the phenomena of sun-stroke are produced by depressed function more or less complete, and varying in degree, of the cerebro-spinal and sympathetic nervous systems. Whilst as yet there are only head symptoms, the derangement is confined to the cerebrum; when the respiration becomes implicated, the medulla oblongata has become involved. In those cases of sudden death by syncope there is an influence, similar to concussion from a blow or a copious cerebral hæmorrhage, which not only destroys consciousness and respiration, but at the same time paralyses the fibre of the heart. In the slighter degrees of syncope it is not improbable that the ganglia or periphery of the sympathetic system are primarily affected; and it is further not unlikely that the slighter degrees of deranged respiration may be caused in some cases also through the same nervous channel by an influence unfavourable to circulation exercised on the pulmonary capillaries, as suggested by Dr. Wood*, or by an influence exercised on the bronchial fibres, leading to some amount of spasm.

In the mixed form there is from the commencement depression to some extent of the nervous influence which regulates the action of the heart; it is in this fact that resides the difference between it and the first form. The nature of the proximate cause of this disturbance of the nervous system will be considered in connection with the etiology.

It has been conceived by several recent observers, that in a large proportion of cases death is caused by asphyxia—apnœa—induced by insufficiency of oxygen in the atmospheric air consequent on rarefaction by heat.

* "Practice of Medicine," vol. ii. p. 108.

The principal fact adduced in favour of this opinion is the engorged state of the lungs, the right side of the heart, and venous system found after death.

The arguments against it, are: — 1. The fact, that when death takes place speedily by coma, that is, when great depression of the nervous influence of the medulla oblongata is coincident with or follows closely upon that of the cerebrum, the post-mortem appearances are identical with those of death by asphyxia, viz. engorged lungs, right side of heart, and venous system. The reason is evident. Failure of the medulla oblongata as effectually puts a stop to respiration as irrespirable air or mechanical occlusion of the air passages; but in correct pathological language this is not death by asphyxia, but by coma*, and it is important that this distinction should be carefully observed.

2. Atmospheric air is in a more rarefied state by elevation at ordinary Hill Sanitaria than it ever is by the heat of the hot season in the plains, in any part of India.† Consequently, asphyxia from insufficiency of oxygen resulting from rarefaction of the air by heat is an untenable proposition.

* I am aware that there may be exceptional cases in which the medulla oblongata suffers first, unpreceded by insensibilty, and that, strictly speaking, in these cases, when fatal, death cannot be said to occur by coma; yet such are few and practically unimportant. It is well to regard the expression "death by coma" as synonymous with death by failure of the nervous influence of the medulla oblongata in respiration.

† To make this assertion more evident, let me state the physical facts which bear upon it, and then suggest certain probable inferences:—(*a*) Normal respiration in man may be assumed to consist of sixteen respirations in the minute, with each of which 30 cubic inches of air are inhaled, which is equivalent to 400 cubic feet in twenty-four hours. (*b*) 400 cubic feet of dry air at 32° F. contains 83·2 cubic feet of oxygen. (*c*) 400 cubic feet of air at 32° F. will, at 80° F., expand to 441·21 cubic feet; and the proportion of oxygen in 400 cubic feet of this expanded air is 75·428 cubic feet. (*d*) 400 cubic feet of air at 32° F. will, at 100° F., expand to 459 cubic feet; and the proportion of oxygen in 400 cubic feet of this expanded air is 72·51 cubic feet. (*e*) In latitudes of temperature 80° F. at the sea level, there is at a height of 5000 feet a decrease of temperature to 60° F.; and 400 cubic feet of this air, rendered less dense by elevation, contains 74·19 cubic feet of oxygen. At a height of 10,000 feet the temperature falls to 40° F., and the proportion of oxygen in 400 cubic feet of this still more rarefied air decreases to 63·294.

From these data it may be inferred:—

1. That as the temperature of the pulmonary air-cells in man is about 100° F., it is improbable, whatever the external atmospheric temperature may be, that air with a larger proportion of oxygen than 72·51 cubic feet in 400 cubic feet ever reaches the air-cells; and therefore the conclusion is erroneous, that the air of a climate at 100° F., when in the *air-cells* oxygenating the blood, contains a less proportion of oxygen than that supplied by a climate at 32° F. 2. In tropical countries, at elevations of 5000 and 10,000 feet, with atmospheric temperatures at 60° F. and 40° F., and proportions of oxygen (in 400 cubic feet) of 74·19 and 63·294 cubic feet, there must, when the air raised to 100° F. reaches the air-cells, be still more rarefaction, from heat, and consequently

3. Air so deficient in oxygen as to asphyxiate would operate generally, not partially, on all the warm-blooded animals exposed to its influence; and there could be no recovery from the asphyxia without removal into a more respirable atmosphere. We have an illustration of this in the blast of the simoom, affecting not a few individuals but an entire kafila.

Rate of mortality. — On this point satisfactory data are wanting, in consequence of the different system of classification, followed by different observers. Some include under the term "sun-stroke" all degrees of the immediate effects of solar heat, others merely the severer forms.

The following are the results taken from the reports before me:—

	Treated.	Deaths.
Mr. Hill's collected Cases	504	259
Dr. Taylor's, Ghazeepore	115	16
Mr. Longmore, Barrackpore, (19th Regiment)	16	7
Mr. Lofthouse, (14th Lt. Dragoons)	80	10
Dr. Simpson (71st Regiment)	89	24
Mr. Ward (3rd Bombay European Regiment)	25	6
Mr. Ewing (95th Regiment)	60	17
Sir Hugh Rose and Dr. Stuart* (25th Regt. B.N.I.)	200	—
Field Hospital, Jhansi	29	10

further decrease in the proportion of oxygen. Hence there is in the air in the air-cells at heights a considerably less proportion of oxygen than in the air in the air-cells in the plains. 3. But in tropical climates there is undoubtedly less oxygenation of the blood, because there is less necessity for, and less generation of, animal heat. At elevations of 10,000 feet the temperature is 40°, and man is found healthy and robust; therefore there must be sufficient oxygenation of the blood—to generate animal heat—to meet the demand of the low external temperature. By what means is respiration so adjusted as to satisfy the different requirements of a tropical climate at the sea level, and of an elevated locality? certainly not by a different proportion of oxygen in the air respired, for that at the elevation where more oxygenation is necessary contains much less oxygen than that at the sea level in the tropics, where the degree of oxygenation is diminished. The adjustment is effected by the varying amount of air received into the lungs at each respiration, and by the varying number of inspirations taken in the minute. In the warm climate at the sea level the respiratory function is reduced by lessened expansion of the lungs. In the elevated locality the respiratory function is increased, to meet the diminished proportion of oxygen and the greater demand for animal heat, by (*a*) augmented pulmonary expansion, (*b*) increased number of respirations: this obtains within certain limits. If there be no longer capacity of air-cells, or increase of respiratory movements to compensate for the diminished proportion of oxygen, then symptoms of *asphyxia* begin.

For the calculations on which this note is based, and for the suggestion that the air in the air-cells must always be at a temperature of about 100° F., whatever that of the external air may be, I am indebted to the kindness of Dr. Forbes Watson.

* The number 200 is from Sir Hugh Rose's dispatch. Dr. Stuart, in his report, says, "Sixteen cases only admitted into hospital, none fatal; but of course many in the field, none of them fatal."

ETIOLOGY. — The documents before me supply the following facts in reference to season, age, period of service in India, and duration of attack. The *months* of prevalence have been almost exclusively April, May, and June, but chiefly May and the first half of June.

In respect to *age*, my only data are derived from twenty-seven fatal cases of the Rajpootana and Central India Field Forces, and ten of the K Battery of Royal Artillery fatal at Baroda.

Age.	Rajpootana, and Central India Field Forces.	K Battery.
19 years and under . .	—	2
20 to 25	12	2
26 to 30	8	6
31 to 35	4	—
36 to 40	2	—
Total . .	26	10

The *period of service in India* of twenty-seven fatal cases was, in ten, six months and under ; in twelve, seven to nine months ; in four, four to sixteen years, and in one it was not noted.

The 71st Regiment arrived in India at the end of February 1858, and had eighty-nine men attacked with sun-stroke, between the 5th May and 15th August. The K Battery had also been only six months in India, when it suffered at Baroda. These corps then illustrate the relation of sun-stroke to recent arrival from colder latitudes.

Death occurred at varying periods from the commencement of the attack, thus: —

	Rajpootana and Central India Field Forces.
Day of admission	19
Following day	4
Upwards of five days . .	3
Not Noted	1
	27

	K Battery.
1 to 3 hours	2
4 to 6 "	1
7 to 12 "	6
13 to 24 "	1
	10

Sun-stroke is not confined to Europeans. In Dr. Don's report on the Medical Topography of Sukkur, there is an interesting account of the sufferings of an escort of Bengal and Bombay Native Infantry, when marching in the latter half of May 1839 from Sukkur to Dadur. The 25th Regiment Bombay Native Infantry, during the campaign in Central India, in 1858, was, as already stated, temporarily crippled by sun-stroke; and I have it from the best authority, that the appearance presented by the corpses of many of the rebel troops opposed to the Central India Field Force showed that death had resulted from sun-stroke and not from wounds. The meteorological observations made during the seasons of prevalence of sun-stroke are very meagre, but the temperature would seem to have ranged from 96° to 120° in the shade. This high atmospheric heat, chiefly observed on the Coromandel coast, Central India, the north-west provinces, Scinde, and the Punjab, may be received as the chief exciting cause.

But predisposing causes are also very influential. There is a very general concurrence of opinion that the sthenic constitution of the recently arrived European predisposes to the cerebro-spinal form of the disease, and this predisposition may be greatly increased by the intemperate use of alcoholic drinks. Then, as predisposing conditions of the cardiac and mixed forms may be named the asthenic constitution of the natives of India, and of long resident Europeans, increased by fatigue and other exhausting causes, also, a diathesis cachectic from malaria, scurvy, or from degeneration of the fibre of the heart or secreting structure of the liver or kidney.

The * high atmospheric heat probably excites the cerebro-spinal form of sun-stroke by increasing the temperature of the blood some degrees above its normal standard; and it produces this effect, not so much by direct conduction to the body, as by impaired evaporation from the cutaneous surface, leading to an undue accumulation of animal heat in the following ways:—

1. A still or moist atmosphere of 94° F. and upwards. Dr. Taylor remarks of sun-stroke at Ghazeepore:—"This epidemic was undoubtedly the direct morbid effect of the high temperature of the season. Instead of the regular hot winds from the N.W. the wind during the month of May had been constantly N.E. and the tatties were consequently of little service. The ther-

* In restricting my observations to the temperature, moisture, and movement of the atmosphere, I by no means wish to express a belief that there may not be other states, electrical, &c., also influential; but on these questions it is idle to speculate. Observation, not speculation, is the desideratum.

mometer at the end of May averaged 105° in the shade, and from the unfavourable direction of the wind for working the tatties, the heat in the barracks could be but little diminished. On the 1st of June the wind was still N.E. and light with the thermometer at 104°. The sensation of heat was intense. On the morning of the 2nd, the day of the outbreak of the epidemic, the wind came round to the N.W. and was strong and scorching. The thermometer in a covered passage facing N.E. showed a temperature of 108° at two P.M."

Mr. Naylor observes of the Field Hospital at Jhansi,—in which, during six weeks, the thermometer ranged at noon from 110° to 120°,—"but it was observable that it was not in the hottest days that the affection showed itself, the most favourable periods of its occurrence being rather those cloudy days, accompanied with a moist condition of the atmosphere, when even the water in the cooja could not be rendered cool." It is to the stillness and moisture of the heated air, favoured by some degree of vitiation, that are due the attacks in barracks and hospitals. Dr. Taylor alludes to the injurious influence of the crowding of masses of infantry, during the march and on parade, compared to what obtains in artillery and cavalry; and Dr. Lofthouse attributes the greater immunity from sun-stroke of the cavalry of the Central India Field Force to the less exhaustion of men on horseback, and to the air currents caused by the rapidity of their movements.

2. The refrigerating effect of evaporation must be lessened when the due proportion of water in the blood is not kept up by a sufficient and regular supply of drinking water. The importance of this consideration is universally admitted. It is stated by Dr. Don that the much greater exemption from mortality in the Bombay than in the Bengal Regiment of the Sukkur escort was attributed by the commanding officer to the men of the former "being supplied, as is the custom in the Bombay army, with canteens of water, with which they refreshed themselves on the march, as well as at all times on duty, when water could not otherwise have been readily procured."

3. If the opinion of physiologists relative to the influence of the vaso-motor nerves on the size of the capillaries, and consequently on the quantity and movement of the blood in them, be correct, then it is very likely that a sequence of the action of direct solar heat on the cutaneous surface may be such diminished secretion by the sudoriferous glands as shall materially lessen refrigeration by evaporation.

In these three ways—the first having reference to still moist hot air, the two last equally to hot dry air—the temperature of the blood may become increased by accumulation of animal heat from defective cutaneous evaporation.* On this point Dr. Simpson makes the following valuable practical remark:—"Every man seized with sun-stroke, and who could answer questions, informed me that he had not perspired for a greater or less extent of time, sometimes not for days, previous to being attacked, and that he had enjoyed good health as long as he perspired, but that on the perspiration being checked he felt dull and listless, and unable to take much exertion without making a great effort."

But there is still another circumstance which favours the increase of heat in the subjects of sun-stroke.

We have already seen that recent arrival from colder latitudes predisposes to the *cerebro-spinal* form. Dr. Crawford, in his "Notes on Coup de Soleil in the 51st Regiment at Rangoon," says, that obesity was present in all the fatal cases. Dr. Taylor remarks: "The subjects of the disease were with few exceptions large-chested, muscular, and fat men." These conditions of the system favour undue generation and retention of animal heat.

It is not, however, only by increasing the heat of the blood, in the manner explained, to a degree incompatible with the maintenance of the functions of the nervous system, that elevated temperature acts as the exciting cause of sun-stroke. In the *cardiac* form, we must look for another explanation; because in these speedily fatal attacks, the sudden violence of the onset, and in the milder attacks, the cold and clammy skin, are inconsistent with the idea of a gradual heating of the blood as the proximate cause. The action must therefore be direct either on the nervous centre near to the origin of the vagus nerve, or on the general periphery of the cutaneous nerves, as supposed by Dr. Alison. His† words are: "The effect of very intense *heat* applied to a pretty large surface of the body, as in an extensive burn, or to the whole body, as in the case of a *coup de soleil*, is also quite similar to that of concussion."

To recapitulate. 1. The cerebro-spinal form, commencing with cerebral symptoms, without much depression of the pulse in the first instance, characterised by pungent heat of skin, and proving

* When evaporation is deficient, and the external air above 100, then there will be increased heat of the body, not only from accumulation of animal heat, but also by conduction from the air.

† "Outlines of Pathology and Practice of Medicine," p. 13.

fatal by coma, is due to increased heat of the blood disturbing and depressing the functions of the cerebro-spinal nervous system. 2. The cardiac form, with small or imperceptible pulse, cold and clammy skin—often suddenly coming on and proving speedily fatal—is due to a direct depressing influence, probably on the entire nervous system, irrespective of the condition of the blood. 3. In the mixed form there are varying proportions of both conditions, viz.—overheated blood and direct influence on the nervous system.

It is at present a favourite doctrine with many pathologists that sun-stroke is in part due to a supposed venous condition of the arterial blood. I am not acquainted with any facts or any sound arguments which go to justify this hypothesis. The explanation of asphyxia given by Kay, and universally assented to by physiologists for the last thirty years, is, that death takes place in consequence of the stagnation of blood in the pulmonary capillaries, leading to general congestion of the vascular system behind, and permitting but a scanty stream of blood to pass to the left side of the heart. Little, if any, of the deranged phenomena can be reasonably attributed to the poisonous influence of the small quantity of venous blood which *for a minute or two* before death passes to the left ventricle, and thence through the systemic arteries.*

Again, it follows from Kay's experiments, that venous blood will not circulate through the pulmonary capillaries, and that therefore the supposed continued circulation of venous blood poisoning the tissues generally is inconsistent with ascertained facts.

The idea of the assumed pathological import of venous blood would seem to have originated—1. In forgetfulness that Bichat's opinion that venous blood is poisonous has been long since disproved; and that the phenomena of asphyxia are little, if at all, dependent on the circumstance of the blood in the arteries being

* It is very remarkable that though there is a universal assent to Kay's theory, and a general dissent from the doctrines of Bichat that the venous blood is poisonous; still, this latter erroneous view is freely applied by pathologists at the present day. I would instance Dr. Watson's fifth lecture, in which, speaking of Dr. Kay, he says, "His experiments tend moreover to prove, that venous blood, circulating through the arteries has no direct poisonous operation" (p. 69, vol. i.). But further on, at p. 73, drawing the distinction between death by syncope and apnœa, he attaches an importance to the venous character of the blood which reaches the left side of the heart more consistent with the theory of Bichat than that of Kay. If in asphyxia the blood stagnates at the lungs, at first incompletely and shortly afterwards completely, we have in the general congestion from venous obstruction, and in the insufficient quantity of blood in the arteries in the first instance, and shortly afterwards its absence altogether, an adequate explanation of the phenomena without attributing anything to the venous condition of the slender and transient stream which for a few minutes may circulate through the arterial system.

venous. 2. In the erroneous inference that persisting diminished respiration, either from elevated temperature, or slight vitiation of the atmospheric air, from small quantities of carbonic acid, as in cities, crowded rooms, &c. leads to a venous condition of the blood in the arteries: there is no evidence of this in an altered colour of any part of the surface of the body. The effect of the diminished respiration is altogether different. The appetite for food, digestion, assimilation, and the quantity of blood, are brought into harmony with the diminished respiration, and there results not venous blood and purple lips, but anæmia more or less, as shown in the pallid countenance of the tropical resident and of the dweller in the impure air of crowded cities.

The passage of venous blood from the venous into the arterial system takes place only when its complete aëration has become impossible, either from an insufficiency of oxygen or defect of the lung, or of nervous influence; and the immediate sequence of this is the commencement of stagnation in the pulmonary circulation. There is no fact, so far as I am aware, which can justify the assumption that venous blood can continue to circulate in the arterial system, and in consequence of its venous character excite derangement. A venous condition of the blood in the arteries must, it seems to me, be always *consecutive* on defective aëration, be *preceded* by pulmonary stagnation, *attended* by the symptoms of apnœa, and, if not speedily removed, followed by death.

The opinion that *malaria* is an exciting cause of sun-stroke appears to rest on no sufficient grounds. The occurrence of death by coma in a proportion of the severer forms of remittent fever is no reason for concluding that sun-stroke is caused by malaria, the more especially as this latter disease prevails most at seasons which hitherto have not been regarded as those in which malaria is chiefly generated.

Prevention and Treatment. — The prevention of sun-stroke by avoiding as far as practicable the predisposing and exciting causes, is of essential importance.

The following influences must be carefully guarded against: — (*a*) Needless exposure to the sun. (*b*) Exhaustion from fatiguing duties, defective commissariat arrangements, and other causes. (*c*) Intemperance from the excessive use of alcoholic drinks.

A full and well-regulated supply of good drinking water, under all the circumstances of military service in the hot season, is an essential measure for the prevention of sun-stroke. It ministers to the cooling effect of evaporation from the cutaneous surface, and materially assists in warding off that state of exhaustion which leads to syncope.

Protection of the body from direct, reflected or radiated solar heat by suitable clothing, is a subject to which of late much attention has been justly given.* The object in view is to devise the best practicable means of obstructing the transmission of external heat to the body without interfering with free cutaneous evaporation. The non-conducting head-dress with ventilating arrangements, and the loose tunics of suitable light wadded material, are constructed on this principle. If the pathological views which attribute much to the implication of the medulla oblongata be correct, the importance of a neck-piece to the head-dress, already established by ample experience, is very intelligible; and a similar observation may be made relative to the spinal cord, the solar plexus and the general nervous periphery, and the necessity of providing for their protection by suitable clothing. The great importance of space, of the interception of external heat, of ventilation, and of means, as wet tatties and punkahs, of reducing the temperature, and of agitating and maintaining pure the atmosphere in tents, barracks, and hospitals cannot be too strongly insisted upon; while the injurious effect of crowding men in masses during the march and on parade should receive its just measure of attention.†

In the *medical treatment* of sun-stroke there is now great unanimity of opinion; and the conclusions so generally admitted are in accordance with the views entertained of the pathology and etiology of the disease. General blood-letting has few supporters.

* I would refer the reader to the following sources among others of much useful information on this and other subjects, relating to the health of the soldier in India: — "The British Army in India," by Julius Jeffreys; "The British Soldier in India," by Dr. F. Mouat; "Reports on Coup de Soleil," by a Board of Medical Officers, and by Dr. Simpson; "Transactions, Medical and Physical Society of Bombay," No. 4. New Series.

† It may happen that troops are so circumstanced, that a slight change of air may exercise a very beneficial effect. The following is an illustration: —

In May 1859, K Battery, Royal Artillery, and two companies of the 4th Regiment were stationed at Baroda, in Guzerat. The atmosphere was still, and the thermometer rose to 110° in the shade. Both corps were housed in equally good barracks, with punkahs day and night. The stable duties of the battery entailed however greater exposure, and the canteen reports showed a large daily consumption of arrack, which increased after sickness commenced on the 27th May; between which day and the 2nd June ten men died of sun-stroke, and there was amongst the men a general dread of the disease. The men were now moved out in tents to Dubka, on the banks of the Myhee, fourteen miles from Baroda, and within the influence of the sea breeze, and with space for recreation and amusement. No more deaths occurred. The health of the men improved, and they returned to Baroda with fewer sick than they

Though it may be admitted that an occasional case occurs in which cautious venesection might be useful, yet the evidence of the great injury usually resulting from it is so conclusive that there should be no hesitation in altogether interdicting this proceeding in the treatment of sun-stroke. The cause of the ill success of blood-letting is not difficult to understand. The proof, occurring more or less early, but certainly at some period or other in all attacks, of a sedative influence on the heart, distinctly contra-indicates its use. The affusion of cold water over the head, neck, and chest has been proved to be the most efficacious means of treatment; and as its power is greater the earlier it is resorted to, well arranged methods of applying it should be always ready at hand. It acts in two ways. 1. By reducing the heat of the body. 2. By stimulating the nervous system through the impression made on the periphery of the cutaneous nerves. The first is the mode of action which is probably most beneficial in the cerebro-spinal form; the second in the cardiac form.

The extent and continuance of the affusion must be regulated by the temperature of the surface of the body and the state of the pulse. While the skin is hot and dry, and the pulse of good volume, water may be freely poured over the head, neck, spine, and chest, and frequently repeated; but when the cold, clammy skin, the sighing respiration, and the small pulse, indicative of syncope, are present, the water should be merely dashed, or sprinkled from time to time, on the face and chest. It should never be forgotten that after the temperature of the body has been reduced, and the skin become accustomed to the impression, the affusion of cold water soon begins to exercise a sedative influence on the heart. In using this remedy, therefore, the distinction between the cerebro-spinal and the cardiac form of the disease should be borne in mind, and the state of the pulse and skin should be carefully watched and noted.

These cautions are very necessary, for if they be disregarded, and a routine system be adopted, it may be safely predicted that cold affusion in sun-stroke will share the fate of all powerful remedies used without discrimination and judgment, and soon cease to maintain the high place to which it is justly entitled in the treatment of this disease.

had had for some time. There was only one death from sun-stroke in the detachment of the 4th Regiment, and little sickness of any kind.

The improvement in the men of the battery was doubtless due to greater temperance, relief from stable duties, the cooler locality, and mental interest and occupation.

When the patient is able to swallow, stimulants and nourishment should be given, with a frequency and in quantities according to the state of the pulse.*

It is, moreover, of great importance in the treatment of sun-stroke to supply the patient freely with good drinking water. Dr. Crawford, of the 18th Royal Irish, in the notes of his experience in Rangoon, attaches more weight to this indication than any other writer with whose works I am acquainted. If the view taken of a deficient supply of good water, as a predisposing cause, be correct, the necessity of diluents in the treatment is self-evident.

When the tendency to death by coma or syncope has been overcome, and febrile reaction and some degree of local congestion remain, the treatment should be conducted on ordinary principles. Moderate local blood-letting, mercurial and other purgatives, and diuretics, may be used with much advantage. But in applying this principle of treatment it should be remembered that the patient has lately passed from a state of which a sedative influence on the heart was a constituent, and that this condition may easily be reproduced by injudicious evacuation and the neglect of appropriate nourishment.

Concluding Remarks. — This important subject has been very inadequately explained by me, but this, in fact, is unavoidable, and only to be remedied by further careful clinical observation and description. The following are the points on which information is chiefly to be desired: —

1. A more careful and precise observation of the symptoms with reference to the different tendency to death in different cases.

2. Carefully conducted post-mortem examinations with the view of determining whether the division into cases fatal by coma and by syncope is correct.

3. Meteorological observations on the temperature, moisture, pressure, movement, and electrical states of the atmosphere.

* In an anonymous letter, dated May 1859, published in the "Lancet," and also in a private letter from a friend whose judgment I respect, it has been suggested that Marshall Hall's ready method might be of use in the treatment of sun-stroke. The idea rests on the belief that death takes place by asphyxia, from defect of the aërating medium. I have already expressed my dissent from this pathology, but nevertheless I think the suggestion ought not to be lost sight of, for, as in some cases of narcotic poisoning, the influence on the medulla oblongata may be so transient in an occasional case of sun-stroke, as not to preclude the idea of advantage from artificially assisting respiration. But, irrespective of this, the change from dorsal decubitus, involved in the acts of the "ready method," is likely to retard the pulmonary congestion, and thus postpone death.

4. Precise facts, bearing on the state of predisposition, having reference to exposure, clothing, diathesis, habits, exhausting conditions, supply of water, accommodation, age, residence in India, and previous disease.

5. Precise clinical notes on the condition of the patient before the use of remedies, and on the effects produced by the remedies.

CHAP. XXVII.

ON DELIRIUM TREMENS.

SECTION I. — *On the Symptoms and Treatment of Delirium Tremens in the European General Hospital at Bombay.*

As my clinical knowledge of this important disease has been chiefly acquired in the European General Hospital at Bombay, I shall confine my present observations, in a great measure, to my experience in that institution.

During the five years, from July 1838 to June 1843, 237 patients were under treatment for delirium tremens, being 3·1 per cent. of the total hospital admissions. Forty-one cases terminated fatally, being 17·8 per cent. of the admissions from delirium tremens, and 7·5 per cent. of the aggregate deaths in the hospital.

Though 17·8 per cent. was the average annual rate of mortality for the five years, it varied considerably in different years, and very strikingly in different months. In the years 1839 and 1841, the deaths were above 20 per cent. of the admissions, whereas in the year 1842 they were only 7. Throughout the five years, there was not a single fatal case of delirium tremens recorded in the months of January and February, though the admissions from the disease were respectively 3·2 and 5·3 per cent. of the total hospital admissions; whereas in the months of May and October the rate of mortality from delirium tremens was above 40 per cent., though the admissions were not above 4·7 and 1·2 per cent. of the aggregate hospital admissions. In the month of May the admissions were also numerically considerably above those of any other month of the year.

The data from which these statements have been made, will be found, with additional statistical details of a similar character, in the tables which are annexed to this chapter.*

* When we compare the statistical facts of these five years with those of the ten which succeed, it is found that in the latter there were 453 admissions of delirium

Persons admitted into the General Hospital, affected with delirium tremens, have belonged generally to one of the following classes:— 1. Engineers and boilermakers connected with the Steam Flotilla, or works in the dockyard—men not long resident in India, and whose ages may range from twenty to thirty-five. 2. Non-commissioned officers and soldiers attached to the different branches of the military department at the presidency—men of various periods of service in India. 3. Seamen belonging to the public service or to merchant ships, who have been on shore on liberty, and have for a succession of days been dissipating in the bazaar; or seamen and others out of employment who have been lodging in taverns.

From the class of seamen, however, the admissions have been considerably the most numerous.

Symptoms and Treatment.—The division of delirium tremens into two species, which has been made by some writers *, is clinically correct. The first in general immediately succeeds the excitement of hard drinking without an intermediate period of abstinence from the accustomed stimulus, and is characterised by a flushed countenance, full pulse, slight tremors, a tongue coated in the centre and frequently florid at the tip, with, generally but not invariably, more or less irritability of stomach. In the second the symptoms come on in the habitually dissipated, after the

tremens into the European General Hospital, equivalent to 3·7 per cent. of the total hospital admissions. Of these thirty-eight died, being a mortality-rate from this disease of 8·4 per cent. Though 8·4 per cent. was the average mortality for the ten years, it has varied considerably in different years, and very strikingly in different months. In the year 1848 the deaths were 20·4 per cent. of the admissions, whereas, in the year 1853, they were only 2·2. Throughout the ten years there is only one death from delirium tremens in the months of January and February, though the admissions were respectively 2·5 and 2·4 per cent. of the total admissions. The month of greatest mortality has been October, viz., 26·6 per cent., when the admissions per cent. of the total hospital admissions were not more than 3·7. Though the great mortality of the month of May does not appear to the same extent in these ten years as in the five which preceded, yet the aggravation in the hot months (April and May) is sufficiently apparent.

The striking difference between these statements and those in the text is the much lower rate of mortality from 1844 to 1853 than from 1838 to 1843. Particular reference will be made to this in the sequel. The tabular returns for these ten years are also annexed to this chapter. On this subject I would further refer to Dr. Stovell's "Decennial Report of the European General Hospital," published subsequently to the 1st edition of this work, in No. 3, new series, "Transactions, Medical and Physical Society of Bombay."

* "Copland's Dictionary of Practical Medicine, and British and Foreign Medical Review," vol. ix. p. 475.

accustomed stimulus has, from some cause or other, been for a time withheld.*

* As my remarks on *delirium tremens* have reference to a particular series of cases, and were written at a time (1843) when the diaries were before me, and the clinical impressions fresh on my mind, I am unwilling to alter the statements made in the text, though I believe that a fuller explanation respecting the division into species is necessary to prevent misapprehension. The *first species* probably includes cases that now would be classed as "ebrietas." The definition of the *second species* leaves it to be implied that it comes on in the habitually dissipated, *only* after the accustomed stimulus has been withdrawn: but this is an error, and not consistent with the toxæmic theory of the pathology. In the "British and Foreign Medico-Chirurgical Review" for October 1859, the subject of delirium tremens is fully considered as respects its pathology and causes, and partially as respects its treatment. The principal doctrines inculcated are:—1. Delirium tremens is a toxæmia from alcohol, and becomes developed when the poisoned condition of the blood and of the nervous matter is sufficient in degree. 2. The idea that the attack comes on in the habitually dissipated, when the use of alcohol has been suddenly discontinued, is an error; and therefore to withhold this stimulus cannot be injurious, but, on the contrary, must be beneficial. (*a.*) The erroneous idea has arisen in consequence of delirium tremens occurring in individuals admitted into hospitals with injuries, and it is maintained that the explanation of this event is not as hitherto supposed—the suspension of the use of alcohol—but the *shock* of the injury, acting as a determining cause in constitutions in which the toxæmia is considerable, but not of itself sufficient to excite the disease. (*b.*) It is argued that the withdrawal of alcohol cannot be the cause, because observation shows that in gaols and houses of correction, into which the dissipated are received in large numbers, delirium tremens rarely occurs in the recently admitted, though, as a matter of course, the use of alcohol has in them been discontinued. 3. Not only is the treatment by free opiates and alcoholic stimulants condemned, but it is maintained that, as the patient is alcoholised when suffering from delirium tremens, to propose the use of more alcohol in the treatment is irrational.

These doctrines are in part correct, but they do not embrace the whole subject, and are therefore, it seems to me, in part erroneous. The following appear to me to be the defects:—1. The distinction between the toxæmic effect on the nervous system of the continued use of alcohol, and the stimulant effect on the heart of regulated quantities occasionally given, is not observed. 2. Though the disease often comes on when the toxæmia is complete, without any suspension of the use of alcohol, yet when the toxæmia is not complete, it may be determined by the sudden withdrawal of alcohol; and the error has consisted merely in a too general application of this occasional fact. (*a.*) The explanation would seem to be, that the removal of the *stimulant* effect of the alcohol by depressing the action of the heart determines the attack, just as the shock does in the case of injury, or depletion in a co-existing inflammatory disease. (*b.*) The argument that delirium tremens is rare in the inmates of gaols, is not of much force; for the evident answer is, that though the use of alcohol was suspended on admission, the disease did not become developed because the toxæmia was insufficient. Indeed, it might be anticipated that delirium tremens would not frequently attack the recent admissions into gaols, for a person on the verge of delirium tremens cannot be said to be in a state well fitted for the commission of general crime. 3. When the toxæmia is great, the withdrawal of alcohol may determine the attack. In this state the general tremor, the small pulse, the damp and coldish surface, indicate the necessity of stimulants, and alcohol, used with this view, will under these circumstances sometimes prevent the attack. But it does not follow that in less degrees of the toxæmia, where the same necessity for a stimulant does not exist, it may not be withdrawn with perfect safety: this measure is, *then*,

Of the *first species*, cases are occasionally admitted into the General Hospital, occurring, usually, in steam-engineers, and not unfrequently terminating by convulsion unexpectedly coming on, passing into complete coma, with rapid pulse, pungent heat of skin, and proving fatal in a few hours after the accession of convulsion. Symptoms of gastric irritation, in this form of the disease, are common, and require to be specially attended to in directing the treatment. Many cases do well under the use of cold affusion frequently repeated, attention to rest and quietness, the exhibition of effervescing draughts with a few minims of tincture of opium, and the application of sinapisms to the epigastrium, or a blister, if the symptoms are more urgent. Six or seven grains of calomel, with one grain of muriate of morphia, and one of ipecacuanha, given at bed-time, preceded by cold affusion to the head and a hot foot-bath, are often beneficial.

It is only in this species that the question of the local detraction of blood, can, with advantage, be entertained; and probably the best guides to its successful use are the diathesis of the individual, — whether plethoric or not — the knowledge of the length of time to which he has been addicted to habits of dissipation, and the duration of the symptoms. In young men of robust constitution, not long resident in India, and not confirmed drunkards, it is often useful, at the commencement of the attack, to detract blood locally by cupping the nape of the neck, or leeching the temples; but it is only under these circumstances that this practice holds out any prospect of benefit. In regard to the general abstraction of blood, it is even in these cases very seldom expedient, and, if ever had recourse to, should be carried into effect with very great caution.

Stimulants (wine, &c.) in this form of delirium tremens are not usually required, — but the state of the pulse and skin sometimes calls for their exhibition. When symptoms of gastric irritation are not present (and such cases occasionally occur), tartar emetic combined with more or less opium, according to the character of the

the only method by which the attack can be prevented. 4. In the treatment of delirium tremens, alcohol should not be used without good reason, because the tendency of its frequent repetition must be to increase the alcoholism; but when the skin and pulse indicate on general therapeutic principles the necessity of stimulants, then they must be used in this as in other diseases, and wine and brandy are the best at our command. Tendency to death by syncope must not be neglected in delirium tremens, because the stimulants used temporarily to avert an immediate and pressing danger are by frequent repetition likely to increase the toxæmia, and lead to a remoter evil. Here as in the practice of medicine generally, the physician's science lies in a correct appreciation of the good and the evil of his remedies; and his art in the skill with which the first quality is sifted from the other, and usefully applied.

head symptoms, in the manner to be subsequently more particularly adverted to, is perfectly applicable.

But the *second species* of the disease is the one of greatest importance, and most frequent occurrence; the other being comparatively rare.

The division of the *second species* into three stages, first, I believe, suggested by Dr. Blake *, is in accordance with the character of the disease as observed in the European General Hospital at Bombay, viz.: — 1. A stage of depression, characterised by tremors (in some cases excessive), a feeble pulse, sleepless nights, but no delirium, anorexia, and frequently irritability of stomach. 2. The stage of active delirium. 3. The third stage, in cases which have gone on favourably, is one of lengthened sleep, followed by recovery; in cases which have progressed unfavourably, it is a state of low muttering delirium, with contracted pupils, tremulous agitation, feeble and rapid pulse, and generally terminates fatally by convulsion and coma, or by coma unpreceded by convulsion. It is to this train of symptoms, that throughout these remarks I shall apply the designation "*third stage.*"

First stage. — By treating this stage with stimulants, wine, brandy, ammonia, and occasionally † an opiate at bed-time preceded by cold affusion to the head, — the occurrence of the second stage is sometimes prevented, and recovery takes place; or, if not prevented, it is much lessened in severity.

When there is irritability of stomach with slimy and florid tongue, effervescing draughts with a few minims of laudanum, sinapisms or a blister to the epigastrium, with stimulants according to the state of the skin, pulse and tremors; also a grain of muriate of morphia, with two or three grains of calomel, and an effervescing draught at bed-time, preceded by a hot foot-bath, — constitute the best method of treatment. In the management of this stage, stimulants ought never to be abruptly stopped, but always gradually lessened, and an adequate diet should be reverted to as soon as practicable.

* "Edinburgh Medical and Surgical Journal for October 1823." I regret that I have not had the opportunity of consulting Dr. Blake's "Practical Treatise on Delirium Tremens," published in 1830; or the second edition of 1840.

† I have said *occasionally* an opiate at bed-time advisedly, because it requires to be given with discrimination; for not unfrequently the first symptoms of the second stage come on after an opiate given at bed-time—whether in consequence of the opiate, or because it has chanced to have been given at the period when the commencement of the second stage was to be looked for in the regular course of the disease, is a question which I do not pretend to resolve. Of the fact as now stated I have no doubt.

The second stage, or that of active mental excitement. — It is unnecessary to enter into any particular description of the delirium of this stage: it is the symptom which most particularly characterises the disease, and is fully and accurately delineated in all the best works on practical medicine.* There are, however, certain particulars which, though noted by some observers, have not received that attention which their importance (as bearing on treatment) seems to me to require; and on these points I shall somewhat extend my remarks.

It has been observed by Dr. Hoeg Guldberg, physician to the hospital at Frederickstadt, that the critical sleep occurs in the greater number of cases on the fourth day; but it does not appear whether he dates from the commencement of the first stage, or from that of the second. In all probability from the former; for, on carefully examining a great many of the diaries of cases treated in the European General Hospital, I find, that of twenty-six cases in which the access of the second stage, and its termination, were distinctly recorded, the average duration of this stage was forty-six hours — the shortest period being twenty-four, and the longest sixty.

It is stated by Dr. Blake, that the mental irritation requires a given time to subside; and it is also the opinion of Dr. Ware of Boston, that this disease runs a certain course. From considering the cases which had passed under my own observation, I had arrived at a similar conclusion, when not aware that the same view had been entertained by previous observers.

The circumstances which suggested this opinion to me, were: — 1. The frequently observed fact, that the quantity of opium which on one day failed to induce sleep, succeeded on the following; a circumstance to be explained, either on the supposition, that the natural tendency of the symptoms was to abate, after a certain course, or that the effect of the opium was cumulative — a conclusion which would be contrary to our experience of the action of this medicine in all other forms of disease. 2. In cases treated with full opiates frequently repeated, I have several times remarked, that sleep was induced for three or four hours, but that the patient afterwards woke up delirious as before; and some of these cases terminated fatally.

It is the circumstance of the second stage running a certain

* Dr. Stovell, at page 68 of his Decennial Report, gives an excellent summary of his observations on the character of the illusions of patients with delirium tremens in the European General Hospital.

course,—which seems to me not to have received its full consideration in relation to treatment. For, if acknowledged, it may be safely affirmed, that the indication of cure is not by full doses of narcotics to force a state of sleep, but to conduct the patient through the period of delirium, by withdrawing all sources of irritation, by moderating or sustaining the circulation, and by calming the nervous excitement. Though a similar opinion is expressed by Dr. Blake in the following words: "It does not appear to me to be of any service to attempt to break the chain of morbid concatenation too abruptly, as the stage of mental irritation seems to require a given time to subside, in proportion to the stage of exhaustion, to the mode of treatment adopted, and to its previous causes," I am not aware that any subsequent writer has given to this feature of the disease that prominence which its importance demands.

The indications of cure, as thus stated, are best effected by cold affusion, tartar emetic combined with opium or other narcotic, and stimulants.

In regard to *cold affusion*, it may be used with excellent effect three or four times in the course of the twenty-four hours,—the most important, however, being that before bed-time,—in all cases in which the circulation is steady, the skin not covered with perspiration, or its temperature not reduced below the natural standard; or, in which there are not present any of the local complications which usually contra-indicate the use of this remedy. In cases in which, from the state of the pulse, there may be doubt of the propriety of the cold affusion, it frequently becomes quite admissible by preceding its application, by a stimulant (as brandy); and in the still more doubtful cases, — even in instances in which the measure may be decidedly contra-indicated, — there is good effect from using cold affusion to the head, and at the same time a hot foot-bath.

There has not been much difficulty experienced in inducing patients to submit to this remedy, and it is hardly necessary to add that the employment of coercive measures to effect it is altogether inadmissible. In considering this statement, however, it must be borne in mind, that I write of the disease in a climate whose mean temperature is about 80°, that the water used has never been artificially cooled, and that the practice of frequent bathing is habitual to many of the patients. The first consideration is important, as bearing on the question of the temperature of the water; and the second, as, in all probability, explaining the little difficulty which has been experienced from the opposition of the patients.

But the exhibition of *tartar emetic with opium or other narcotic,* first introduced into practice by Dr. Law, of Dublin *, and followed by Dr. Graves †, Dr. Clendinning ‡, and others, constitutes the most successful means of controlling the symptoms of this stage of the disease. This mode of treatment was, during the five years to which my remarks apply, much followed in delirium tremens, in the European General Hospital at Bombay; and there was also, during the same period, ample opportunity of comparing it with that by free opiates frequently repeated.

Tartar emetic and opium, in proportions modified according to the symptoms, and associated with the use of cold affusion and stimulants, is, in my judgment, a much more successful and satisfactory method of treating the second stage of delirium tremens than the more common plan of giving free opiates uncombined, or in combination with stimulants alone; and is moreover devoid of the risk of positive injury, which more or less attends the latter system of treatment.

Tartar emetic was given in doses from half a grain to a grain in an ounce and a half of camphor mixture, with from twenty to thirty minims of tincture of opium or tincture of hyosciamus, repeated every hour, second, or third hour §; the variations in the dose, and the intervals, being dependent on the state of the circulation, the condition of the skin, and the degree of mental excitement. Though in determining these variations, there is room for the exercise of discretion in each particular case, still, it will be found, that the greater number are sufficiently controlled by three quarters of a grain of tartar emetic and thirty minims of tincture of opium or tincture of hyosciamus every second hour, continued till sleep is induced, — with intermissions of several hours, at times, if the sinking of the pulse or reduction of

* "London Medical Gazette for 2nd July and 30th July, 1835."

† "The Dublin Journal of Medical Science for May, 1836."

‡ "London Medical Gazette," January 14th, 1842.

§ In regarding the proportion of opium here recommended, in reference to my objections to an exclusive opiate treatment of delirium tremens, the clinical student must bear in mind the well-established therapeutic fact, that the narcotic effect of opium is lessened by antimony. But I would add, that Dr. Stovell, in applying these principles, has usually reduced the quantity of tincture of opium to ten minims; and in the expediency of this modification I am disposed to concur. I would therefore recommend it, as the rule, instead of the larger quantity stated in the text to have been given in the series of cases to which these remarks specially refer.

the temperature of the skin, should indicate the expediency of this measure. The tincture of opium is the more useful; the tincture of hyosciamus was used in milder cases, and chiefly with the view of avoiding the constipating effect of the opium. Tartar emetic thus combined and repeated every hour, very seldom, even in grain-doses, causes nausea or vomiting. In fact, it has seemed to me that in the second stage of delirium tremens, there is as complete a tolerance of the emetic action of tartar emetic as in pneumonia; and this I have remarked, even in cases in which there had been irritability of stomach during the first stage,—an observation which accords with Dr. Law's experience.*

In cases treated in this manner for about twenty-four hours, without tendency to sleep, it is often useful to intermit the medicine for a few hours before bed-time, then to use cold affusion, preceded, if the pulse and skin indicate the expediency, by a stimulant; and after the affusion to give one dose of the antimonial with a drachm of tincture of opium. By this means, sleep is often induced in cases in which, without this fuller opiate, it might have been still postponed for several hours. It is, however, very generally of no avail to adopt this course within the first twenty-four hours of the second stage.

Stimulants, as wine, brandy, ammonia, are more or less required throughout the treatment of this stage of the disease; and their use is perfectly compatible with that of cold affusion, tartar emetic, and opium. The degree to which these stimulants are required in individual cases, must vary according to what may be known of the previous history of the patient; and the state of the pulse and skin at different periods ought to be the principal guide. From six to eight ounces of port wine in the twenty-four hours will generally be sufficient, though the necessity of adding brandy to the extent of from four to six ounces, not unfrequently occurs; and it follows, that the cases in which there is the greatest necessity for stimulants, are those in which the utility of tartar emetic is least apparent, and in which it is most frequently necessary to intermit its use. But cases of this nature constitute a small proportion of the admissions, and occur for the most part only in those whose career of dissipation has been protracted, and who have suffered from several former attacks of the disease.

* On this point Dr. Stovell writes:—"I am in the habit of giving antimony without reference to the presence or absence of irritability of stomach; for not only is there marked tolerance of this medicine in those cases in which there is no irritability of stomach, but its use has often appeared to allay this irritability in cases where it existed."

It has been well remarked by Dr. Budd*, that in the management of the second stage of delirium tremens, it is of consequence to attend to the diet of the patient, with the view of encouraging any desire for solid animal food that he may evince. This suggestion is very important; and it will frequently be found that there is during this stage no great disinclination for food on the part of the patient,—such being rather a feature of the first stage.

The not unfrequent injurious effects of opium, too often repeated, or given in doses too large, in the treatment of the second stage of delirium tremens did not escape the observation of Dr. Pearson † and Dr. Blake; and has been brought forward of late years very prominently by Dr. Wright, of Baltimore, and Dr. Ware, of Boston.‡ On no point of practice is my conviction more decided, than that opium in full doses requires to be used in delirium tremens with very considerable caution,—much more, indeed, than is generally believed;—and that it is liable, under some circumstances, to hasten a fatal result by convulsion and coma, or to aggravate and modify the train of symptoms which characterise the third stage. The following have seemed to me the leading objections which may be urged against the treatment by opium, as frequently followed.

1. If there be good grounds for supposing that the tendency of the second stage is to run a certain course and terminate in sleep, then the indication of cure is, surely, not to attempt to cut short this stage abruptly, by large doses of narcotics; for it would be as sound practice to attempt to obviate the hot stage of an intermittent fever, or the febrile or eruptive stages of the exanthemata.

2. In support of the opinion that the treatment of the second stage, by free opiates, may tend to interfere with its regular course, I would state that in selecting from the cases treated in the General Hospital those which illustrated the duration of this stage §, I confined myself to those in which the change from the first to the second stage was well marked, and in which the occurrence of sleep was critical and followed by recovery; and almost without exception, these cases proved to be instances in which the treatment with tartar emetic and opium, or hyosciamus, cold affusion, and stimulants had been used. In those in which the treat-

* "London Medical Gazette," May 13th, 1843.

† "Copland's Dictionary of Practical Medicine."

‡ "British and Foreign Medical Review," vol. vii. p. 268.

§ The result of which is stated at page 629.

ment by free and frequently repeated opiates had been followed, and in which the issue had also been successful, I experienced a difficulty in determining the commencement and termination of the second stage; because opium had very generally been given more or less freely during the first stage, and had plainly masked the period of transition; and again, very frequently during the course of the second stage, sleep had been produced for some hours, but been succeeded by a recurrence of delirium, again to be checked, and perhaps again to return. It is not disputed that a full opiate given during the period of excitement is frequently followed by sleep, but if the law as stated be just, the probability of this result depends on the time of the stage at which the remedy has chanced to be given; and then it acts favourably merely in conformity with the natural tendency of the disease, and, not because there has been an accurate adaptation of the quantity to the degree of excitement.

3. It has seemed to me, that in cases treated with free opiates there is a greater tendency to pass into the third stage, and that a greater number terminate by convulsion and coma. I have not attempted, by a scrutiny of the cases, to offer a numerical statement in support of this opinion; for, in all questions of medical treatment, such data are open to evident sources of fallacy,—the principal of which is, that there are many important circumstances bearing on success which do not admit of expression by numbers. Still, however, the opinion, as stated, is the result of the impression left on my mind by the cases when under observation, strengthened by a careful review of a great many of the diaries.

4. As has already been remarked, it was the opinion of Dr. Pearson, that after a certain time it is injurious to persist in the use of opium, for the action of the medicine confuses the symptoms of the disease; and a similar conviction is still more strongly expressed by Dr. Wright, of Baltimore. My suspicion on this point was excited — when it was not known to me, that such views had been already entertained — by the following circumstances:—A man under treatment for delirium tremens in the second stage, took one grain of tartar emetic, and one drachm of tincture of hyosciamus, every hour for ten successive times, after which there succeeded convulsive agitation of the hands, which moved about as if in search of objects; there was a rolling motion of the tongue about the teeth and the cheeks, as if in search of something in the mouth; the pulse was 108, of moderate strength;

there was constant incoherent low muttering; the pupils were *very much dilated.* Under the use of blisters, tartar emetic in smaller doses, with spiritus ætheris nitrici, this patient recovered. The symptoms just detailed are those of the commencement of the third stage of the disease, with the exception that the pupils were much *dilated* instead of being *contracted.* It is hardly necessary to observe that henbane in poisonous doses *dilates* the pupils, and opium *contracts* them.

The mode of exhibiting opium to which these remarks are intended to apply is, not only the unusually large quantities recommended by some American practitioners, but — 1. The use of tincture of opium in doses of one drachm or one drachm and a half, with stimulants, given every hour or every two hours for many times. 2. The exhibition of from a drachm and a half to three drachms of tincture of opium at bed-time, followed by a half dose every hour or second hour, for two, three, or more times. 3. One and a half-grain doses of muriate of morphia with a few grains of blue pill at bed-time, repeated every second hour in grain doses for two, three, or more times, if required. The first mode I have witnessed, the second and third I have frequently practised, using at the same time cold affusion.

Before proceeding to consider the symptoms characteristic of the *third stage* of the disease, there are signs which mark as it were, in unfavourable cases, the approaching transition of the second into the third stage; and which, as bearing on treatment, it has seemed to me of much moment carefully to note. After the second stage has gone on for some time, without sleep, the pulse begins to increase in frequency, rising above 100 and becoming more compressible, the skin is damp, the expression of countenance vacant, and the pupils begin to contract*;

* Dr. Barlow, in his "Manual of the Practice of Medicine," p. 541, writes:— "The diagnosis of delirium tremens, in its perfect form, is not difficult; from phrenitis it may be distinguished by the softer pulse, the moist tongue, perspiring skin, scanty urine, and, by what is perhaps a still more important sign, the dilated pupil." That dilatation of the pupil is characteristic of delirium tremens, is, I apprehend, not a usual belief. Copland and Wood state that it is contracted in the second stage. My own opinion is that it presents no peculiarity in the second stage, but that its contraction is to be viewed as a sign of the impending dangers of the third stage.

On my return to India, I requested Dr. Leith, who had succeeded to the surgeoncy of the European General Hospital, to favour me by noticing the state of the pupil in the second stage of delirium tremens. The following is his reply, dated 21st January, 1858:—"With reference to the question whether or not the pupil is contracted or dilated during delirium tremens, I find I have noted the symptom in eighteen of the cases treated in my wards during last year without any opium, and find that in nine the tremors increase and assume more the character of subsultus tendinum than in the earlier period of the disease, and the patient catches at objects, not so much, apparently, from fancying them present when not so, as from miscalculating the distance when they are really before him.

On the occurrence of these symptoms, danger impends either from the sudden access of convulsion with succeeding coma and death, or the passing of the disease into the third stage, characterised by still increased frequency (120), and feebleness of pulse, constant agitation, low muttering delirium, contracted pupils, rolling of the tongue within the lips and cheeks as if in search of objects in the mouth,—passing gradually into coma, and terminating fatally in a few hours.

When these symptoms which indicate the transition of the second stage into the third become developed, then all narcotic medicines should be completely intermitted; the head should be

it was dilated, in seven it was of natural or moderate size, and in none was it stated to be contracted. With regard to the statement 'natural' size, or 'moderate' size, it is indefinite; and, latterly, I have compared the size during the attack with the size after recovery."

Dr. Leith, in his report of the hospital for the year 1858–59, published in No. 5, new series, "Transactions, Medical and Physical Society of Bombay," thus states his latest conclusions:—"For some time past I have attended to the state of the pupil of the eye in all cases of delirium tremens that have come under my care, and the result of my observations is, that the pupil is dilated in this disease, but that at the same time the iris is sensitive, readily obeying the stimulus of light; the pupil oscillates about a mean diameter abnormally large." Dr. Leith also explains "a diagram, in which there is a row of disks of uniform size, each having in its centre a smaller black disk which represents the pupil of the eye," by means of which he gave precision to his observations. He further states,—"With the aid of this diagram or scale, I estimate and note the relative size of the pupil on admission and during delirium; and again, after all signs of delirium have for some time ceased,—the patient being also free from the influence of opium or other medicine. I take care that the circumstances as to light are the same at each observation; and to secure this, I find it best that the patient's eyes should be directed to the sky and not to the observer, and that the time of day be always the same."

The inference which I draw from these statements, though it is not distinctly stated, is, that the dilatation of the pupil, observed in the second stage of delirium tremens, was not great in degree. The following circumstance (doubtless not overlooked by Dr. Leith) renders additional caution necessary in conducting an inquiry of this nature in this hospital. During my time, the cases of delirium tremens were treated in the ordinary light wards; they are now treated in darkened cells, badly constructed and situated in the basement floor. I still incline to the opinion, that in patients in the *second stage* of delirium tremens, undrugged with narcotics, and not secluded in small darkened rooms, but placed in ordinary light, the diagnosis is not assisted by an abnormal state of the pupil, dilatation or contraction, but that the pupil is usually what may be fairly termed natural. Further inquiry is, I think, still necessary.

shaved, a blister should be placed on the nucha, the hot foot-bath should be used, and if the scalp be hot, cold cloths should be applied to it; camphor mixture should be exhibited every second hour, either with a small portion of tartar emetic or spiritus ætheris nitrici, according to the state of the pulse and skin; wine should also be given, and the importance of mild nourishment, as beef-tea and chicken soup, is very great. These means, if adopted at the proper time, and assiduously pursued, are not unfrequently successful,—the patient falls asleep, and awakes comparatively well. It is under these particular circumstances, and also at times earlier in the disease, while *all* these conditions are not yet present, that the application of a blister to the nape of the neck is of great utility. This is a point of practice which, so far as I know, has not been estimated according to its just importance; for it is generally stated, that blisters ought to be confined to the first stage of the disease, a remark in all probability correct as regards their application to the epigastrium, but not to the nape of the neck or to the head.

In the course of these observations, I have anticipated the description of the symptoms; but it remains that a few words be said of the treatment of the third stage. Supposing that the course above recommended has been gone through, a blister should now be applied to the scalp, camphor mixture one ounce and a half with half a drachm of spiritus ætheris nitrici, should be given every second hour with wine and light nourishment. Under this treatment, in instances in which the symptoms of the third stage were fully formed, I have known recovery to take place; but in them there was frequently room for suspicion that the symptoms had, to a certain extent, been caused by the free exhibition of narcotics;—and the fact of recovery from a combination of symptoms which, resulting in the natural course of the disease, is usually, if not always, followed by death, is an additional argument in support of the opinion that the too free use of narcotics is apt to complicate and modify the symptoms of the third stage.

It has been stated by Dr. Blake that when the pulse rises above 100, there is room for apprehension. This remark is in accordance with my experience; care however being taken not to mistake a frequency of pulse caused by muscular exertions which the patient in his excitement may have been just undergoing, — for that frequency which is permanent, and which takes place when the disease is progressing unfavourably.

General Remarks on Treatment, Blood-letting, general and local,

Purgatives, Emetics, &c.—It is unnecessary to notice particularly the use of general or local blood-letting in the treatment of delirium tremens, for with the exception of local depletion, in a few cases of the first species, I believe that all are agreed in considering it inadmissible. It is not often, indeed, (so rarely is it had recourse to), that there exists the occasion of witnessing positive injury from general or local blood-letting in the second species of the disease. The opportunity, however, sometimes occurs, when the application of leeches may have been thought necessary, in consequence of the complication of local inflammatory disease, as dysentery; and it may be very safely affirmed, that this measure is never adopted without a positive aggravation of the characteristic symptoms of delirium tremens.

Laxatives or *purgatives* have not been used by me in the second species of delirium tremens, except with the view of removing existing constipation. Given with this object they are of course frequently required, but further than this, their exhibition does not constitute any part of the treatment, for free purging in this form of the disease must generally be injurious. I am aware that these opinions are opposed to the statements of several very excellent writers*; but it must be recollected that I write of the disease as observed in a climate in which affections of the bowels are common, and easily excited; and in which that free use of purgatives, often safe, and perhaps necessary, in the management of the diseases of extra-tropical countries, is generally injurious.

Emetics may occasionally be useful in the first stage, when the tongue is coated and white, and symptoms of gastric irritation are not present. Cases of this nature are, however, rare, and therefore the utility of emetics, in the treatment of delirium tremens, is very limited.

There are other points of general management on which I have thought it unnecessary to dwell, because it may be presumed that there is little difference of opinion in regard to them. They are—1. The advantage of secluding the patient in a quiet, and partially darkened room, under the care of a trustworthy attendant. 2. The injurious effects of strait-jackets, or bonds of any kind, and the extreme rarity of any necessity for their use, when the management of the patient is conducted with ordinary intelligence and tact. 3. The necessity of guarding against the risk of injury to the patient, either from the suicidal tendency, which is not unfre-

* "Copland's Dictionary of Practical Medicine," &c.

quently present, or from the efforts made by him to escape from some imaginary danger.*

This account of the symptoms and treatment of delirium tremens was presented to the Medical and Physical Society of Bombay, in 1843, and published in the Transactions of the Society †, in the form in which it is now reproduced. I expressed myself then, with confidence, on the superiority of the treatment here recommended, over that with opium and stimulants, because my opportunities of forming an opinion had been ample, and because I felt the practical question to be one of very great importance in the treatment of European Hospital sick in India. It has therefore been to me a source of great satisfaction, to find these views fully corroborated, during the last ten years, by the experience of the medical officers who have succeeded me in the European General Hospital, more especially by Dr. Stovell, who has borne repeated ‡

* The fulfilment of these indications ought never to be aimed at by the construction of darkened, barred, and secluded cells in the basement or other parts of a building not deemed suitable for other sick. The necessary protection of the patient from self-injury, and of the other inmates of an hospital from disturbance, ought to be effected without adding to the alarm characteristic of the disease—the idea of imprisonment and forcible restraint.

† No. vi. p. 139.

‡ "Transactions, Medical and Physical Society of Bombay," No. 9, p. 53; No. 10, p. 861; Second Series, No. 2, p. 66; and No. 3, p. 70.

Since these remarks were written, I have seen two reports, in which a different system of treatment has been advocated. Dr. Laycock, in the "Edinburgh Medical Journal" for October 1858, recommends an almost exclusive expectant treatment—by food, occasional cold affusion, and the soporific influence on the mind of a placebo, given at bed-time as an anodyne. Dr. Leith, in his report of the European General Hospital, Bombay, for the year 1857-58, published in the fourth number of the new series of the "Transactions of the Medical and Physical Society," states:—"The treatment of delirium tremens during the year has been chiefly expectant, and in the uncomplicated cases that have been under my own immediate care no medicine whatever has been given. The patient is secluded, and kept as quiet as the present imperfect hospital accommodation will allow; and where there is any heat of head, the cold affusion is used, and sometimes along with it the hot pediluvium. In many cases, however, even these remedies are not employed. Attention is always paid to alimentation, and strong broth is given at regular intervals. I had followed this plan for many years in the cases that from time to time came under my care, and now that I have had trial of it in a more abundant field of observation, I continue to be satisfied with it." On referring to the return, I find that the mortality was 8 per cent.

These two reports are of much interest, for they confirm the toxæmic view of the pathology of the disease, and the correctness of the general principles of treatment recommended in this chapter. But it no more follows that an expectant treatment is the best in delirium tremens because cases very generally recover under it, than that an expectant treatment is the best in all other forms of toxæmic disease. In treating delirium tremens there is not merely the question of recovery, but—1. Can the duration

testimony to the success of the system here advocated. Though, as I have elsewhere remarked, figured statements, as data from which alone to judge of the success of medical treatment, are open to very evident sources of fallacy, and must be used with much caution, yet I feel satisfied that I run no risk of misleading others, when I point to the statistics of the European General Hospital, in proof of the greater efficacy of the treatment of delirium tremens, by the means, and in accordance with the principles, here inculcated. From 1838 to 1841—the years during which I became convinced, from careful clinical observation of the evils of an exclusive opiate and stimulant treatment—the mortality from delirium tremens was 24·5 per cent. Whereas, from 1842 to 1853—a period during which I know that the disease was chiefly treated in the manner recommended by me — the mortality was 9·4 per cent. Why, the year 1848, in which the mortality again rose to 20·4 per cent., is the single exceptional year of these twelve, I am unable, from the data before me, to explain; but it would be interesting to inquire, by examination of the diaries of the cases of that year,

of the delirium be shortened? 2. Can the delirium be moderated, and thus the general management be much facilitated, and exhaustion in a measure obviated? The answer to these questions is affirmative. It is these objects which the treatment by tartar emetic and small opiates with alimentation effects; and the neglect of which is the objection to an exclusive expectant method.

It may be gathered from Dr. Laycock's cases, that the average duration of treatment was seven days; and allusions to strait-jackets show that in cases there was much violence, for which restraint was used. Dr. Leith gives no details either in respect to the duration of the attack or the character of the delirium, but seclusion in the small barred rooms of the hospital of necessity supplied restraint.

The tartar emetic treatment tends to shorten the attack, and so to moderate the delirium as very materially to facilitate the control and management of the patient without strait-jackets, and small, barred, darkened rooms. But the chief advantage of moderating the delirium is not the convenience to the attendants, but the protection of the patient from direct injury, and, above all, from the exhausting effects of the constant muscular exercise which attends the unmitigated delirium of this disease. Of the importance of this, any one who feels the pulse and skin of a patient affected with delirium tremens, after a paroxysm of restless movement and great alarm, may satisfy himself. Alimentation is a very essential part of treatment, but surely much of its value is lost if the patient be allowed to exhaust himself by uncontrolled excitement. Tartar emetic with small opiates, proportioned to the degree of excitement, prevent much of the exhaustion which results from muscular waste, and does not interfere with the taking of food: hence its utility in the treatment of delirium tremens.

I have dwelt at length on this question, because, not only is it of great importance in reference to the treatment of delirium tremens, but also to those general principles which are unfortunately gaining ground — that because recovery follows, expectant treatment is necessarily the best. This conclusion is neither logical nor consonant to rational pathology or therapeutics.

whether there had not been a backsliding into the old, and I fear, still too common, system of treatment.*

SECTION II.—*On the Pathology, the Principles of Treatment, and Diagnosis.*

I propose in this section to extend the observations of my original paper, in the hope of reconciling the discrepancies which exist in the treatment of delirium tremens. The following statements relative to the general pathology of the brain, may be received as probably true.

1. The functions of the brain may be deranged by toxœmia. It is very likely that the symptoms peculiar to this disease — the busy, apprehensive delirium, the sleeplessness, the muscular tremors—are of this nature. The poison may be "alcohol accumulated slowly in the blood, incorporated, if we may so speak, with the nervous matter of the brain," as suggested by me in 1848†, or a "compound formed of alcohol, and perhaps some morbid matter generated in the system," as advanced by Dr. Todd, in 1850.‡

* On my return to Bombay, in August, 1856, I requested Dr. Leith to have the kindness to cause the diaries of the cases of delirium tremens for the year 1848 to be examined, with the view of ascertaining whether the surmise hinted in the text was correct or not. The following is the reply:—"I at last have got the diaries of the delirium tremens cases of 1848 searched out, and I have gone over them, and the following is the result: of those entered in the register, the diaries of eight cannot be found—of these two died, six recovered; of the thirty-six that have been by me examined, thirty were treated with free use of opiates and brandy—of these six died and twenty-six recovered; six were treated with mist. antimon. c. opio chiefly—of these one died and five recovered." It is evident that the treatment with free opiates and stimulants was the ruling system of the year 1848.

† "Transactions, Medical and Physical Society of Bombay," No. 9, p. 127.

‡ "London Medical Gazette," vol. xiv., new series, p. 1078.

As bearing upon this subject, I may allude to the cases of poisoning with *Datura* which are from time to time received into the Jamsetjee Jejeebhoy Hospital. The symptoms are in many respects allied to those of delirium tremens. The delirium is more muttering, not so busy as that of delirium tremens; but there is the same rambling of the mind on subjects not present to the senses. There is the same power of controlling the thoughts for a few moments, the same desire to appear rational, and, above all, the same picking at small objects, as if they were indistinctly seen, which is often observed in the advanced stages of delirium tremens.

Where the quantity taken has been large, there is coma with agitated movements of the hands and lips, and picking movements of the fingers: in fact, the same class of deranged nervous actions which characterise the third stage of delirium tremens. There is, however, this great difference in these latter phenomena when caused by datura; they are very generally recovered from, not by a return from coma to a state of health, but the coma ceases, and then succeed the delirium and the other phenomena which attend those slighter cases which have never passed into coma.

What is the indication of cure in these cases of datura poisoning after the time has

2. The functions of the brain may be deranged from excess or defect of blood in the cerebral capillaries, without reference to its quality.

3. Determination of blood in the capillaries of the brain is of common occurrence in Europeans in India, characterised by sense of fulness or pain in the head, flushed countenance, injected conjunctivæ, heat of scalp, confusion of thought, or some degree of delirium, liable in its more aggravated forms to pass into convulsion and coma. The appearances found in fatal cases are more or less vascular turgescence of the membranes and substance of the brain, with more or less serous effusion. The more ordinary exciting causes, are elevated temperature, and immediate excesses in drinking. As proof of the influence of these causes, it may be stated, that of twenty-nine cases, with head symptoms, noted by me in the European General Hospital,* in which there was found after death, increased serous effusion in the cavity of the cranium, with or without increased vascularity, twenty-six occurred in the hot months of the year, and twenty-one in individuals addicted to drinking.

4. The subjects of the toxœmia which induces delirium tremens, are very likely to be exposed to the causes of, and to be affected

passed for the exhibition of emetics and purgatives, with the view of removing the poison from the alimentary canal? Certainly not an attempt to destroy the delirium of datura by the sopor of opium, or to remove the coma of datura by the means of treatment applicable to idiopathic apoplexy.

They are viewed as deranged states of the nervous system, caused by the presence of a poison in the blood, and which will not cease till time has been given for its elimination. If the delirium be troublesome and active, and the pulse does not contraindicate, antimonials and cold affusion are appropriate means for moderating these deranged actions. If the pulse be feeble and the skin cold, which is often the case, then stimulants are used to counteract this tendency to death by syncope. If coma comes on, then it is recollected that the suspended action of the brain, consequent on narcotic poisons, is attended by a degree of congestion, and (the state of the pulse and skin permitting) a few leeches, cold douche, and a blister to the nucha are used to lessen this congestion. It is not to be doubted that these means of treatment are often very useful and conducive to the successful issue of many of these cases.

The similarity of many of the phenomena of poisoning by datura and those characteristic of delirium tremens is a circumstance which seems to me to afford a reasonable confirmation of the idea that delirium tremens is nothing but one form of poisoning by alcohol; and to explain the practical fact, that we most successfully treat the disease when we observe the same indications of cure, *i. e.* moderate the symptoms, oppose the tendency to death, and allow time for the elimination of the poison from the blood, before we hope for perfect recovery.

A very interesting account of datura poisoning, as observed in the Jamsetjee Jejeebhoy Hospital, has been published by Dr. Giraud in the Ninth Number of the "Transactions of the Medical and Physical Society of Bombay."

* "Transactions, Medical and Physical Society," No. ix. pp. 120 and 121.

with, cerebral determination. In them we may expect to find symptoms indicative of both deranged states — that is, symptoms of delirium tremens, and of cerebral determination — combined in varying proportions, according as the one or the other predominates. Allusion has been made to this fact, in reference to the pathology of cerebral complication in remittent fever (p. 57), and it is an important consideration in the pathology and treatment of delirium tremens. It is because there is some amount of this combination of cerebral determination, in by far the larger proportion of cases of delirium tremens met with in European hospitals in India, that tartar emetic and cold affusion are so valuable, and the free use of opium and stimulants so dangerous, in the treatment.

5. In the *early* stages of the mixed cases, the danger is from the cerebral capillary derangement; there is seldom risk from failure of the action of the heart: therefore antimony and cold affusion may be freely used, but opium very cautiously. But as the duration increases, the cerebral danger may still continue, and indications of exhaustion begin to appear; and now we must be still cautious with opium, use antimony and cold affusion with more reserve, and direct our attention to stimulants and nourishment.

6. In pure unmixed delirium tremens, the danger is from exhaustion, therefore stimulants, nourishment, and opium are indicated. But they should be used in that moderate expectant manner, which is a therapeutic rule in the treatment of all forms of toxœmic disease. The coma, and serous effusion of unmixed delirium tremens, are probably related to general anæmia with watery blood, and not to local hyperæmia. It is because this form of disease is rare in Europeans in India, that the treatment exclusively appropriate to it is generally inapplicable. This remark must be viewed in connection with what has been written at the concluding part of the preceding head — that in the advanced stages of the mixed cases, there is also hazard from exhaustion. It is probably because unmixed delirium tremens occurs more frequently in the asthenic inmates of civil hospitals in the large cities of Europe, that the exclusive treatment with opium and stimulants still finds acceptance in these institutions.

In these statements I have endeavoured to explain the principles of the treatment which I have advised, and to account for the apparent discrepancy in the results of clinical experience in India and in other countries, in respect to this disease. The same doctrines will be found to pervade the more desultory observations of my original paper.

Morbid Anatomy. — The appearances found after death are sometimes trifling and insufficient to explain the phenomena of the disease. There is in a proportion of cases, but not in all, some degree of vascular turgescence of the membranes of the brain, with frequently more or less serous effusion between the arachnoid and the pia-mater, into the ventricles, or at the base of the skull, and occasionally slight opacity of the membranes. 2. There is often dotted redness at the cardiac end of the mucous lining of the stomach, frequently without alteration of texture, but sometimes with a mammillated state at the pyloric end or body of the organ. Admitting, however, the frequency of this appearance, it does not support the view originating with Broussais, and subsequently supported by Dr. Hannay * of Glasgow and others, that delirium tremens is caused by gastritis. On the contrary, this appearance of the mucous coat of a stomach exposed to the habitual action of the strong stimulus of alcohol, is what might be expected, and doubtless exists in individuals with these habits, even when delirium tremens is absent. The circumstances most important to remember as bearing on the prognosis, are the cerebral determination, the frequency of previous attacks, and the existence of some local complication — dysentery being that which is most common in delirium tremens in India.

Diagnosis. — The diagnosis between simple delirium tremens and cerebral determination or inflammation is easily stated. The characteristic delirium, the tremors, the pale countenance and the compressible pulse of the one; the flushed face, hot head, active delirium, headache, and firm pulse of the other, are sufficiently in contrast. But I have already explained that this picture does not represent the realities of practice. At the bedside of the sick we may readily recognise the peculiar delirium and the tremors of delirium tremens, but we shall generally find something more; and the practical question which ought always to arise is, does any derangement exist *in addition* to the toxœmia which causes the symptoms peculiar to delirium tremens, if so, what is its nature? On the frequency of cerebral determination I have already enlarged. The complication of inflammations, — as pneumonia, pleuritis, dysentery—has been often the subject of comment. Dr. Wood † alludes to the complication of meningitis and delirium

* "London Medical Gazette," March 3, 1838.

† "Treatise on the Practice of Medicine," by George B. Wood, M.D., vol. ii. p. 737.

tremens; this is important and very liable to be misunderstood. The following is an illustrative case.

246. *Meningitis.—Effusion of lymph and serum in the sub-arachnoid space.—Symptoms of delirium tremens.*—John Rechlin, a discharged European soldier, destitute, drinking in the bazaar, and exposing himself to the sun, came to the Jamsetjee Jejeebhoy Hospital in a state of intoxication on the 15th April. The stomach was irritable, and he was delirious in the evening. He was bled to twelve ounces; three dozen leeches were applied to the temples, and a purgative given. The delirium continued, and the illusions were of the character of those of delirium tremens. The conjunctivæ were yellow. On the evening of the 17th, the 18th, and 19th he was treated with potassio-tartrate of antimony, and tincture of opium in repeated but moderate doses. After this there was drowsiness and picking at objects without sleep. The yellowness of the conjunctivæ continued. He was now treated with moderate mercurial purgatives, diuretics, a blister to the nucha, and afterwards to the scalp. The drowsiness continued, with twitching of the arms, and the pulse lost strength. He died on the evening of the 22nd.

Inspection fifteen hours after death.—There were about four ounces of serum in the cavity of the cranium, chiefly at the base. There was also some serous effusion in the sub-arachnoid space at the convex surface of the brain. The vessels of the pia mater were somewhat congested. The pia mater and arachnoid were in parts opaque, and much thickened, chiefly from lymph deposit between them: this was most marked near the longitudinal fissure about its middle. The substance of the brain was healthy. There was no increased effusion in the ventricles. The cerebellum, pons Varolii, and medulla oblongata were healthy. The lungs and heart were normal. The liver was nearly of natural size, of pale yellow colour from biliary congestion; under the microscope the cells were visible here and there, they contained many fat globules, and were surrounded by granular amorphous matter and free fat globules. The structure of both kidneys was healthy.

Section III.—*Delirium Tremens in the natives of India.*

During the six years from 1848 to 1853, forty-one cases were admitted into the Jamsetjee Jejeebhoy Hospital; of these, two proved fatal, one being a European whose case has just been detailed. The classes chiefly affected were Hindoos and native Christians. Though the lower classes of the Parsee community drink spirits to great excess, and though I have often seen them tremulous, and exhibiting other indications of intemperance, I have never witnessed one in the second stage of delirium tremens: the cause of this fact I am unable to explain. In respect to the treatment of the disease in natives, I have followed the principles which have been so fully set forth in this chapter, and found them as applicable to natives as to Europeans.

Section IV.—*Statistics of Delirium Tremens.*

Table XXXVIII.—*Admissions and Deaths, with Per-centage, from Delirium Tremens, in the European General Hospital at Bombay, for the Five Years from* 1838 *to* 1843.

	1838 to 1843.		Monthly Average.		
	Admissions.	Deaths.	Deaths on Admissions.	Admissions on total Admissions.	Deaths on total Deaths.
January . .	18	—	—	3·2	—
February . .	22	—	—	5·3	—
March . . .	11	2	18·1	2·1	6
April . . .	26	1	3·8	4·4	2·4
May . . .	42	18	42·8	4·7	22·4
June . . .	24	2	8·3	3·1	3·9
July . . .	17	2	11·7	2·3	5·4
August . . .	12	1	8·3	1·9	2·8
September . .	18	6	33·3	3·3	11·5
October . .	9	4	44·4	1·2	14·8
November . .	16	1	6·2	2·3	2·1
December . .	22	4	18·1	3·5	·6
Total . .	237	41	17·8	3·1	7·5

Table XXXIX. — *Admissions and Deaths, with Per-centage, from Delirium Tremens, in the European General Hospital at Bombay, for the Five Years from* 1844 *to* 1848.

	1844 to 1848.		Monthly Average.		
	Admissions.	Deaths.	Deaths on Admissions.	Admissions on total Admissions.	Deaths on total Deaths.
January . .	17	1	5·8	2·7	2·2
February . .	14	—	—	2·7	—
March. . .	23	3	13·0	4·8	10·0
April . . .	23	2	8·7	4·5	6·4
May . . .	18	1	5·5	3·1	3·3
June . . .	22	—	—	3·1	—
July . . .	18	2	11·1	2·7	5·6
August . .	18	2	11·1	3·3	13·3
September . .	18	2	11·1	3·9	9·1
October . .	15	5	33·3	2·5	1·3
November . .	13	2	15·4	2·3	6·4
December . .	16	2	12·5	3·1	5·0
Total . .	215	22	10·2	3·2	5·6

TABLE XL. — *Admissions and Deaths, with Per-centage, from Delirium Tremens, in the European General Hospital at Bombay, for the Five Years from* 1849 *to* 1853.

	1849 to 1853.		Monthly Average.		
	Admissions.	Deaths.	Deaths on Admissions.	Admissions on total Admissions.	Deaths on total Deaths.
January . .	11	—	—	2·4	—
February . .	8	—	—	2·2	—
March . . .	23	—	—	5·2	—
April . . .	22	5	22·8	4·2	·0
May . . .	23	1	4·3	4·4	4·2
June . . .	29	1	3·4	5·1	3·4
July . . .	17	1	5·8	3·2	3·0
August . .	15	2	13·3	3·0	5·3
September . .	14	—	—	3·9	—
October . .	20	4	20·0	5·1	17·4
November . .	24	1	4·2	4·6	3·3
December . .	32	1	3·1	5·2	2·5
Total . .	238	16	6·7	4·1	4·5

CHAP. XXVIII.

ON CEREBRAL DISEASE AND PARALYSIS.

SECTION I. — *General Preliminary Remarks on the Pathology and Treatment of Cerebral Disease.*

THE situation of the brain and spinal cord and the nature of their physiological actions prevent our ascertaining the morbid states of these organs by physical signs. It is therefore on derangement of function that we are mainly dependent for a knowledge of their diseases; and the investigation is materially assisted by the variety of the actions in which these nervous centres are engaged, and by the distinctness of the phenomena which attend them. In order to facilitate this inquiry it may be well to state in general terms, the kind of symptoms which indicate deranged function, and then attempt to relate them to conditions of the nervous matter. In following this course, I shall, with the view of simplifying the subject, confine my observations to the brain.

It may be sufficient for clinical purposes, to divide the symptoms of cerebral disease into (*a*) Those which indicate excess of action. (*b*) Those which indicate defect of action. Under the first, may be ranged active delirium, convulsion, pain of head, and of periphery of nerves, intolerance of light and of sound. Under the second, may be included muttering delirium, drowsiness, coma, irregular spasmodic action, paralysis, anæsthesia, blindness, and deafness.

When death takes place from cerebral disease, it is usually preceded by the passage of the first class of phenomena into the second. When we investigate the pathological states of the brain —that is, the proximate causes—in these two classes of symptoms, our practical knowledge is advanced, by simply remembering that they are generally related to different conditions of the capillary circulation, as respects the quantity and quality of the blood, and its rate of movement through the vessels.

In the *first* set of symptoms, there is probably always either that active state of capillary circulation termed determination of blood, present also in the early stage of inflammation; or the quality of the blood is altered by the introduction of some external agent of which alcohol may be taken as a type.

In the *second* set there is probably a state of capillary circulation, in which the blood moves imperfectly, in which, therefore, the processes between the blood and the nervous tissue are inadequately carried on,—as obtains in passive congestion, in the stasis-stage of inflammation, in anæmia, also when the cerebral substance is partially unfit for function from organic lesion, hæmorrhage, laceration, exudation and degeneration of lymph, &c. Or the imperfect action between the blood and nervous tissue may depend on the quality of the former being altered by foreign agents, as narcotic poisons, or the materies of cachexiæ. This class of symptoms also often co-exists with evident pressure on the cerebral mass, as from depressed fracture, considerable effusion of blood, or other fluids. Without denying that the nervous matter itself may, in some manner or other, be affected by these mechanical influences, still I would suggest that the primary effect of pressure is exercised on the capillary vessels, obstructing the passage of the blood through them, and therefore impairing the functions of the brain from deficiency of the processes between the blood and tissue, just as obtains in passive congestion and anæmia.

This reference to the general pathology of the brain would be incomplete without an allusion to the influence of concussion, as evincing my belief that a condition distinct from that of disordered capillary circulation, or changed states of the blood, may be operative in some of the deranged actions of the brain. But it is not my intention to enter into the discussion of this question.

Assuming that these general pathological doctrines are correct—what is their bearing on principles of treatment?

1. If it be true that the first class of symptoms—those of excess of cerebral action—tend to pass into the second, and then to end in death, it is very evident that the prompt recognition and treatment of these symptoms must be very important. Setting aside for the present toxœmic cases, they are caused by active determination, or commencing inflammation, and are to be controlled by the appropriate use of blood-letting, cold to the head, tartar emetic, and purgatives.

2. In the treatment of the second class of symptoms much discrimination is requisite. When they depend on general cerebral

congestion—apoplexy—blood-letting, and purgatives are often useful. When they depend on destruction of structure from extravasated blood or the results of inflammation, on anæmia, or cachexia, remedies which reduce the action of the heart and lessen the quantity of blood are no longer applicable, because these conditions of cerebral disease are always characterised by failing action of the heart, and require the use of tonics and stimulants.

The treatment of narcotic poisoning is a consideration apart from my present inquiry.

The remarks in this chapter are classed under the heads:— 1. Apoplexy; 2. Meningitis; 3. Acute Hydrocephalus; 4. Chronic Hydrocephalus; 5. Morbid growths within the cranium; 6. Hemiplegia; 7. Facial Palsy; 8. Paraplegia; 9. Paralysis from arsenic.

Section II. — *Apoplexy.* — *Meningitis.* — *Acute and Chronic Hydrocephalus.* — *Morbid Growths within the Cranium.* — *Paroxysmal Headache.*

In pathology, the term cerebral *apoplexy* is only correctly applied to sudden coma, caused by general cerebral *congestion*, with or without serous effusion or hæmorrhage. But in hospital returns, it is sometimes used to designate sudden coma, caused by general cerebral *determination*, with or without serous effusion, excited by elevated temperature or alcoholic excess. In this looser acceptation, the term must be understood in the following statistical remarks.

The admissions from apoplexy, into the European General Hospital during the fifteen years, from 1838 to 1853, amounted to twenty-nine, and of these twenty-five proved fatal. The subjects of these attacks were chiefly seamen, or others who had been leading lives of dissipation and exposure to the sun, and who had been brought to hospital some hours after the access of the attack. These circumstances explain the great mortality.

Of the 311 fatal cases of European officers so frequently alluded to, eighteen deaths took place from sudden coma, viz., seven from true apoplexy; nine from elevated temperature, and two from alcohol. It has already been shown (p. 76) that of ninety fatal cases of remittent fever, thirty-three took place with coma, preceded by delirium or convulsion. A scrutiny of all these cases, both febrile and idiopathic, would doubtless show a relation between this train of symptoms and imprudence of one kind or other. Thus, it appears that of the European officers who have died in the Bombay Presidency, from 1830 to 1850, death has been caused in one sixth by forms of cerebral disease, towards the prevention of which ordinary prudence and care exercise an undoubted and considerable influence.

The admissions from apoplexy into the Jamsetjee Jejeebhoy Hospital during the six years from 1848 to 1853 amounted to forty-five, and the deaths to forty-three.

In the following table the admissions in different months in both hospitals are shown.

	European General Hospital.		Jamsetjee Jejeebhoy Hospital.	
	Admissions.	Deaths.	Admissions.	Deaths.
January	—	—	4	5
February	1	—	1	1
March	3	2	5	6
April	1	1	3	3
May	9	9	4	4
June	5	4	4	4
July	1	1	3	3
August	1	1	2	2
September	2	2	6	5
October	1	1	3	3
November	3	3	4	4
December	2	2	6	3
Total	29	26	45	43

Though it is well to abstain from drawing conclusions on the causes of apoplexy from numbers so limited as these, and stated with so little pathological precision, yet we cannot fail to notice the striking contrast in the months of seizure of Europeans and natives. In the former, one-half of the attacks took place in the hot months May and June; whereas in the latter, the admissions are pretty equally distributed throughout the year. The inference from this fact is, that of the admissions into the European General Hospital a proportion was not true congestive apoplexy, but sudden coma, related to elevated temperature, in other words, sun-stroke.

With respect to the symptoms and pathology of true apoplexy, I would refer the clinical student to Abercombie's classical work for information equally applicable to India as to European countries.*

* I would venture to counsel the graduates of the Indian colleges who are fixing the foundations of medical science and of rational medical practice in a new and great country, to study well the writings of this eminent physician, not only on account of the numerous valuable facts with which they are enriched, but also on account of the

I have nothing to add to the lucid descriptions and philosophic deductions of this distinguished pathologist.

Meningitis.—Inflammation of the pia mater and arachnoid, marked by opacity and thickening of these membranes, by deposits of lymph, or by serous effusion containing flaky flocculi, existed in cases 10, 11, 29, 30, 31, 133, 246; and the notes of others, some caused by injuries of the head, might have been added. On the whole, then, it would appear that this form of disease has not very frequently come under my notice in hospital practice in India. In the present defective state of hospital medical statistics, there are no records calculated to show whether meningitis is of more frequent occurrence in hospitals in European countries than it seems to be in India. Of the 311 fatal cases of sick officers, meningitis was the reputed cause of death in six.

Acute Hydrocephalus.—During the four years that I held medical charge of the Byculla Schools, the number of children was about 235, and with exception of 25, their ages ranged from five to fifteen, yet case 29 is the only one of cerebral inflammation which came under my observation. During the succeeding eight years, when the medical charge of these schools had passed into other hands, and during which there had been a considerable increase in the number of children, the only case with symptoms of acute hydrocephalus which has come to my knowledge, was one which occurred to Mr. Carter, who has kindly favoured me with the following statement of the symptoms and the morbid appearances found after death.

simplicity and accuracy of the diction, and the correct application of principles of reasoning to medical science and observation. The "Pathological and Practical Researches on the Diseases of the Abdomen," though meagre on several subjects of great interest to the Indian practitioner, still contain very much that is valuable to the student of medicine in all countries. The work more particularly alluded to here, "Pathological and Practical Researches on the Diseases of the Brain and the Spinal Cord," is not open to the same objection; for,—if we except the microscopic discrimination of inflammatory from degenerative softening, a more precise knowledge of the pathological changes in diseased cerebral arteries, speculations relative to the influence of cardiac and renal disease, and the correction by Dr. Burrows of Dr. Kellie's faulty experiments relative to the cerebral circulation,—I am not aware of any great addition to our knowledge of the pathology of the brain since Abercrombie wrote.

The little allusion to diathetic conditions, and the activity of the treatment, are to be in a great part attributed to the fact that the subjects were not hospital patients, but from classes of the community less influenced by diathetic states, and more likely to be benefited by depletion. The hospital physician, in comparing his own results with Abercrombie's statements, should bear this fact in recollection.

247. *Acute Hydrocephalus.*—A boy, twelve years of age, after being under treatment with febrile symptoms from the 8th to the 23rd August, 1848, complained of pain increased by pressure at the margin of the right ribs. On the 26th he had headache, became drowsy, and screamed occasionally. On the 27th and 28th there was more or less delirium; there was drowsiness, slight strabismus, impaired vision, and a pulse ranging from 68 to 80, and a remission of febrile heat of skin. During the 29th, 30th, and 31st, the drowsiness increased, the heat of skin was more marked, the pulse became very frequent, and lost strength; and he died comatose on the 1st of September.

Inspection.—The arachnoid membrane over the hemispheres of the brain presented rather an opaque appearance; it had also, where investing the cerebellum, an opaque, lymphy, almost puriform character, and was much thickened at the base of the brain. The lateral ventricles were much distended with serum, and the cerebral substance in contact with the ventricles was softened. The fourth ventricle was also much distended, and the membranes about it and around the spinal cord were opaque. The peritoneal surface of the liver was opaque, and studded chiefly at its lower edges with granular lymphy deposit.

Thus it would seem that in Bombay, during twelve years, in a body of children, in number from 255 to 350, partly Indo-British, partly descended from European parents, and the greater number ranging in age from five to fifteen, only one case of undoubted strumous meningitis has been observed. How far this result accords with, or differs from, that of similar circumstances in other countries I am unable to judge.*

When my attention is turned to the other fields of practice, in which I have been engaged, only one case of acute hydrocephalus in a European child of about ten months old, of strumous parents, who died in the Jamsetjee Jejeebhoy Hospital, comes to my recollection. There was no examination after death.

* In regard to the eight years during which I did not hold medical charge of the Byculla Schools, my statement must be looked upon as an accurate approximation to the truth. A reference to the Returns and Registers of Disease in the Schools for this period, does not show any fatal case referable to hydrocephalus. I have referred to two of the medical officers who have been in medical charge during the period adverted to. Dr. Leith, in reply, observes, "I am certain I did not see a case of acute hydrocephalus in the Byculla Schools"; and Dr. Coles states, "I do not recollect any case of any description of hydrocephalus happening whilst I was in attendance in the schools." Dr. Graham, who has also been in charge of the schools during this period, has returned to England, and I have been unable to make a similar reference to him.

The question of the comparative greater or less degree of prevalence of acute hydrocephalus in the children of these schools, is probably part of a more general question of the degree of prevalence of the strumous diathesis. I do not know what might be the result of the application of the test suggested by Mr. Phillips in his work on Scrofula—viz., "Enlarged Cervical Glands discoverable by touch"; but I believe that I am correct in saying that scrofulous disease of the joints, suppurating lymphatic or tubercular mesenteric disease, is of infrequent occurrence. On the other hand, if the history of these children be traced after they have grown up and left the schools, it will be found that phthisis pulmonalis is a cause of death sufficiently common: I can bring to my recollection several cases in proof of this.

Chronic Hydrocephalus, I have seen only two cases, both patients of Dr. Peet. In one the head was three times tapped: the particulars of the case, which terminated fatally, have been reported by Dr. Peet.*

Morbid Growths within the Cranium.—The following is the only instance of this pathological state in my notes.

248. *Amaurosis of both eyes, headache, fatuity, convulsions, tumour in the brain, with much softening of the cerebral substance.*—Joshua Paterson, aged twenty-five, seaman of the ship *Don Pascoa*, was admitted into the European General Hospital on the 25th April, 1841, affected with complete amaurosis of both eyes, and complaining of pain of the right side of the head, fixed at the temple and shooting in different directions. He was somewhat reduced in flesh and strength. He stated that about fifteen months before, he became affected with headache, and had continued subject to it ever since. About seven months before admission the pain was confined to the left temple, and was followed by amaurosis of the left eye. Whilst at sea, about two months since, the pain affected the right side of the head, and the amaurosis of the right eye took place about a fortnight before admission. He continued in hospital till the 2nd December, 1842, (a period of nineteen months,) when he died. During the first month or two there was more or less pain of head. Leeches, blisters, &c., were used. During the greater part of his residence in hospital, he was in a fatuous state, and made little complaint. On two occasions he experienced convulsive fits, followed by sopor, and twice extensive sloughing ulcers formed on the sacrum. Some days before his death he lay in a drowsy state, with twitching movements of the fingers, and refused all food.

Inspection eight hours after death.—Head.—The lower part of the anterior lobes and the anterior part of the middle lobes of the brain adhered to the calvarium, and were separated from it with difficulty. The brain in these sites, but chiefly the anterior part of the middle lobe of the left side, was in a very pulpy state; in the latter site there was imbedded a tumour, the size of a small walnut, partly schirrous and partly tubercular in its character. The rest of the brain appeared to be normal.

Paroxysmal Headache.—There is a circumstance relating to the symptomatology of cerebral disease, to which my attention was directed at a very early period of my service in India, and to which a brief allusion may be useful. Cases of paroxysmal headache related to malarious influence, mercurial or syphilitic cachexia, came under my observation from time to time;† but others in which organic cerebral disease was apprehended were also of occasional occurrence: of the latter I may instance three, in which this suspicion proved ultimately correct. The first, an officer seen by me on the Mahubuleshwur Hills, whose case is quoted by Mr. Murray, in his first report on the climate of that sanitarium‡: this officer died of hypertrophy of the brain at Sholapore. The second, a much esteemed officer, who, after suffering

* "Transactions, Medical and Physical Society of Bombay," No. 7, p. 97.

† Such cases have certainly been of less frequent occurrence of late years, and this I attribute to the greater caution observed in the use of mercury in the general treatment of disease in India.

‡ "Transactions, Medical and Physical Society of Bombay," No. 1, p. 143.

for a considerable time from attacks of acute periodic headache, became subject to occasional convulsion, and ultimately died, also of hypertrophy of the brain. The third, an officer of the royal army, under my care at Mahubuleshwur, subsequently died in Dublin of cerebral disease, of the precise nature of which I have not been informed.

In the year 1836, a communication on this question of diagnosis was submitted by me to the Medical and Physical Society of Bombay, in which I brought together the doubtful cases which had occurred in my own practice; and then quoted a series of instances of cerebral disease characterised, with one exception, by paroxysmal pain of head, extracted from the Fifth Volume of Andral's Clinique Medical, and Abercrombie's work on Diseases of the Brain. The diagnosis of functional from organic paroxysmal headache is sometimes difficult, and depends on a careful consideration of the history, and of the associated symptoms. The beneficial effect of treatment directed under a belief in the functional character of the headache is not always to be relied upon as a means of diagnosis: in two of the three cases above adverted to — those of hypertrophy of the brain — the headache was at times alleviated by the use of antiperiodic remedies.

The cases of fatal cerebral disease characterised by paroxysmal pain of head, reported by Andral and Abercrombie, submitted by me to analysis, amount to thirty-four, and the conclusions which were drawn from them may now be briefly stated. The following were the lesions found after death: —

1. Softening of some part of the brain or cerebellum	9
2. Tumours, chiefly encephaloid and scirrhous	13
3. Hypertrophy and induration of the whole cerebral mass	3
4. Tubercles in different parts of the brain and cerebellum	8
5. Patch of effused lymph on the arachnoid membrane	1
Total	34

1. *Softening of some parts of the Brain or Cerebellum.* — The duration of these cases was generally very much under a year, dating from the commencement of the illness. In one it was only ten days, and in another twenty.

The pain was usually confined to a particular part of the head, and in eight of the cases it existed on the side in which the lesion was found after death. In all the pain was persistent, in some obtuse, in others severe, but in all acuter paroxysms took place from time to time. In one case there was no pain of head, but pain of the extremities of the side opposite to that in which the lesion was found after death: the pain was followed by spasmodic twitching and paralysis. In one case there was pain of head at the site of lesion, and also pain of the neck and of the upper extremity of the opposite side, which gradually ended in paralysis.

After the pain of head had persisted for some days a sense of diminished power of the extremities of the opposite side began to be experienced. This generally commenced in the upper extremity, then extended to the lower, and ended in complete paralysis. Sometimes the diminution of power was preceded by spasmodic twitching, or permanent contraction, of some of the joints; and in these cases the spasms were preceded by paroxysmal pain of the extremities. In none of the cases under notice did spasm precede the paralysis, without itself having been preceded by paroxysmal pain of the affected parts.

After paralysis had existed for some time, spasmodic contractions again recurred in some cases, but in these there was reason for believing that there had been aggression of fresh inflammatory action.

It was usually observed in these cases that with the gradual access of the paralysis there was remission of the pain of the head.

In these nine cases the fatal result took place in the following manner:—

By sudden apoplexy from cerebral hæmorrhage	2
By gradual exhaustion	1
By pneumonia	1
By gradual coma	2
By convulsion	1
By access of general inflammation of brain and membranes	2
Total	9

From this statement it would appear that there is not much likelihood of mistaking pain of head symptomatic of inflammatory softening of the brain for functional headache. When the pain — obtuse or severe — is confined to a particular part of the head, is permanent but liable to occasional acute paroxysms, there are grounds for apprehension. When, after the persistence of such headache for some days, there is sense of tingling or pain, spasmodic twitching or awkwardness in using the arm of the opposite side, the existence of serious cerebral disease becomes almost certain, unless the individual affected is evidently the subject of malarious cachexia. I make this latter reservation, because I have witnessed at least one very striking case, in which recurrences of intermittent fever with occasional periodic headache were followed by spasmodic twitching of one of the arms and of the muscles of the face. In this case, in consequence of the history, the periodic character of the headache, the cachectic state of the patient, and the choreic character of the muscular action, the affection was attributed to malaria and not to cerebral disease. This patient quite regained his health after return to England.*

In the relation just stated between inflammatory softening of the brain and pain of head, it will be understood that my observations apply to a certain series of cases; for it must be well known that softening of the brain often runs its course without pain of head, and is then indicated by the kind of symptoms which have been here described as having taken place in succession to headache.

2. *Tumours in the brain.* — In the thirteen cases classed under this head the duration of the disease was considerable. In seven it extended to two or three years, in one to ten, and in another to fifteen. The ages of the individuals affected with encephaloid degeneration ranged from thirty to sixty years. The pain in these cases was more decidedly intermittent than in those of softening; but it generally became permanent towards the close of the affection. When paralysis of the opposite extremities was present, it generally occurred in the advanced stages, and after the headache had existed for a length of time. The manner of termination was, in several, by the aggression of varying degrees of inflammation of the membranes or substance of the brain.

3. *General hypertrophy of the brain.* — The three subjects of this lesion were under thirty years of age, and the duration of illness, dating from the commencement of cerebral symptoms to

* I have, since this passage was written, seen another case in which the diagnosis was still more doubtful, because there was no influence of malaria to explain it. An officer of about twenty-one years of age, of good constitution, with whom I had travelled to India in July and August of 1856, not long after his arrival accompanied the force to the Persian Gulf, whence he returned about May 1857, after suffering from headache and pain of limbs, looked upon as rheumatic. I saw him at Poona in June, when he was affected with irregular spasmodic movements somewhat choreic in character. They commenced in the right side, became less there and passed to the left side, but subsequently became general, and were sometimes to such a degree as to seem to threaten an attack of general convulsion. The articulation was imperfect, and there was slight facial twitching. The pulse was of good strength, the face flushed, and no notable periodicity of the symptoms. I apprehended organic lesion probably of the cerebellum. He was leeched, and an attempt made to affect the system with mercury without success. There was no marked effect from the treatment, but after upwards of a month he began gradually to improve, and the irregular movements had ceased before the middle of September. He subsequently came to England, and has quite recovered his health. I saw him last in July 1860.

the period of death, was respectively fifteen, twelve, and ten years. In all, paroxysmal headache had been present for some years; it did not, however, present the fixed and limited character of that usually related to other lesions, but extended over the whole head. In one case there was complication of epilepsy from the commencement, and in the other two convulsion towards the close. The headache related to hypertrophy of the brain was frequently attended with irritability of stomach.

4. *Tubercles in different parts of the brain and cerebellum.*—The eight subjects of this morbid state were under thirty years of age, and tubercles were generally found present in other organs. In one death took place from pulmonary phthisis. The symptoms which attended the development and progress of tubercles in the brain in these cases were very similar to those already stated in regard to the formation of tumours.

SECTION III.—*Paralysis.—Hemiplegia.—Myelitis.—Paraplegia.—Paralysis from Arsenic.—Facial Palsy.*

The admissions from paralysis into the Jamsetjee Jejeebhoy Hospital, during the six years from 1848 to 1853, amounted to 288, and the deaths to forty-two. They exhibit a mortality of 14·6 per cent., and a ratio of 0·01 per cent. of the total hospital admissions, and 1·02 per cent. of the total hospital deaths. The admissions are pretty equally divided throughout the year.

In my brief remarks on this class of disease, I shall allude to—1. Hemiplegia; 2. Paraplegia; 3. Paralysis from arsenic; and 4. Facial Palsy.

HEMIPLEGIA.—Of the 288 cases of paralysis, by far the greater number have been hemiplegia. I regret, however, that my notes do not supply data for determining with precision the proportion of hemiplegia to the other forms of paralysis. The diaries of forty-seven cases of hemiplegia treated in the clinical ward are before me, and the few practical observations about to be offered have reference to these cases, and are arranged under the heads—1. Causes; 2. Pathology; 3. Symptoms; 4. Treatment.

Causes.—The ages of the forty-seven clinical patients were:—

20 to 30 years	22
31 „ 40 „	13
41 „ 50 „	6
51 „ 60 „	5
Upwards of 60 years	1
	47

In this statement, we find that three-fourths of the affected with hemiplegia were below the age of forty. Whether a result so different from that which is usually asserted of the relation of age to this disease is sufficiently explained by the fluctuating character of the population of Bombay, and the probable abnormal proportion of individuals in the prime of life; or whether the influence of advancing years is less operative in causing hemiplegia in the natives of India than of European countries, is a question which, for the present, must be left *sub judice.*

The *caste* of these clinical patients is stated in respect to forty-five; viz: —

Hindoos	19
Mussulmans	12
Parsees	10
Native Christians	4

In the chapter on Pericarditis and Endocarditis it is shown (p. 565) that the proportion of Parsees to the total hospital inmates is only about one-twelfth; but this statement makes the proportion of Parsees affected with hemiplegia only a little less than one-fourth. Though, from arrangements connected with my clinical ward, the proportion of Parsees affected with hemiplegia to the other castes is here represented in excess, still, from hospital experience and from cases seen in consultation with the College Graduates, I entertain the belief that Parsees are more subject to hemiplegia than the other native classes in Bombay.

The record of the *habits* of these clinical patients has not been sufficiently attended to. Seven are mentioned as addicted to the use of spirits, opium, or bhang.

Of late years it has been maintained by pathologists, that structural disease of the heart, and Bright's disease of the kidney, play an important part in the causation of hemiplegia as well as in that of other forms of cerebral disease. The condition of the heart, judged of by physical signs, is distinctly noticed in thirty-three of these cases, and in thirty of them the organ was considered healthy.* In Chap. XXV., twenty-eight cases of heart-disease are treated of, and cerebral affection was absent in all. In twenty-five of the forty-seven clinical cases of hemiplegia, the condition of the urine was carefully observed, and in none did it present traces of albumen. It has been already shown in Chap. XIX., p. 481, that

* The remaining three cases are narrated in this chapter, 251, 254, 255. If my results were arrived at from fatal cases alone they would conform more nearly to those usually stated; but on a question open to clinical as well as to post mortem observation is it not an error to generalise exclusively from the records of the dissecting room?

my cases of Bright's disease do not tend to confirm the etiological relation usually supposed to exist between affections of the brain and albuminuria.

On these results it may be remarked that they at least suffice to justify a suspicion that it will ultimately be proved that pathologists have, on these questions, indulged in a premature and hasty generalisation. The investigations of others have doubtless shown that a coincidence of the diseases is not uncommon; but that the relation is one of cause and effect, is, I would submit, as yet problematical.

Pathology. — As hemiplegia depends upon a deranged condition of a limited portion of the nervous matter of the brain, it may be assumed that the derangement is generally of a kind which involves structural lesion. The destruction of tissue may be caused by laceration, by a blood-clot, by inflammation ending in softening or abscess, or by degeneration from mal-nutrition consequent on deficient blood-supply from mechanical arterial obstruction or from a general cachectic state. Twenty-nine of my clinical cases were considered to be dependent on cerebral hæmorrhage, fourteen on structural lesion from inflammation, and one on degenerative softening. The diagnosis of the hæmorrhagic cases chiefly rested on the suddenness of the seizure, the absence of headache, febrile disturbance, soreness of the affected side, and contraction of the joints; that of the inflammatory cases, on the presence of more or less of these symptoms, preceded sometimes by pain of head and febrile excitement. The single case of degenerative softening was proved by inspection after death (255).*

Of the cases about to be narrated, six † illustrate inflammatory softening; and one (255) degenerative softening. Case 256 shows well the obscurity with which abscess in the brain may form, and case 94 also illustrates this truth. Of the nine cases just referred to, the lesion in four was in a corpus striatum, and in the others was situated elsewhere in a hemisphere. In the eight in which hemiplegia had been present, the lesion was, it need hardly be observed, on the side of the brain opposite to the paralysed extremities. In case 257, not examined after death, there was hemiplegia of the right side, caused as was supposed by hæmorrhage; but the occurrence of gangrene of the left leg, from obstruction of the femoral artery, afterwards suggested the suspicion that

* The reader will bear in mind that Gluge and Bennett have lately pointed out that the distinction of inflammatory from degenerative softening, may be facilitated by the detection with the microscope of exudation corpuscles in the former.

† Cases 249 to 254.

the paralysis might have been produced by obstruction of a cerebral arterial branch by a blood-clot or fibrinous coagulum. In case 258 there had been hemiplegia of the left side for four years, followed by transient palsy of the muscles, ruled by the portio dura, on the right side; so that the case formed no exception to the almost universal, but not well-explained, fact, that in hemiplegia, the portio dura of the affected side remains intact.

249. *Hemiplegia of the right side.—Softening of the left corpus striatum.*—Crushna Govind, a Hindoo cart driver, of thirty years of age, after twelve days' illness, was admitted into the clinical ward, on the 24th September, 1849. There was paralysis of the right side, face included, indistinct articulation, and deviation of the tongue to the affected side. The right elbow and wrist were permanently flexed. There was no anæsthesia. The right side of the chest moved less than the left on inspiration. He was leeched on the temples, a small blister applied, and diuretics and laxatives exhibited. He was comatose on the 2nd October, and died on the 3rd.

Inspection nine hours after death.—Head.—There was some degree of turgescence of the vessels of the dura mater; and those of the pia mater were very turgid with blood even to their minute ramifications. The cortical substance of the brain was of darker colour than natural; and the white substance, when incised, presented numerous bleeding points. There was dark-red softening in the centre of the anterior and the posterior parts of the left corpus striatum. The posterior softened portion was the size of a small bean: the anterior was considerably larger. There was no increased serous effusion in the ventricles, nor at the base of the skull. The cortical substance of the cerebellum was also darker than natural, and the white substance presented numerous bleeding points on incision. No coagulum of effused blood, old or recent, could be detected in any part of the brain. The kidneys were healthy.

250. *Apoplexy.—Hemiplegia of the right side.—Death.— General congestion of the membranes of the brain.— Red softening of the left corpus striatum.* — Munchee, a Portuguese sailor, of forty-four years of age, was brought to hospital on the 11th December, 1848. He was in a comatose state. The pupils were contracted. There was paralysis of the right side, with tremors of the left leg and arm. After excesses in drinking, he had been found on board ship in this condition, two days before he was brought to hospital. He died on the 12th.

Inspection twenty hours after death. — Head. — On separating the skull-cap from the dura mater, dark-coloured blood oozed in small quantity from the vessels. The glandulæ Pacchioni were more developed in parts, and caused a firmer than natural adhesion between the surfaces of the arachnoid, where it dips between the hemispheres to line the falx. The vessels of the pia mater were congested, and a thin veil of serum was here and there effused between the arachnoid and pia mater on the convex surface of the brain. The anterior part of the left corpus striatum was, compared to that of the other side, considerably softened, pulpy, and of dark-red colour, but there was no trace of distinct extravasation of blood. The substance of the brain and cerebellum did not present any other appearance worthy of note. The vessels at the base were healthy. There was no increased effusion of serum in the ventricles. Slight dotted vascularity of the mucous membrane of the stomach existed. The liver and the kidneys appeared healthy.

251. *Hemiplegia of the right side.—Softening of the left corpus striatum.—Disease of the mitral valve.*—Mahomed-Avad, a Mussulman beggar, of thirty years of age, was brought to hospital by a police peon. He was paralytic of the right side, and very drowsy. He died a few hours after admission.

Inspection. — The upper portion of the left corpus striatum was reduced to a creamy consistence, and was of darker colour. The ventricles of the heart were dilated. The mitral valve was thickened, and on its surface near the attachment of the chordæ tendineæ, there were two or three indurated granular bodies.

252. *Symptoms of inflammation of the brain, followed by hemiplegia of the right side, and death by coma.—Red softening of the left corpus striatum found after death.* — Pandoo-Souza, a washerman, of twenty-five years of age, a native of Goa, was brought to the Jamsetjee Jejeebhoy Hospital, on the 30th September, 1830, in a state of coma. His friends stated that he had been ill fourteen days with fever attended with headache — that eight days before admission the extremities of the right side had become paralysed. The coma had existed for three days. The pulse was small and slow. He died on the 4th October.

Inspection made by Mr. Lesboa. — Head. — An ounce of serum oozed out on separating the calvarium, and an ounce and a half were found at the base of the skull. The vessels of the pia mater were turgid, and a small point of the superior surface of the left hemisphere at its middle part, and near to the longitudinal fissure, was opaque from slight lymph effusion into the sub-arachnoid tissue, and a similar spot was observed in the left Sylvian fissure at its commencement. Numerous bloody points appeared on incising the brain. The left corpus striatum when cut into was found darker than the right, and broke down readily into a soft pulpy substance on pressure. There was no surrounding redness. The texture of the right corpus striatum and thalamus was healthy. The other cavities of the body were not examined.

253. *Hemiplegia of the right side. — Meningitis and softening of the anterior and middle lobes of the left cerebral hemisphere. — The premonitory symptoms well marked.* — An officer, of forty-two years of age, of corpulent and plethoric habit, after twenty-five years' residence in India, became, in April 1834, suddenly affected with giddiness, general but not severe pain of head, tingling sensation in the ring and little finger of the right hand, and subsequently slight impairment of articulation. The senses were undisturbed. He was actively treated and resumed his duties, which were frequently of a harassing description. During one or two months subsequent to the above attack, there was occasional numbness and tingling of the fingers of the right hand, also at times a dragging of the right leg, and a constant and irresistible inclination to sleep after dinner. In the course of the following monsoon all these symptoms were removed, with the exception of the strong inclination to sleep. On returning to Bombay in the ensuing cold season, from the Deccan, where the events above detailed had occurred, the somnolency was still experienced, and there was frequent pain over the left temple, with giddiness and feeling of numbness of the right arm. The somnolency he attributed to increasing corpulence, the headache and other symptoms to biliousness, aggravated by the harassing duties of his office; and by the action of a smart purgative, they were in general temporarily removed. This officer arrived on the Mahabuleshwur Hills, on the 4th May, 1835, to appearance in robust health. After having felt an increase of headache and giddiness for two days, he was seized in the morning of the 12th with hemiplegia of the right side and loss of speech without suspension of consciousness. He continued without any improvement, and died on the 14th, after having been comatose for only two hours.

Inspection. — Head. — There was much vascularity of the pia mater, with here and there turbid lymph effused under the arachnoid. The substance of the brain, on being sliced, showed a surface crowded with bloody points. A large portion of the central part of the anterior and middle lobes of the left hemisphere was very markedly softened and reduced to a pultaceous mass. There was no effusion into the ventricles. The heart was healthy, but commencing deposit existed at the beginning of the aorta.

Remark. — I am indebted to Mr. Murray for the notes of this case, and the opportunity of witnessing the examination after death,

254. *Incomplete paralysis of left side.— Improvement.—Disease of heart and valves. — Death hastened by diarrhœa. — Puriform softening of part of anterior lobe of right*

cerebral hemisphere. — Bhao, a Hindoo liquor-seller, of thirty-five years of age, habitually using spirits in moderate quantity, while evacuating the bowels at midnight, suddenly fell down insensible. On becoming conscious he found the left extremities deficient in power, and on the following day his speech was indistinct and he was affected with headache. Four days afterwards he was admitted into the clinical ward, on the 13th October, 1851. There was incomplete paralysis of the extremities and face of the left side and indistinct articulation. He complained of pain of the right temple, and suffered from febrile accessions coming on with chills at midnight. The præcordial dulness extending from the third intercostal space was continuous with the hepatic dulness, and was bounded externally by a vertical line dropped from the left nipple. There was a systolic murmur at base and apex, but of different tones, also a slight diastolic murmur, most distinct at the apex. The systolic murmur was loudest and roughest at the third right costal cartilage and continued so to the top of the sternum. The pulse was of moderate volume and distinctly jerking in character. The urine was frequently tested and gave no trace of albumen. The bowels tended to be relaxed. He was treated with small blisters to the nucha and diuretics, and on the 5th November the paralysis of the limbs was reported to be removed, but that of the face still to continue. The diarrhœa increased, became dysenteric in character; he lost strength, and on the morning of the 22nd November hs was found comatose with dilated pupils, stertorous breathing, cold and clammy and imperceptible pulse, and died an hour afterwards.

Inspection seven hours after death. — *Brain.* — There was increased vascularity of the membranes of the brain, and on the convex surface considerable increased effusion of serum into the sub-arachnoid space. There was slight opacity here and there of the arachnoid, and firmer adhesion than usual between the surfaces at the dipping down of the falx. There was about an ounce of serum at the base of the skull. At the anterior part of the right anterior lobe of the brain there was a portion near the under surface about the size of a pigeon's egg, soft, pulpy, and yellow, and in parts consisting almost entirely of pus. There was no cyst and no traces of inflammation of the pia mater or of the arachnoid in the neighbourhood of the abscess. *Chest.* — The heart reached from the second to the seventh rib, and transversely almost to the junction of the right costal cartilages with the ribs. About an ounce and a half of clear serum was found in the pericardium. On the external surface of the heart there were three or four opaque patches of organised lymph. The right auricle and ventricle were distended with blood. The left ventricle contained a considerable quantity of dark coagulated blood, was dilated, and its walls were somewhat thicker than natural. The mitral valve was considerably thickened from firm warty-looking deposit, and there was similar deposit on the chordæ tendineæ, which were rendered more friable. The aortic valves were also thickened at their edges and the diameter of the aortic opening increased. The right ventricle was also somewhat dilated. The tricuspid valves and those of the pulmonary artery were healthy. The ascending aorta was considerably dilated, and its inner surface and that of the arch was irregular and very rough from firm organised deposit, which had become ossific just above the aortic orifice. The coats of the aorta much thickened. The lungs were spongy and crepitating. *Abdomen.*—There was no morbid appearance of the mucous membrane of the intestines. The liver was healthy. There was a little encroachment on the tubular portion of the left kidney. The right kidney was healthy.

Remark.—The examination after death confirmed the diagnosis of the heart disease, as noted on admission, viz., "hypertrophy with dilatation of left ventricle, disease of the mitral and aortic valves, the latter permitting regurgitation, dilatation of the aorta, and roughing of its inner surface."

255. *Hemiplegia of the left side.* — *White softening in the right cerebral hemisphere.* — Nickus, aged sixty, a beggar, an infirm old man, paralytic, and frequently in hospital, was admitted on the 1st August, 1852, in a state of debility. On the 25th there

were convulsive movements of the left side, except the face, which was calm. Both feet were flexed, pupils unaffected, skin above natural temperature; pulse rather frequent: was perfectly sensible, but spoke with difficulty, and could not protrude the tongue beyond the lips. He said that he felt pain in the head and nape of the neck, chiefly the latter. On the 27th there was continuance of the symptoms, with, however, towards evening, the convulsive movements affecting both sides. On the 28th the convulsive movements were confined to the left side. He continued to sink, and died on the 4th September.

Inspection by Mr. Lesboa, fifteen hours after death. — *Head.* — There were about seven ounces of turbid fluid at the base of the skull. In the substance of the posterior lobe of the right hemisphere, immediately behind, and to the outer side of the posterior cornu of the right ventricle, there was softening to the extent which would be occupied by a pigeon's egg. The softened substance was very pulpy, and of yellowish white colour. The surrounding parts of the brain were healthy. The right lateral ventricle was considerably enlarged, but there was no unusual quantity of fluid in it or in the left. The arachnoid membrane, covering the cerebellum, was somewhat thickened and opaque in some points, chiefly around and over the vermiform process. No other morbid change in the brain was detected. *Chest.*— The lungs were healthy. The aortic semi-lunar valves were thickened at their attached margins by some hard deposits. In other respects the heart was healthy. The liver was smaller than natural; the fibrous capsule was thickened, and the surface irregular and lobulated; the substance was firm and indurated, and when cut into presented a distinct nodulated appearance. The nodules about the size of a small pea, with bands and streaks of white fibrous tissue crossing between.

256. *Abscess in the left hemisphere of the brain; for some time general febrile symptoms.—Hemiplegia of the right side some days before death.*—Jeremiah Merit, an African, aged twenty-four, after a month's illness was admitted into the European General Hospital, on the 2nd September, 1842. He suffered from a mild attack of dysentery, and was discharged well on the 9th October. Re-admitted on the 19th October ill with quotidian fever, associated with pain of the left hypochondrium: he was discharged well on the 1st November. Re-admitted on the 24th November, suffering from irregular febrile accessions, but to no great extent: he made no complaint of local uneasiness, and the suspicion was entertained that he was disposed to make more of his ailments than their apparent importance justified. On the 20th December his bowels were relaxed, and he complained of cramps of the limbs. On the 21st the right arm and leg were weak. On the 22nd there was complete hemiplegia of that side, with occasional twitching of the arm. There was heat of skin, and he was manifestly losing flesh and strength; no headache complained of. He continued in this state, with generally a febrile accession towards evening. He died on the 28th.

Inspection seven hours after death.—*Head.*—There was considerable thickening with an opaque state of the arachnoid membrane of the upper surface of the brain, with yellow points here and there. In the left hemisphere of the brain, above the lateral ventricle, there was an abscess, the size of a large walnut, filled with pus, and surrounded by a pulpy state of the cerebral substance. The right side of the brain was healthy. *Chest.*—Old adhesions of the lungs and pearly deposit on the surface of the heart.

257. *Apoplexy, followed by hemiplegia of the right side.—Gangrene of the left foot and leg, apparently from obstruction of the femoral artery.*—Kasoojee, a Hindoo, of forty years of age, a native of Kattywar, but for many years resident in Bombay, following the occupation of sandal-wood seller, and temperate in his habits, was admitted into the clinical ward on the 28th October, 1853. There was complete hemiplegia of the right side, face included, attended with anæsthesia and absence of reflex action on tickling the sole of the affected foot. He was drowsy and unable to speak, but seemed

to apprehend what was said to him; was unable to protrude his tongue. He was of spare habit, but the pulse was full. The sounds and impulse of the heart were normal. It was reported that, three days before admission, he had been much exposed to the sun, making preparations for an entertainment; and that subsequently, after having been for some time in a stooping posture serving his guests, he assumed the erect position, then fell down suddenly in a state of complete coma, with stertorous breathing, but without convulsion of any kind. After a time he vomited, recovered his consciousness, but remained in the state present on admission. He continued in the hospital till the 5th November, when he was removed by his friends. On the 30th there was febrile heat of skin, and he began to complain of pain of the left leg; and on the 31st the pulse of the paralytic side was somewhat fuller than that of the left side. On the 2nd November the upper part of the left leg was still painful, but the lower part and the foot were cold and livid, somewhat swollen, and without sensation. No signs of cardiac disease. No change in the paralytic symptoms of the right side. On the 4th, absence of pulsation of the femoral artery at the left groin was noted. The gangrene increased in degree, but not in extent. He suffered from epistaxis two or three times, was restless, and at times wandering. The pulse lost strength and increased in frequency, and in this state he was removed from hospital by his friends. Treated with leeches to the head, a blister, and purgatives.

Remarks.—The history and the symptoms seemed clearly to point to general cerebral congestion, with partial hæmorrhage, as the proximate cause of the attack. The gangrene of the unparalysed foot and leg, apparently from obstruction of the femoral artery, suggests the question,—whether the apoplectic and paralytic symptoms might not also have been due to fibrinous coagula obstructing branches of the cerebral arteries.

258. *Hemiplegia of left side, persistent.—Facial palsy of the right side, consecutive and transient.*—Moorarjee, a Hindoo shopkeeper, of fifty years of age, was admitted into the clinical ward on the 8th August, 1852. There was incomplete hemiplegia of the upper and lower extremities of the left side; but the portio dura of the right side was also affected, as indicated by the open state of the right eye. The sounds and impulse of the heart were normal. His statement was that the hemiplegia of the left side had existed for four years, but that two days before admission, when cooking his food, he suddenly fell, and that since then giddiness and the facial distortion had been present. He remained under observation till the 15th September, using occasional laxatives, diuretics, and small blisters to the nucha, and electro-galvanism to the affected limbs. The urine, frequently tested, gave no trace of albumen. On discharge he could close the right eye, and the distortion of face was almost gone; but the hemiplegia of the left side remained unchanged.

Symptoms.—The hemiplegia in these clinical cases has been nearly equally divided between the two sides: there were twenty-four of the right, and twenty-three of the left side. The face of the same side was affected in thirty-six, articulation impaired in twenty, and deviation of the tongue to the affected side, was usually observed in the cases in which the face shared in the disease. There was anæsthesia of the paralytic side in ten; and in some it disappeared under treatment, though no alleviation of the paralysis had been effected.

There was a state of flexion more or less rigid of the elbow joint of the affected side in seventeen cases; sometimes accompanied with a similar condition of the wrist or finger joints. This event generally occurred in cases which had been considered inflammatory from the commencement, or in which the after symptoms indicated the probability of inflammation having affected the cerebral tissue around a blood-clot.

Dr. Todd, in his clinical lectures on paralysis, has adverted to great muscular rigidity, occurring both early and late. The first related to inflammatory action. The second attributed to the contraction of the cicatrices consequent on absorbed blood-clot acting on the neighbouring healthy tissue, and keeping up a slow and lingering irritation.

The presence or absence of reflex action in the affected limbs was noted in some of the cases, but not with sufficient regularity to merit notice here.

I have confined my remarks on hemiplegia to the desultory suggestions, which my own observations have prompted, and have made no attempt to enter upon a full consideration of this important subject. The work of Abercrombie, abounding with interesting facts and philosophic deductions, should be in the hands of every clinical student of this branch of pathology.

Treatment. — It is sufficiently easy to lay down abstract principles of rational treatment for the different forms of hemiplegia. The difficulty is in the diagnosis, and consequently in the application of the principles to particular instances. For example, if the hemiplegia is due to recent cerebral hæmorrhage, and symptoms of general excess of blood in the cerebral capillaries are present, it may be necessary to reduce this by general or topical blood-letting, cold to the head, position, and purgative medicines. If, on the other hand, general cerebral congestion is absent, these means are not required, and the removal of the clot, by absorption, must be a work of time: in the management of such a case we must be careful not to reduce the system too much, for this reparative process is dependent on a certain vigour of the vital actions; while, at the same time, we must be watchful for the access of inflammation of the surrounding cerebral tissue, in order that the appropriate remedies may be used.

Should, however, the hemiplegia be attributable, not to hæmorrhage, but to inflammation leading to lymph exudation and softening, then the remedies appropriate for this morbid action, in relation to stage and constitutional state, must be had recourse to. It has been usual — on a therapeutic principle generally acknowledged and elsewhere fully explained — to give, in this state of cerebral disease, *mercury* to the induction of its influence on the system: it has generally been used in my clinical cases of this nature; but benefit consecutive on ptyalism has not occurred in a single instance of paralysis under my care. I am unwilling to express with confidence a dissuasive opinion on this point of practice, but I may avow my belief that benefit from mercury in inflammatory hemiplegia is improbable, simply because the paralysis does not in all likelihood occur till after degenerative softening of the lymph, and of the tissue around, has already taken place. Recovery from this state can only be effected by absorption of the softened substance, with subsequent cicatrisation and contraction: in processes of this kind mercury is not even theoretically indicated; for, to be useful in inflammation of the brain, it should be given in those early stages of the lymph-exudation which precede softening, and in which, unfortunately, the symptoms are often obscure. I make no reference to the use of mercury in the hæmorrhagic cases with the view of favouring absorption of the clot, for I am not aware that an idea so irrational has been entertained by any physician.*

Electro-galvanism and strychnine have been used in the advanced stages of many of my cases, but without results calculated to inspire confidence in their efficacy.

It may, in conclusion, be assumed, that suspension of part of the function of the brain consequent on *destruction of structure* is a state from which complete recovery can seldom be looked for, that we should be satisfied with endeavouring to limit and to stop the lesion, and then to favour its repair; and should always recollect that time, and judicious regimen—not medicines—conduce most to this end.

I am very sensible that these observations on hemiplegia add little or nothing to existing knowledge, and that there is much in respect to this disease to which the medical inquirer in India may turn his attention with interest and advantage,—as the relation of hemiplegia to period of life, to heart and kidney-disease, to particular diathesis and habits, to hæmorrhage, inflammatory and degenerative softening, disease and obstruction of cerebral arterial branches, to the frequency and import of reflex action and of rigidity of the joints of the affected limbs, the existence of anæsthesia, and the discrimination of the cerebral nerves which are involved in the deranged processes.

MYELITIS.—Idiopathic inflammation of the membranes or sub-

* I need hardly say that when symptoms indicate that inflammation is commencing in the nervous matter around the clot, that mercury may be indicated; but on a principle quite distinct from that of absorption of the clot.

stance of the spinal cord is a rare form of disease. I have notes only of two cases. One a Hindoo, of thirty-five years of age, admitted on the 19th February, 1857, under Dr. Ballingall's care,—with pain in the dorsal and lower cervical regions of the spine, paralysis and anæsthesia of the lower extremities, heat of skin, hurried and oppressed breathing, bronchitic rales and cough. He had been ill four days, and attributed the attack to exposure to cold at night in a boat. The paralysis had commenced in the feet, and the evening after admission it had extended partially to the right arm, with sense of formication in the left. There was retention of urine. He continued with failing pulse, occasional fever, no convulsion, till the 26th, when he died.

The upper part of the spinal cord, as far down as one fourth of the dorsal portion, was healthy; but from this to its termination it was diffluent, mottled pink and yellowish in parts, and exhibited under the microscope the exudation corpuscles of inflammation. No trace of spinal meningitis.

The other case was under my own care. It occurred in a Persian Parsee, who was admitted into hospital on the 14th December, 1856, ill, as it seemed, with gastric remittent fever. After six or seven days he complained of pain about the sixth dorsal vertebra, also of the chest and abdomen. The breathing was hurried; then succeeded paralysis of the upper and lower extremities, with impaired sensation, and a flexed state of the fingers. No retention of urine. He continued thus till the 1st January, when an attack of general convulsion, followed by coma, supervened. After recovery, there was more or less incoherence. On the 5th the convulsion returned, and he died on the 6th. The catheter had not been required. No inspection permitted.

Paraplegia.—Cases of paraplegia, consequent on injury of the spine and caries of some of the vertebræ, have from time to time come under my observation; as well as paraplegia in females, without cognizable spinal disease, and referable, in all probability, to hysteria. I cite only the following case, in which there was division of the left half of the spinal cord by a stabbed wound, followed by paralysis and anæsthesia of the lower extremity of the same side. This case is of interest in reference to the functions of the cord, and to the opinions of M. Brown-Sequard, that division of one segment of the cord causes paralysis of the side of section, but loss of sensation on the opposite side not on that of the section.

259. *Division of the left half of the spinal cord by a wound.—Paralysis and anæsthesia of the left lower extremity.*—Joseph Gomez, aged forty-five, a painter, was on the evening of the 2nd December, 1851, when sitting quietly in his house at Mazagong, stabbed and wounded in three places by a Malay seaman. The wounds were about the level of the fifth and sixth dorsal vertebræ; one was a foot in length, and extended transversely across the middle of the back, reached to the muscles, and partly divided some of them. A little above this and to the left of the backbone there was a deep stabbed wound, about an inch in length, directed inwards towards the spine; its depth was not ascertained. There was a third small wound on the back of the arm. When brought to the hospital shortly after the injury, there was paralysis and anæsthesia of the left lower extremity. The anæsthesia extended downwards from the angle of the scapula. There was retention of urine, much diarrhœa and involuntary discharge of fæces. He lingered in this state till the 12th December, when he died.

Inspection.—The punctured wound had sliced off the left transverse process of the fourth dorsal vertebra, and the point of the knife had penetrated the spinal canal and divided transversely the left half of the cord, reaching almost to its median line. Here there was no softening or lymph effusion. About two inches lower down, for about the length of an inch, the cord seemed shrivelled, and to consist of little else than the pia mater and vessels; and below this it again became of natural appearance.

Remark.—This case was the subject of inquiry before the coroner, and the above are the notes from which my evidence was given. I am unable to understand the shrivelled appearance of the cord below the injury. The difficulty occurred to me at the time. There was therefore no apparent explanation, such as laceration of the parts, in making the examination.

But paraplegia is of still further interest in India and other tropical countries. Bontius, Lind, Clark, and Marshall have described a form of it under the name "Barbiers." It is thus defined by Copland: "Tremor with pricking, formicating pain; numbness of the extremities, principally of the lower, followed by contractions and paralysis of the limbs; inarticulation and hoarseness of voice, emaciation, and sinking of all the vital powers." This disease has been viewed as related to cachectic states, and exposure to wet or cold, as predisposing and exciting causes. Bontius confounded barbiers with beri-beri, and Marshall has accurately pointed out the distinction of the two affections. But the affection described under the former title, and answering to Copland's definition, has of late years been lost sight of. That paralysis, chiefly paraplegic, related to cachectic diathesis and exposure to cold, and independent of spinal structural disease, does occur in the natives of India, is true: it is not common, but I have met with occasional instances. The subject requires investigation; but no advantage can result to science by retaining the name barbiers. It is sufficient for the clinical inquirer in India to be aware that paraplegia, related to cachexia, cold, and wet as causes, and independent of structural lesion of a nervous centre, is an occasional occurrence, and that its pathology and etiology are imperfectly understood.*

Paralysis from Arsenic.—Paralysis caused by arsenic is not merely a subject of interest, as a toxicological fact, but also from its bearing on the general pathological question of the toxœmic causation of some forms of disease of the nervous system.

The case which I now quote is a good illustration of this effect from arsenic.

260. *Paralysis from arsenical poisoning.—Pneumonia also present.*— Cazee Ahmud, a Mussulman, of seventeen years of age, was brought to the Jamsetjee Jejeebhoy Hospital, on the 20th April, about noon. It was stated that having eaten of curds at nine o'clock the previous night, he became affected two hours afterwards with vomiting, which recurred several times during the night; also with purging. On admission into hospital, the pulse was seventy-two, feeble; the skin of natural temperature, the respiration hurried, and rather thoracic, and the tongue somewhat florid at the tip. There was no recurrence of vomiting after admission. The bowels, however, were relaxed, but to no great extent, and on one occasion the evacuations consisted in part of mucus. The tongue continued florid, and there was uneasiness at the epigastrium. He was treated with leeches; and sinapisms to the epigastrium, and effervescing draughts. He was discharged on the 30th April. He was re-admitted on the 7th May. He had become considerably emaciated, and there was partial paralysis of both upper and lower extremities. The hands dropped from the wrists, and the fingers were bent somewhat backwards, and the hands were closed feebly and with difficulty. He was able to bend the knee joints but imperfectly, and he lay stretched with the feet extended, and the toes pointing downward. He was also affected with cough, the breathing was somewhat short and hurried, and the left side of the chest, both anteriorly and posteriorly, was dull on percussion, and the respiratory murmur was inaudible. The pulse was 100, and feeble, the skin cool, the tongue whitish in the centre, not florid at the edges, but there was tendency to diarrhœa, and the evacuations were passed in bed. He stated that after his discharge from hospital on the 30th April he attended several successive days at the police office. On the third

---

* In No. 12, of the "Indian Annals of Medical Science," published at Calcutta, July 1859, and received while these sheets are passing through the press, there is a very interesting notice of this form of paralysis by Dr. J. Irving. It is stated that in Pergunnah Barra, in the district of Allahabad, situated on the right bank of the Jumna, 3·19 per cent. of the population are affected with this form of disease, and that it is attributed by the people to habitual use of the kessaree dal (*Lathyrus sativa*) as an article of food, and to exposure to wet chiefly in the monsoon season between July and October. The Pergunnah is described as swampy, and intersected by numerous jheels and tanks. Males suffer more than females, and different villages are affected in different proportions.

Dr. Irving further calls attention to notices of this form of paralysis, attributed to kessaree by other observers, viz., by Dr. K. W. Kirk, in Upper Scinde, in his "Topography of Upper Scinde;" by Col. Sleeman, in the Saugor territories, in "Rambles and Recollections of an Indian Official;" and by Dr. Thomas Thompson in Thibet, in his "Travels in the Himalayas." The subject is of great interest and calls for further careful investigation. The native opinion on the influence of the Lathyrus sativa is worthy of every attention, but it must be regarded as still *sub judice* till submitted to logical and systematic inquiry.

day he had a febrile accession, attributed to having lain on the ground at the police office. The accession came on in the evening, ceased the following morning, recurred the subsequent night, continued three days without distinct intermission, and left his legs in the state in which they were on re-admission. During his residence in hospital he complained, at times, of pain of the arms and legs, and there was a good deal of desquamation of the cuticle of the hands, and about the shoulders. The pneumonia was treated successfully, with Dover's powder and quinine, and a blister to the affected side. He was discharged on the 4th September. The paralysis, though less, still existed in considerable degree. He was unable to walk. The emaciation was less, but still considerable. There had been no return of diarrhœa.

It appeared in evidence that the milkman had purchased arsenic, he said, at the boy's request, for killing rats. The opinion of the judge was that the milkman's story was true, and that the boy had taken the poison with suicidal intent. The milkman was acquitted.

Facial Palsy.—Paralysis of the portio dura, first discriminated by Sir Charles Bell and now well understood, occurs in India as in other countries, presenting its usual characteristic phenomena, and frequently traceable to exposure to cold. The cases which have passed through the clinical ward during the six years do not, however, exceed three in number, and do not suggest anything worthy of notice.

Section IV. — *Statistics of Paralysis.*

Table XLI.—*Admissions and Deaths, with Per-centage, from Paralysis, in the Jamsetjee Jejeebhoy Hospital, at Bombay, for the Six Years from* 1848 *to* 1853..

	1848 to 1853.		Monthly Average.		
	Admissions.	Deaths.	Deaths on Admissions.	Admissions on total Admissions.	Deaths on total Deaths.
January . .	25	3	12·0	1·2	0·7
February . .	22	2	9·1	1·1	0·7
March . . .	26	4	15·4	1·2	1·04
April . . .	20	2	10·0	0·9	0·6
May . . .	28	2	7·1	1·3	0·7
June . . .	23	6	26·1	1·1	1·9
July . . .	24	6	25·0	1·18	1·9
August . . .	19	1	5·2	0·9	0·3
September . .	19	3	15·8	0·9	0·9
October . .	24	5	20·7	1·1	1·5
November . .	29	6	20·7	1·3	1·2
December . .	29	2	6·9	1·2	0·5
Total . .	288	42	14·6	1·11	1·02

CHAP. XXIX.

ON TETANUS.

SECTION I.—*The prevalence of Tetanus in certain classes of the community in India.*

THAT tetanus is a disease of frequent occurrence in certain classes of the community in India, is sufficiently apparent from Dr. Leith's Register of Deaths in Bombay, and from the records of the Jamsetjee Jejeebhoy Hospital.

During the five years from 1848 to 1852 there took place in Bombay 1716 deaths from tetanus, which is in the ratio of 2·5 per cent. of the total deaths during the period.

During the nine years from 1845 to 1853 the admissions from tetanus into the Jamsetjee Jejeebhoy Hospital amounted to 289, and the deaths to 186, or 64·3 per cent. The ratios of admissions and deaths from tetanus to the total hospital admissions and deaths may be learned in respect to six of the nine years, by reference to the tabular statement at the end of the chapter: they are respectively 0·8 and 3·9 per cent.

But it would be an error to conclude from the statements which have just been made, that tetanus is a disease which will necessarily come frequently under the observation of every practitioner in India.

Between the years 1829 and 1838, while doing duty with European and native troops, and at the sanatory station on the Mahubuleshwur Hills, and habitually putting myself in the way of observing disease, wherever it was to be witnessed, I did not meet with a single case of tetanus.

Between the years 1838 and 1845, while attached to the European General Hospital at Bombay, and in medical charge of the Jail, House of Correction, and Byculla Schools, only three cases of tetanus came under my notice. Two of them were idiopathic: one the son of the marshal of the House of Correction, a European boy of about twelve years of age; the other a sailor in the European General Hospital. The third case occurred in a young English merchant, consequent on a lacerated wound over the tibia, caused by a carriage wheel.

Thus during the first sixteen years of my service in India, though actively engaged in varied fields of practice, I met with only three cases of tetanus; but during the last nine years 289 have come under my observation in one institution, and a considerable number of them have been under my immediate care.

I have no data before me to show the proportion of tetanus in the European and native armies of India, but it is probably small. On referring to my notes of fatal cases of European officers, I find two instances in a total of 311: both were traumatic, consequent on lacerated wounds of the leg, by carriage wheels. The death of a young English merchant in Bombay, from traumatic tetanus, has already been alluded to; another instance occurred a year or two afterwards in the same class of the community from a wound close to the tibia, caused by the shaft of a buggy. Thus all the instances of tetanus in the higher classes of Europeans, of which I have notes, were consequent on injuries to the leg by carriages. The only other case which I can bring to recollection is that of a medical officer at Vingorla, after a compound fracture of the leg from a fall.

The brief practical remarks which I have to make on this important disease will have reference to my experience in the Jamsetjee Jejeebhoy Hospital. In addition to notes of my general impressions, the diaries of thirty-three cases, of which about one half was treated in the clinical ward, are before me; also a very valuable report* on tetanus, as observed in the same hospital by my able and experienced colleague, Dr. Peet.

I shall arrange my remarks under the heads:—1. Pathology. 2. Causes. 3. Symptoms. 4. Treatment.

SECTION II.—*Pathology.—Nature of the deranged action with reference to the Physiology of the Spinal Cord.—Division into Idiopathic and Traumatic, Acute and Chronic.—Morbid Anatomy.*

In the preliminary observations on the pathology of the brain, I stated that it was sufficient for clinical purposes to divide the symp-

* "Transactions, Medical and Physical Society of Bombay," No. 1, new series.

toms of cerebral disease into, 1st, those which indicate *excess* in the actions of the brain; 2nd, those which indicate *defect*.

A similar classification may be made of the symptoms of disease of the spinal cord. But when we confine our attention to the spinal cord as a nervous *centre*, it is necessary to limit the inquiry to the symptoms which indicate excess of action; because those which imply defect may be caused by change in the medullary portion which conducts, as well as in the vesicular portion which originates, nervous influence. In other words, we cannot separate the defect of action of that part of the cord, which exercises the function of a nervous centre, from that which exercises merely the function of a nervous conductor.

Defect of action of the spinal cord has been already noticed in that section of the preceding chapter which treats of Paralysis. I would therefore now advert to the spinal cord as a *nervous centre*, and confine my remarks to the symptoms which indicate excess of action, and to the conditions on which this depends.

It is assumed that the clinical student is familiar with the functions of the grey nervous matter of the spinal cord, as at present taught by physiologists—that it receives impressions – excito-motor—made upon the peripheral extremities of afferent fibres, and in respondence generates motor impulses—reflex—which are conveyed by efferent fibres to muscular tissue; and that the resulting action may be altogether irrespective of sensation and volition. That in addition to the contraction of muscular fibre induced by volition and reflex action, there is a permanent slight degree, to which the terms antagonistic, muscular tension, tonicity have been applied: it probably depends upon a continuous supply of nervous influence, proceeding from the spinal cord as its centre of generation.

Excess of action of the spinal cord will then necessarily be indicated, — 1. By forcible involuntary muscular contractions, often originating without evident excito-motor impression, but always readily excited by the slightest peripheral irritation. 2. By excess of muscular tension, that is, by permanent rigidity of more or less of muscular structure.

It is to phenomena of this kind that the term *Tetanus* has been applied: they bear the same relation to the spinal cord as a nervous centre that active delirium and excessive sensation do to the brain as a nervous centre.

The subordinate phrases, *trismus*, *opisthotonos*, *emprosthotonos*, *pleurosthotonos*, merely express the fact that the phenomena are prominently displayed in certain sets of muscles: they are unimportant in reference to pathology, and may be altogether set aside.

When inquiring into the *proximate* cause of excess of action of the brain, I remarked that it probably always consisted either of that active state of the capillary circulation termed determination of blood, or of an altered quality of the blood from some external agent, of which alcohol might be taken as a type.

It is reasonable and consistent to entertain the same views of the pathology of the spinal cord and to relate tetanus to determination of blood, or to toxæmia. Strychnia may be named as a typical agent of the latter.

But we experience a difficulty which was not felt in the instance of the brain. Tetanus has been divided into *idiopathic* and *traumatic*, *centric*, and *eccentric*. The conditions of the nervous centre just stated are sufficient for the explanation of the idiopathic or centric; but the traumatic or eccentric would seem to imply that altered states of the periphery of afferent fibres may so affect the quality of excito-motor impressions, as to lead to excessive reflex action, irrespective of actual derangement of the centre itself.

Without pretending to assert that injured periphery of nerves may not be adequate, in some circumstances, to cause the phenomena of tetanus, I would express my belief that derangement of the spinal cord, similar to that in idiopathic tetanus, always plays an important, often the principal, part in the pathology of traumatic tetanus also; and for the following reasons:—

1. The rarity of tetanus after, compared with the frequency of, injuries. 2. Tetanus after wounds is most frequent in countries in which the idiopathic disease is not unusual. This fact seems to imply that there exists something common in the causation of the two forms. 3. Tetanus has been frequently observed after trifling injuries; but this has been chiefly, if not exclusively, in countries, and in classes, in which the idiopathic form is of frequent occurrence. 4. Tetanus after wounds has not been usually noticed as an early sequence of their infliction, but as an event coming on after an interval of several, sometimes many, days, and in association with quiescent as well as irritated conditions of the wound.*

* Dr. Peet mentions a circumstance which bears on this question. The only four cases in which tetanus followed the operation of amputation, were, in persons affected with traumatic gangrene; in one, tetanus came on in ten hours after the operation; in the second, in twenty hours; in the third, in forty-eight hours; in the fourth, in between three and four days.

Dr. Peet, referring to the first three cases, very justly remarks: "Are they not

These facts are more accordant with the idea of a diathetic influence extending to the spinal cord than of a mere respondence to excito-motor impressions. 5. Permanent rigidity of muscular structure is a symptom of traumatic as well as of idiopathic tetanus; and though we might admit that the paroxysms of spasmodic action may be due to peripheral derangement alone, there is no reason for believing that the action of the spinal cord in respect to muscular tension is dependent on the reception of peripheral impressions, or likely to be increased by alterations of their quality.

The statement very generally made by writers on tetanus, that the idiopathic form is not so severe and fatal as the traumatic, is not supported by experience in Bombay. My belief is that on these points there is no difference in the two forms.* If there be little, if any, difference in the pathology of idiopathic and traumatic tetanus, and none in the severity of the symptoms or in the principles of general treatment, then there is little to be practically gained by dwelling on the distinction: it is perhaps sufficient to say, that when a wound or other injury co-exists with tetanus, it should be treated on ordinary surgical principles.

Tetanus has also been divided into *acute* and *chronic*.

By the first is understood severity of form, and a fatal result generally within nine days. By the second, less severity of symptoms, a protracted course, and often a successful termination.

These terms, which have been objected to by some writers, may be viewed as synonymous with *severe* and *mild*, and as indicating the influence of different degrees of the predisposing and exciting conditions. In cases which terminate favourably, — whether they have been mild from the commencement, or severe at first and subsequently mild,—the course is always protracted, and recovery slow and gradual: this fact seems to imply the influence of a diathetic state.

In regard to the *morbid anatomy* of tetanus, the appearances

calculated to favour the idea that there is in this disease, as in most others, a period of incubation; a stage during which the efficient cause, or more correctly, perhaps, the disease itself, is actually in existence, without its presence being manifested by any appreciable signs or symptoms?" He further relates the tetanus to the original injury, not to the surgical operation.

* Dr. Peet, in his interesting report, has already pointed out the discrepancy between the result of observation in Bombay and recorded statements, and has narrated cases illustrative of the severity of the idiopathic form of the disease. His opinion is that the idiopathic form is more severe than the traumatic. My impression, as just stated is, that there is no difference in this respect.

found in the spinal canal after death are analogous to those found in the cranium, when death has followed close upon symptoms of excessive action of the cerebral functions, viz., more or less increased capillary turgescence, with or without increased serous effusion. These are in fact the only anatomical changes which may be looked for after death in organs which have been the seats merely of active determination.

The question—whether inflammation of the membranes or substance of the cord is the proximate cause of tetanus, has been discussed.

In cases which have terminated fatally after a few days' illness,—and of such the records of morbid anatomy may be held exclusively to consist,—the presence of only increased vascularity is not conclusive against the idea of recent inflammation during life, for in encephalitis, quickly fatal, no other appearance may be found. But the improbability of tetanus being dependent on inflammation seems to me to rest on facts of another kind.

1. When inflammation of the cranial contents becomes protracted to those stages when blood-stasis or lesions of structure take place, then excess of action of the brain ceases to be indicated; but muttering delirium, drowsiness, coma, irregular muscular contraction, and paralysis—the symptoms of defective action—come on.

2. In chronic tetanus, though protracted for weeks, the symptoms of excess of action continue to the close. There is never muscular relaxation or paralysis.

For these reasons, I believe that inflammation is not the proximate cause of tetanus.

In death from cerebral disease, the suspended function of the sensorium—coma—extends to the medulla oblongata, and death by apnœa takes place. But in many forms of cerebral disease, depressed action of the heart is also very evident, and a tendency to death by syncope is thereby created.

In fatal cases of tetanus, death takes place partly by apnœa, not caused by paralysis of the muscles of respiration, as in cerebral disease, but by their excessive contraction. I have said partly by apnœa, because in tetanus a depressed action of the heart, with tendency to death by syncope, is also a prominent symptom, and one which it is most important to regard in treatment.

The syncope may be due to paralysis of the muscular fibre of the heart, but in all probability is most generally caused by spasm. On this question my data are limited; but I have before me the notes of three cases observed by me subsequent to my return to India, in which the heart was firmly contracted—in a state of the so-called concentric hypertrophy. In all these cases there was general rigidity of the muscles, and a flexed condition of the fingers at the time of examination, made, in one three hours after death, in another twelve, and in the third nineteen.

There is still an observation to make relative to the pathology of tetanus. It would seem that the reflex actions of the spinal cord, which affect muscular fibres concerned in organic functions, and little controlled by volition, are usually exempt from derangement in tetanus. In this respect the contrast with hydrophobia is very striking; for in this latter disease the nervous circle of the eighth pair is remarkably involved. Or this feature in tetanus may be described by saying, that the muscular structures on which the excess of action of the spinal cord is expended, are, in the normal state of the system, also subject to contraction from volition.

SECTION III.—*Etiology.—Diathesis, Cold, Entozoa?—External Injuries.*

The etiology of tetanus is beset with difficulty and obscurity.

1. It is most probable that there are diatheses influential in the production of both idiopathic and traumatic tetanus. But the nature of the agencies which induce these diatheses, whether akin to malaria, or other climatic conditions, or related to habits and regimen, has yet to be determined.

Though the disease shows itself most frequently in the native classes who seek relief in civil hospitals, yet it has not been observed by me to be particularly related to asthenic and cachectic states, for many of the affected have been in good condition. Again, when we reflect on the possible relation of tetanus to toxæmia, we naturally turn to the pathology of hydrophobia, a kindred affection of a limited section of the spinal cord; and also to the fact, that tetanus is never recovered from by a sudden cessation of the symptoms, but always by gradual and slow restoration.

2. Is *cold* a common exciting cause of idiopathic tetanus? My general impression is, that in a considerable proportion of the cases the attack has been attributed to such causes as sleeping on the damp ground or exposure to the night air. But when we inquire into the seasons of admission and death from tetanus generally, the influence of cold is not very evident.

The following is a statement of the monthly deaths from tetanus of all kinds recorded by Dr. Leith:—

	1848.	1849.	1850.	1851.	1852.	
	Deaths.	Deaths.	Deaths.	Deaths.	Deaths.	Total Deaths.
January	34	24	31	18	21	128
February	27	17	25	28	32	129
March	29	28	45	26	35	163
April	18	24	52	26	36	156
May	24	31	44	28	22	149
June	25	28	50	21	34	158
July	27	24	37	27	21	136
August	17	27	30	29	24	127
September	16	24	27	31	28	126
October	17	24	35	30	24	130
November	27	27	34	29	35	152
December	22	35	37	39	29	162
Total	283	313	447	332	341	1716

From this we find that the deaths from December to May amounted to 887, and those from June to November to 829, giving an excess of 58 in favour of the first half-year, which includes the cold months.

Of the 289 admissions into the Jamsetjee Jejeebhoy Hospital, in nine years—164 took place from December to May, and 125 from June to November, which gives an excess of 39 in favour of the half year which includes the cold months. Though it may be reasonable to attribute part of the excess of tetanus in both these instances to the influence of season, yet it must be borne in mind, that the period referred to is that during which the fluctuating population of Bombay is at its maximum, and during which there is consequently the greatest absolute amount of sickness and death.

We saw reason to relate excess of action of the nervous matter of the brain to *elevated temperature* as an exciting cause, and the question naturally arises, may not tetanus—excess of action of the spinal cord—be related to the same exciting cause? There is no good reason for entertaining this opinion; for it must be remembered that heat as an exciting cause of cerebral disease was most frequently exhibited in the European constitution; but tetanus is far more common in the native.

3. *Entozoa* in the intestinal canal have been suggested as an occasional exciting cause of tetanus. The lumbricus teres is very

common in natives of Bombay, and doubtless may be found frequently present in patients affected with tetanus. But to infer from this fact that there has been relation of cause and effect, would be illogical, just as it would be to regard entozoa as the cause of pneumonia, cholera, or the many other diseases with which in the same classes they co-exist with equal frequency.

4. In *traumatic tetanus** what part does the wound or injury play in the causation of the disease? I have already (p. 676) stated my belief, that in the pathology of the two forms there is probably little difference. In all likelihood, the degree of a wound's influence as a determining cause varies in different circumstances—considerable when the wound is severe, trifling, if existing at all, when the injury is slight. Indeed, it is sufficiently common to find that the history of cases of tetanus with slight external injury, points as distinctly to cold as an exciting cause, as that of many in which injury does not co-exist. In a word, when the wound is trifling, its influence in the causation of tetanus is, I apprehend, very problematical. If this opinion be correct, then the inference may be drawn, that of the cases registered by Dr. Leith, or admitted into the Jamsetjee Jejeebhoy Hospital, the proportion of cases *truly* traumatic was very limited.†

5. Tetanus, excited by strychnia or other poisons, if such there be, is related to toxicology, and does not come within the scope of this work. I have witnessed one case of the effect of an over-dose of strychnia taken by mistake by a medical apprentice, and recovered from.

SECTION IV.—*Symptoms.—Muscular Rigidity and Spasms.—Respiration.—Pulse.—Febrile Disturbance, &c.*

Here, as in respect to most of the diseases which have been treated of in this work, it will be taken for granted that the clinical student is acquainted with the descriptions of systematic writers.

* I make no special reference to the term *puerperal*, which has been applied to tetanus occurring in puerperal women. It is sufficient to be aware of the fact that the adverse conditions in which puerperal women, natives of India, are placed, are predisponent of tetanus. I would class the disease arising under these circumstances with idiopathic not traumatic tetanus. A similar remark may be applied to *trismus nascentium*, as the history of the Dublin Lying-in Hospital amply proves.

† The train of reasoning which I have followed in this section, will explain why I have not dwelt upon an inference drawn by Dr. Peet, from an analysis of a portion of his cases; viz. that idiopathic tetanus was most common in October, November, December, and traumatic in April, May, and June.

I shall, therefore, merely notice those symptoms which seem to me the most important. Tetanus commences with excess of muscular tension, which leads to that permanent rigidity which is one of the characters of the disease. This state comes on more or less quickly in different cases, and involves more or less of the muscular structures. The muscles of the neck, the jaws, and abdomen are those which are earliest and most universally affected. This excess of tension is accompanied with sense of stiffness and pain, and leads to more or less permanent closure of the mouth, and rigidity of the anterior abdominal walls.*

Dr. Peet has called attention to a peculiarity in the expression of the countenance which he correctly thinks is often the earliest indication of tetanus. He says:—

> "But, even before pain is complained of, there is often something very peculiar in the expression of the face: it is not easy, perhaps, to describe exactly in what this change consists, — it has seemed to me to depend upon an apparent increase in breadth, the angles of the mouth being, in some degree, drawn outwards, the lips compressed, and the eyelids slightly corrugated. This expression is very different from that present at a later period, in which the skin is wrinkled, the furrows of the face highly developed, the angles of the mouth depressed, and the whole appearance that which has been so well designated by the term '*risus sardonicus*.' The length of time over which the change in the expression of face first noticed may extend I am unable to state: I have witnessed and pointed it out ten hours before any other symptom of tetanus was present." †

The greater or less permanent rigidity is followed, sooner or later, and sometimes very speedily, by spasmodic contractions, which vary in force, frequency, duration, extent, and preference for particular muscles. In these variations consists the difference in severity in different cases. The extent and force of the permanent rigidity are always in proportion to the force, frequency, duration, and extent of the spasms. The spasms may recur at intervals, ranging from two or three minutes to half an hour or more, and may endure from a second or two to half a minute or a minute. The preference given to one set of muscles over another occasions the varieties which have been previously alluded to (p. 674).

The spasms may recur without any appreciable excito-motor impression, but they are generally very readily excited by trifling

* The fact that the permanent muscular rigidity — the excess of tension, and the subsequent spasmodic contractions — excess of reflex actions — are distinct, seems to me to complete the proof, that normal muscular tension is maintained by nervous influence generated in the spinal cord. This is a point on which physiologists have not always agreed.

† "Transactions, Medical and Physical Society at Bombay," 2nd Series, No. 1, p. 13.

causes, as the sound of the voice, the motion of the observer's hand, the slightest touch, &c.

I concur with Dr. Peet in believing that it is not always possible to say from the symptoms at the commencement whether the course of the disease will be rapid and fatal, or prolonged and recovered from. I have seen cases that gave every promise of being mild, become suddenly and unexpectedly aggravated, and others which threatened to be severe become unexpectedly moderated.

The statement usually made that the fatal result from tetanus occurs for the most part within nine days from the commencement of the attack, is on the whole correct. Yet exceptional cases are by no means uncommon. I have seen several in which death took place as late as the twentieth day, under recurrence of an aggravation of the symptoms, or in consequence of increasing asthenia. And I entertain the opinion that more frequent recoveries, and a more protracted course in fatal cases would result, if depressing remedies and full narcotism were abandoned, and moderate anodynes, with tonics, stimulants, and support, substituted.

The abnormal muscular contraction and spasm interfere with the right performance of the function of respiration: hurried respiration is always an unfavourable symptom. The marked depressed action of the heart is practically a very important feature of the disease, and one which becomes apparent at a very early period in severe cases; the pulse becomes small and very compressible. Dr. Peet dissents from Dr. Parry's remark that, "if the pulse by the fourth or fifth day does not reach 100 or 110 beats in the minute, the patient almost always recovers." It is true that fatal cases, with a pulse considerably below 100, for a longer period than five days, and recovered cases, with a pulse of 100 from the commencement, may be observed. Such cases I have witnessed, but still the general clinical fact remains that a frequent pulse is a bad symptom in tetanus, and that when the pulse becomes small it is generally also rapid.

On the co-existence of febrile symptoms with tetanus, Dr. Peet remarks:—

"The mode of commencement of the disease has presented a good deal of variety. In a certain number of cases the manifestation of muscular derangement has been preceded by distinct febrile symptoms, not attributable to the state of the wound. These have reached over a period varying from a few hours to two days. I was at one time under the impression that such cases were invariably *acute*; but further experience has thrown a doubt upon the accuracy of this opinion. Within the last two years I have witnessed at least three cases of recovery where the premonitory febrile disturbance was distinctly marked.

"Febrile symptoms at or previous to the accession of the tetanic symptoms have, however, been by no means general. In the larger number of cases they were altogether absent."

In these opinions I concur; and from having witnessed one case of cured remittent fever succeeded by fatal tetanus, and one case of improved tetanus followed by fatal fever, it has seemed to me not improbable that the co-existence of febrile symptoms with tetanus may be sometimes best explained on the supposition of a co-existing malarious influence acting on the affected individual.

The bowels are usually constipated. The condition of the expellent abdominal muscles, and the small quantity of food taken, are sufficient to explain this symptom. I am not acquainted with any fact which countenances the idea that the muscular fibre of the intestinal canal is in a state of spasm: indeed, it is very doubtful whether there is much abnormal contraction of the sphincter ani. Retention of urine very rarely takes place in tetanus, from which it may be inferred that undue contraction of the sphincter of the bladder is not common. It has been already remarked that the phenomena of the disease point chiefly to implication of muscular fibres normally under the control of volition as well as excito-motor impression.

Section V. — *Treatment of Tetanus.*

The most important clinical facts relative to the treatment of tetanus are: — 1. The evident failing action of the heart. 2. That recovery never takes place except through a protracted course and a gradual subsidence of the deranged actions.

From the first fact it may be inferred that remedies sedative, as blood-letting, tobacco, digitalis, tartar emetic, purgatives, mercury, are contra-indicated. This inference is sustained by clinical experience. Such means have been freely and often used, and, it may be added, are now universally condemned.

From the second fact, two inferences may be drawn: — 1. That as recovery is always gradual and slow, it cannot be a safe system of treatment to use remedies which, while they make a decided impression on the tetanic symptoms, tend to derange and materially injure other actions important to life. Such remedies are narcotics given to the degree of frequently inducing or maintaining a state of marked narcotism. With this view opium, extract of hemp, belladonna, inhalation of ether and chloroform, have been used. The tendency of this treatment is, while it relieves the spasm, to cause death by coma. Nay, more, associated with narcotism, there is always a failing action of the heart; therefore, under narcotics used to this degree, the tendency to death by syncope, already distinct in tetanus, becomes seriously increased. Further, if in cases thus treated, the narcotics be intermitted, it will be found that the spasms will recur with greater frequency and severity than before the exhibition of these remedies had commenced. The explanation is this: the general powers of resistance of the system will have been lowered, and the influence, whatever it may be, which causes the tetanus will, being less resisted, be more free to act.

These statements are not grounded on the observation of the bad effects of the excessive use of opium or hemp, for I have always felt that the injurious action of the first especially had already been proved; but they rest on my own experience of the inhalation of sulphuric ether or of chloroform to the extent of frequently inducing or maintaining a full narcotic influence. The effect of the inhalation of chloroform in relaxing the spasms and relieving the suffering of tetanus is most striking, and the temptation to use it freely is consequently great. But it is treacherous and unsafe. The influence passes off in two or three minutes, and the spasms recur. If the chloroform be frequently repeated, increasing failure of the pulse becomes very evident; if the remedy be intermitted, it will be found that the frequency of the spasms has been augmented by its use; if it be continued to the close, it will be found that death is preceded by some degree of muttering delirium and coma, which are not symptoms of the termination of tetanus when unmodified by narcotics.

A system which leads to results such as these cannot with propriety be designated the curative treatment of tetanus. It is euthanasia through chloroform, and if tetanus were an invariably fatal disease, the question of its adoption might perhaps be entertained. Such, however, is not the character of this disease, and this would become still more evident if the second inference were more generally acknowledged, and practically applied, viz., that as recovery is always gradual and slow, the indication is to sustain the strength. This we effect by such moderate use of narcotics as shall somewhat relieve pain and lessen spasm, and thus ward off part of that exhaustion which follows the continuance of great suffering; and by tonic remedies, nourishment, and stimulants. A combination of quinine with extract of hemp may be used: the former in doses of from three to six grains, the latter from one to two grains, given at intervals of from two to six hours, with animal broths, and other nourishment in small quantities frequently repeated, and from ten to twenty ounces of wine in the twenty-four hours. By this system of treatment not only are the protraction of the disease and the chances of recovery increased, but the suffering is alleviated — a fact which the protraction of the disease necessarily implies. I have also used chloroform, on the principle of merely allaying the pain and lessening the spasm, every third or fourth hour. For this purpose the inhalation of thirty or forty minims will generally be sufficient. The practical objection to chloroform is the risk of over dose and the temptation to push it beyond the limits of safety. But the relief of pain is not the only practical advantage gained by the moderate and safe use of narcotic remedies as now recommended: the relaxation of spasm is useful by materially facilitating the ingestion of food, wine, and medicines. Recovery in one case, in which the trismus was complete, seemed to me to be due to the use of thirty minims of chloroform inhaled before each time of administering food: this was sufficient to unlock the jaws to the necessary extent without causing injurious narcotism.

In February 1853 I had the opportunity of witnessing several cases of tetanus in the native hospital at Calcutta through the kindness of Dr. J. Jackson; and it was satisfactory to me to find that observation in that institution had led to conclusions on the principles of treating tetanus very similar to those which have just been detailed, and which had for some time been entertained by me. Dr. Jackson has since published the results of his experience in the first number of the "Indian Annals of Medical Science." There is, I apprehend, very little difference in the principles of treatment respectively advocated by us. Dr. Jackson, perhaps, attaches more value to chloroform than I am disposed to accord to it.

Blisters, cold affusion, &c. — have been used: of these I have not any experience; but when we consider the readiness with which the spinal cord responds to the most trifling peripheral impressions, it seems to me unreasonable to expect any result but harm from remedies of this class.

To remove constipation, occasional recourse may be had to combinations of castor oil and turpentine, sometimes with addition of croton oil, or the latter alone given with mucilage. Dr. Jackson has used aloes in small doses from time to time, with the hemp and quinine.

The five following cases will serve to illustrate some of my statements. The first three show the good effect of the treatment recommended; the fourth proves the striking influence of chloroform in relaxing the spasms, but as the urgency of the symptoms was great, and the course rapid, the injurious effects of the agent are not apparent; the short continuance of the relief from the chloroform is, however, shown. The last case is an instance of the difficulty which not unfrequently arises in determining the idiopathic or traumatic character of the disease.

261. *Tetanus.—Treated with quinine, extract of hemp, wine, and nourishment.—Recovered.*—Mahomed Azim Khan, a Beloochee horse-dealer, of stout frame, was admitted into hospital on the 26th April, 1853. He had been the subject of guinea-worm for fifteen days. Symptoms of tetanus had come on the day before admission, subsequent to sleeping, exposed to the open air, on the ground. The spasms were frequent, the trismus incomplete, the breathing hurried, and the pulse, not above 100, tended to become weak. He was treated freely with quinine and extract of hemp, and twenty-four ounces of wine were given daily. After this treatment was commenced, the improvement was striking. The spasms lessened, the pulse improved in strength, and the breathing became calm. He was removed on the 7th May by his friends, who wished to take him to Kurrachee. When discharged, there was still some stiffness and pain of the legs, with occasional spasms; but he was otherwise well, and the pulse good. This case was treated by Dr. Forbes Watson.

262. *Idiopathic tetanus.—Treated with quinine, hemp, wine, and nourishment.—Recovery.*—Runnee Ram, a Marwaree labourer, of twenty-six years of age, was admitted into the Jamsetjee Jejeehoy Hospital on the 29th March, 1853. He had suffered from tetanic symptoms for ten days unpreceded by injury. Four days before admission the actual cautery had been applied to the spine and calves of the legs, There was opisthotonos, incomplete trismus, frequent spasms, much sweating, and the surface of the body was covered with sudamina. He remained in hospital till the 7th May, slowly improving; but on his discharge he was considerably reduced in flesh, and there was still a good deal of rigidity of the muscles of the legs and abdomen. He was treated with quinine, forty grains in the twenty-four hours, given with extract of hemp; wine sixteen ounces daily, and soup frequently. While under treatment, the pulse was never above 100, and he took the wine and nourishment well.

263. *Tetanus in a child.—Though fatal, the good effects of treatment with quinine, hemp, and attention to nourishment were very apparent.*—Chund Bux, a Mussulman boy, three years of age, residing with his parents at the Lighthouse, Colaba, in a cold exposed situation, was admitted into the Jamsetjee Jejeebhoy Hospital on the 5th December, 1851, on the fifth day of illness, with tetanus. He had a superficial, small, suppurating, but healthy-looking wound on the forehead, caused by a fall ten days before admission. The spasms were frequent, the trismus complete, the pulse feeble, and the child was constantly moaning. Ten minims of the tincture of hemp were given every second hour, and soup, wine, and milk, in small quantities frequently. The spasms were lessened in severity, and then two grains of quinine were added to the dose of hemp, and the medicine continued every third hour with the same attention to nourishment. The child seemed to be slowly improving. The spasms were not so frequent, and the permanent rigidity of the abdomen was less. The trismus, however, continued. Nourishment was taken frequently in small quantities, and the pulse improved in strength. This was the state of the patient on the 14th and the morning of the 15th. But on the evening of the latter day there was again increase

of the spasms, and he died in the course of the night. The treatment had been unchanged till the evening of the 14th, when the intervals were lengthened to four hours; but three hours were reverted to on the evening of the 15th.

264. *Tetanus treated with chloroform.* — *Fatal.* — Suttoo, a Hindoo labourer, was admitted into the Jamsetjee Jejeebhoy Hospital on the 3rd November, at 4½ P.M., after three days' illness with tetanus. There was opisthotonos, with constant short spasms of the abdominal and other muscles, causing general agitation of the body. The pulse was barely perceptible. There was a superficial abraded wound at the lower part of the calf of the left leg, caused by a box falling on it. A drachm of chloroform was inhaled with relaxation of the spasms and development of the pulse, which continued for about three minutes. The spasms and rigidity then recurred. The chloroform was then repeated with similar effect; it was again used at 5¼ P.M., at 6¼ and at 8 P.M.: in all five times. In each instance the spasms ceased, continued absent about four minutes, then recurred. The pulse lost strength. He refused sago and wine, and died at 9½ P.M.

Remark. — The utmost that can be said in favour of the chloroform is, that twenty minutes' relief from suffering resulted from its use. But whether the fatal result was postponed or hastened, or not influenced by it, is an open question.

265. *Tetanus fatal on the twenty-first day.* — *Whether traumatic or idiopathic, doubtful.*—*Treated with quinine, hemp, nourishment, and stimulants.*—*Fatal.*—*Spinal veins congested.*—Deen Mahomed, aged thirteen, a Mussulman buggy driver, was admitted into the clinical ward on the 25th November, 1853. There was tetanic expression of countenance. The mouth could be opened only to the extent of a quarter of an inch, and the tongue protruded about half an inch. The corners of the mouth were drawn outwards. There was rigidity of the muscles of the back, abdomen, and neck. There were also general tetanic spasms, which lasted about half a minute, and returned after an interval of about three minutes. The skin of natural temperature. The pulse, small and compressible, was about 80 during the intervals, and rose to a 100 during the spasms. There was a small wound covered with a scab on the inner side of the left heel, and a pustule on the anterior surface of the lower third of the right leg. He had been received into the hospital with trismus four days previously, but had deserted, and was now brought back by his friends. His statement was, that the wound on the heel was caused by a stroke from a horse-shoe twelve days before, but of the pustule he could give no account. The night before his first admission he slept in the open air in his buggy. Was temperate in his habits. From the 27th November to 4th December the spasms were not quite so severe, the intervals were somewhat longer, the mouth was not quite so closed, and the pulse had improved in volume. The bowels were generally slow, and the urine passed freely. He became, however, notably thinner, and increased heat of skin was at times observed. Thus he continued, still losing flesh, but with the pulse of pretty good volume, till the morning of the 13th, when he was found bathed in perspiration, with the pulse just perceptible. There had been increase of spasms during the night, and he had been unable to swallow the medicine regularly. He died during the visit at which this report was taken. The wound on the heel was nearly well on the 8th. The treatment consisted of quinine four grains, extract of hemp one grain, or one grain and a half, every third hour, chicken soup two ounces every fourth hour, sago two ounces, and arrack half an ounce every fourth hour; and after the 5th forty minims of chloroform were inhaled every sixth hour, and the bowels were opened by an occasional dose of castor oil and turpentine oil. The wound was poulticed. There was no drowsiness from the hemp. The effect of the chloroform continued for about twenty minutes.

Inspection three hours and a half after death. — The body was much emaciated and rigid. On examining the wound on the left heel nothing abnormal was detected in the neighbouring blood-vessels and nerves. *Head.*—On removing the calvarium, the vessels of the membranes of the brain were seen congested. About three ounces of clear serum were found at the base of the skull, but none in the ventricles. The substance of the brain was in a healthy condition. *Spinal Cord.*—Spinal veins were turgid. The structure of the cord was healthy. *Chest.*—On opening the chest, the lungs were found collapsed. The structure was healthy, with exception of emphysematous patches here and there, chiefly on the anterior thin edges of both lungs. The cavities of the right side of the heart were filled with dark fluid blood. The left ventricle was contracted and contained no blood. *Abdomen.*—The liver was normal. The spleen was about three inches long, and an inch and a quarter in breadth, and was somewhat firmer than usual; but the structure was healthy. The kidneys were normal, the distinction between cortical and medullar portions being well marked.

Section VI.—*Statistics of Tetanus.*

Table XLII.—*Admissions and Deaths, with Per-centage, from Tetanus, in the Jamsetjee Jejeebhoy Hospital at Bombay, for the Six Years from* 1848 *to* 1853.

	1848 to 1853.		Monthly Average.		
	Admissions.	Deaths.	Deaths on Admissions.	Admissions on total Admissions.	Deaths on total Deaths.
January	12	9	75·0	1·6	2·0
February	17	9	52·9	0·9	2·8
March	25	14	56·0	1·2	3·7
April	21	14	66·6	0·9	4·1
May	23	14	60·9	1·1	4·8
June	15	12	80·0	0·7	3·9
July	13	5	38·5	0·8	1·6
August	8	6	75·0	0·4	1·8
September	12	11	91·7	0·6	3·5
October	17	9	52·9	0·8	2·6
November	18	10	55·6	0·8	3·0
December	23	14	60·9	1·0	3·5
Total	204	127	62·3	0·8	3·9

CHAP. XXX.

ON HYDROPHOBIA.

SECTION I. — *Short allusion to Symptoms and Pathology. — Illustrative Cases detailed.*

I HAVE witnessed ten cases of this fearful disease, — one in a little girl of the Byculla Schools, and the other nine in the Jamsetjee Jejeebhoy Hospital.

I have not any notes of the first case, but the child was bitten so severely in the palm of the hand that the excision of the parts was impracticable: nitrate of silver was freely applied. Symptoms of hydrophobia came on in about six weeks, and proved rapidly fatal. Of the other nine cases four occurred from September, 1848, to September 1849, one in 1850, and three in 1851. Of one the year is not given. Among the European officers in the Bombay Presidency I recollect the occurrence of three cases in twenty-five years. There is so little in common in the symptoms of tetanus and hydrophobia that an error in the diagnosis ought to be very rare. In the latter disease there is none of the permanent muscular rigidity, increased by paroxysms of tonic spasm, so characteristic of the former. The deranged muscular action in hydrophobia is confined chiefly to the neck, pharynx, and larynx, and is more clonic in character. An accumulation of viscid mucus about the pharynx, larynx, and mouth, and a consequent hawking and spitting, would seem to be invariably present. I have observed these phenomena only once in tetanus, in slight degree, but with the other symptoms of the disease so well marked as to leave no room for doubt. The sensorial derangement and the agitated actions consequent on excitement and alarm are always, more or less, present in hydrophobia. Symptoms of this kind do not occur in tetanus.

On the pathology of hydrophobia it is sufficient to remark that the morbid poison, the cause of the disease, chiefly expends its force on the nervous circle of the eighth pair, and extends its influence to the sensorium.

I shall best describe the phenomena of hydrophobia by narrating the four* cases treated by me in the Jamsetjee Jejeebhoy Hospital.

266. *Hydrophobia: three months after the bite.*—Camillo Pereira, a native Christian, from Goa, following the occupation of cook, of fourteen years of age, was admitted into the clinical ward on the 24th December, 1850. It was said that he had been bitten by a strange dog at Karlee on the 26th September. At about the middle of the outer side of the right leg, there were three cicatrices resembling those caused by a bite. He stated that on the night of the 21st December he awoke feeling chilly and uncomfortable, but he fell asleep again, and was able next day to attend to his avocations. On the following night he was again restless, and alarmed with dreams; and at noon of the 23rd, he was found by a friend in a state of agitation and excitement, increased by the sight of water. He passed the night in an excited state, and was with difficulty controlled by his friends. On admission into hospital the following day, he was agitated, and constantly talking to himself. He made no complaint of pain, but when approached or touched he shrieked as if from fear. There was no marked spasm of muscles observed. The tongue was protruded with effort and with a jerk. He did not seem to be affected by currents of air, but when water was brought, he became more excited, and was unwilling to drink or even to touch it. Noises distressed him, and he seemed anxious to be left alone. The skin was of natural temperature, the pulse frequent, small, and easily compressed. The bowels had not been opened for two days. He died at half-past 10 P.M., about six hours after admission. The excitement and alarm had continued; the latter was chiefly indicated by an outstretching of the hands, as if to protect himself. The mouth became filled with adhesive saliva, which excited coughing, and was constantly trickling down from the right angle of the mouth. The lower extremities became cold, the pulse scarcely perceptible, and the breathing laborious. Pills of extract of hemp and muriate of morphia were prescribed, but he had been able to take only two.

267. *Hydrophobia, treated with chloroform.*—Mussoojee Govinda, a Maratha, aged fifty, was admitted into the Jamsetjee Jejeebhoy Hospital on the 28th August, 1849, at 5 A.M. He had been bitten on the calf of the left leg, two months before, by a dog believed to be rabid. The wound healed, and he remained well till two days before admission, when he suffered from fever; and the day before admission, at noon, he became excited and anxious. On admission, there was constant hawking and spitting of frothy mucus, with a frequent ringing scream; and these symptoms were increased in paroxysms from time to time. He seemed anxious and distressed, somewhat delirious, and maintained a sitting posture, grasping the tapes of the cot. The pulse was very feeble. One drachm of chloroform was placed on a sponge, and slowly brought near to the face: it was inhaled with apparently partial relief. It was repeated every half hour, and in all ten drachms were used. He died at 2 P.M., nine hours after admission.

268. *Hydrophobia.—Chloroform used, but obliged to be discontinued.*—Succaram Bappoo, aged twenty-eight, a Bundari, was admitted into the Jamsetjee Jejeebhoy Hospital on the 2nd September, 1849, at half-past 4 P.M. Two months before, he had been bitten on the right leg by a dog supposed to be rabid. Some native remedies had been used. The wound had not completely cicatrised, but it was granulating

* The other five cases, though seen by me, were treated by Dr. Peet, and have been fully reported by him in the ninth and tenth numbers of the "Transactions of the Medical and Physical Society of Bombay."

and healthy. The occurrence took place at Girgaum, and the dog was the property of a Parsee. The patient had continued at his occupation as a day labourer till four days before admission. He was brought to the hospital exposed to the rain, and all his sufferings had become aggravated. He was agitated and alarmed, and constantly talking incoherently, and in a supplicating manner. He lay on the abdomen, hawking, and at times making a barking sound; but there was no great spitting of frothy mucus. The attempt to swallow fluid, or a current of cold air from opening the window, or the approach of the sponge with chloroform to the face, all excited violent general spasms, of short duration, but which seemed to cause much distress. The attempts to give the chloroform were discontinued. The pulse was very feeble on admission, and by degrees became more so; and shortly before his death, at eight P.M., four hours after admission, was imperceptible.

269. *Hydrophobia in a Parsee boy.*—Gorabjee Dhunjebhoy, a Parsee boy, of nine years of age, was admitted into the Jamsetjee Jejeebhoy Hospital about midnight of the 4th.* About a month before he had been bitten on the calf of the right leg by a dog on the road. The bite bled freely: it was dressed with plaster, and got well in three or four days. He continued well till four days before admission into hospital, when he became affected with febrile symptoms, but without spasms. On the afternoon of the 4th, he first showed signs of alarm when water was brought to him, and since then he has continued in an agitated state, talking much and incoherently, and in a supplicating manner. He complained of thirst, but when water was offered to him he became violently agitated, and said that he was unable to swallow. He pointed to the throat, the head, and the thigh, and the bitten limb as the seat of pain, but there was no pain experienced in the cicatrix. There was sense of chilliness and annoyance from the presence of people around him. The pulse was thready and barely perceptible. An attempt was made to give him some of a native remedy in the form of a pulp, which had been sent from Rutnagherry by Captain Haselwood; but he was able to swallow only a small part of it, and that with great effort. He shortly afterwards began to hawk and spit, and to make attempts to retch, and some of the medicine was vomited. He continued with increasing anxiety till 11 A.M. of the 5th, when he was removed by his friends and died half an hour afterwards.

* The month and year are not mentioned in my note, but it must have been in 1849 or 1850.

CHAP. XXXI.

ON BLOOD DISEASES.

SECTION I. — *Object of the Chapter explained.*

AN altered state of the blood has been regarded as forming part of the pathology of several of the diseases which have already been considered. To discuss the important subject of the pathology of the blood, is not my present object. The title prefixed to this chapter, has been adopted simply as a convenient one for enabling me briefly to notice several blood diseases, which the time, space, or data at my command, do not admit of my treating in a manner commensurate with their importance. They are: — 1. Pyæmia. 2. Leprosy. 3. Elephantiasis. 4. Scurvy. 5. General Dropsy, including Beriberi. 6. Rheumatism. 7. Snake Bite.

SECTION II. — *Pyæmia. — Short notice of Symptoms and Pathology. — Illustrative Cases.*

I use the term *Pyæmia*, to signify the concurrence of several collections of pus in the subcutaneous and intermuscular areolar tissue, frequently associated with puriform cysts in the substance of internal viscera, and generally attended with more or less febrile disturbance always adynamic and often remittent in type. The term, however, is objectionable, for it implies a relation between the development of the abscesses and the pre-existence and circulation of pus in the blood. The previous presence of pus in the blood is however hypothetical.

Ten cases of this affection are before me: for eight of them I am indebted to Mr. S. Carvalho, who, at my request, directed his attention to this subject, during the period that he officiated as one of the medical officers of the Jamsetjee Jejeebhoy Hospital. Mr.

Carvalho submitted his notes to Grant College Medical Society, and subsequently kindly placed them at my disposal.

Five cases proved fatal, and five recovered. Of the former, an examination after death was made in four. Small puriform cysts were found in the lungs in three, associated in two with similar collections in the kidneys. In none were abscesses found in the liver. In the fourth case no pus was discovered in any of the internal viscera. In none were there traces of phlebitis. In all, the small abscesses had evidently formed consecutive on inflammation.

In each of the five recovered cases, there were several large subcutaneous collections of pus, in such situations as the thigh, the chest, over the scapula, the leg, the neck, &c. In all, two or three abscesses were opened; but in some there was, in addition, the formation of swelling and hardness, which threatened to pass on to suppuration, but which nevertheless subsided: this latter event, however, only took place towards the close of the disease, after the general health had manifestly begun to improve. These abscesses were all preceded by the ordinary signs of inflammation — some degree of pain, heat, swelling, and hardness.

The cause of the affection was not apparent in any of the cases. A suppurating wound was noticed in only one instance: it was situated on the heel, and after death the veins leading from it were carefully examined, but showed no trace of inflammation. In all the cases there was some degree of febrile disturbance. In the worst, the type was adynamic, with brown dry tongue, failing pulse, and delirium; and remissions and exacerbations were generally well marked. Irregularity in the period of remission, and the early access of adynamic phenomena, served to raise the suspicion that the febrile symptoms were not those of malarious remittent fever, and to direct attention to the early detection of suppuration.

The character of the fever, and the nature of the local phenomena, are sufficient to indicate that the disease is one of the blood. In the milder instances, important internal viscera escape, in the severer they are involved. The existence of pus corpuscles in the blood, entangled in and obstructing capillaries, is unproved. But even if these bodies had been detected in the blood there is surely so little in common between the constitution of a pus corpuscle and a globule of mercury, as to destroy the force of the asserted analogy between pyæmia and Cruveilhier's frequently quoted experiments.

I shall conclude these brief and desultory remarks with a short summary statement of five of Mr. Carvalho's cases: viz. four fatal, and one recovered.

270. *Fever.—Several abscesses.—Small puriform cysts in lungs.—No trace of phlebitis.*—A Hindoo, of forty years of age, after eight days' illness, was admitted into hospital with febrile symptoms, enlarged glands of the left side of the neck, and an abscess in the left dorsal region, succeeded by dyspnœa, with subcrepitous rhonchus. He died five days after admission. There was purulent infiltration about the pectoral muscles and neck of the left side. The lungs were of dark-red colour and œdematous, and contained numerous puriform cysts, from the size of a hemp-seed to a small bean, and many of them immediately beneath the pleura. No puriform cysts in the liver; no trace of phlebitis in the axillary and brachial veins of either side.

271. *Adynamic fever.—Several abscesses.—Puriform cysts in the lungs.—One in the kidney.—Small suppurating wound of heel.—No trace of phlebitis.*—A Hindoo labourer, of twenty-five years of age, was admitted into hospital with a small wound in the sole of the left heel discharging pus, caused by a thorn twelve days before. An abscess formed above the left knee, and further purulent collections took place, preceded by pain, in both axillæ, and about the pectoral muscles, accompanied with adynamic febrile symptoms, and hurried breathing. He died five days after admission. There was no trace of phlebitis in the left saphenous and femoral veins, or in the axillary and brachial veins of the right side. There was purulent infiltration in the anterior and lateral parts of the chest, and extending up the neck, situated in the subcutaneous and intermuscular areolar tissue. There had been recent pleuritis on both sides. There were numerous hepatised nodules in both lungs, from the size of a pin's head to that of a pea, chiefly situated immediately under the pleura, with a small deposit of pus in the centre of each. No trace of purulent deposit in the liver or spleen; but a small one immediately under the capsule of the right kidney.

272.—*Adynamic remittent fever.—Small abscess on the forehead.—Carbuncle on the back.—Numerous puriform cysts in the lungs and kidneys.*—A Brahmin, of twenty-three years of age, was admitted into hospital, after fifteen days' illness with fever. The type, as observed after admission, was distinctly remittent, and of adynamic character. On the twelfth day after admission, a small abscess was noted on the forehead; and two days afterwards a carbuncle on the back. He died the following day with hurried breathing. There was recent pleuritis of both sides. The posterior parts of both lungs were in a state of red engorgement, with many collections of pus, each about the size of a small pea, and situated immediately under the pleura. No deposits in the liver. After removing the capsule of the kidneys, dark-red spots were observed, which, when incised, showed pus deposit in the centre; there were also two or three similar collections of pus deep in the cortical substance.

273. *Many abscesses.—Fever.—Death by exhaustion.—No puriform deposits in the internal viscera.*—A Hindoo sepoy, of thirty years of age, was admitted into hospital with a small abscess over the left olecranon, which was attributed to a fall sustained eight days before. Other abscesses formed: one over the left trochanter, another at the posterior fold of the right axilla, a third in the left lumbar region, and a fourth on the left natis. The febrile disturbance, slight at the commencement, increased with the progress of the affection. Diarrhœa came on and he died, exhausted, seventy days after admission. No deposits of pus found in the internal viscera.

274. *Adynamic fever.—Several abscesses.—Recovery.*—A horsekeeper, of thirty years of age, was admitted into the Jamsetjee Jejeebhoy Hospital with febrile symptoms of adynamic type attended with delirium. On the sixth day an abscess over the left pectoral muscle was detected, which he attributed to a kick from a horse. Subsequently, three other abscesses formed: one in the left lumbar region, a second in

the left thigh, and the third in the posterior part of the left leg. The abscesses were all opened, and discharged red-tinged pus. There was at one time some hurry of breathing and bronchitic rales. He also became affected with cholera; yet he recovered, and was discharged twenty days after residence in hospital.

SECTION III.—*Leprosy—Tubercular and Anæsthetic.—Short Account of the Symptoms and Pathology.*

The disease, which forms the subject of the present section, is the Elephantiasis Græcorum, the Lepra Arabum—but the term *Leprosy* is preferred by me, as sufficient and not likely to mislead. *Elephantiasis* I shall restrict to Bucnemia — the Barbadoes or Cochin leg, the Elephantiasis Arabum — as an appellation more appropriate to this affection than to leprosy. This application of the words leprosy and elephantiasis to these two diseases is in accordance with usage in India. It is unnecessary to add that leprosy is altogether distinct from the genus Lepra, of the order Squamæ of cutaneous diseases.

On the historical interest of leprosy in Europe throughout a series of centuries, I shall not enlarge. It still prevails in Norway; and the Report of a Royal Commission appointed some years since by the Norwegian Government, and drawn up by Drs. Danielssen and Boek, is, I believe, the best practical account of the disease as yet published.*

Leprosy is common in India. The numbers received into the Leper establishment at Calcutta are unknown to me, but I visited this institution in 1853, and found the accommodation and arrangements altogether inadequate for the comfort and well-being of those afflicted with this sad disease. Through the kindness of Dr. A. Hunter, the reports of the Madras Leper Hospital for the years 1851 and 1852 are before me. The admissions in these years amounted to 212, and the deaths to thirty-two. The system followed in this institution, at the time of my visit, when under the judicious management of Dr. Hunter, formed a pleasing contrast to that of Calcutta. The patients were classified according to their previous habits and position in life. Books were provided for the educated; and gardening and other light occupations conducive to health and cheerfulness were encouraged. The arrangements for

* I have not had the opportunity of consulting the original work of the Norwegian Physicians, "Traité de la Spedalskhed, ou Elephantiasis des Grecs," &c. It is fully referred to by Mr. Erasmus Wilson in a series of interesting papers in the "Lancet," April 1856, and was noticed some years since in the "British and Foreign Medico-Chirurgical Review."

lepers in Bombay, inferior to those of Madras, are superior to those of Calcutta. There is accommodation allotted for them in the Jamsetjee Jejeebhoy Dhurmsala, and under exacerbations of the disease they are received into a ward of the Jamsetjee Jejeebhoy Hospital appropriated for the purpose.*

During the six years from 1848 to 1853, 391 cases of leprosy were admitted into the hospital, and of these ninety-nine died. Under the system which obtains of transferring the patients from the dhurmsala to the hospital on exacerbations of the symptoms, and retransferring them to the dhurmsala on remissions, there must necessarily be a considerable number of re-admissions included in the 391 cases above adverted to.

Though visiting the leprous patients in the hospital almost daily, the various other subjects which pressed upon my attention prevented me from entering upon the careful clinical study of this disease. I, however, requested Mr. Lisboa, an intelligent graduate of Grant Medical College, during the period of his service in the hospital, to investigate the subject, and supply my deficiencies. His researches formed the subject of an interesting communication to Grant College Medical Society.†

Leprosy in Bombay occurs both in the tubercular and anæsthetic form, and occasional cases are observed in which the characters of both varieties are combined; but in this brief and imperfect notice I must confine my remarks to a summary statement of the characteristic symptoms of the two forms, and to a passing allusion to the pathology and treatment. I trust, however, that at no remote period, the clinical history and pathology of leprosy may be investigated in a manner commensurate with the opportunities enjoyed by many practitioners in India, and worthy of comparison with the careful inquiry of the Norwegian Commission.

Tubercular Leprosy.—The characteristic phenomena of this form of leprosy are sometimes preceded by a sense of languor and depression, and occasionally by distinct febrile accessions. More generally, however, the symptoms come on gradually and slowly, without premonitory indications. Irregularly disseminated patches of the skin become discoloured, and present a dark reddish or livid

* Before leaving India in September 1859, I placed the reports of the Madras Leper Hospital in the hands of Dr. Bhao Dhajee, and proposed to him as an object worthy of his well-known zeal and philantrophy the establishment and endowment, with the aid of his fellow-countrymen, of an institution in the proximity of Bombay, arranged in such manner as to minister to the comfort and the cheerfulness of this unfortunate class of sufferers.

† Extracts have been published in the "Transactions of the Medical and Physical Society of Bombay," No. 2, New Series, p. 290.

appearance, with a surface shining as if oil had been applied to it. The skin in these situations has, for the most part, its sensibility blunted; but this state is sometimes preceded by a stage of tenderness and pain. Then the vivid colour fades, the skin is left brown and tawny, and becomes thickened and tubercular. The morbid deposit is in some cases confined to the cutis, in others it extends to the subjacent areolar tissue. The cutaneous tubercles thus formed are small, soft, reddish or livid, and vary in size from a pea to an olive. They appear on every part of the face, but particularly on the nose and ears, and on the legs. In some rare instances they are confined to the legs. The disease may remain stationary in this state for some time; then the tubercles become affected with inflammation, and either suppurate or pass into states of foul ulceration, and those about the toes and fingers may lead to sphacelus and sloughing of the phalanges. The mucous membrane of the mouth, the fauces, the uvula, the tonsils, the pharynx and the nasal fossæ, become also studded with tubercular elevations, and these may degenerate and ulcerate, and give rise to sero-puriform and sanious discharges. The disease may now extend to the cartilages, and bones of the nose, and affect internal organs, as the lungs.

Anæsthetic Leprosy.—Large bullæ are often the first sign of this form of the disease. They lead to the formation of spots or patches of lighter shade than the surrounding skin in the darker races, and of a tawny brown colour in the white races. They appear first on the feet, hands, legs, and arms, seldom on the face and trunk till an advanced period. They are sometimes slightly prominent, and the hair on affected parts falls off. These patches are insensible, and extend slowly over the legs and arms to the trunk, and are unattended with swelling. As the disease advances the toes and fingers become shining and slightly swollen and stiff. The soles of the feet and palms of the hands present deep ragged furrows; ulcers form on the metacarpal and metatarsal articulations in the lines of flexion, enlarge by sphacelation, and the fingers and toes drop off, and the parts that are left cicatrise. At this stage the lobes of the ears and alæ of the nose become thickened and enlarged, and ultimately ulcerate. The voice now becomes hoarse, ulceration attacks the throat; and after a period of years, more or less prolonged, during which these morbid processes have been going on, diarrhœa or dysentery supervenes, and hastens the fatal result.

General Pathology of both forms.—Leprosy is a striking instance of a cachexia causing structural change of organs, by exudation-deposit from the blood, with subsequent degeneration of the deposit, and more or less of the adjacent structures. Drs. Danielssen and Boek have stated, that in the anæsthetic form, much of the deposit takes place about the spinal cord, as between the arachnoid and pia mater, and that the cord becomes hard, tough, and reduced in size.

The morbid anatomy of leprosy has been altogether neglected in India. Mr. Lesboa reports only one case in which an examination after death was made, and in this, though of the anæsthetic form, the appearances described by the Norwegian physicians were not present.

On the nature of the altered condition of the blood, and of the causes which induce it, I am unable to offer any useful practical suggestion; and the same remark may be made on the treatment. I am not acquainted with any medicines capable of controlling this disease, beyond what obtains in all cachectic diseases from a well-adjusted tonic regimen and suitable tonic remedies.

SECTION IV.—*Elephantiasis.*—*Symptoms.*—*Pathology.*—*Causes.*—*Treatment.*

As explained in the last section, I apply the term *Elephantiasis* to that disease which has been described under the names Elephantiasis Arabum, Bucnemia, Barbadoes leg, Cochin leg, Egyptian Sarcocele. It is not uncommon in Bombay, but occurs still more frequently in other parts of India, as in Bengal and on the coast of Malabar.

Symptoms.—The parts of the body most generally attacked are the extremities—the lower more frequently than the upper—the scrotum, the labia pudendi, and the mammæ. The affection is very often ushered in with rigors, nausea, headache, and febrile excitement; then the part which is to suffer becomes red, swollen, with a sense of smarting heat, and sometimes tenderness and hardness in the course of the lymphatics leading to the nearest glands: similar phenomena also occasionally occur in the course of the veins. These general and local symptoms, with exception of a certain degree of tumefaction of the part, disappear in a few days. Then, after irregular intervals, the same train of symptoms recurs from time to time; and after each attack, the affected part is left more tumefied and indurated, till finally it attains that great increase of bulk, to which it owes the designation elephantiasis. The cutaneous surface is left of a pale yellowish or livid colour; it is often scaly, rough or fissured, and covered with soft vegetations or horny excrescences, and more rarely is ulcerated. In other cases the surface is traversed by enlarged veins. In the advanced stages, deep-seated suppuration, with offensive discharge and sphacelus, may take place in different parts of the diseased mass, or in the enlarged lymphatic glands in its proximity: sometimes a milky-like fluid oozes in considerable quantity from the hypertrophied papillæ of the skin, and generally coagulates spontaneously into a gelatinous mass.

Pathology.—From the circumstance of the local affection being preceded by febrile excitement*, being liable to frequent recurrences,

* Since these remarks appeared in the first edition of this work, a report on "Elephantiasis as it exists in Travancore," has been published in the ninth number of the "Indian Annals of Medicine," by Mr. Waring, in which the primary character of the fever and the secondary character of the deposits is advocated. Dr. Ballingall, in the fourth number of the new series of the "Transactions of the Medical and Physical Society of Bombay," dissents from Mr. Waring's views, and regards the local affection as the primary morbid state, and the fever as symptomatic, and he thinks that the solution of this question has an important bearing on the surgical treatment of elephantiasis. Dr. Ballingall justly does not attach much importance to conclusions drawn from the mere statement of native patients, and he states that his own experience, which he admits to have been limited, does not support the view of periodicity of the attacks of fever and deposit. The fact that fever has ceased to appear in his cases of elephantiasis of the scrotum, after removal of the tumour, seems to him also a valid reason for concluding that the affection is local.

I still retain the opinion indicated in the text, that the disease is endemic, the fever primary, and the deposit secondary—just as the albuminous deposits in the liver and spleen are secondary on recurring intermittent fever. Further, that by preventing the fever in its early stages by suitable treatment and change of air, the deposits may be prevented in a great many cases. The argument in favour of a local origin from the circumstance of fever not returning after removal of the tumour, must, it seems to me, be received with much reservation. First, there should be a complete history as to the duration of the local affection, the locality of its origin and progress, as bearing on the likelihood of the return of fever at the locality of operation. Second. The existence of a large scrotal tumour is sufficient in a malaria-tainted constitution to determine recurrences of fever, with a frequency that may admit of being materially lessened by removal of the tumour, irrespective of considerations relating to changes in the locality of origin, progress, and surgical operation.

Mr. Waring also, it seems to me, attaches too much importance to the likelihood of return as an argument against surgical interference; for though the treatment of the constitutional state cannot receive too much attention after the operation, still it must be remembered that, in the instance of the scrotum, the deposit has probably selected that part in consequence of the favouring influence of anatomical conditions of structure and position, and that, when the tumour is removed, the conditions which favoured its origin have also ceased to exist, and therefore the return of the tumour becomes improbable. Why elephantiasis of the leg is common in some places, and that of the scrotum in others, I do not know. But the fact is so, and is practically important in forming an estimate of the chances of return of elephantiasis in other parts after the removal of a scrotal tumour.

There is still room for further accurate clinical research in this disease.

consisting of inflammatory action in particular tissues, and leading to peculiar results, elephantiasis may be regarded as a blood disease. An exudation of liquor sanguinis takes place into the interstices of the affected structure, and the lymph becomes formed into fibrous tissue of low organisation. On examining the diseased parts after death, the epidermis and the cutis are found thickened, sometimes to the extent of half an inch and more. The subcutaneous areolar tissue is either hypertrophied in a less degree than the cutis, or it has a semi-liquid gelatinous matter deposited in its areolæ. The microscopic appearances of this abnormal fibrous and elastic tissue are described and figured in an interesting account of this disease published by Professor Allan Webb.* The muscles are in general pale, thin, or softened.

By some pathologists, as Dr. T. A. Wise†, elephantiasis is supposed to originate in inflammation of the veins, preventing the free return of blood from the affected part; but this opinion is not generally concurred in. The more probable view is, that the thickening of the coats of the veins, the state sometimes of dilatation, at others of contraction of these vessels, are due to the influence of the lymph exudation and organisation, and the varying necessity, hence arising, for freer channels for the return of an abnormal quantity of blood. A marked difference between the pathology of Leprosy and Elephantiasis is, that in the former there is a more general and extensive exudation deposit, and a greater deviation in it from the blood plasma, as is shown by its readiness to undergo softening, ulceration, and gangrene.

Causes.—Elephantiasis would seem to be related to particular localities; to be most common in damp, low situations, near to the sea, in warm climates. It has also been supposed that the use of fermented toddy is favourable to its production, just as wine and beer are to that of gout.

Treatment.—It is of great consequence to note the earliest indications of this disease; to treat the febrile symptoms on ordinary principles with emetics, purgatives, diaphoretics, and rest, and the local inflammation by evaporating lotions and position. After the febrile attack and the coincident local phenomena have been removed, then the indication of cure is to elevate the general health, to prevent recurrences of fever by the use of quinine, and,

* "Indian Annals of Medical Science," No. 4.

† The very instructive observations on Elephantiasis by Dr. Wise, will be found at p. 156, of the seventh volume of the "Transactions of the Medical and Physical Society of Calcutta."

when practicable, to have recourse to change of locality. It is very important to follow this course of treatment, for when considerable hypertrophy of these fibrous tissues has taken place, their restoration to a normal state is beyond the resources of medical art. By compression with bandages, friction, and iodine applications, the bulk of the affected part may become diminished to some extent; but this result is consequent on the absorption of the liquid inter-areolar effusions, not the removal of any part of the abnormal fibrous tissue.

The question of the removal by surgical operation of parts affected with elephantiasis, is the only remaining practical consideration. Elephantiasis of the scrotum has of late years been very frequently the subject of surgical operation, and much success has attended the proceeding. It is to Brett, Esdaile, Allan Webb, Shircore, and Baboo Permanand Sett, that we are chiefly indebted for the elucidation of this department of surgery in Bengal *, and to Dr. Ballingall in Bombay.

SECTION V. — *Scurvy.* — *Prevalence in India.* — *Short practical Remarks.*

The admissions from scurvy into the European General Hospital at Bombay, during the fifteen years from 1838 to 1853, amounted to 618, and the deaths to nine. Those of the first five years of this term, the period of my service in the hospital, were 182 in number, being 2·4 of the total hospital admissions: of these, none proved fatal. These cases were almost exclusively of seamen from merchant ships, generally small class vessels, badly found, having made long voyages, and belonging to English or Scotch provincial ports. But, in all probability, it will be found that of all ships which trade to our Indian ports, scurvy appears most frequently in coal ships — of these many arrive yearly at Bombay as well as Aden — and this result might have been anticipated, for their voyages are generally long, and cleanliness is out of the question.

* It was in the removal of these scrotal tumours that mesmerism was practically applied by Dr. Esdaile, and afterwards by Professor Allan Webb, and a small hospital was established for the purpose in Calcutta. The Mesmeric Hospital still existed at the time of my visit in 1853, but chloroform as an anæsthetic had displaced mesmerism; and, though endeavours were made, with much courtesy and kindness, to show me the mesmeric effects, they proved unsuccessful. I witnessed the dexterous removal of these tumours by Mr. Shircore and Baboo Permanand Sett, and several successful cases in various stages, after the operation. For details relative to the operation, I would refer to Mr. Webb's and Dr. Ballingall's papers already adverted to.

In the report of the European General Hospital for the year 1851 *, Dr. Stovell makes somewhat similar observations on the cases of scurvy for that year.

During the six years from 1848 to 1853, 364 admissions of scurvy took place into the Jamsetjee Jejeebhoy Hospital: of these, sixty-four died. A considerable proportion of this class of patients had been labourers on the public works at Aden; and among these many deaths occurred from extensive scorbutic, sloughy ulceration, chiefly of the lower extremities. Consequent on improvement in the regimen of these public servants at Aden, there was, during the last three years of the term, a considerable diminution in this great but remediable evil.

In the years 1853 and 1854 admissions of scurvy began to take place from a quarter altogether different.

In consequence of the desertion of European crews from ships at Melbourne, for the Australian gold diggings, Lascars were shipped in numbers from Calcutta to supply the deficiency. Arriving at Melbourne, after a voyage of two or three months, they were transferred to the deserted ships, and again soon sent to sea. Ships with these Lascar crews, in a very scorbutic state, have arrived at Bombay, and doubtless at other ports also. I am not aware whether these events continue to occur, but if so, it is clearly the province of the magistrate to enforce the regulations relative to the shipment of Indian Lascars to other countries, or, should these be insufficient, to bring about their revision and change.

The general historical details of scurvy are of great interest, but they need not be repeated here; nor is it necessary to detail the symptoms.

In regard to the *pathology*, I would only observe, that scurvy escaped the solidism of Cullen, and has always been regarded as a blood disease. The particular nature of the changes in the blood are now very little better understood than in the days of Huxham and Lind. The water and fibrine are in excess, the red corpuscles defective, and the other constituents within the normal range. These, I apprehend, are all the positive facts which chemists, at the present time, can advance in respect to the blood in scurvy.

I shall conclude my notice of this disease with the following practical observations: —

* "Transactions Medical and Physical Society of Bombay," November 10.

1. Scurvy is caused by defects in diet, which involve deficiency in the quantity and variety of the alimentary principles, essential to the healthy constitution of the blood.

2. The defect is by some attributed to absence of organic vegetable acids; by others, to insufficient proportion of sulphur, phosphorus, potash, or vegetable albumen.

3. Whatever the explanation may be, the practical fact remains, that a diet with a just proportion of azotised nutritive principles and succulent vegetables, is that which prevents scurvy, and effects its cure. The curative effect of a suitable diet is increased by the use of acid fruits or vegetable acids, of which the citric is the best. The bad effects of an unsuitable diet are lessened by the use of vegetable acids or fruits.

4. Dr. Christison attributed the occurrence of scurvy in the jails of Scotland, in 1845 and 1846, to a reduction in the proportion of milk in the dietaries. That milk is a necessary part of an anti-scorbutic diet for the adult, is sufficiently disproved by the fact, that it does not form a part of the dietary of the British navy. On the other hand, that milk is an efficient anti-scorbutic under certain circumstances, is evident: were it otherwise, scurvy would be very common in children under two years of age.

5. A review of all these facts seems to justify the practical statement, but nothing more, that a diet adequate to prevent and to cure scurvy, should consist of a suitable and varied combination of the albuminous, saccharine and oleaginous principles, with the salts usually associated with them. Milk, as was first observed by Prout, is a typical combination of these principles appropriate for the early periods of life; therefore it is not improbable that Christison's statement is correct, that the reduction of the proportion of milk in a particular dietary is likely to affect its anti-scorbutic properties.

6. The phenomena of scurvy are well marked, but it is reasonable to infer that the changes in the blood take place gradually, and that they are present in some degree, before they attain to that which occasions the well-known scorbutic symptoms. This consideration is practically important, from the wide range which it justifies us in giving to a scorbutic taint as a condition predisposing to various forms of disease.

7. I have frequently adverted to certain debilitating influences as predisposing causes of disease generally. The influences alluded to are exposure to cold or wet, elevated temperature, malaria, vitiated atmosphere, inattention to cleanliness, over fatigue of body,

anxiety and depression of mind, previous diseases, &c. These are also predisposing causes of scurvy, and as such are often influential in favouring the development of the disease; but it will not occur under their influence without the exciting cause of unsuitable diet.

8. If the conditions just enumerated predispose the system to attacks of scurvy, it may readily be understood that the opposite conditions — viz. absence of cold, wet, heat, malaria, and defective ventilation, with attention to cleanliness, cheerful occupation of mind, and avoidance of bodily fatigue, must fortify the system against the influence of the exciting cause when operative, must tend to keep off the disease for a time, and to lessen its severity and hasten its cure.*

9. It is very useful, with reference to a right understanding of the etiology and prevention of scurvy, to appreciate justly this distinction between *predisposing* conditions and the *exciting* cause of scurvy, and to estimate truly their relative importance.

Section VI. — *General Dropsy. — Beriberi. — Symptoms. — Pathology. — Treatment. — Illustrative Cases.*

The occurrence of general dropsy in connection with renal and cardiac disease, has been already considered, but the affection is not confined to these circumstances. Cases of dropsy related to a very asthenic state, as that proceeding from frequently-recurring malarious fever, are not unfrequent in India. But my principal object, in this section, is to describe a train of dropsical symptoms to which writers on tropical disease have for a long time applied the term "Beriberi."

Beriberi. — The unnecessary introduction of this word into Indian nosology has served to retard and obscure our knowledge of the pathology and treatment of general dropsy, as it presents itself to our notice in the natives of India. In the month of February 1851 I called the attention of the Medical and Physical Society of Bombay to this subject, and explained the opinions on beriberi which I had been in the habit of stating to the students of Grant Medical College. In June 1853 several cases of beriberi were admitted into the Jamsetjee Jejeebhoy Hospital, and were carefully observed by me. They confirmed

* A large proportion of the men of the German Legion, sent from the Cape of Good Hope to India, were on arrival at Poona in November and December 1858, tainted with scurvy, from unsuitable food at the Cape. Some of them improved during the voyage, and all did so very rapidly at Poona, under the influences adverted to in the text.

the opinions which I had previously expressed on the pathology of this affection.*

I shall first describe the symptoms of beriberi, then explain the views on its pathology which I have long entertained, and finally narrate the circumstances connected with the hospital cases above adverted to.

The *symptoms* sometimes advance gradually, but at other times suddenly appear. When they have been gradual in their approach, the individual experiences for several days a sense of weakness, and inability, or unwillingness to exert himself, and shortly afterwards pain, numbness, stiffness, with more or less œdema of the lower extremities. There is also some degree of dyspnœa present, with a sense of oppression and weight at the epigastrium. The œdema is not confined to the extremities, but extends to the trunk and face, and occasions a puffed and bloated appearance. The weakness of the limbs and the dyspnœa are particularly complained of on motion. As the disease advances, the difficulty of breathing increases, the face becomes more swollen, and the lips livid. The limbs become almost paralytic, the oppression at the epigastrium is aggravated, frequent vomiting takes place, and the ejected matters are sometimes mixed with blood. The urine is scanty and high-coloured, sometimes almost suppressed, the thirst is great; the pulse, at first quick and small, or unaffected, becomes irregular, intermittent, and fluttering. Palpitations are experienced, attended with a sense of suffocation, a sinking pulse, and death. These symptoms may run their course in from two to three weeks; or the progress may be much more rapid, and when so, the numbness, the stiffness, and œdema of the lower extremities become quickly followed by the dyspnœa, the palpitation, and the sinking pulse.

These are merely the usual phenomena which attend on serous effusion into the connecting areolar tissue of the extremities, the cavity of the abdomen, the pleura, the pericardium, or into the air cells of the lungs, and their connecting areolar tissue — in other words, the symptoms of general dropsy more or less extensive, more or less quickly forming. Dr. Watson, in his excellent lectures, thus writes of dropsy: — "Now from whatever cause this watery condition of the whole body may arise, the effects resulting from

* In August 1853, "Remarks on the Pathology and Treatment of Beriberi," were presented by me to the Medical and Physical Society, and published in the 2nd Number of the "Transactions," New Series.

the presence of the *water* are the same: and of what do patients in this state usually complain? Why, of shortness of breath and palpitation of the heart; of a sense of impending suffocation if they attempt to lie down or actively to bestir themselves; of tightness and distress across the epigastrium, relieved somewhat by eructation, augmented by food and drink; of weight and stiffness of the limbs, and sometimes of drowsiness."

The morbid appearances found after death in fatal cases of beriberi are anasarca, œdema of the lungs, hydrothorax, hydropericardium, ascites, and cranial effusion. In some cases, traces of old or recent inflammation of internal viscera exist; but these constitute no essential part of the disease. It was the opinion of Dr. Malcolmson, entertained chiefly on account of the supposed paralytic symptoms, that the chief part of the disease was in the spinal cord or its membranes. This idea, however, cannot be sustained. Beriberi is a general dropsy; and in order to understand its *pathology*, let us call to mind the circumstances in which general dropsy usually occurs.

There is one form to which the name active has been given: it arises when the surface of the skin, after free exhalation, has become suddenly exposed to cold. The excretion of water by the skin is checked, the blood is driven inwards, and the kidneys from some cause or other do not take on their compensating action — they become congested, and general dropsy with scanty urine is the result. Active dropsy, under these circumstances, implies a certain amount of fulness of the vessels. There are several varieties of passive general dropsy, depending on different deranged conditions — on congestion of blood, local or general, on disease of the heart or of the lungs, or perhaps merely on feeble action of the heart, and also on disease of the kidneys. Passive dropsy, more particularly when related to diseased kidney, more surely occurs when cold or wet is applied to the surface of the body, and the excretion of water by the skin thereby impeded. Again, dropsy may arise, not from disease of the heart or lungs or kidney favouring congestion, but from blood deteriorated and abounding in watery constituent; and here, too, the onset of the dropsy will be favoured by the action of external cold upon the cutaneous surface. If diseased heart, or lungs, or kidneys, or blood too dilute, or vessels too full of blood, in their separate influences, lead to dropsical effusion, — how much more surely will this result take place if two, three, or more of these conditions are associated together — if, for example, we have disease of the kidney and of the heart combined; or if we have the vessels tolerably full of blood, with excess of watery constituent, circulated by a feeble heart, and the sufferer in both instances be exposed to the influence of external cold.

Beriberi is, in my opinion, a general dropsy of this complicated character. A state of the system in which the blood is sufficient in quantity, and its water in undue proportion, is the predisposing condition; and cold or wet is the exciting cause: no doubt in some instances the effusion is further favoured by co-existing heart, lung, or kidney disease. But how does this state of the blood arise? It is present in the scorbutic diathesis, and this constitutional condition may exist to some extent before the phenomena characteristic of *scurvy* appear. Let it further be remembered, that impaired irritability of muscular fibre, that of the heart included, is among the early derangements of the scorbutic state. We have thus as predisposing conditions of dropsy, not only watery blood, sufficient in quantity, but also propelled by a feebly acting heart. Let us suppose an individual in this state to have the surface of the body exposed to an atmosphere cold and damp, or to the chilling influence of piercing winds, and we have a combination of circumstances surely adequate to predispose to and excite general dropsy — the more certainly if the skin has been previously actively perspiring, and the kidneys, from congestion or structural defect, do not readily assume a compensating action.

The circumstances in which beriberi has usually appeared justify this view of its pathology. The disease always attacks many of a community, and has been chiefly observed in Ceylon, on the Malabar Coast, in the Circars, and among Lascars in ships on the adjacent seas. There has been much written on it by army surgeons in Ceylon, and by medical officers of the Indian army—Dr. Malcolmson and others, and more lately Mr. Carter;—but, on the whole, there is a want of fulness in the descriptions on the points on which accuracy is chiefly desirable. There is too much dwelling on symptoms, not difficult to understand, and too little of precise statement on important etiological conditions. I would except, however, Mr. Carter's excellent paper*, which contains much useful information. Notwithstanding these general defects there is still sufficient in the narratives to countenance the opinion that beriberi, more particularly in its acute form, occurs usually in persons favourably circumstanced for the development of a

* "Transactions, Medical and Physical Society of Bombay," No. 8.

scorbutic taint, and subsequently exposed to cold dry or moist winds, or to lying on the ground wet with rain or dew, while the body has been inadequately protected with clothing. The practical view to take of each separate case of beriberi is to regard it as a general dropsy, and to investigate it in the method observed in other cases of general dropsy. We should inquire into the state of the heart, the lungs, the kidneys, the condition of the blood; and carefully review the circumstances in which the individual has been placed, with the object of ascertaining whether he has been exposed to predisposing and exciting causes of dropsy. It is by keeping distinctly in view the general pathological principles involved in this inquiry that we may hope to reconcile the seeming contradictions of the confused details of which the accounts of this disease are for the most part composed. To me then it seems that beriberi is a general dropsy, and that in regard to each instance, the question ought to be, what is the pathology of this case of general dropsy? Generally it will be found that a scorbutic diathesis and external cold or wet are the determining conditions.

The symptoms, the pathology, the causes of beriberi have been discussed. The *treatment* need not detain us long. It resolves itself into prevention and cure. If it be true that a scorbutic diathesis is the predisposing condition, then attention to the means which are preventive of scurvy will also prove preventive of beriberi; and if external cold be the ordinary exciting cause, then attention to clothing and avoidance of exposure are most important sanitary measures.

The treatment of the disease when fairly formed should accord with the principles observed in general dropsy. In the acute forms of dropsy in a sthenic habit, with excited vascular action, there may be scope for general blood-letting, but it can be only under such conditions of the general system and of the circulation that this measure can be admissible, and these will not, I apprehend, be often found present in beriberi. In other cases of dropsy in which vascular action is not depressed, in which there is no irritation of the gastro-intestinal mucous lining, we may endeavour to reduce the effusions — by active purgatives, as elaterium, or other members of this class. Then there are other instances in which cathartics are unsafe, and diuretics are the chief remedies to be trusted to. Cases also occur in which the action of the heart is depressed, and in these stimulants must be given at the same time with diuretics. Nor may we forget that the skin is sometimes an appropriate channel by which to lessen the water of the blood, and favour the absorption of dropsical effusions. The vapour bath, or the hot air bath may be used with this view. In the treatment of beriberi general blood-letting, purgatives, diuretics, and stimulants have been recommended. But if the pathology and therapeutics of dropsy have been rightly explained, then there is no special method of treating beriberi. The means which are the best in one case may be the worst in another.

Beriberi as observed in the Jamsetjee Jejeebhoy Hospital in June 1853.—In the month of June 1853, four cases of beriberi were received into the Jamsetjee Jejeebhoy Hospital. The sufferers were Lascars, belonging to a ship which had just arrived from sea. Many others of the crew had also suffered. One individual died on his way from the ship to the hospital, and an inquest was held on the body. The expediency of eliciting information relative to the length of the voyage, and the management of the crew, was suggested by me to the coroner. I shall first quote the deposition of the captain of the ship; then state the important facts of the cases admitted into hospital; and finally inquire whether they confirm or not the view which has already been taken by me of the pathology of the disease:—

William Eames, on being duly sworn, says:—I am master of the ship *Faize Allum*, of the port of Bombay, and have been constantly commanding, or been chief officer of vessels trading out of Bombay, with a Lascar crew, since the year 1838. I last left Bombay on the 3rd day of June, 1852, with a Lascar crew of sixty-five men and boys; and the deceased, Bhana Moorar, aged about forty years, and deceased Jadow Dewa, aged about twenty-five years, both Hindoos, formed part of the crew. We proceeded from Bombay to Singapore, and from thence to Siam, and returned from thence to Singapore, and so back again to Siam; and from thence to Singapore, which place I quitted for Bombay on the 3rd March this year, expecting to make the voyage in seven weeks, the average passage being about two months. I had on board curry-stuff, rice-water, dall, ghee, salt, &c., as prescribed by the regulations, with a good supply of water; and during such time as the ship was in harbour always supplied the crew with greens, fresh fish, and fresh provisions. The crew all remained healthy till about the 21st day of May last, in latitude 10° N., longitude 64° W. We had then been two months and eighteen days at sea. On the 15th day of April I was within about seventy miles or thereabouts of the island of Ceylon; but being unable to stand the strong current and west winds then blowing, after consulting with my Serang and chief officer and passengers, I determined on relinquishing the attempt to get round Ceylon, and bore away for the line, to come up to Bombay by the southern passage, round the Laccadives and Chagos, and ran to the south of the line as far as 8° 49′, and then to the westward as far as 63° W., and crossed the line again, running north, about the 6th or 7th May, and during most of the time had rain and squalls. Most of the water having been consumed, we filled up the water casks with rain water, collected on the surface of a clean awning. After making the line on the 6th of May, we had light weather, with occasional squalls and constant rain, and came on with the S.W. monsoon up to 16° N. latitude on or about the 2nd June, and arrived in the harbour of Bombay on the 6th June, I consider that I first fell in with the S.W. monsoon about three degrees north of the line. The crew were all healthy up to the 21st of May. When in latitude 10° N., longitude 64° W., symptoms of disease first showed themselves. The deceased Jadow Dewa complained of pains in his feet, and loss of strength down the legs, and pain in the chest, with difficulty of breathing, and constipated bowels. I gave him jalap and cream of tartar, and to rub on the chest hartshorn, laudanum, and sweet oil. The crew since the 15th of April had been on reduced allowance of about ten pounds in ninety pounds of rice, fish and water full allowance, the latter being rain water. Between the 21st day of May and 6th June, eight other men were seized in the same manner, and all died; the average suffering about four or five days; a Portuguese sepoy died in three days. The deceased Jadow Dewa appeared to be recovering fast, and left the ship on the evening of the 6th of June. Bhana Moorar also appeared convalescent, and left the ship in my dingy. All the survivors of the crew are landed, the voyage being completed. The passengers, twelve in number, natives, and myself and officer, and the majority of the crew, are well. We drank the rain water very freely, and I believe the deceased died of a disease called the beriberi of Ceylon. I had a good medicine chest on board, and treated those taken ill according to the instructions laid down in Dr. Thomas' book of medicine. We had no liquor on board the ship. I offered the crew pickles and vinegar, and also sugur, but they refused to eat it. The passengers and myself used pickles, sugar, and vinegar freely, but the crew declined till latterly. The whole number who were attacked were about thirty-five, of whom ten have died. We were in the latitude of Cochin when the disease first appeared, and were about 10° to the westward of the coast of India, with light N.W. and N.E. winds. The crew were protected from wet as far as possible. The disease attacked persons of all ages, but principally the old and more infirm of the crew. Further I know not. The cargo consisted principally of sugar in bags, of Malling ivory, teak wood, plant and sapan wood, and raw silk. The hatches were kept constantly open when the weather would permit, the forecastle well cleansed and fumigated with powder burnt and benjamin."

The jury returned the following verdict:—"Deceased died of beriberi."

275. *Beriberi.—Recovery.*—Purshotum Zeena, a Hindoo kalasee, of the ship *Faize Allum*, twenty-five years of age, a man of stout frame, was admitted into the Jamsetjee Jejeebhoy Hospital on the 7th of June, 1853. He had been ill sixteen days. The feet, legs, and thighs were œdematous, and, in consequence of the stiffness of the thighs and groins from the swelling, he walked with a waddling gait. The pulse was easily compressed. There was no abnormal dulness of the præcordial region, and the sounds of the heart were normal. The bowels were rather confined, and the urine scanty. He complained of uneasiness at the epigastrium and the hypogastrium. There was no vomiting; the tongue was not coated, but was rather florid. There was no sponginess or discoloration of the gums. He continued in hospital till the 27th June, when he was discharged well. For some days after admission he complained of uneasiness and sense of weight at the epigastrium, and there was abnormal dulness on percussion, to within two inches of the umbilicus. The urine showed no trace of albumen. He was treated with occasional doses of compound powder of jalap, the anti-scorbutic mixture of the hospital, a diet with fresh vegetables, and lemonade, and a small allowance of arrack. Under this treatment the dropsical symptoms and the fulness at the epigastrium disappeared, and he left the hospital quite well.

276. *Beriberi.—Slight discoloration of the gums.—Recovery.*—Bhowan Rama, a Hindoo kalasee, of the ship *Faize Allum*, thirty-five years of age, and of stout frame; ill for fifteen days. The legs, thighs, and feet were very anasarcous, and his gait waddling from the stiffness of the legs and groins. The pulse was very feeble, and the urine scanty. He had uneasiness at the epigastrium, but no dyspnœa, except after walking. The sounds of the heart were normal, and there was no dulness of the præcordial or other regions of the chest, and the respiratory murmur was distinct; the tongue moist and without fur; the gums discoloured, but not swollen; the teeth felt tender on

eating; urine not albuminous. The treatment followed was the same as in the first case, with the addition of the occasional use of the warm bath. He was discharged well on the 27th June.

277. *Beriberi.—Anasarca.—Death.—No kidney disease.—Liver congested.—Cavities of the heart full of thin blood,*—Visram Narrayen, a Hindoo kalasee, of the ship *Faize Allum*, twenty years of age, ill fourteen days, was admitted into the Jamsetjee Jejeebhoy Hospital on the 7th June, 1853. There was general anasarca. The pulse was feeble. There was no abnormal præcordial dulness; the sounds of the heart were normal; there was slight fulness of the abdomen; no swelling of the gums. On the 8th and 9th the pulse became feebler, and the breathing oppressed; the urine was very scanty, but showed no trace of albumen. He died on the afternoon of the 9th. He was treated with stimulants—ammonia and arrack. The body was examined two hours after death, and Mr. Lisboa has favoured me with the account of the appearances.

Head.—On opening the cranium, about five ounces of serous fluid oozed out. The structure of the brain, cerebellum, pons Varolii, and medulla oblongata was healthy. The ventricles of the cerebrum contained the normal quantity of fluid. *Chest.*—The cavity of the chest contained only two ounces of thin transparent fluid. Both lungs collapsed freely, and their structure was healthy; they showed no appearance of œdema. The heart appeared slightly enlarged. On opening both the right and left cavities, they were found to contain a thin red fluid and a few soft red coagula of blood; the fluid in the right ventricle was frothy. *Abdomen.*—The abdominal cavity did not contain more than two ounces of thin transparent serous fluid. The peritoneal surface of the intestines was of reddish colour from congestion; all the abdominal viscera were more or less congested, but their structure was healthy. The liver presented appearances of congestion more than any other organ; from its incised surface fluid blood flowed freely.

278. *Beriberi.—Anasarca.—Gums discoloured.—Hydrothorax.—Fatal.—Cavities of the heart full of fluid blood.*—Jadow Dewa, a Hindoo kalasee, of the ship *Faize Allum*, twenty-five years of age, ill sixteen days, was admitted into the Jamsetjee Jejeebhoy Hospital on the 7th June, 1853. There was general anasarca, the abdomen was rather full, and distinctly fluctuating; the breathing was oppressed; there was no abnormal præcordial dulness; the sounds and action of the heart were irregular. He complained of pain at the epigastrium; the pulse was very small, and the skin coldish; the gums were discoloured, but not swollen. He died on the morning of the 8th. The body was examined five hours after death; and I am indebted to Mr. Lisboa for the account of the appearances.

Head.—On removing the calvarium, about five ounces of thin serous fluid oozed out. The structure of the brain, and of the other contents of the cranium, was healthy. The ventricles of the cerebrum contained a little more than the normal quantity of thin transparent serum, with a few bubbles of air. *Chest.*—Both cavities contained about twelve ounces of serous fluid. The right costal pleura adhered to the visceral, by means of old bands of areolar tissue, which was also infiltrated with serous fluid, except at the lower part of the chest, where there was a sort of sac, holding about four ounces of serum. The left lung collapsed freely. The structure of both was healthy, except that it appeared to be slightly compressed. On pressing the incised surface, a small quantity of frothy serous fluid oozed out. The heart was apparently enlarged (dilated); both auricles and both ventricles were distended with fluid blood, and some few soft red coagula. The fluid in the right ventricle contained a few bubbles of air. The structure of the heart was healthy. All the abdominal viscera were more or less congested, but otherwise they were healthy. The peritoneal lining of the abdominal cavity, and that covering the intestines, presented a reddish appearance. The blood, examined under the microscope, showed a normal state of the corpuscles.

The circumstances in which beriberi made its appearance in the ship *Faize Allum* were certainly confirmatory of the view which I had taken of the pathology of this disease. The ship had been two months and eighteen days at sea. The crew were for the last month on somewhat diminished rations, and at no period did anti-scorbutics form part of the dietary. The weather was bad, and there was exposure to fatigue. The disease appeared on the 21st May. The weather during the fifteen days preceding had been wet and squally. Of a crew of sixty-five, thirty-five were attacked, and ten died. The officers and passengers of the ship did not suffer from the disease: they used antiscorbutics freely, and we may assume, at least as regards the passengers, that they were not exposed to the inclemencies of the weather; and as regards the officers, that they were by clothing better protected than the Lascars.

It is true that in the four cases which came under my observation in hospital, the external phenomena of scurvy were not present: in two the gums were discoloured, but not swollen and spongy. But in order to explain the pathology of the disease the actual presence of scorbutic phenomena is not necessary. The diathesis is doubtless of gradual formation, and requires, in all probability, the influence, for a considerable time, of the conditions which induce it, before the characteristic symptoms of scurvy appear. Nor can it be questioned that the changes which the blood is slowly undergoing in the gradual development of the scorbutic state must predispose to derangements of various kinds, — must, for example, be favourable, on the surface of the body becoming chilled, to the occurrence of internal congestions with dropsy and occasional hæmorrhage. It is, indeed, only when the diathesis is partially formed, that we are likely to meet with beriberi, for it is not probable that sailors really scorbutic will be fit for duty, and exposed to wet and squally weather.

Though the acknowledged characters of scurvy were absent in these cases, still there were facts which showed that the diathesis existed in some degree. In both the fatal cases the blood was found more or less fluid after death. In all the cases the feeble action of the heart was very remarkable: in three—the two successful cases, and one fatal—this could not be attributed to thoracic dropsical effusions, for in none of them was there œdema of the lungs, or effusion into the pleura or pericardium. Again, in the two fatal cases, all the cavities of the heart were dilated and filled with blood, showing that the circulation had ceased from failure of irritability of the muscular fibre — that death had been by syncope. This defective irritability of the heart points to something in the pathology of the disease, in addition to the dropsical effusions; and, perhaps, there is no condition of the system more generally characterised by impaired irritability of muscular fibre than the scorbutic. There is no fact more familiar in the history of disease than occasional sudden death by syncope in patients affected with scurvy.

There are other considerations of interest in these cases. A sense of weight and uneasiness at the epigastrium is a common symptom of beriberi: in one of the successful cases enlargement of the liver was evident on percussion, and in both the fatal cases a congested state of this organ was well marked. This symptom, then, is probably due to congestion of the liver. This congestion, with the altered state of the blood, also explains the occasional occurrence of hæmatemesis in beriberi. In these cases there was no disease of the heart or kidney.

The principles of prevention and treatment are sufficiently clear. By suitable dietaries, to prevent the formation of the scorbutic diathesis; by suitable clothing, as far as practicable, to protect the crew from inclement weather. In regard to treatment: (*a.*) the use of antiscorbutic regimen and remedies; (*b.*) to regard the feeble pulse as a condition independent of the dropsical effusions, and to give stimulants more or less freely; (*c.*) to remove the dropsy by purgatives or diuretics, being guided to the use of the one or the other by the state of the pulse; (*d.*) to increase the cutaneous capillary circulation by friction and warm clothing. The hot air bath or warm water bath requires caution, in consequence of the increased depression of the heart's action which follows transient excitement from these means. They had better not be regarded as part of the regular treatment of the disease. I attach great importance to the fact, which these cases clearly establish, that the feeble pulse is not consequent on the functions of the heart or lungs being interfered with by serous effusions, but is dependent on impaired irritability of the fibre — one of the phenomena of the scorbutic diathesis. We shall therefore be disappointed if we expect the power of the heart to improve by the mere removal of the dropsy by purgatives or diuretics. The use of stimulants must go hand in hand with that of these evacuants; indeed must in many cases, in advanced stages, be the only safe measure. While we keep up the action of the heart, and remove the effusions, it is, if these pathological doctrines be correct, also a very important indication to improve the diathesis by antiscorbutic means.

In the statistical report of the health of the royal navy for the year 1856, ordered to be printed by the House of Commons, on the 26th July, 1858, mention is made of an epidemic dropsy which prevailed in the ship *Juno* in the Australian seas, and the cause of which appeared to be wrapped in mystery. There is no clinical description of the dropsical symptoms—but from the terms "epidemic ascites" and "peritoneal dropsy" being used—it may be inferred that the effusions were chiefly abdominal. The only account of symptoms is the following:—

> "In general the patients, amongst whom were a large proportion of the strongest men in the ship, exhibited little or no constitutional disturbance, and, with the exception of a sallow complexion or paleness of the whole surface, they presented no unusual appearance. They, however, complained of mental depression, a feeling of uneasiness, and a troublesome barking cough, which generally existed for some days or even weeks previously to the attack."

The prominent facts were these:—The ship's company had been victualled for a considerable time on salt provisions during the last quarter of 1855. The ship returned to Sydney about the beginning of January 1856, from a lengthened cruise amongst the islands in the Pacific; left Sydney on the 8th of March, reached Hobart Town on the 13th; sailed again for Sydney on the 28th, and arrived on the 6th April.

During the stay of the *Juno* at Sydney, from January to 8th March, three cases occurred. From the 16th to the 28th March, at Hobart Town, eighteen cases. From the 6th April to 2nd June, at Sydney, eight cases. There is a slight discrepancy between the total of these figures, extracted from the report, and the following summary:—

> "The total number of cases of this singular malady put on the sick list between the 3rd January and the 2nd June, amounted to thirty: of these eleven were invalided and nineteen returned to duty. Though no case terminated in death, they were all exceedingly protracted, and the recovery in most instances imperfect."

The holds were free from offensive effluvia, and to the eye appeared to be thoroughly clean; but in cleansing the lower deck, the wooden shot-racks, placed close to the sail lockers, were found to be in a rotten state, and a quantity of dark, slimy matter was discovered beneath. Notwithstanding the occurrence of cases, long after the removal of these offensive matters, the surgeon continued of opinion that the disease originated from "a malarious poison arising from the putrefaction of the vegeto-animal accumulation on the lower deck, which had been imperfectly going on, and injuriously affecting the health of the ship's company." The reporter objects to this view, that the persons most constantly engaged in cleaning the holds were not attacked in greater number than the rest of the ship's company; and that offensive effluvia, or malaria, arising from similar collections of matter, have existed in innumerable instances, both in houses and in ships, without producing any disease of the same nature.

The two following further extracts from the report are, it seems to me, conclusive as to the etiology and pathology of this disease:—

"The assistant surgeon, in a well written report, observes, 'That although the bad effluvia arising from the dirt and moisture under the shot racks might have had a predisposing influence, he considered that the disease depended on causes producing a morbid state of the fluids, which most resembled their condition in scorbutus.'"

The surgeon remarks:—

"A certain reduction of temperature appeared to be necessary for the development of the disease; for while the men in warm weather continued in the enjoyment of tolerable health, on getting into cooler weather at Sydney and Hobart Town, the disease broke out in consequence of the cold rendering the poison more active, or the people more susceptible, or probably from both causes."

The disease was clearly dropsy, excited by external cold in a scorbutic diathesis — in other words *Beriberi*.

Section VII. — *Rheumatism.* — *Prevalence in India.*

The admissions under this head into the European General Hospital at Bombay, during fifteen years, from 1838 to 1853, amounted to 1457, and the deaths to six.

Of these 528, with four deaths, took place during the five years of my service in this hospital, being 6·8 per cent. of the total hospital admissions. The admissions were pretty equally divided throughout the year: the greatest proportion, in the month of February, 12·1 per cent., and the least, in the month of October, 3·6. By far the largest number were of chronic rheumatism, traceable, in many cases, to a scorbutic taint or previous venereal affection. In the treatment of rheumatism in India, as well as in temperate climates, it is necessary to recollect the great tendency to pericarditis and endocarditis.

Metastasis to the testicle was observed in several cases of chronic rheumatism,—swelling and hardness of the organ coming on, followed by cessation of the pain and swelling of the joints, which, however, recurred on the alleviation of the orchitis.

In my remarks on pericarditis and affections of the heart, it was explained, that though acute rheumatism is not of such frequent occurrence in India as in European countries, yet that it is sufficiently so to command our careful attention, more especially as its relation to cardiac disease is quite as important in the one country as in the other; chronic rheumatism, however, is much more common in India, particularly in natives. The term is applied to pain in the muscles and joints, often without much or any swelling of the latter, frequently attended with irregular febricular disturbance, and very generally related to scorbutic, malarious, syphilitic, or mercurial cachexia.

The admissions from rheumatism into the Jamsetjee Jejeebhoy Hospital for four years, from 1848 to 1852, amounted to 1384: of these 574 were registered as acute, and 810 as chronic. The following tabular statement shows the prevalence in different years and castes;—

Admissions and Deaths, from Rheumatism, in the Jamsetjee Jejeebhoy Hospital at Bombay, from 1848 *to* 1852, *arranged according to Caste and Sex.*

	Hindoos.		Mussulmans.		Christians.		Parsees.		Females.		Total.	
	Admitted.	Died.	Admitted.	Died.	Admitted.	Died.	Admitted.	Died.	Admitted.	Died.	Admitted.	Died.
1848-49	83	4	95	—	58	1	13	1	39	—	288	6
1849-50	72	1	112	3	53	—	17	—	32	1	286	5
1850-51	120	2	151	3	64	—	43	—	57	1	435	6
1851-52	114	1	129	1	71	—	35	—	26	—	375	2
Total .	389	8	487	7	246	1	108	1	154	2	1384	19

SECTION VIII. — *On Snake-Bite.*

My experience in snake-bite is exclusively confined to one species, and to one period of my service in India. The observations which follow were published nearly in their present form, in the year 1850.*

* "Transactions, Medical and Physical Society of Bombay," No. 10.

In the years 1834 and 1835, while in medical charge of the Convalescent Station on the Mahabuleshwur Hills, I made some observations on the effects resulting from the bite of the phoorsa, a small snake common on the hills, and known to the natives by that name. The phoorsa snake is about a foot in length, the tail tapers suddenly from about an inch from the end; the colour is olive brown, of different shades, variegated with white: on the back and sides there are olive brown lozenge-shaped patches; the belly is white, with brown spots, and the transverse plates under the belly and tail are single; a small isolated fang is distinct in the upper jaw.

279. *A small dog bitten by the phoorsa snake: fatal.*—About the month of January 1834, a small puppy dog was brought to me, said to have been bitten on the upper lip by a phoorsa snake,—but, as the animal seemed lively and well, I thought that there might be some mistake: the snake, however, was shown to me, and the dog had been found playing with it. In a short time the lip swelled slightly, and was painful on being touched; it was rubbed with ammonia, and some was also given internally. During the course of the day the animal appeared sufficiently lively, took food and ran about; but the swelling continued to increase, and caused much pain. On the following day the face and neck were very much swollen, especially under the lower jaw. The dog died in the course of the day, about thirty hours from the time it had been bitten.

On dissection, the swollen face and neck were found much infiltrated with bloody serum; and in some places, especially in the neighbourhood of the bitten part, there was extravasation of blood. The larynx, trachea, and lungs were healthy; no congestion of the mucous lining. The other organs seemed healthy.

280. *A horsekeeper bitten by the phoorsa snake: fatal.*—At 11 A.M., on the 20th March, 1834, a horsekeeper, in the service of Colonel Lodwick, was brought to me. On the middle finger of his left hand there was a small punctured wound, caused by the bite of a snake. The occurrence took place about half an hour before I saw him. He made no complaint of pain; there was no swelling around the wound; the pulse was natural: the bitten part was excised, caustic applied, and a ligature tied round the wrist. At 3 P.M., appearance unchanged; no complaint but of pain in the hand, which was somewhat swollen. This I attributed chiefly to the ligature, and removed it. On the morning of the 21st, he was reported to have slept well. The hand was considerably swollen—the swelling was tense, painful, and extended above the wrist; the tongue natural. He made no complaint but of the hand. Cold lotion was directed to be applied. At 1 P.M. it was observed, that over the right tibia, here and there, on the right foot, and also between the fingers of the right hand, the skin had cracked, or rather had assumed an abraded appearance; and from these points fluid and florid blood oozed and trickled slowly. One of these points had existed on the previous day, but the others had only been noticed within an hour or two. The skin was natural in temperature; the hand was more swollen; pulse 64, full and firm; and he had a sense of weight in the forehead. The saliva was tinged slightly with blood, the tongue expanded, but not furred; breathing slow. About ten ounces of blood were abstracted from a vein in the right arm, by which the uneasy sensation in the head was relieved and the pulse reduced; the blood did not flow very freely, the orifice in the vein being small. At 4 P.M. I found that there was hæmorrhage from the arm in which he had been bled; it had been necessary to renew the compress twice, and three or four ounces of blood had been lost. About the right elbow joint, principally ante-

riorly, extending down the fore-arm and up the arm, there was tense, elastic, painful swelling, very similar to that of the bitten hand; the blood, dark and thin, trickled down the arm from the orifice made in the vein. It was impossible, from the swelling and hæmorrhagic tendency, to stop the bleeding in the ordinary way; it was in part effected by pressure with the finger, afterwards by means of a cork compress and adhesive plaster. The pulse had become small, the skin cold; he was restless and distressed looking, but answered questions freely when spoken to. The tongue was expanded, and its edges deeply marked with indentations from the teeth. The blood taken from the arm had not coagulated in the slightest degree; it was a dark red-brown liquid. Stimulants of brandy and ammonia were given in full doses, and frequently; he continued restless and drowsy, but was always roused when spoken to. The pulse continued barely perceptible; he complained chiefly of the pain of the swelling of the arm in which he had been bled. At 10 P.M. the swelling of the bitten hand had become much reduced, and softer; that of the opposite arm, in which he had been bled, had increased. He continued pulseless, restless, and drowsy, but answering questions when roused, till 5 A.M. of the 22nd, when the breathing became difficult, and he died at 7 A.M. There was nothing peculiar in the appearance of the body; the bitten hand was much less swollen than it had been. No examination of the body permitted after death.

281. *Parsee woman bitten by a phoorsa snake.—Recovery.*—On the 20th April, 1835, at 10 A.M., a Parsee woman, resident in the bazaar at Malcolm Peth, was bitten by a phoorsa on the dorsum of the last phalanx of the ring finger of the right hand. I saw her half an hour afterwards; a ligature had been applied to the finger; I excised the bitten part, and applied caustic, and continued the ligature till the afternoon, when it was removed, in consequence of the pain which it occasioned. She complained once or twice of her head, and took some doses of eau de luce. There was swelling of the finger, and the hand, but to no great extent. There was constant oozing of blood from the excised part, which on the 22nd increased to a constant dropping of blood, and continued so during the night. On the 24th the bleeding continued, and the pulse was feeble; the actual cautery was used, and stopped the bleeding, which was absent on the 25th, but recurred on the 26th, and was stopped by pressure. On the 1st of May she was quite well. Ammonia was the only internal remedy used.

282. *Dog bitten by a phoorsa snake.—Fatal.—Post mortem examination.*—A full sized dog, on the morning of the 24th May, 1834, at 10 A.M., was bitten over the right false ribs by a large phoorsa snake. He continued well all day, took food and water freely. In the evening slight diffused swelling about the bitten part, but the animal did not cry on pressure of the part. On the morning of the 25th the dog seemed dull, and did not take his food, the swelling was slight and diffuse, and did not seem to cause pain on pressure. At 2 P.M. the sluggishness was found to have increased, and near to the animal there was some dark fœtid pitch-looking fluid, which must have been either vomited or passed by stool. About eleven o'clock at night he was heard to howl, and probably died at midnignt; he was found dead early in the morning of the 26th having lived about forty hours; and more of the dark pitchy fluid was found on the ground, and as it covered the legs and tail of the animal, it seemed to have been passed by stool. The body was not at all swollen.

Inspection.—The body was carefully examined after death. Around the bitten part there was infiltration of the subcutaneous cellular tissue, for an extent of eighteen inches in a longitunal direction, and six in a vertical. The fibres of the tissue seemed thickened and condensed, so that the fluid did not run freely nor in quantity from the cut surfaces. Where the infiltration was greatest the thickness was about a quarter of an inch, and formed a dark red fleshy-looking substance. Towards the periphery of the infiltrated portion the colouring matter of the fluid was much less in quantity. In no situation did the infiltration pass the mesial line to the left side of the thorax.

It was not an ordinary infiltrated cellular tissue, such as is seen in anasarca; the organisation of the tissue seemed to have undergone a change, so that a portion macerated in water lost its dark red colour, but retained the other physical properties —its thickness and firmness. *Thorax.*—The heart was empty and pale. The arterial system empty and contracted. The jugular veins contained some thin fluid blood. The lungs were much collapsed, and perfectly pale, with the exception of a few superficial red patches; when incised they were perfectly dry. I never saw lungs so devoid of anything like congestion of blood, or so absolutely without serous infiltration, or the natural secretion of the mucous lining. The mucous membrane of the trachea and bronchial tubes was perfectly pale. *Head.*—The brain firm, healthy, pale, ex-sanguine. *Abdomen.*—The liver healthy, but with some red serous congestion. The stomach and intestines were externally natural; there was no discoloration nor vascular congestion; they were laid open from the pharynx to the rectum. The œsophagus was natural; the stomach contained yellow fluid, mixed with food; its coats were natural. About two feet of the upper part of the small intestine contained mucus, deeply tinged with bile; descending the bowels the mucus became tinged with blood, like red currant jelly. Descending still further, this state of the secretion increased in quantity, and deepened in colour; in the large intestine, extending to the anus, there was a thick coating of it, very fœtid, and in colour and consistency resembling pitch. Wherever this secretion was scraped from the lining tunic the appearance of the latter was natural, no discoloration, no vascularity, no alteration of condition; in every point it was a pale healthy mucous tissue. The bowels were not distended, and, take away their contents, they could not have been more healthy or natural, in colour, structure, and relations. The kidneys were healthy. The bladder was filled with healthy urine; its lining membrane presented one faint discoloured patch.

CHAP. XXXII.

ON DRACUNCULUS.

Section I. — *Prevalence of, in Bombay Presidency. — Relation to Season. — Allusion to Theories respecting its mode of origin. — Short notice of Symptoms and Treatment.*

Dracunculus, or guinea-worm, from its great prevalence in many parts of the Bombay Presidency, has, during the last thirty years, engaged the attention of several medical officers* of that establishment.

The inquirers have generally assumed that there probably exists some connection between guinea-worm and an external existing species. Therefore a leading object of their research has been to determine whether any relation subsists between the prevalence of this affection, and particular seasons, soils, and sources of water supply; and to discover whether the soil or water of affected localities constitutes the habitat of any species of worm zoologically allied to this entozoon. These investigations, as well as those relating to the manner of entrance into the human body of the ova of the assumed external related species, have not led to positive or satisfactory results. In fact, the obscurity in the natural history of entozoa generally, is well illustrated in the instance of dracun-

* 1. Dracunculus, as prevailing in the Artillery while stationed at Matoongha in the Island of Bombay, has been described by Mr. Smyttan and Dr. Bird, in the early volumes of the "Transactions of the Medical and Physical Society of Calcutta."

2. There are two papers by myself in the 6th and 8th volumes of the "Calcutta Transactions," on Dracunculus in the 4th Light Dragoons, at Kirkee, published in 1833 and 1835.

3. A communication by Mr. Duncan, on Dracunculus at Bhewndy, in the 7th volume of the "Calcutta Transactions," in 1834.

4. A Report by Mr. D. Forbes, on Dracunculus at Dharwar, in 1836 and 1837, in the 1st Number of the "Transactions of the Medical and Physical Society of Bombay."

5. Note on Dracunculus in the Island of Bombay, by Mr. H. J. Carter, in the 2nd Number of the 2nd Series of the "Transactions of the Medical and Physical Society of Bombay," in 1853.

culus. , I shall briefly notice some of the statements which have been recorded, and allude to the principal inferences which have been drawn from them.

Annexed to this chapter are tabular returns of dracunculus, as observed by me in Her Majesty's 4th Light Dragoons, in the Jamsetjee Jejeebhoy Hospital, and as prevailing generally in the Bombay army in 1832 and 1833. The total number recorded in these tables amounts to 2926. The ratio of admissions from dracunculus to the total strength of the Bombay army was, for these two years, 3·055 per cent.* During the six years from 1848 to 1853 the ratio to total admissions into the Jamsetjee Jejeebhoy Hospital was 2·2 per cent. In considering these tables with the view of determining whether this affection is more prevalent in some months than in others, I have arranged the months in three groups of four each, with the following result:—

ADMISSIONS IN—

May	448	March	165	November	123
June	480	April	273	December	93
July	428	September	246	January	46
August	337	October	224	February	64
	1693		908		326

It was in the hospital of the 4th Light Dragoons at Kirkee, in 1832, that I first had an opportunity of studying this disease. The secondary trap formation of the part of the Deccan in which Kirkee is situated, suggested to me the idea of following out the opinion formed by Chisholm, from observation in Grenada, that there was a relation between dracunculus and the use of water taken from wells sunk in rocks of igneous origin. This inquiry forms the subject of my communication in the eighth volume of the Calcutta Transactions.

Through the courtesy of the Zillah collectors I obtained a series of official reports, made by the village or district native functionaries, relative to the absence or presence of Guinea-worm in the villages of the Northern and Southern Concan, and the sub-collectorate of Bagulcotta. The results have been published in the paper just adverted to, but they lead to no satisfactory conclusion, and need not be reproduced. The following extract of the general summary will suffice:—

* In 1857, there were admitted into the Hospitals of the several Police Corps in the Deccan, viz., at Poona, Sattara, and Ahmudnuggur, 1260 cases of Guinea-worm, being a ratio to the strength of 3·4 per cent. Poona was the highest,—5·7 per cent.

"1. In four talookas * Guinea-worm does not occur, and in all the upper crust is of laterite rock. The water used is not specified, but, from the physical features of the districts, it must be chiefly that of wells.

"2. There are reports from 494 villages in which Guinea-worm does not occur. Of these 364 are in a district the upper crust of which is of laterite rock: the nature of the water is not mentioned; but, from the physical features of the district, it must be chiefly that of wells. Of the remaining villages, in 109 the water of rivers of considerable size is used (of these 102 being situated in districts where primitive rocks, chiefly marble and clay-slate, constitute the geological features, and seven in secondary trap districts), and twenty-one villages use the water of nullahs, wells, and tanks.

"3. Of 991 villages in which Guinea-worm prevails, 309 are in districts of secondary trap formation; 451 in districts in which there is a probable alternation of geological structure, but in which the secondary trap formation prevails to a considerable extent; 215 are in districts in which primitive rocks prevail: in 120 limestone and clay-slate are the principal members of the series.

"4. Of the 991 villages in which Guinea-worm occurs, in 479 the nature of the water is not stated; but, from the physical features of the districts, it must be chiefly of wells. Of the remaining villages, 276 use the water of wells; 131 the water of nullahs or tanks, and 58 the water of rivers; but in a great proportion of these villages, in which nullah water or river water is used, the disease is stated to occur every second, third, or fourth year, and not annually."

The anatomy of dracunculus has been adverted to by Mr. Duncan and Mr. Forbes, but only minutely and carefully investigated and described by Mr. Carter. Mr. Duncan first called attention to the fact that the greater part of the interior of the mature Guinea-worm is occupied by an ovisac filled with myriads of minute vermiform young. This observation has been confirmed by Mr. Forbes and Mr. Carter, and all three observers describe minutely the appearance of the young Guinea-worm and the nature of its active movements.

When the period for the extrusion of the Guinea-worm from the human body has arrived, the young are emitted in large numbers from the orifice of the protruding end of the worm. Both Duncan and Forbes found that the young died in about six days when placed in water; but the latter observer noticed that when placed in moist red clay they survived for about twenty days, but did not increase in size. Mr. Duncan states, that the soil and pools about Bhewndy abound, in the rainy season, with a worm smaller and more slender, but otherwise exceedingly like the Guinea-worm: it does not, however, appear whether this resemblance refers to the mature or young dracunculus. Mr. Forbes found that in the months of August and September the tanks in the neighbourhood of Dharwar were abundantly supplied with animalcules, some of which very much resembled the young Guinea-worm, and others were eight times the size: they inhabited

* A talooka is a subdivision of a district.

the half-dry beds of the tanks, and appeared to live longest when partially covered with water.

Mr. Carter discovered that minute worms, having a great resemblance to the young dracunculus existed in great abundance in confervæ of some tanks in Bombay. He describes the size of the young Guinea-worm to be, length $\frac{1}{33}$ inch, breadth $\frac{1}{633}$; that of the tank-worm to be length $\frac{1}{54}$ inch, breadth $\frac{1}{1900}$. He believes in the identity of these animalcules, notwithstanding the fact, that the specimens taken from the ovisac were double the size of those which were born and leading an independent existence; and the additional fact, recorded by Duncan and Forbes, that the young of the Guinea-worm invariably die in the course of five or six days when placed in water. The further opinions of this able microscopic inquirer are also very improbable, viz., that Guinea-worm is produced by the small tank-worm working its way into the human body through the tubules of the sudoriferous glands, and that the spread of the affection may be best obviated by preventing those affected with it from bathing in tanks and contaminating the water with the young issuing from the protruding end of the parent entozoon; — an idea conceived in forgetfulness of the fact, that the young of the Guinea-worm die in water.

Dr. Helenus Scott remarks, "It is well known that the men who in India are employed in camps or elsewhere to carry water in leathern bags on their backs, are infested by this animal over all that part of the skin that has often been wetted."* And this statement has generally been used as an argument for the entrance of the ovum through the skin. I am ignorant of the nature of the facts on which this observation, with which I have long been familiar, is grounded; but I can affirm, after ample opportunity, and on little attention bestowed on the study of dracunculus, that I am unable to bring to my recollection a single instance of a water-carrier affected with it at that part on which the water-bag rests, nor have I any reason for supposing that they suffer more than other classes.

The manner of propagation of the Guinea-worm, its mode of entrance into the human body, and the question of its relation to an external species, are at the present moment, I believe, no more positively determined than the same propositions in respect to other entozoa. They are all, with one exception—tænia—involved in equal obscurity.

Symptoms.—The presence of Guinea-worm is often discovered by a corded substance being felt beneath the skin before any indi-

* Johnson and Martin, on Tropical Climates, 1841, p. 370.

cation from sense of itching, swelling, or the formation of a bulla has been given.

The extraction of the worm is sometimes attended with much inflammation and suppuration; at others it gives rise to little disturbance. The first result is influenced by the state of constitution of the individual affected, the situation of the worm—whether entwined round tendons or not—and the care with which the proceeding is conducted.

Both Duncan and Forbes are of opinion that the diffusion of the young of the Guinea-worm, consequent on rupture of the parent, among the human tissues, is the cause of the inflammation. It is true that this result is often consecutive on the worm being broken; but whether the explanation just adverted to is correct or not, I am unable to decide.

The presence of dracunculus, however, does not necessarily entail its extrusion: the worm may shrivel, become cretified and enveloped in areolar tissue. It is not very uncommon to find them thus changed in the dissecting-room of Grant College; and I have already detailed a case (215) in which a cretified Guinea-worm was found between the pericardium and the inner aspect of the right lung.

Treatment. — There has been a good deal written on the treatment of this affection. It has been a favourite subject for nostrums and special applications. It is best managed on simple surgical principles. The question of extraction when the worm is quiescent and felt only under the skin first arises. This practice I saw followed extensively in the 4th Dragoons. The worm was cut down upon with a lancet, and a probe passed underneath, and extraction cautiously made. The method followed by native barbers, of digging a small hole down to the worm with a needle and razor, I have also frequently witnessed. By these means extraction is often successfully and speedily effected. At other times it is followed by all the evils of inflammation and suppuration. If the worm be over a fleshy part, the operation will generally succeed. If, on the other hand, the worm be situated near tendons — as in the foot, near the ankle, or the popliteal space — the risk of injury from inflammation will be great. On the whole, as a rule of practice, I incline to non-interference.

When, after the formation of the usual bulla, the end of the worm protrudes, the extraction should be very gently and gradually effected, care being taken, by means of rest of the part and ordinary simple surgical appliances, to prevent or moderate inflammatory action. The only caution necessary in respect to water applications, is not to allow them to come in contact with the worm, lest, by softening its structures, they lead to its rupture. Should, unfortunately, much inflammation with suppuration take place, then the only safe course is to be guided by sound principles of surgery, and not to be led away by an unwise credulity in the asserted efficacy of special plasters and cataplasms, many of which are irritating and injurious.

SECTION II. — *Statistics of Guinea-Worm.*

TABLE XLIII. — *Admissions of Guinea-Worm in the 4th Light Dragoons at Kirkee.*

	1827.	1828.	1829.	1830.	1831.	1832.	1833.	1834.	Total.
January	—	—	—	1	—	—	1	—	2
February	—	—	1	—	—	1	2	1	5
March	—	—	2	5	—	5	3	2	17
April	—	—	—	5	1	7	7	6	26
May	—	3	3	2	2	57	3	31	101
June	—	3	—	1	—	64	1	29	98
July	—	2	—	3	1	48	3	20	77
August	—	—	—	1	—	26	1	13	41
September	—	—	—	—	—	3	1	7	11
October	—	—	—	—	—	—	3	3	6
November	—	—	—	—	—	1	—	1	2
December	—	—	—	—	—	3	3	—	4
Total	—	8	6	18	4	215	26	104	390

TABLE XLIV.—*Guinea-Worm in Jamsetjee Jejeebhoy Hospital.*

	1848 to 1853.		Monthly Average.		
	Admissions.	Deaths.	Deaths on Admissions.	Admissions on total Admissions.	Deaths on total Deaths.
January	18	1	5·5	0·9	0·2
February	13	—	—	0·7	—
March	22	—	—	1·02	—
April	49	—	—	2·3	—
May	71	—	—	3·2	—
June	66	1	1·5	3·1	0·3
July	82	—	—	4·06	
August	70	—	—	3·5	—
September	48	1	2·1	2·3	0·3
October	43	—	—	2·01	—
November	39	1	2·6	1·8	0·3
December	31	1	3·2	1·3	0·3
Total	552	5	0·9	2·2	1·2

TABLE XLV.—*Admissions from Dracunculus in the Bombay Army in the Year* 1832.

Presidency Division.

Stations in the different Divisions.	Bombay.	Colaba.	Severndroog.	Bombay.	Bhewndy.	Tannah.	Surat.	Broach.	Baroda.	Dapoolee.
Kind of Troops.	Europeans.			Natives.						
Average Strength.	287	878	29	2747	894	190	1004	321	1400	1761
January	0	0	0	3	0	0	0	0	1	0
February	0	2	0	2	1	0	0	0	0	0
March	2	0	0	8	0	0	3	0	2	1
April	2	0	1	20	0	2	3	1	0	1
May	2	2	0	10	3	1	2	0	3	2
June	2	2	0	14	5	0	1	0	4	0
July	2	4	0	5	6	2	4	0	1	1
August	0	4	1	8	3	0	4	0	1	0
September	0	3	0	5	3	0	3	2	6	1
October	1	4	0	4	5	1	1	3	5	1
November	0	1	0	0	1	0	1	1	4	1
December	0	0	0	4	0	0	0	2	0	4
Total	11	22	2	83	27	6	22	9	27	12

Northern Deccan Division.

Stations in the different Divisions.	Poonah.	Kirkee.	Ahmednugger.	Poonah.	Seroor.	Ahmednugger.	Malligaum.	Asseerghur.	Candeish.
Kind of Troops.	Europeans.			Natives.					
Average Strength.	1665	616	638	1605	337	1680	1611	858	327
January	0	0	0	1	0	1	2	0	0
February	0	1	0	2	0	4	3	0	0
March	0	5	0	6	2	7	8	0	0
April	5	7	0	5	2	5	10	0	0
May	6	57	2	8	6	13	6	0	0
June	2	64	0	11	2	14	8	0	0
July	0	48	1	15	1	7	4	0	0
August	0	14	0	20	0	5	9	0	0
September	0	3	0	19	0	0	1	0	2
October	0	2	0	8	1	0	4	0	0
November	0	2	1	7	0	1	4	0	0
December	0	3	0	4	0	0	2	0	0
Total	13	206	4	106	14	57	61	0	2

Southern Deccan Division.

Stations in the different Divisions.	Belgaum.	Sholapoor.	Belgaum.	Dharwar.	Kalladghee.	Sholapoor.	Sattarah.	Himgaul.	Warree.	Ram Ghaut
Kind of Troops.	Europeans.		Natives.							
Average Strength.	864	118	667	962	1592	1461	921	"	"	"
January	0	0	0	0	0	2	1	0	0	0
February	0	0	0	3	0	10	1	0	0	0
March	0	0	0	1	2	18	2	0	0	0
April	1	0	0	1	0	31	6	0	0	0
May	0	0	0	4	1	46	1	0	0	0
June	0	1	0	2	2	59	7	0	0	0
July	0	1	0	2	0	54	5	0	0	0
August	1	1	0	1	1	39	3	0	0	0
September	0	0	0	0	0	19	9	0	0	0
October	0	1	0	1	0	11	7	0	0	0
November	0	1	0	1	0	5	2	0	0	0
December	0	0	0	1	0	1	0	0	0	0
Total	2	5	0	17	6	295	44	0	0	0

North-West Division of Guzerat.

Stations in the different Divisions.	Bhooj.	Deesa.	Ahmedabad.	Kaira.	Rajcote.	Bhooj.	Total of each Month throughout the Army, 31,933.
Kind of Troops.	Europeans.	Natives.					
Average Strength.	89	139	1736	534	1771	771	
January	0	0	0	0	0	0	11
February	0	0	0	0	0	0	29
March	0	0	0	1	1	0	69
April	0	0	0	0	0	0	103
May	0	0	1	1	1	0	178
June	0	0	1	0	0	0	201
July	0	1	2	0	0	0	166
August	0	1	0	0	0	0	116
September	1	0	0	1	2	0	80
October	0	0	0	2	1	0	63
November	0	0	0	2	0	1	36
December	0	0	0	0	2	0	23
Total	1	2	4	7	7	1	1075

* For this and the following table I was indebted to the kindness of Mr. Kemball, who was at the time President of the Bombay Medical Board, and who was always ready to encourage and promote medical inquiry.

TABLE XLVI. — *Admissions from Dracunculus in the Bombay Army for the Year* 1833.

Presidency Division.

Stations in the different Divisions.	Bombay.	Colaba.	Severndrog.	Bombay.	Bhewndy.	Tannah.	Surat.	Broach.	Baroda.	Dapoolee.
Kind of Troops.	Europeans.			Natives.						
Average Strength.	878	798	19	2743	577	181	992	342	2006	1602
January	0	0	0	2	0	0	0	1	1	2
February	1	1	0	2	0	0	0	0	0	0
March	1	2	0	9	2	1	1	0	3	0
April	0	4	0	19	1	3	1	2	13	1
May	3	1	0	6	1	0	2	1	3	1
June	3	0	0	12	6	1	0	3	12	1
July	0	2	0	9	11	8	0	4	14	0
August	1	3	0	43	4	1	0	0	7	0
September	1	6	0	20	5	3	0	3	5	0
October	0	0	0	24	4	0	0	0	9	2
November	0	0	0	9	2	0	0	0	2	0
December	0	0	0	8	0	0	0	0	1	0
Total	10	19	0	163	36	17	4	14	70	7

Northern Deccan Division.

Stations in the different Divisions.	Poonah.	Kirkee.	Ahmednugger.	Poonah.	Seroor.	Ahmednugger.	Malligaum.	Asseerghur.	Candeish.
Kind of Troops.	Europeans.			Natives.					
Average Strength.	1574	669	584	1623	475	1558	1683	817	655
January	0	1	0	0	0	0	1	0	0
February	1	0	0	2	6	1	0	0	0
March	0	3	0	0	15	1	1	0	0
April	1	0	0	7	19	4	1	0	0
May	1	7	0	29	4	3	1	2	1
June	1	3	2	25	3	1	1	0	1
July	0	1	1	16	3	2	1	0	3
August	0	3	2	14	3	3	4	1	2
September	0	1	1	25	7	4	2	0	0
October	0	1	0	37	10	5	1	0	0
November	0	3	1	12	4	2	4	0	1
December	0	1	0	14	2	4	2	0	0
Total	4	24	7	181	76	30	19	3	8

Southern Deccan Division.

Stations in the different Divisions.	Belgaum.	Sholapoor.	Belgaum.	Dharwar.	Kalladghee.	Sholpor.	Sattarah.	Himgaul.	Warree.	Ram Ghaut
Kind of Troops.	Europeans.		Natives.							
Average Strength.	832	94	1135	896	895	2285	794	"	228	31
January	0	0	1	1	0	4	0	0	0	0
February	0	0	0	1	1	1	0	0	0	0
March	0	1	1	3	1	11	0	1	0	0
April	0	0	0	4	0	8	2	0	0	0
May	0	0	2	9	4	7	0	0	0	0
June	1	0	0	6	2	13	0	0	1	2
July	0	0	0	5	0	9	1	0	1	1
August	0	0	0	5	1	8	2	0	0	0
September	0	0	0	5	0	12	3	0	0	1
October	0	0	1	0	1	8	3	0	0	1
November	0	0	0	1	0	2	1	0	0	0
December	0	0	1	1	0	1	0	0	0	0
Total	1	1	6	41	10	84	12	1	2	5

North-West Division of Guzerat.

Stations in the different Divisions.	Bhooj.	Deesa.	Ahmedabad.‡	Kalra.	Rajcote.	Bhooj.	Total of each Month throughout the Army, 33,030.
Kind of Troops.	Europeans.	Natives.					
Average Strength.	80	1351	1696	530	1323	1064	
January	0	0	0	0	1	0	15
February	0	0	0	0	0	0	17
March	0	0	0	0	0	0	57
April	1	0	1	0	2	1	95
May	0	1	5	3	0	1	98
June	0	0	14	0	1	0	115
July	0	2	8	0	0	0	103
August	0	0	2	0	1	0	110
September	0	0	2	0	1	0	107
October	0	0	1	0	4	0	112
November	0	0	1	0	1	0	46
December	0	0	0	0	0	0	35
Total	1	3	34	3	11	2	909

CHAP. XXXIII.

ON THE HILL SANITARIA * OF THE DECCAN.

It will save unnecessary repetition and the risk of misapprehension if the sense in which certain terms are used is first explained: —

1. By "*Deccan Hill climate* or *station*" is meant an altitude of from 4000 to 4500 feet on the Western Ghaut range or its easterly projecting spurs, between about 20° and 15° N. latitude.
2. The term "*Deccan table land*" is restricted to that portion of it between 20° and 15° N. latitude which is within about sixty miles of the eastern side of the Western Ghauts, and has a general elevation of from 2300 to 1700 feet. It is necessary to be thus precise in indicating the sense in which the term Deccan is used in this report, because at localities more remote from the Ghauts the extremes and the range of temperature are greater at all seasons, and the atmosphere during the rainy season is drier.
3. The "*cold season*" is understood to extend from the middle of November to the end of February.
4. The "*hot season*" from the beginning of March to the middle of June.
5. The "*rainy season*" from the middle of June to the end of September.
6. October, which has been excluded from this division of the seasons, presents much of the character of the hot season months.

There are two recognised Sanitaria in the Deccan, Malcolm Pait on the Mahabuleshwur Hills, established in 1828, and the Hill Fort of Poorundhur in 1852.

Mahabuleshwur Hills. — On the medical topography and

* Written early in 1859, and communicated to the Bombay Government.

meteorology of these hills there are full and excellent reports * by Mr. Murray, published in the first, second, and seventh numbers of the Transactions of the Medical and Physical Society of Bombay, from which the following summary statement of some of the leading qualities of the climate has been compiled: —

Malcolm Pait.	Mean Temperature.	Mean Range.	Mean depression of Wet Bulb Thermometer	Rain-fall, Inches.	Direction of the Wind.
Cold Season .	64·5	13·	10·2	0·11	Easterly.
Hot Season .	72·8	13·6	13·5	1·09	NE., NNW.
Rainy Season .	64·4	3·6	2·2	243·28	WSW.
Month of October .	66·6	9·8	6·4	4·58	Variable.
† Annual Means .	66·6	9·7	7·8	254·05	

The station Malcolm Pait is situated on the western slope of the table-land in 17° 56″ N. latitude and 73° 30″ E. longitude, and has a general elevation of about 4,500 feet. The accommodation

* Mr. Murray is unquestionably still the best authority on the hill climates of India, though it is now sixteen years since he last wrote on the subject; and he will undoubtedly continue to be so, so long as the present rule of changing the medica officers in charge of hill stations every two years continues in force.

Mr. Murray was resident at Mahabuleshwur about twelve years, and thus ample opportunities were afforded for the exercise of his intelligent and enquiring mind, and for arriving at useful and safe results.

The biennial tour of duty came into operation when Mr. Murray left Mahabuleshwur in 1844, and since then at least six different medical officers have been in charge of the station, but without contributing the most fragmentary addition to our knowledge. Indeed, it is impossible to conceive a system better calculated to cramp and check inquiry than that now in force, not only at Mahabuleshwur, but, I believe, in all the hill stations in India, and this, too, with reference to sanitary questions ill understood and of great moment to the State.

On this point I write with confidence and from experience. About twenty-five years ago I was for two years in medical charge of Mahabuleshwur during Mr. Murray's absence at the Cape of Good Hope, and I left the station just as I had acquired that preliminary knowledge which further experience of the hill climate might have enabled me to mature and usefully apply. Such, I apprehend, is the process through which every medical officer in charge of a hill station on the biennial system must pass, and such the reason for the backward state of our knowledge of the meteorology and the action on the human body of the hill climates of India.

Officers should be selected with reference to their qualifications and tastes for the kind of investigation required, and should be left in charge so long as their efficiency and zeal remain unimpaired. The principle, that it is just to extend the benefit of the hill climates to a number of officers, and to effect this by biennial removal, is very considerate; but it is not one by which scientific objects are likely to be advanced, and this is the paramount end which should be kept in view in medical appointments at hill stations in India.

† As the month of November has been excluded from the summary, the annual means here given, taken from the original tables, will be found to differ slightly from the means calculated from the sums of the columns of the summary.

at present consists of Government quarters for sixteen sick officers, and seventy-seven private bungalows. In the year 1829 a party of invalid soldiers was sent to this Sanitarium, but the selection of cases and of the season was unsuitable. The result was unfavourable, and the experiment has not been repeated. Since that period, however, the annual resort of an average of about 300 visitors—civilians, military officers, and others, with their families—has afforded ample opportunity of determining the qualities of this hill climate and its influence on the European constitution in health and disease.

Poorundhur.—The hill on which the Fort of Poorundhur is placed is an offshoot from the easterly side of the Western Ghaut range. It is situated in 18° 22″ N. latitude and 73° 54″ E. longitude, and is distant nineteen miles from Poona. It is a saddle-backed mountain. The altitude of the highest part of the ridge is 4570 feet, but that of the lower fort, in which the Sanitarium is located, is 4200 feet. The lower fort occupies a narrow table about a mile in length, projecting from the northern slope of the mountain. There are two barrack rooms, which afford accommodation for one hundred men, and a very good hospital, adapted for forty sick. There are ten private bungalows, generally occupied in the hot season by officers and their families. A patchery for ten families and a small female hospital are in course of erection. The Sanitarium may, therefore, at present, be considered sufficient for 130 soldiers and ten families. A good foot-road has been carried round the hill on the level of the Sanitarium, as well as round Wuzurghur, an adjoining hill connected at the same level by a narrow ridge to Poorundhur. This foot-road is about seven miles in extent, and in consequence of its circular character, its position 230 feet below the highest ridge, and the general form and direction of the mountain, there is space for exercise shaded from the sun till nine or ten in the morning. The *climate* of Poorundhur compared with that of Malcolm Pait has a temperature about three degrees higher, and, in consequence of its more inland position, there is greater atmospheric dryness in the months of March, April, and May. The great difference, however, is in the rainy season: at Poorundhur the rain-fall is seventy-two inches; at Malcolm Pait it is 254. The rain and fog are so incessant at Malcolm Pait that the station is uninhabitable during the rainy season. The Hill of Poorundhur is also frequently enveloped in mist, and though the convalescents remaining there at this season have in general benefited, yet the climate is gloomy, and out-door exercise is often prevented by rain and dense fog. About 650 sick and convalescents have been received into the Poorundhur Sanitarium since its establishment. The greater number have belonged to regiments stationed in the Deccan. A proportion, however, has been sent from Bombay, Guzerat, and Scind. The selection of cases and of season has been sometimes suitable, at other times the reverse. It is this mixed experience, both at Poorundhur and Mahabuleshwur, not again we may hope likely to occur, which has created data from which the medical inquirer is enabled to ascertain with confidence the right sanitary use of these hill climates.

Panchgunnee. —Malcolm Pait is rendered uninhabitable from the middle of June to the end of September by incessant rain and fog, consequent on its position on the western side of the mountain; but it is to this position also that are due a greater coolness and softness of the climate in March, April, and May. There are localities on the eastern side of Mahabuleshwur which possess a climate nearly resembling that of Poorundhur, in which the temperature is about three degrees higher than that of Malcolm Pait, the fog less constant during the rainy season, and the rain-fall about fifty inches. Panchgunnee, distant ten miles from Malcolm Pait, overlooking the valley of Wye, at an elevation of 4000 feet, is the locality on the eastern side of which the character of the climate is best known. Notes on the monsoon climate of Panchgunnee were published by me in the year 1840.*

Singhur, &c. — The Hill Fort of Singhur, distant fourteen miles from Poona, is placed on a table about 4200 feet above the sea. It has an irregular surface, with a circuit of about a mile and a quarter. There are fifteen private bungalows, usually rented during the hot season by officers and their families from the Poona and Kirkee Brigade. The climate of Singhur cannot differ much from that of Poorundhur.

Between the river Taptee on the north and the fifteenth degree of north latitude on the south, there are probably many situations more or less spacious on the easterly side of the Western Ghaut range, or on the spurs projecting inland from it, with an elevation from 4000 to 4500 feet, which present the same characteristics of climate in the dry and rainy seasons as Panchgunnee, Poorundhur, and Singhur. But it must be borne in mind, for reasons which will presently appear, that the hot-season climates of such localities are two or three degrees warmer and are drier than Malcolm Pait and other similar positions on the western or seaward side of the Ghauts.

* "Transactions, Medical and Physical Society of Bombay," No. 3.

The conclusion to which these several statements lead is, that the soldier in this Presidency has not as yet derived much benefit from the Deccan Hill climates; and the practical question which has now to be determined is, by what system this benefit, if real and important, may be extended.

The practice hitherto has been to select from among the sick and convalescents in Hospital those men who are not regaining health, or are progressing slowly to recovery. But the climate of these Hills is by no means suited at any season for all cases which come under this description, and at some seasons is unsuitable for them all. It is therefore of the utmost importance that medical officers on arrival in India should early familiarise themselves with the principles relative to the sanitary application of the Deccan Hill climates which past experience has enabled us to advance with tolerable certainty. With the view of facilitating this necessary preliminary object, a memorandum * was prepared by me in May, 1858, when Superintending Surgeon of the Poona Division, relative to the Poorundhur Sanitarium, and the doctrines inculcated in it may be regarded as equally applicable to other Hill stations of similar altitude and climate. It will be sufficient to state here as the general result of past experience, that the debilitated soldier, who in the plains of the Deccan, the Concan, Bombay, and Gujerat regains his strength and efficiency slowly, will after the removal of positive disease be much benefited by a Deccan Hill climate in the month of October and in the hot season; and at those Hill stations (as Poorundhur) in which the rain-fall is not more than seventy inches, and the mists, though frequent, by no means continuous, there will be still further advantage to many of this class of convalescents by—after a hot-season residence—their stay being prolonged throughout the rainy season and the month of October. The benefit which may be looked for is this:—The soldier will have become fitted for duty, he will be less liable to fresh attacks of disease, and when attacked the disease will be of milder type. Whereas had he continued exposed to the exhausting hot season of the Deccan or of the coast, he would have remained inefficient, and have become very predisposed to attacks of the severer forms of tropical disease—those forms which swell the mortality and invaliding rates of European troops in India. The ultimate effect of these Hill Sanitaria applied as now explained must be, in proportion to the degree in which they are used, to reduce mortality and invaliding.

* See Appendix.

But a large proportion of the class of convalescents just adverted to, if sent to the Hills in the *cold* or *rainy* seasons, would run the risk of being injured by the return of their former diseases or by the access of others of similar character. It is therefore necessary that caution and judgment should be exercised, not only in the selection of the cases, but also in determining the season. There are cases of imperfect recovery from some forms of organic disease which, if the opportunity of a sea voyage and change to colder latitudes is not available, may be sent to the hills in the hot season, if the facilities of carriage are good, with temporary advantage from avoiding the heat of the plains. But for all cases of imperfect recovery from all forms of organic visceral disease the cold and rainy seasons of the Hills are altogether unsuited, and are generally positively and markedly injurious. The evils which result from the neglect of this now well-ascertained truth were apparent at Mahabuleshwur in the experiment of 1829. They have occurred also from time to time at Poorundhur, and have been very frequently observed at the Neilgherry and Himalayan Hill Sanitaria.

The superiority of the Deccan Hill climate is in the month of October, and from March to early in June.

The Deccan *table-land* has, during the cold season, a mean temperature of 70°, and a range of 25°. Its climate at this season exercises no injurious influence on the European constitution, and is less likely to be prejudicial in the conditions described above than the climate of the Hills at the same period of the year.

The Deccan table-land has, in the rainy season, a mean temperature of 73·70°, a range of 14·6°, and a rain-fall from about 30 to 20 inches. The climate is genial and refreshing. Though the lower temperature of Poorundhur (67·3°) at the same season is an advantage to some convalescents, still in others it is counterbalanced by the gloom and confinement to quarters consequent on the frequent fog and rain. It may therefore, under existing data, be concluded that the Hill climate in the rainy season has no advantage over that of the table-land in the neighbourhood of the Ghaut range.

In the hot season the mean temperature of the Deccan table-land is about 80°, the range 25°, the dryness 22·5°, and a hot wind blows throughout a considerable part of the day. At this season the European constitution is apt to suffer from the influence of elevated temperature, and to become more or less debilitated; and convalescence from all forms of disease is tardy and unsatisfactory.

In the 9th Number of the Transactions of the Medical and Physical Society of Bombay there is a paper by Mr. Murray on the climate and diseases of Sattara. It contains much valuable information on the meteorology and general characters of the different seasons in the Deccan, and may be consulted with much advantage with reference to the subject under consideration.

In Bombay the mean temperature of the hot season is 82°, and the range 11°. The mean temperature of the rainy season is 80·8°, and the range 6·2°; the rain-fall is 75 inches; and the atmosphere from the middle of June to the end of September is humid, and often not far from the point of saturation. The hot and the rainy seasons in Bombay are exhausting to the European, and a similar remark may be applied to the same seasons on the Western Coast generally, and the low southern portion of the province of Guzerat.

It appears, then, that the hot season of the Deccan table-land and the hot and rainy seasons of Bombay, the Coast, and Guzerat are inimical to Europeans, the degree being in proportion to the previous state of debility of those who are exposed to their influence.

The value of the Deccan Hill Sanitaria is restricted to the hot season. The weakly soldier of the Deccan stations with the cold and rainy season on the table-land, and the month of October and the hot season at a Hill station, has every advantage which the climate of this part of India is capable of affording. The weakly soldier of the Coast and Guzerat stations with the cold season of his own locality and the rainy season of the Deccan table-land and the month of October and the hot season at a Hill station, has also every benefit from climate which his circumstances admit of.

Hitherto the improvement to health which results from a judicious use of the climates at our command has, in the instance of the soldier, been confined to the small number of hospital cases for which a change to Poorundhur has been considered suitable. In order to extend the advantage, a modification of system would seem to be all that is necessary. In *addition* to the hospital cases a percentage of the men in barracks and of their families, say of the former from 10 to 25 per cent. (varying according to the necessities of service), should be selected at Deccan, Coast, and Guzerat stations. The selection should be made by the medical officer with reference to constitution, medical history, and service in India. The men thus selected should leave their stations towards the end of February, so as to reach the Hills at the beginning of March. The Deccan soldiers should return to their stations in the first week of June, if within the salubrious limit, but if belonging to more inland stations, they with those of the Coast and Guzerat should be sent to a well-selected Deccan table-land Sanitarium; and all should return to the Hills in the first week of October, remain there till the middle of November, and then proceed to rejoin their respective stations for duty, so as to reach them early in December.

In this view the Hill stations are regarded merely as hot season Sanitaria, and the establishments and arrangements should be organised with reference to this limited object. For the Sanitarium of the rainy season a suitable locality on the Deccan table-land would require to be selected.

By this system the Deccan soldier, whether in hospital or at duty, would have the advantage every fourth or fifth year of a hot season on the Hills; and the Coast and Guzerat soldier of a hot season on the Hills and a rainy season on the table-land. It may be confidently anticipated that a sanitary measure of this scope and nature, in connection with a never-failing attention, under all circumstances, to barrack accommodation and the various other matters of detail which relate to the health and welfare of the soldier, would in a few years have a marked effect in reducing the proportion of sick, of mortality, and of invaliding. It cannot be too often repeated that, by maintaining the general health of troops at as high a standard as the conditions of service in a tropical climate permit, not only is present efficiency increased, but the predisposition to disease, and particularly to disease of bad type, may be so diminished as most materially to reduce mortality and invaliding. To what degree this advantage may ultimately be found to reach, future experience must determine; but there can be no doubt that the principles are true, and that a sanitary system founded on their strict observance, and faithfully and judiciously followed for a series of years, must prove of very great advantage to the European soldier in India, and consequently to the State.

The method now proposed of applying the Hill and Deccan climates for the preservation and improvement of the health of the soldier rests on no new or untried doctrines. The proposition merely aims at extending to the soldier, and to the families of soldiers, a system which has for the last thirty years been successfully followed by civilians and officers and their families; and which by them has been found to include all the benefit which these climates are capable of conferring.

It now remains to state briefly the means by which these views may be, under existing circumstances, most readily reduced to practice. The Sanitarium at Poorundhur should be continued on its present scale and plan for the reception of convalescents on sick certificate from regiments in the Deccan. It should be continued as now during the rainy season, so as to admit of further observation of the effects of this season, and of careful comparison of the results with those of the hospital cases from the Coast and Guzerat, whom, as will presently appear, it is proposed to locate on the Deccan table-land during the rains. Though there can bè little doubt that the monsoon climate of the Deccan table-land is on the whole preferable to that of Poorundhur, still it is very expedient to take advantage of the already organised establishment at this Sanitarium for prosecuting the enquiry further, and finally settling the question to the satisfaction of those who may still entertain doubts on the subject. Poorundhur does not admit of extension as a Sanitarium for *all* seasons, but a *hot* season site may be found on Fitzclarence Point. Considering, however, the limited space on the mountain, even this extension is inexpedient as a permanent arrangement.

For the men selected from barracks from all stations, whether in the Deccan or elsewhere, and for the hospital cases from Bombay, the Coast, Guzerat, and Scinde, a hot season Sanitarium should be established on the Mahabuleshwur Hills in the proximity of Malcolm Pait. The Deccan soldiers should return to their stations at the beginning of June, and those from elsewhere should be moved to Sattara for the rains, return to Mahabuleshwur in October, and thence proceed to their respective stations in the latter half of November.

Should it on further experience at Poorundhur, and on comparison with the results at Sattara, appear that there is greater advantage from the monsoon residence on the Hills than existing data seem to suggest, then instead of moving the Coast and Guzerat and Scinde soldiers to Sattara for the rains, let monsoon barracks and a suitable hospital be built at Panchgunnee, which would thus become the rainy season position of the military Sanitarium on the Mahabuleshwur Hills. There would in this arrangement be merely the cost of original erection. The establishment of the hot season would be available for the rains, whether passed at Sattara or at Panchgunnee. As the barracks at Panchgunnee would not be required for men belonging to Deccan stations, they would necessarily be on a smaller scale than those at Malcolm Pait. Considering the proximity of Bombay, Poona, and Sattara to Malcolm Pait the many advantages possessed by the western side of the mountain, and the fact that a well-proved Sanitarium has long existed there, and assuming that the views expressed in this report on the true use of these Hill stations are accepted as just, then there need be no delay in erecting barracks at Malcolm Pait. For should it afterwards be proved that there are advantages in a residence during the rains at such positions as Panchgunnee, which it is desirable to secure, no unnecessary outlay will have been incurred in erecting barracks at Malcolm Pait, for it must be always remembered that the western side of the mountain has advantages in the hot season over the eastern side, which it would be unwise to throw away; and as respects the cost incurred at Sattara in carrying out the measures suggested for immediate adoption, it cannot under any circumstances be lost, for there is little risk of barrack accommodation proving excessive at a station healthy like Sattara, and otherwise not unimportant.

Should, however, the distance to Mahabuleshwur be found inconvenient to regiments in the southern Mahratta country or in Kandeish, or, after the railway lines are completed, to those in Central India, then other Hill stations may be sought for, north and south of Mahabuleshwur, in the Ghaut range itself, or on the spurs that project inland from its easterly side; it being borne in mind that if the Sanitarium is for the hot season alone, a westerly position is very important, but that if the rainy season is to be included, then a station on the eastern side of the Ghauts, or more inland on the projecting spurs, must be selected, and the full advantages of the Deccan Hills in the hot season be in some measure sacrificed.

Though the sanitary advantages to be derived from the Deccan Hill climates, and the means by which they may be effected, have now been considered, there yet remains an important question to discuss with reference to the full benefit attainable from change of climate within the limits of the Bombay Presidency.

It has been argued in this report that the chief use of these Hill Sanitaria is confined to the hot season, and to the acceleration of convalescence from disease that has been removed, or of recovery from disease which is merely functional; but that for individuals affected with chronic organic disease benefit from the hot season at a Hill station is only occasional, and at other seasons in such cases the climate is generally positively injurious. It is from organic visceral disease, primary, or complicating or consecutive on the various types of fever, that the greater part of ordinary mortality in India results. It is from these same forms of disease, after they have passed into a chronic state, and also from chronic rheumatic affections, that the great proportion of invaliding in India proceeds. The climate of the Hills in the cold and rainy seasons is injurious in all these forms of disease, and the climate of the Deccan table-land in the cold season is also often unsuitable. It is therefore important to inquire whether in such cases, stationary or retrograding in the cold season in the Deccan, there is any prospect of advantage from change of climate, short of a voyage to sea and return to colder latitudes. It may be with confidence replied that the climate of the coast, about the latitude of Bombay, from the middle of November to the end of February, with a temperature of 74·8°, and range of 14°, and without the atmospheric dryness of the inland upland stations, affords this advantage.

A cold season Sanitarium suitably placed on the coast, and accessible with little fatigue, would be frequently of much utility in the management of cases of organic disease which are retrograding or stationary or slowly convalescing in Deccan hospitals in the cold season. They would recover more rapidly, and become more surely fitted for transference to a Hill station in the hot season, and, in some cases, life might be saved, and invaliding prevented. A sea-coast Sanitarium, then, on a small scale, may be regarded as an important part of the sanitary system of this Presidency. But in order to the safe application of the principle on which its utility rests, it will be very necessary that medical officers, on arrival in India, should early become well acquainted with the state and stages of disease for which it is appropriate, and that the locality be selected with reference to accessibility, facility, and comfort of transport.

On the subject of a coast Sanitarium it may be useful to remark that, under the improved state of general health which will accrue to the soldier in India from an improved sanitary system, including the avoidance in the hot season of the heat of the plains by resort to Hill stations, the proportion and severity of visceral organic disease and of rheumatic affections will, after a time, become so diminished that gradually the necessity for change to the sea-coast will be lessened. This result may be expected for the same reasons that it is anticipated that mortality and invaliding will, by these same means, become very materially reduced.

Though this report has reference to the Deccan, and to troops for which the Deccan Hill Sanitaria are available, still it may not be altogether inappropriate briefly to allude to other Hill climates and troops in other parts of India.*

* For information on the Hill stations of the sub-Himalayan range, the reader is referred to the first, second, and fourth volumes of the "Indian Annals of Medical

The general principles which have been advanced are applicable to all localities and to all European troops in India, for they tend to one leading practical object, viz. the maintenance of the greatest degree of health and efficiency for the ordinary contingencies of service in a tropical country. This end is to be attained by avoiding, as much as possible, unhealthy localities and seasons, such as localities with malarious characteristics, the hot season all over India, and the rainy season in many parts of it.

The advantages which are, in some measure, peculiar to the Bombay Presidency are :—

1. Hill stations which, from elevation (4000 to 4700 feet), proximity to the sea, and safe approach at all seasons, afford a cool retreat from the heat of the plains in the hot season, without the risk of injury from cold and wet.
2. A considerable extent of country on the Deccan table-land possessing in the rainy season a climate salubrious and refreshing.
3. Facilities for the establishment of Sanitaria on the sea-coast in suitable latitudes.

Whereas the sub-Himalayan Hill stations, with elevations from 4200 to 7400 feet, are of unsafe approach at some seasons, and present, in greater degree than Mahabuleshwur and Poorundhur, the disadvantages of the cold and rainy seasons; while during the hot season, owing to distance from the sea and other causes, their climates are not so temperate, equable, and dry. Thus the unfavourable hot and rainy seasons of the adjoining plains are ill provided against by these Sanitaria. There is no healthy monsoon climate, and no facility of access to a suitable sea-coast.

The approach to the Neilgherries is, at some seasons, unsafe, but there are stations at different elevations and on different sides of the mountain, which, with the Mysore table-land and a sea-coast, though of low latitude, give to the Madras Presidency in considerable degree the advantages stated to appertain chiefly to that of Bombay.

The problem which has been kept in view in preparing these observations has been, how to fit the European soldier for the

Science," also to the eleventh number of the same work, in which the subject is treated fully in Mr. Chever's elaborate paper, "On the means of preserving the health of the European soldier in India."

Mr. M'Clelland's "Medical Topography of Bengal" contains very useful information on Hill climates and allied subjects.

The climate of Mount Aboo on the Aravalli range is described in the third number, new series, "Transactions, Medical Society of Bombay," by Dr. Lownds.

maximum of efficient service in India with the minimum sacrifice of health and of life. The attempt has not been made to inquire by what means he may attain to the full physical constitutional vigour of his native land and of the other countries of the colder latitudes of the globe—simply because this condition is incompatible with the circumstances in which he is placed. The question has at different times been proposed, whether a regiment fresh from Europe located at an elevation of 7300 feet, and in a climate such as that of Ootacamund on the Neilgherry Hills, would not retain much of its European vigour. Doubtless it would, a deduction, however, being made on account of the rarefied atmosphere. But this regiment would not be efficient for the contingencies of service in India. If suddenly called to the plains for service in the hot season, it would soon show a heavy sick list, and a rapid loss of vigour and stamina would ensue. Let us suppose the service to be concluded, and the regiment, exhausted by heat and fatigue and sickness, moved back to Ootacamund, and the result would be much mortality and invaliding from congestive, inflammatory, and organic visceral disease. The proof that this is no fancied picture will be readily found in what takes place under the ordinary circumstances of troops fresh from Europe arriving at the commencement of the hot season; and in what has taken place between the years 1840 and 1850 on the transference to the Himalayan Hill stations of several European regiments weakened by service, climate, and disease.

There is no antagonism between the Hill climates of India and a voyage to sea, followed by a residence in the higher latitudes. The states of disease for which the latter is required are usually unsuited for the former. The Hill climates can never be regarded as a substitute for a voyage to Europe or to Tasmania, but their judicious use will render the greater change less frequently necessary, will improve the general health, minister to the comfort and happiness, and increase the efficiency of the European soldier in India.

APPENDIX.

A.

Notes and Tables on the Meteorology of Bombay.

(Prepared by T. M. Lownds, Esq., M.D., Assistant Surgeon, Bombay Establishment.)

These tables * of the meteorology of Bombay, for the six years from 1847 to 1852, have been compiled from the Colaba Observatory Reports, from the published reports for four years; and for 1851-52, I am indebted to Dr. Leith, to whom the daily observations are furnished from Colaba.

Temperature. — *The monthly mean* is calculated from the daily observations taken each hour in the twenty-four. A very cursory examination will show how slight are the differences in one year from the mean of six as recorded. The greatest differences from the mean of six years are only as follows, the greatest difference in any of six months being taken: —

Thus, of six months of			January, greatest difference from mean is			+ 2·1°
"	"	"	February	"	"	− 1·4
"	"	"	March	"	"	+ 0·7
"	"	"	April	"	"	+ 0·7
"	"	"	May	"	"	+ 1·5
"	"	"	June	"	"	+ 1·6
"	"	"	July	"	"	+ 1·1
"	"	"	August	"	"	+ 0·8
"	"	"	September	"	"	− 1·3
"	"	"	October	"	"	+ 1·2
"	"	"	November	"	"	+ 3·3
"	"	"	December	"	"	+ 0·9

January is the coldest month of the year, December and February almost the same, as also November and March; October forms a mean between March and April. April and May are the hottest months. The monsoon months vary little in mean temperature, and, as might be expected, the range in them is very small. The great difference between hot and cold months is not so much in greater temperature during day, but in cool nights, and hence the range forms a distinguishing character between the

* These tables and memorandum, kindly prepared, at my request, with much care, are published in the form in which they were communicated by their zealous and able author.

hot and cold season; of course the range being much greater during the cold than in the hot months. A considerable degree of correspondence will be found relatively between the mean daily and monthly range, and the range of the Wet-bulb Thermometer. The extremes call for no remark.

The daily temperature is at its minimum at sunrise, almost without exception. It then rises rapidly for the first two or three hours, until 9 A.M., when it rises slowly, and attains its maximum at noon; occasionally at 11, or even 10 A.M., but this is rare; still more rarely it is delayed till 1, or even 2 P.M., declines slowly till 5 P.M., or sunset, when it again takes a stride or two rapidly downwards till about 7 P.M., when it continues slowly declining till sunrise. The mean daily monthly variation is well represented in the table. The daily variation is sometimes very great, as much as from 20° to 23°, but this is comparatively rare, and only occurs in cold months. In the monsoon, on the contrary, the range is very slight.

WET-BULB THERMOMETER. — I have preferred giving the temperature of wet-bulb, to the calculated dew-point, as some difference of opinion exists about the proper calculation. It will be seen that the temperature of wet-bulb does not differ much from year to year, and that the range in each month corresponds pretty closely. The mean temperature of *humidity* represents the point of saturation. Full saturation is supposed to be unity. This enables us to compare the atmospheric moisture pretty exactly. It does not vary much.

BAROMETER. — Of the barometer I have only given the mean height for each month, and this may be said to be almost without variation in the series of years. It descends with great regularity from its highest in January to its lowest in June, and the height varies little during the monsoon. The average range of the barometer during the whole year is very slight, 0·110 inch, or 0·112 inch, representing it. The extreme range is highest in the cold months, occasionally the daily variation is as much as 0·2 inch, or a little more. The variation is least in the monsoon months.

RAIN FALL. — The rain table is given so fully, that it seems unnecessary to add anything to it.

The *evaporation* in Bombay is excessive, and by the accounts published, almost equals the average fall of rain. (Vide tables for 1849 = 72 inches.

DIRECTION AND FORCE OF WINDS. — The wind usually sweeps round the horizon every day, blowing, as the tables quoted show, chiefly from the sea, and with a force usually of about half a pound, for an hour or two daily, generally less. In the monsoon, the force is greatly increased, and reaches as high as 8 or 10 lbs. The account of the wind must only be taken as approximative, as often there is not wind enough to move a feather.

I have not said anything of particular variations, as I conceive the purpose of the table to be, to give a correct idea of the general climate of Bombay, and such as may easily be referred to for practical purposes. For minute investigation, the Observatory Reports are most admirable.

I. *Observations on the Temperature at Bombay.*

	MEAN TEMPERATURES.							EXTREMES.												MEAN DAILY RANGE.					
	1847.	1848.	1849.	1850.	1851.	1852.	Six Years' General Average.	1847.		1848.		1849.		1850.		1851.		1852.		1847.	1848.	1849.	1850.	1852.	Average of Five Years.
								Maximum.	Minimum.	Maximum.	Minimum.	Maximum.	Minimum.	Maximum.	Minimum.	Maximum.	Minimum.	Maximum.	Minimum.						
January . .	75·2	75·5	73·3	72·4	72·2	71·9	73·4	90·5	61·0	86·5	65·0	88·2	58·5	86·5	64·4	90·0	57·3	89·6	57·4	15·4	16·2	13·3	13·3	16·0	14·8
February .	73·7	75·1	75·8	75·1	75·5	75·8	75·1	89·5	53·3	91·1	57·0	92·6	67·0	95·5	60·0	93·3	63·5	88·2	63·0	12·4	14·3	12·1	16·3	14·8	14·0
March . . .	79·4	75·7	79·2	79·3	79·8	80·1	79·4	93·0	70·5	98·0	67·0	94·0	69·7	92·5	68·5	91·4	70·0	95·0	69·0	11·0	12·4	11·7	11·7	14·1	12·2
April. . . .	82·1	83·1	82·1	82·0	83·3	83·1	82·6	94·2	73·6	92·7	69·3	91·0	72·4	97·0	-	92·6	75·3	92·5	71·2	10·1	10·2	11·0	10·3	13·2	10·9
May	83·9	84·6	85·2	84·4	84·7	86·3	84·8	91·6	75·7	94·5	-	93·0	76·8	-	-	93·0	77·5	94·2	77·3	9·1	9·7	9·3	9·5	11·8	9·9
June . . .	81·0	81·5	81·3	83·8	82·5	83·9	82·3	89·0	72·5	90·1	75·6	91·0	74·4	-	-	91·7	74·0	95·5	76·0	4·2	5·8	5·3	7·4	9·3	6·4
July	80·4	81·1	80·1	81·7	80·1	82·0	80·9	-	-	90·5	74·0	88·0	73·5	-	-	90·4	74·5	89·5	76·3	4·6	4·9	4·8	5·1	7·5	5·4
August . . .	79·8	80·2	80·1	81·0	79·9	80·4	80·2	-	-	85·8	73·0	87·0	75·0	-	-	88·0	74·5	88·0	75·6	5·7	4·4	5·0	6·3	7·2	5·7
September .	78·9	81·0	78·8	80·7	80·4	80·6	80·1	-	70·5	87·6	73·3	85·5	75·6	95·7	-	88·5	72·8	88·4	75·4	7·0	8·3	4·4	7·3	8·0	6·6
October . .	82·1	80·9	81·2	83·0	81·5	82·2	81·8	93·5	73·9	88·7	73·2	95·0	71·5	95·7	76·2	89·6	71·0	92·0	74·2	10·9	10·0	10·3	10·4	11·1	10·5
November .	75·9	79·3	81·3	79·3	79·5	80·2	79·2	87·6	62·7	93·2	67·8	96·5	75·5	91·5	67·6	93·0	68·4	91·2	70·8	14·0	13·7	13·2	14·4	15·2	14·1
December .	75·7	76·6	76·5	75·8	75·0	75·7	75·9	91·2	65·5	90·5	61·7	94·0	68·3	90·5	67·0	89·5	66·0	91·6	66·0	14·4	13·2	14·2	13·2	12·9	13·6
Annual. . .	79·0	79·8	79·6	79·9	79·5	80·2	79·6	-	-	-	-	-	-	-	-	-	-	-	-	9·4	10·4	9·5	10·4	11·7	10·3

II. *Observations with the Wet Bulb Thermometer, at Bombay.*

	WET BULBS.											HUMIDITY.						
	MEAN TEMPERATURE.					Average of Five Years.	DAILY RANGE.				Mean of Four Years.	1847.	1848.	1849.	1850.	1851.	1852.	Average of Six Years.
	1847.	1848.	1849.	1850.	1851.		1847.	1848.	1849.	1850.		Mean.	Mean.	Mean.	Mean.	Mean.	Mean.	
January .	68·8	69·2	66·8	65·8	65·3	67·2	7·1	7·1	6·6	7·0	6·9	0·90	0·90	0·89	0·88	0·87	0·84	0·88
February	67·3	68·6	69·9	67·7	69·1	68·5	6·8	7·4	5·4	6·5	6·5	0·89	0·89	0·91	0·88	0·90	0·89	0·89
March .	73·7	72·6	72·8	72·7	73·4	73·0	5·3	5·4	5·2	5·5	5·3	0·90	0·91	0·91	0·91	0·91	0·89	0·90
April .	76·4	77·4	75·7	75·1	76·9	76·3	4·1	3·4	4·3	3·5	3·8	0·93	0·93	0·92	0·91	0·92	0·91	0·92
May .	78·5	78·5	78·0	78·4	77·8	78·2	3·5	3·5	3·5	3·9	3·6	0·94	0·93	0·92	0·93	0·92	0·90	0·92
June .	78·7	78·4	79·6	79·6	78·9	79·0	2·1	2·8	3·3	3·8	3·0	0·97	0·96	0·98	0·96	0·96	0·95	0·96
July .	77·9	78·1	78·0	78·9	77·9	79·2	3·4	2·5	2·6	3·5	3·0	0·97	0·97	0·98	0·97	0·98	0·96	0·97
August .	77·2	77·0	77·4	77·6	77·3	77·3	3·0	2·9	2·5	3·7	3·0	0·97	0·96	0·97	0·96	0·97	0·96	0·97
September	76·1	77·0	76·6	76·7	75·8	76·5	3·1	3·4	2·8	3·5	3·2	0·96	0·95	0·97	0·95	0·94	0·96	0·96
October .	77·8	78·0	76·8	78·1	77·0	77·5	4·1	4·8	3·4	3·9	4·1	0·95	0·96	0·95	0·94	0·94	0·94	0·95
November	70·8	72·9	75·5	71·8	72·9	72·8	5·3	4·8	3·6	5·4	4·8	0·92	0·91	0·92	0·89	0·91	0·88	0·91
December	69·1	70·5	68·3	69·5	67·5	69·0	6·4	5·7	5·0	5·4	5·6	0·90	0·91	0·87	0·90	0·88	0·89	0·89
Annual .	74·4	74·8	74·6	74·3	75·8	74·4	4·5	4·5	4·0	4·6	4·4	0·93	0·93	0·93	0·92	0·92	0·91	0·92

III. *Barometric Observations at Bombay.*

	BAROMETER.						
	1847.	1848.	1849.	1850.	1851.	1852.	
	Mean.	Mean.	Mean.	Mean.	Mean.	Mean.	Mean Average of Six Years.
January	29·917	29·927	29·958	29·891	29·958	29·929	29·930
February	29·903	29·916	29·919	29·939	29·901	29·903	29·914
March	29·872	29·830	29·880	29·898	29·857	29·829	29·861
April	29·791	29·770	29·792	29·830	29·779	29·794	29·793
May	29·722	29·741	29·727	29·776	29·740	29·746	29·742
June	29·621	29·649	29·637	29·652	29·631	29·630	29·637
July	29·651	29·654	29·686	29·656	29·598	29·660	29·650
August	29·707	29·706	29·713	29·750	29·697	29·731	29·717
September	29·748	29·812	29·741	29·800	29·783	29·756	29·773
October	29·825	29·826	29·853	29·799	29·828	29·856	29·831
November	29·892	29·909	29·902	29·905	29·838	29·905	29·892
December	29·897	29·821	29·923	29·962	29·946	29·923	29·912
Annual	29·796	29·805	29·811	29·821	29·805	29·805	29·806

IV.—*Observations on the Rain Fall and the Direction and Force of the Winds at Bombay.*

	RAIN.												Average of Six Years.		Comparison of Average of Six Years of Mean Temperature, with Wet Bulb.		1851. Wind.		1852. Wind.	
	1847.		1848.		1849.		1850.		1851.		1852.									
	Inches.	Number of Rainy Days.	Inches.	Number of Rainy Days.	Inches.	Number of Rainy Days.	Inches.	Number of Rainy Days.	Inches.	Number of Rainy Days.	Inches.	Number of Rainy Days.	Inches.	Number of Rainy Days.	Dry.	Wet.	From Sea. Hours.	From Land. Hours.	From Sea. Hours.	From Land. Hours.
January .	0·22	1	-	-	0·30	2	-	-	-	-	-	-	-	-	73·4	67·2	15	9	17	7
February	0·02	1	-	-	-	-	-	-	-	-	-	-	-	-	75·1	68·5	19	5	19	5
March .	-	-	-	-	-	-	-	-	0·04	1	0·01	1	-	-	79·4	73·0	22	2	19	5
April .	0·27	1	0·58	2	-	-	-	-	-	-	-	-	-	-	82·6	76·3	22	2	22	2
May .	1·13	6	4·27	7	-	-	-	-	0·52	4	0·30	2	-	-	84·8	78·2	21	3	23	1
June .	36·52	29	40·76	21	23·17	27	12·62	23	24·50	20	21·76	22	-	-	82·3	79·0	22	2	20	4
July .	15·99	29	14·61	25	48·14	26	19·22	30	47·02	26	22·17	23	-	-	80·9	79·2	23	1	24	-
August .	8·29	30	7·07	25	12·13	21	4·71	22	20·01	25	11·15	26	-	-	80·2	77·3	23	1	24	-
September	5·21	19	2·50	6	27·77	20	4·83	20	3·89	12	12·69	20	-	-	80·1	76·5	22	2	22	2
October .	0·29	1	5·39	6	0·80	3	4·29	8	0·04	2	0·17	1	-	-	81·8	77·5	20	4	18	6
November	5·71	5	0·19	2	0·61	2	0·22	1	0·07	1	-	-	-	-	79·2	72·8	16	8	11	13
December	-	-	-	-	-	-	-	-	-	-	1·01	4	-	-	75·9	69·0	15	9	12	12
Annual .	73·65	122	75·37	94	111·39	101	45·89	104	96·09	91	69·26	99	78·61	102	79·6	74·4				

B.

MEMORANDUM ON THE SANITARIUM AT POORUNDHUR, 19 MILES DISTANT FROM POONA, LATITUDE N. 18·12, LONGITUDE E. 73·54, ALTITUDE 4200 FEET.—ESTABLISHED IN 1852.

1. TABLE *showing the Atmospheric Pressure, the Temperature, the Dryness, the Rain-fall, and the Direction of the Winds at Poorundhur.*

	Barometer.	Thermometer.			Dryness, Difference between Dry and Wet Bulb Thermometers.	Rain-fall, average of Six Years.	Direction of Winds.
		Mean.	Mean Maxima.	Mean Minima.		Inches.	
January . .	26·022	66·8	71·0	61·8	17·3	0·5	SE. NW. W. NE.
February . .	26·023	73·3	76·6	66·6	24·4	0·30	Variable.
March . . .	25·940	76·7	81·0	69·6	26·4	0·20	NW.
April . . .	25·958	78·1	83·0	70·6	28·3	0·50	NW.
May . . .	25·883	72·9	78·4	68·0	12·1	5·70	NW.
June . . .	25·795	69·8	80·0	65·4	3·2	10·18	NW.
July . . .	25·806	66·9	70·8	65·2	1·1	22·98	SW. and NW.
August . . .	25·837	65·4	68·2	64·4	0·7	16·34	SW. and NW.
September .	25·844	67·4	72·6	65·4	2·1	7·39	NW.
October . .	25·946	71·2	74·2	67·0	10·6	6·54	SE.
November . .	26·041	69·3	73·2	65·2	18·8	0·67	SE.
December . .	26·011	64·1	69·8	59·2	13·2	1·36	E. and SE.
Mean . .	25·925	70·1	74·9	65·7	13·2	72·21	Total inches.

The Pressure, Temperature and Dryness are taken from the Report for the years 1852-53, and are therefore to be regarded merely as an approximation. The Rain-fall is the average of six years' observation: the greatest was in 1854, viz. 97·24 inches; the least in 1856, viz. 44·76 inches. The hill is more or less covered with fog in June, July, August, and September; in greatest degree in July and August.

2. The object of this Sanitarium is to promote the restoration to health and strength of soldiers who have become debilitated from the effects of climate, or from recurrences, or from long duration of various forms of disease, and thus to increase their efficiency, lessen their liability to suffer from severe types of disease, and add to the probabilities of lengthened service.

3. These beneficial results occur with greater certainty in convalescents, in whom there exists no internal organic disease, or marked tendency to it. It will, therefore, be found that the young soldier derives more benefit from the climate of Poorundhur than the soldier of ten years' service and upwards in India.

4. From the commencement of the month of March to the middle of November is the season during which these advantages will be gained. The period of residence required for complete restoration of strength will vary in different cases, and its determination should be left to the discretion of the Medical Officer in charge of the Sanitarium.

5. Though in the class of invalids adverted to in the 3rd paragraph, the hill climate from the middle of November to the end of February might not prove injurious, still it possesses no advantages over that of Poona, and the season is suitable for return to this latter station and to duty.

6. The class of convalescents hitherto referred to as likely to be benefited by this climate, are: 1st.—Those who have become reduced in strength from recurrences of intermittent or remittent fever at Poona, or other adjacent stations, in June, July, August, and September, may, with advantage, reside at Poorundhur from the beginning of September to the middle of November. After this period, however, such cases had better be returned to Poona; for, from the middle of November to that of February, there will be a greater liability to re-attacks of fever in the hill climate than at Poona. 2nd.—Those who have suffered from recurrences of malarious (intermittent or remittent) fever in October, November, December, January, and February, may be sent to the hill with every prospect of benefit, in the month of March; the duration of residence in each instance being prolonged or not according to necessity. 3rd.—Young recruits debilitated from attacks of common continued fever (febricula) in March, April, and May, will, after convalescence has fairly commenced, be benefited by the climate of Poorundhur. 4th.—Those whose health and strength have become enfeebled from the general effects of a tropical climate or from strumous or allied diathesis, and in whom chronic lymphatic glandular swellings, or indolent external ulcerations are present, are likely to derive advantage from a residence, more or less prolonged, between the beginning of March and middle of November.

7. The months in which invalids may resort to Poorundhur are: 1st.—From the commencement of September to the middle of November,—regard being had to the character of the monsoon weather, in different years, in the first named month. From the middle of November till towards the end of February, convalescents of all kinds are probably better in Poona than at Poorundhur; and, as already stated, it will generally be expedient to return to the former station invalids who have been sent to the hill in the September and October immediately preceding. 2nd.—Though invalids already at Poorundhur, and who have been resident there for some time previously, are generally improved by the climate of July and August, it is, nevertheless, unadvisable to send them there in these

months. 3rd.—March, April, and May are the months most suitable for the transfer of convalescents to Poorundhur. A greater variety of cases may be sent at this period, and they can have the advantage, if necessary, of a continued beneficial residence of eight months and a half, viz. to the middle of November. In many cases more or less of the climate of March, April, and May is necessary to fit the constitution for deriving benefit from the monsoon months.

8. The more precise application of the climate of Poorundhur will be best explained by reference to some of the chief forms of disease.

I. Fevers. The convalescent, from all forms of uncomplicated fever, will be benefited from March to the middle of November. Individuals who have suffered from frequent attacks of *malarious* fever are liable to have the disease re-excited—chiefly in the tertian form—by external cold in the months of December and January; this liability (the degree of predisposition in both instances being assumed equal) is greater at Poorundhur than at Poona; therefore the former locality should, under these circumstances, be avoided in these months. Such individuals are also liable to re-attacks in July, August, September, and October; this liability would seem to be greater at Poona than at Poorundhur, probably in consequence of the great equability of temperature of the latter not favouring cold as a determining cause, and the more continuous moisture preventing the generation of malaria. Therefore, the predisposed to intermittent fever may pass the rains with advantage at Poorundhur, provided he has resided there a month or six weeks of the hot season just preceding. Convalescents from malarious fever, in whom some degree of *splenic enlargement* is present, may resort to Poorundhur at the suitable seasons without risk of injury, and with every prospect of advantage, provided appropriate care and management be at the same time adopted. A similar remark may be applied to those in whom, with the febrile recurrences, there has been tendency to *hepatic congestion*, provided the disease has not been of long duration, nor the subject of it long resident in India. For it is reasonable to infer that where congestion of the spleen or of the liver is coincident with, and in a measure consequent on, the febrile recurrence, and diminishes or ceases with its intermission, the tendency of a climate which prevents the return of the febrile paroxysm must be gradually to remove the dependent congestions and their consequences, if appropriate medical treatment and management be at the same time had recourse to. It follows, then, from these observations, that benefit from the climate of Poorundhur to convalescents from fever will be contingent on accuracy of diagnosis as respects absence, nature, and degree of organic complications.

II. Dysentery and Diarrhœa. The convalescent from uncomplicated dysentery or diarrhœa may with propriety be sent to Poorundhur in March, April, and May, and his stay there prolonged or not according to circumstances.

III. Hepatitis. Individuals who have recently suffered from attacks of acute hepatitis, and who are consequently predisposed to recurrence, should, as a general rule, avoid this climate at all seasons, though probably there is still room for experiment as to whether the monsoon season at Poorundhur may not, under these circumstances, be useful in young, previously sound, and at the time thoroughly convalescent constitutions.

IV. Cirrhosis. The hill climate is unsuitable for the soldier in whom this condition of the liver is suspected to be present.

V. Dyspepsia. When the symptoms to which this term is applied are related to debilitated states of constitution, or to chronic irritation of the mucous membrane of the stomach, the climate of Poorundhur, with due attention to diet and medical treatment, is in general very useful. When, however, they are dependent on cirrhosed liver, or other allied visceral change, benefit is not to be looked for: such cases, indeed, have been erroneously classed.

VI. Pulmonary Affections. In the incipient and early stages of phthisis, good will probably result negatively in March, April, and May from avoidance of the debilitating influence of the heat of the plains. The soldier, generally of some length of service in India, suffering from chronic bronchitis or asthma, is not likely to be improved by a residence at Poorundhur; on the contrary, these affections are liable to be increased.

VII. Affections of the Heart. Organic disease of the walls or valves of the heart will, it need hardly be observed, derive no benefit. The symptoms consequent on the embarrassed action of the organ will generally become aggravated. Yet there are cases of disease, occasionally erroneously named *Carditis*, characterised chiefly by palpitation, often distinctly traceable to frequent exposure to the sun, or to alcoholic or other intemperance, which may be improved by avoidance of the hot season of the plains. In selecting such cases, however, careful attention to diagnosis is essential.

VIII. Cerebral Congestive, Inflammatory, or Structural Disease is liable to be aggravated by the climate of Poorundhur.

IX. Rheumatism.—Cases of pain, with or without slight swelling of the joints, occurring in cachectic constitutions, provided the cachexia is not decidedly syphilitic, often derive benefit if sent to the hill after the beginning of March; and if the improvement has been considerable in the months of April and May, it will probably be increased and perfected by a residence continued during the monsoon months.

X. Secondary Syphilis.—There is no quality of the climate of Poorundhur calculated to aid in the eradication of the syphilitic virus. Still, in cases in which treatment has been inefficacious in the plains, and in which the cachexia is rapidly advancing, it may be reasonable enough to expect greater benefit from treatment conducted at Poorundhur in March, April, and May. In some instances syphilitic eruptions have improved during the monsoon months. This climate will also be useful to the debilitated convalescent from syphilis, just as it is in similar conditions of constitution consecutive on other forms of disease.

9. It may be inferred from the general tenor of these observations, that complete restoration to health and strength from a residence at Poorundhur will be chiefly found to occur in the soldier of a few years'

service in India, in whom a proclivity to attacks of malarious fever has not become firmly established, and organic disease is as yet slight and remediable in character. If such as respects previous disease be also the conditions of the soldier of ten years' service and upwards, then to him also the climate of Poorundhur will prove beneficial. The tendency of the advantage thus gained, will be to maintain and increase the vigour of the constitution, to render it less predisposed to the severer forms of disease, and thus prolong the period of the soldier's efficient service in India. But when the soldier has served in India ten years and upwards, and during that period has frequently suffered from disease, and the question of invaliding has arisen, then, though it may be of advantage to him to pass at Poorundhur the period that it may be necessary for him to remain in India; still it is not to be expected that residence there will be in any respect, under these circumstances, a substitute for invaliding, or will lessen the number of unfits of this class.

10. The transfer of sick in states and stages of serious disease at the time requiring care and medical treatment, in the hope that these may be conducted with more advantage at Poorundhur, was not in contemplation when the Sanitarium was established; and there has been nothing in experience there since to justify this proceeding, but much to dissuade from it. It is, doubtless, disheartening and unsatisfactory to watch disease progressing, notwithstanding our best efforts to remove it; but this evil is not to be prevented by the heedless transfer of sick from station to station. It is to be lessened: 1st.—By such sanitary measures in regard to barracks, hospitals, dress, rations, duties, amusements, and judicious use of hill and other Sanitaria, as shall maintain the health and vigour of the soldier at as high a point as practicable, and, therefore, less prone to the severer types of disease. 2nd.—By such careful study of the pathology and rational principles of treatment of disease in India as shall teach us to distinguish, at the earliest periods, all serious forms, and to conduct the cure with watchful care and steady judgment.

11. There are diseases, as recurring malarious fevers with or without splenic and hepatic complication, idiopathic affections of the liver and bowels, pulmonary, cardiac, nephritic, and rheumatic affections, for which the climate of Poona from the middle of November to the end of February is not favourable, and for which that of Poorundhur at the same season is still more adverse. For these a Sanitarium on some well-selected site on the sea-coast would be a great boon to the suffering soldier, and, consequently, a great advantage to the Government. It would, further, be useful in those forms of hepatic disease for which both Poona and Poorundhur are unsuited also in the hot months of the year.

*** This Memorandum was prepared by me, when Superintending Surgeon of the Poona Division, after full consideration of the Reports of the several Medical Officers, and careful personal inspection of the Sanitarium and of the Invalids at the time (May 1858) resident there, in the hope that it might be useful to Medical Officers in charge of European troops, more especially those who had recently arrived in the Poona Division. It makes no pretension to having exhausted or fully developed the subject, and was intended to be suggestive, not dogmatic.

LIST OF CASES.

*** *The Numeral at the end of the Title of each Case is that of the Case in the First Edition, and is now added to facilitate Reference from one Edition to the other. Those without a second number are published for the first time in this edition.*

CHAPTER III.

INTERMITTENT FEVER.

1. Abnormal præcordial dulness from enlarged spleen, 8. . . . Page 36
2. Abnormal præcordial dulness from enlarged spleen associated with systolic murmur, 9. 37
3. Abnormal præcordial dulness from splenic enlargement. Systolic murmur present, 10. 37
4. Abnormal præcordial dulness from enlargement of the spleen. Systolic murmur present, 11. 37
5. Extended præcordial dulness, with systolic and venous murmurs, without splenic enlargement from anæmia alone, 12. 38
6. Intermittent fever complicated with hepatitis. Death from cholera. Liver in a state of vascular turgescence, 17. 44
7. Intermittent fever with enlargement of the liver, 18. 44
8. Intermittent fever with gastric irritation treated with quinine, 19. . 49
9. Intermittent fever, 20. 50
10. Intermittent fever, with chronic meningitis. Symptoms chiefly during accession. Death from unexpected collapse, 21. 51
11. Intermittent fever: some of the paroxysms complicated with convulsive fits, one of which terminated fatally. Thickening and opacity of the arachnoid membrane, 22. 51
12. Intermittent fever complicated with pericarditis and pneumonia. Recovery, 23. 54
13. Intermittent fever complicated with asthma, 24. 55

CHAPTER V.

REMITTENT FEVER.

14. Remittent fever fatal from unexpected collapse, 25. . . . . Page 68
15. Great collapse in the course of remittent fever. Recovery by stimulants, 26. 69
16. Exhaustion taking the place of exacerbation in remittent fever, 27. . . 70
17. Remittent fever. Death by coma. Bright's disease of both kidneys, 28. . 77
18. Remittent fever, with adynamic symptoms. Serum underneath the arachnoid and at the base of the cranium. No coma. The liver much enlarged. Dark rosy tint of the mucous coat of the stomach, 29. 78
19. Remittent fever with irregular symptoms in an intemperate man of very corpulent habit, and in whose head, heart, liver, and kidneys there was extensive old organic disease, 30. . 78
20. Remittent fever in a person of very intemperate habits, with symptoms in some respects resembling delirium tremens. Death by coma. Three ounces of serum at the base of the skull; liver much enlarged. Commencing degeneration of the kidney. Mucous coat of the colon softened, with here and there red patches, with a mucous follicle in the centre of each discoloration. Softening of the mucous coat of the stomach, 31. 79
21. Remittent fever with adynamic symptoms. Obscure pneumonia. Death without coma. Bright's disease of both kidneys, 32. 80
22. Remittent fever. Death by convulsion and coma. Vascular congestion of the

vessels of the pia mater. Rosy tint of the substance of the brain. One ounce of serum at the base of the skull. The heart dilated and its tissue pale and flabby. Partial redness, thinning, and softening of the mucous coat of the stomach. Peyer's glands enlarged. The spleen enlarged and softened, and the kidneys congested, 39 . . Page 82

23. Remittent fever in a man of intemperate habits. Fatal with convulsion, coma, and tumultuous action of the heart. Considerable effusion of serum in the head. Streaked redness and softening of the mucous membrane of the stomach. Deep red tint of the endocardium and muscular tissue of the heart, 33. 83

24. Remittent fever in a man of intemperate habits. Death by coma. Increased vascularity of the membranes of the brain and considerable effusion of serum. Softening and vascularity of the mucous coat of the stomach and large intestine. Commencing degeneration of the kidneys, 34. 83

25. Remittent fever. Simulating delirium tremens. Pia mater very vascular, with bullæ of air between the arachnoid and pia mater and in the vessels, 35. . 84

26. Remittent fever proving fatal by collapse and coma at the close of an exacerbation. No serous effusion in the head. Dotted redness and softening of the mucous membrane of the stomach. Enlargement of the mucous follicles of the colon and of Peyer's glands. Lumbrici in the small intestine, 36. .. . 85

27. Remittent fever. Drowsiness and coma. Considerable quantity of serum effused in the head. Vascularity and thickening of the mucous membrane of the stomach, 37. 86

28. Remittent fever. Coma from exhaustion, 38. 86

29. Remittent fever. Meningitis. Effusion of serum in the cavity of the arachnoid and sub-arachnoid space. Opacity and thickening of the arachnoid membrane, 40. 87

30. Remittent fever admitted after a week's illness. Head symptoms chiefly marked by unsteadiness of manner, and latterly drowsiness. Arachnoid membrane opaque and thickened. Increased serous effusion, 41. 87

31. Remittent fever admitted in an advanced stage. Death by coma. Extensive lymph and serous effusion in the sub-arachnoid space. Hepatisation of both lungs, 42. 88

32. Remittent fever with adynamic symptoms. Slight vascularity of the membranes of the brain with air in the vessels and beneath the arachnoid. Turgescence and ulceration of Peyer's glands at the end of the ileum, 43. . Page 89

33. Remittent fever. Symptoms adynamic and badly-developed. Serous effusion and slight vascular congestion in the head, also air in the vessels. The colon distended and in part displaced, 44. 89

34. Remittent fever, with head and gastro-enteritic symptoms; two or three ounces of serum in the cranium. Firm granular exudation on the mucous surface of the colon. Dark redness of the end of the ileum. The subject of a large hydrocele, 45. 95

35. Remittent fever. Peyer's glands enlarged and ulcerated. Head symptoms with moderate turgescence of the vessels, 46. 95

36. Remittent fever with jaundice. Drowsiness. Biliary congestion of the liver. Enlarged lymphatic glands in the course of the common duct. Slight dilatation of the hepatic duct. Gastro-duodenitis. Granular exudation on the mucous surface of the ileum and colon. Nodules of pulmonary apoplexy; one softened into a cavity, 47. 98

37. Remittent fever with jaundice. Tenderness at margin of right ribs. Coma. Gastro-duodenitis. Enlarged lymphatic glands in the course of the common duct. Biliary congestion of the liver, 48. 99

38. Fever with jaundice. Tenderness at the margin of the right ribs. Drowsiness. Biliary congestion of the liver. Obstruction of the hepatic duct by a lumbricus, of which there were many in the duodenum and stomach. No gastro-duodenitis. Enlargement of the lymphatic glands in the course of the common duct. Hepatic cells distinct, 49 . . . 99

39. Remittent fever with jaundice. Tenderness at the margin of the right ribs. Drowsiness. Enlarged lymphatic glands. Enlarged head of the pancreas. No duodenitis. Biliary congestion of the liver, 50. 100

40. Remittent fever with jaundice. Tenderness at the margin of the right ribs. Death from exhaustion. Enlargement and biliary congestion of the liver. Gastro-duodenitis. Hepatic cells distinct, 51. 101

41. Remittent fever with jaundice in an opium-eater. Tenderness at the epigastrium. No coma. Death from exhaustion. Enlargement and biliary congestion of the liver. No duodenitis. No enlargement of the lymphatic glands, 52. , ... 101

42. Remittent fever with jaundice. Ten-

derness at the margin of the right ribs. Death from exhaustion. Cirrhosis. Gall bladder distended. Enlarged lymphatic glands around the common duct. Duodenitis. Granular exudation on the mucous membrane of the ileum and large intestine, 53. . . . . Page 102

43. Fever with jaundice. Died exhausted. Biliary congestion of the liver. No enlargement of the lymphatic glands. Contraction of the cystic duct. Distention of the gall-bladder, mucous membrane of gall-bladder and ducts normal, with exception of slight vascularity of common duct at point of entrance into duodenum. Hepatic cells distinct, 54. . . 103

44. Remittent fever with jaundice. Drowsiness. Enlarged lymphatic glands in course of common duct. Constricted cystic duct. Gall-bladder full, 55. . 104

45. Remittent fever with jaundice. No tenderness at margin of ribs. Drowsiness. No enlargement of lymphatic glands. Dark-redness of mucous membrane of duodenum, 56. . . 104

CHAPTER XIV.

DYSENTERY.

46. Under treatment nine months. Dysentery alternating with rheumatism, probably syphilitic; terminating in general cachexia with febrile symptoms. The lungs, liver, mucous coat of stomach and intestines presented morbid appearances of various characters, 131. . 239

47. Chronic dysentery, discoloration with thickening of parts of the mucous membrane of the large intestines. Commencing degeneration of kidneys, 133. 239

48. Melanosis of the colon. No ulceration. Tubercles in the liver, 134. . . 240

49. Membranous mucous exudation on the inner surface of the large intestine, 240.

50. Chronic dysentery in an opium-eater. The mucous coat of the colon lined with a firm granular layer. The lungs tubercular. Cartilaginous contraction of the pyloric orifice of the stomach, 135. 241

51. Diarrhœa tedious. Granular yellow exudation on the mucous surface of the large intestine with thickening of the tunic, 136. 242

52. Dysentery with adynamic febrile symptoms. Granular exudation on the mucous coat at the end of the ileum. Sloughy ulceration of the large intestine, 141. 246

53. Granular exudation on mucous surface of ileum and colon, with irregular ulceration of the latter. No disease of the liver. Displacement of the colon, 162. . 247

54. Dysentery alternating with febrile accessions. Bands of granular deposit at the end of the ileum. Sloughy ulceration of the colon, 143. . . . Page 247

55. Dysentery. Sloughy ulceration of large intestine. Granular deposit in transverse bands in the ileum. Peritonitis and matting of the omentum. An opium-eater, 144. 248

56. Probable scorbutic taint. Dark, irregular, ragged, internal surface of the colon, with thickening. Granular deposit on mucous membrane of ileum, with thickening, 145. 249

57. Thickening and sloughy ulceration of large intestine, with here and there a small encysted abscess in the thickened tissue. Granular deposit on inner surface of ileum. Peritonitis. Old pericarditis and heart disease, 146. . 249

58. Dysentery. Sloughy ulceration in transverse bands, and the follicles of the colon in different stages of disease. Insensibility for an hour before death. Two ounces of serum at the base of the skull, 147. 250

59. Dysentery neglected for thirteen days, attended with abscess in the liver. Sloughy ulceration of the mucous coat of the colon, with fringe of granular exudation, 148. 250

60. Acute dysentery. The large intestine ulcerated in transverse ridges. The mucous follicles enlarged. Considerable effusion of serum in the head without symptoms, 149. 251

61. Acute dysentery. The ulceration in transverse ridges. Considerable effusion of serum in the head, without symptoms, 150. 251

62. Dysentery in an advanced state obscured by secondary peritonitis. Granular deposit on the mucous surface of the large intestine, 151. . . 252

63. Several attacks. Colon thickened. Sloughy ulceration, with granular deposit on other parts of the mucous surface of the colon. Slight peritonitis, 152. 252

64. Dysentery admitted in the last stage. Peritonitic inflammation. Sloughy ulceration of the mucous coat of the colon, 153. 253

65. Patches of submucous puriform infiltration in colon, 161. . . . 255

66. Sloughy patches of mucous membrane of colon, with submucous œdema, 162. 255

67. Numerous small follicular ulcerations of the colon, 163. 256

68. Chronic dysentery in a person of broken constitution. Numerous follicular ulcers in the large intestine, many of them cicatrising. Serous effusion in the head without symptoms, 164. 256

69. Dark-grey discoloration, with some degree of thickening of mucous membrane of colon, with numerous circular ulcers, 165. . . . Page 257
70. Circular and transverse ulcers of the large intestine. Matting of the omentum over the colon, with displacement. Liver healthy. Distention of the urinary bladder, 167. 257
71. Dysentery. Death in early stage by cholera. Gangrenous patches of mucous membrane of large intestine, but no separation 258
72. Dysentery. Sloughs of the mucous coat passed before death. Much displacement of the colon to the left side. Abscess in the liver, 169. . . . 258
73. Acute dysentery. Extensive sloughy ulceration of the inner surface of the large intestine. Dark-red grumous discharges, 170. 259
74. Dysentery. General peritonitis before the fatal termination. Serous effusion in the head; no head symptoms. The mucous coat of the colon in process of separation from the other tunics, 171. 260
75. Sloughy state of mucous membrane of the colon. Submucous puriform infiltration, forming little cavities. General peritonitis. Matting of omentum. Retention of urine, 172. . . . 260
76. Mucous membrane of colon sloughy and separating in shreds. General peritonitis and matting of the omentum, 174. 261
77. Dysentery attended by general peritonitis. The ulcers in different stages of progress, some cicatrised, one perforating, but patched up, 176 . . 263
78. Chronic dysentery. Enlarged mesenteric glands. Mucous coat of the colon firm and thickened. The cicatrices of ulcers, 177. 264
79. Pleuritis cured, succeeded by hydrocele radically cured; followed by rheumatism, succeeded by dysentery, cachexia, and recurrence of dysentery. Colon ulcerated, 178. . . . 264
80. Sloughy ulceration of colon. General peritonitis and matting of the omentum, 181. 266
81 Sloughy ulceration of large intestines without thickening. Commencing abscesses in the liver. Peritonitis, 182. 266
82. Sloughy ulceration and thickening of large intestine. Matting of omentum. Dysuria. Peritonitis of bladder, 183. 267
83. Much sloughy destruction of the colon. Peritonitis and matting of the omentum. Former attack of hepatitis. Puckered fibrous bands in liver, 184. 267
84. Thickening of the colon. Numerous deep ulcers. Matting of the omentum. Liver with fibrous puckered bands, 185. . . . Page 267
85. Thickening and sloughy ulceration of large intestine. Matting of omentum. Congestion of the liver, 186. . . 268
86. Habitual constipation. Colon contracted in parts and strictured by a band of the omentum. Tubercular infiltration of the lungs. Ulceration of the ileum and cœcum, probably from softening of tubercles, 187. 268
87. Chronic dysentery. A palpable tumour of the cœcum. The lungs studded with tubercles not suspected during life. Considerable effusion of serum in the head, 188. 269
88. Dysentery. Perforation of the cœcum, with consequent formation of a circumscribed sac, with gangrene of the muscles and integuments, 189. . 270
89. Circular ulcers with sloughs in mucous membrane of colon and stomach. No thickening, 190. . . . 271
90. Grey softening, with a few ulcers of the mucous lining of the stomach and colon. Cicatrices of ulcers in the former, 191. 272
91. Dysentery. The use of purgatives too much abstained from. The lower end of the ileum distended from thin feculence, 192. 301
92. Good effects of opium, in the treatment of some states of dysentery, illustrated, 199. 303
93. Acute dysentery in a child. Treated with ipecacuanha and blue pill, 194. 315

CHAPTER XV.

HEPATITIS.

94. Abscess in the brain not suspected during life. Abscess in the liver, with pneumonia of the lowest lobe of the right lung, revealed by symptoms. Vascular turgescence of liver, 195. . . 330
95. Hepatitis. Several abscesses in the right lobe. Nodules in the left lobe. The mucous coat of the colon ulcerated. Serous effusion in the head without symptoms, 196. 331
96. Dysentery complicated with delirium tremens. Milkiness of the arachnoid. Matting of the omentum over the colon. Numerous sloughy ulcerations of the mucous coat of the cœcum. Many abscesses in liver, 179. 331
97. Illustrates formation of abscesses from breaking down of lymph deposit. Pus tinged with bile. The corpuscles granular and broken down. Surrounding turgescence, 198 331

98. Hepatitis. Abscesses, in one, breaking down of the parenchyma; in the other the deposit in the interstitial tissue had not yet broken down into pus. Mucous coat of the colon dark-red, and covered, with firm granular exudation, 199. . . . Page 332

99. Hepatitis. An abscess lined by firm membrane in the right lobe. Several nodules in different places of the liver; in some suppuration commencing at the centre. Traces of ulceration in the colon. Granular exudation on the mucous coat of the rectum, 200. . 332

100. Hepatitis. Two large abscesses from degeneration of lymph and tissue. The liver mottled buff. The mucous coat of the colon dark-grey with red patches, and several ulcers. The kidneys malformed, 201. 333

101. Abscess in the liver. Sac smooth without flocculi. Large intestine, with sloughy ulceration of the mucous coat. Complicated with intermittent fever, which, at the commencement, was the prominent feature. Several lymph nodules, 202. 333

102. Large hepatic abscess, with shreddy flocculent walls and surrounding vascular turgescence. No intestinal ulceration, 204. 334

103. Abscess in liver discharged by the lung, followed by convalescence. Proceeded to England, and died shortly after arrival. No account of the post mortem appearances, 205. 336

104. Hepatic abscess attributed to blows. Opening into the lung. Improvement. Record as to the issue incomplete, 206. 336

105. Hepatic abscess opening through the lung. Result of the case not recorded, 207. 336

106. Hepatic abscess communicating with the lung (?). Result not known, 208. 337

107. Dysentery. Secondary hepatic abscess forming obscurely. Opening into the lung. No ulceration of the intestine, 209. 337

108. Large hepatic abscess with brick-red pus. Smaller one opening into lung. Brick-red sputa. No diarrhœa till just before death. Intestines not examined. A spirit-drinker, 210. 338

109. Hepatic abscess opening through the lung. Causing pleuritis and effusion. Also presenting externally, but not opened, 211. 339

110. Hepatitis, ending in abscess discharged through the lung. An abscess in the third lobe of the right lung, communicating freely through the diaphragm with the abscess of the liver. Mucous coat of the large intestine ulcerated. Many of the ulcers cicatrised, 214. . . 340

111. Two hepatic abscesses. One opening into the lung, with expectoration of deep bile-tinged puriform sputa, Page 215. 340

112. Abscess in the liver opening through the diaphragm into the sac of the pleura, and causing purulent effusion there, 217. 341

113. Abscess in the left lobe of the liver opening into the stomach. No vomiting. No detection of pus in the intestinal discharges. No intestinal ulceration, 221. 343

114. An abscess of the liver communicating with the colon. Others in process of repair by absorption, 223. . . 344

115. Hepatic abscess, recovered from, by probable opening into the colon, 222. 344

116. Hepatic abscess opening into the colon (?). Recovery. . . . 345

117. Hepatic abscess opening into the colon and stomach (?). Recovery. . . 345

118. Two hepatic abscesses in process of absorption. Death from cholera. Painful decubitus on right side explained by the situation of one of the abscesses. Ulceration of colon, 224. . . . 346

119. Four hepatic abscesses. General peritonitis, but no evidence of abscess rupture. Two of the abscesses in process of cure by absorption, 225. . . 347

120. Hepatic abscess in process of cure by absorption. 348

121. Hepatic abscess. Absorption (?). Recovery. 348

122. Purulent sac between the liver and the diaphragm, communicating with the left lung. No hepatic abscess. . . 349

123. Amputation of the right hand, followed by general bad health and chronic hepatitis. A purulent sac between the liver and the ribs filled with fœtid pus. Hepatisation of the lower part of the right lung, 226. 349

124. Abscess in the liver. Also one external and circumscribed communicating with former. Dark-red colour of mucous surface of large intestine, which contained much clotted blood, 227. . 350

125. Hepatitis. Abscess bounded beyond by a firm sac. A circumscribed abscess in the peritoneal cavity over the edge of the liver. Substance of the liver mottled red and white, 228. . . . 350

126. Abscess in the liver communicating with purulent deposit in the right iliac region. Habitual constipation. The sigmoid flexure of the colon much contracted, 230. 351

127. A circumscribed sac between the liver and the ribs. An abscess in the substance of the right lobe. The mucous coat of the colon studded with circular ulcers, 231. 351

128. Abscess in the liver. Empyema of the right pleura. Symptoms not well marked. Dejection of a pint of clotted blood before death. Mucous coat of the colon dark-red, with ulceration, 232. Page 353
129. Abscess in the liver. Effusion of four pints of serum, with lymph in the right pleura. Ulcerated colon. No coma. Serum between the pia mater and arachnoid, and two or three ounces at the base of the skull, 233. . . 353
130. A small purulent sac circumscribed in part by the base of the right lung and by the diaphragm, and extending to the fissure between the second and third lobes of the right lung, mistaken for hepatic abscess, 235. 354
131. Hepatitis. Abscess in the liver. Five pints of pus in the sac of the right pleura. A layer of lymph on the surface of the heart and inner surface of the pericardium. General peritonitis, with effusion of lymph and sero-purulent fluid, 236. 354
132. Pericarditis. The inner surface of the pericardium and the outer side of the heart covered with a thick layer of irregular lymph. Also effusion of serum and displacement of the liver, partly caused by the distended pericardium. Abscess of the liver, 237. . . 355
133. General peritonitis. Abscess of the liver following head symptoms. Serous effusion in the head with thickening of the arachnoid membrane. The kidneys had undergone yellow degeneration, 239. 356
134. General peritonitis. Matting of the omentum over the cœcum. Round ulcers in the colon, and an abscess in the liver, 240. 357
135. General peritonitis, with sero-purulent effusion and abscess in the liver, 241. 357
136. Probably small superficial abscess of under surface of lobulus Spigelii, leading to puriform sac in gastro-hepatic omentum, and this by rupture to general peritonitis. Jaundice, 245. . . 358
137. Large abscess in right lobe, flocculent walls, communicating with branch of hepatic vein. Lumbricus in the abscess. Pus orange-coloured. No ulceration of large intestine. Jaundice, 249. . 364
138. A large abscess in the liver. No dysenteric symptoms. No ulceration. No projection of liver below the ribs, 260. 366
139. Hepatitis. Abscess in the right lobe. Mucous coat of the large intestine dark red without ulceration, 261. . 366
140. Chronic pneumonia of upper part of left lung. Secondary hepatitis and abscess, with flocculent walls, and peritonitic inflammation. No intestinal ulceration, 265. . . . Page 367
141. Three abscesses in different stages of progress. Pus bile tinged. General peritonitis without rupture. No ulceration of the intestine, 269 . . . 367
142. Hepatic abscess. No ulceration of the intestine 368
143. Hepatic abscess. No ulceration of the intestine 368
144. Slight dysenteric symptoms of some days' duration, followed by febrile symptoms. Those of hepatic inflammation coming on obscurely, and ending in abscess, 281. 379
145. Diagnosis doubtful: whether right pleuritic effusion, or large hepatic abscess, or both conjoined, 282. . . 381
146. Hepatic abscess. Mistaken for pleuritic effusion 382
147. Asthenic pneumonia mistaken for communicating hepatic abscess, 283. 384
148. Whether asthenic pneumonia or communicating hepatic abscess. Doubtful, 284. 384
149. Hepatic abscess pointing at the epigastrium and successfully punctured. Trocar used, 285. 393
150. Hepatic abscess pointing at the epigastrium, punctured successfully, 286. 394
151. Hepatic abscess pointing between the eighth right rib and umbilicus, successfully punctured, 287. . . . 394
152. Hepatic abscess, punctured. Recovery, 288. 394
153. Hepatic abscess, punctured at the point of the right ninth rib. Recovery, 289. 394
154. Hepatic abscess pointing between the right ninth rib and umbilicus, punctured. Case not followed to the close, but in all probability successful, 290 . . 395
155. Hepatic abscess pointing at the epigastrium, punctured. Result not known; probably successful, 291. . . 395
156. Chronic hepatic abscesses. One was punctured and healed, but there was no adhesion to the abdominal wall at site of puncture found after death. Ulceration of colon; but dysentery clearly secondary. Second abscess and death, 292. 396
157. Abscess in the liver pointing between the right seventh and eighth ribs. Opened into the lung and also externally. Gangrene of the integuments around the orifice, also of the intercostal muscles, and necrosis of a rib, 293 397
158. Hepatic abscess punctured over the last right false rib. Gangrene and sloughing around the wound. Death. No inspection, 294. . . . 398

159. Large hepatic abscess punctured. Death from exhaustion, with sloughing of the wound. No examination after death, 295. . . . . . Page 398
160. Superficial abscess of right extremity of the liver leading to circumscribed sac between the organ and lateral abdominal walls. Punctured between the tenth and eleventh rib. Sloughy state of wound. Necrosis of rib, and death from hectic fever, 296. 398
161. Abscess in the liver punctured. Carious ribs projecting into the abscess. At first superficial and leading to circumscribed sac between liver and diaphragm. Also empyema of right pleural sac without communication, 297. . . . 399
162. Two large hepatic abscesses. One deep, the other a sac between the surface of the liver and abdominal walls, originating probably in rupture of a small superficial abscess, there being lymph nodules in the part of the liver adjoining. This abscess punctured. Sloughing. No ulceration of intestine, 298. 400
163. Hepatic abscess punctured at the epigastrium. Gangrene and sphacelation around the orifice. Death. No inspection, 299. 401
164. Hepatic abscess pointing at the epigastrium, punctured. Extensive sphacelus around the opening. Death, 300: . 401
165. A single abscess at the thin edge of the left lobe of liver existing for five months, punctured. Gangrene of the orifice. Dysenteric symptoms latterly. Ulceration of mucous membrane of the colon, 301. 402
166. Two hepatic abscesses. One punctured with increase of febrile symptoms. Attributed to fist blows. Habits temperate. Diarrhœa, with redness of mucous membrane of colon. No ulceration. Commencing gangrene at the opening in the abscess, 302. . . 402
167. Hepatic abscess pointing at the epigastrium, punctured. Sloughing around the wound. Death, 303. . . 403
168. Cirrhosis of liver. Abscess in thin edge of liver punctured. Purulent sac between liver and diaphragm. Ulceration of large intestine. Death, 304. 403
169. Hepatic abscess in epigastric region, punctured; very little discharge. Dysenteric symptoms, secondary. Died. No examination, 305. 404
170. Abscess partly of right and left lobe, punctured. Death from dysentery clearly secondary. Ulceration of large intestine. Effusion in both pleural sacs, 306. 405
171. Pleuritic effusion. Abscess in the liver punctured. Attributed to a blow. Death the day after the abscess was opened. No examination after death, 307 . . . . . Page 406
172. Large abscess of right lobe of liver punctured with trocar. Several abscesses in left lobe in different stages. Also lymph nodules, 308. . . 406
173. Large abscess in the right lobe. The liver free of abnormal adhesions. The cicatrices of former ulcers in the colon. Jaundice. Enlarged glands in the course of the ducts, 309. 413
174. Aneurism of the abdominal aorta. Acute pain of right hypochondrium and shoulder. The edge of the liver distinct. Treated four times for disease of the liver, 310. 416
175. A tumour, situated between the edge of the liver and the transverse colon, 311. 416

CHAPTER XVI.

CIRRHOSIS, ETC.

176. Cirrhosis, with enlargement. Ascites. No kidney or heart disease. Jaundice, 312. 422
177. Ascites. Liver small and indurated. Cirrhosis. Considerable effusion of serum in the head, 313. . . . 423
178. Abscess in the liver. Cirrhosis. Sloughy perforations, patched, of large intestine, but no thickening of its coats noted, 314. 424
179. Abscess in liver with cirrhosis, notwithstanding ptyalism. Displacement of colon. Adhesion of it to the left side of diaphragm. Sloughy ulceration of large intestine, without thickening, 315. 425
180. Abscess in liver, notwithstanding ptyalism. Cirrhosis. Cœcum and ascending colon thickened and ulcerated, 316. 425
181. Dysentery complicated with delirium tremens. Abscess and cirrhosis of the liver, 318. 426
182. Remittent fever. Œdema of the liver 428
183. Treated for supposed dyspeptic symptoms. Numerous cancerous tubera disseminated throughout the liver. One had opened into the stomach, 320. 429
184. Phthisis pulmonalis. Lungs tuberculated, hydatid sac in the abdomen, also in the liver. Peritoneum studded with miliary transparent tubercles, 321. 430
185. Hepatitis. Abscess. Inflammation of the external and internal surface of the gall-bladder. Sudden collapse, continuing with varying symptoms for several days, 322. 431

186. Fever with jaundice. Gall-bladder distended, seemingly, from inflammation of the common duct. Little improvement from treatment, 323 . Page 432
187. The gall-bladder, distended, reached to the umbilicus. Gastritis. Colon contracted, 324. 432

CHAPTER XVII.

PERITONITIS, ILEUS AND COLIC.

188. General peritonitis from a penetrating wound of the liver and effusion of blood into the abdomen. Considerable effusion of serum in the head without symptoms, 325. 444
189. Fracture of both thigh bones. Abdomen bruised by a fall. Death in fifty-four hours, under symptoms of peritonitis. General redness and effusion of lymph on the peritoneal surfaces. A pint of turbid serum in the cavity, 326. 444
190. Wound of the abdomen with protrusion of intestine. Vascularity of, and lymph-exudation on, the peritoneum, and the protruded intestine, 327. . . 445
191. Peritonitis. Purulent effusion into the cavity of the abdomen. Lymph general on the peritoneal surfaces, 328. . 446
192. Peritonitis after parturition, but probably caused by blows, 329. . . 446
193. Partial peritonitis leading to formation of a large circumscribed purulent sac, 330. 446
194. General peritonitis. The lungs studded with crude tubercles. The mesenteric glands tuberculated. The end of the ileum, the cœcum, and colon ulcerated. Considerable effusion in the head, 331. 448
195. Extensive ulcer on the groin. Miliary tubercles in the lungs and underneath the peritoneum throughout its whole extent. Follicular ulceration of the large intestine. Three ounces of serum in the cavity of the cranium. No head symptoms, 332. 449
196. Chronic peritonitis. Tubercular. Much effusion and complete dulness on percussion, 333. 450
197. Effusion in chest and abdomen. Access of cholera. Disappearance of the effusion. Bright's disease of the kidney and tubercular peritonitis, 99. . 451
198. Ileus, with granular effusion on the inner surface of the ileum. Biliary calculi, 334. 454
199. Ileus. Strangulation of part of the intestine by old peritonitic adhesions, 335. 454
200. Colica-pictonum. The colon was much distended and displaced. Death with head symptoms. Only slight serous effusion at the base of the skull, 336. Page 456

CHAPTER XVIII.

AFFECTIONS OF THE STOMACH.

201. Poisoning by arsenic, admitted in the stage of collapse, after the active symptoms of gastritis were passed, 337 . 458
202. Poisoning from arsenic in which symptoms of narcotism were prominent at the commencement, 338. 459

CHAPTER XIX.

BRIGHT'S DISEASE OF THE KIDNEY.

203. A diver by occupation. Anasarca ascites. Urine of low density and albuminous. Dilatation of the right ventricle of the heart. Hypertrophy, and dilatation of the left. Kidneys enlarged, lobulated, in a state of yellow granular degeneration, 340. 468
204. Dropsical symptoms. Urine of low density and albuminous. Bronchitis, diarrhœa, periostitis, erysipelas, as secondary affections. Kidneys large, and in a state of yellow granular and fatty degeneration. An opium eater, 341. 469
205. Gastro-enteritis, anasarca, and ascites. Urine of low density and albuminous. Paracentesis. Death from peritonitis. Kidneys small, in a state of yellow granular degeneration, 342. . . 470
206. Anasarca and ascites. Urine of low density and albuminous. Was eight times tapped. Kidneys in a state of yellow granular degeneration, 343. 471
207. Anasarca and ascites. Urine of low density and very albuminous. Sunk under diarrhœa. The kidneys in a state of yellow granular degeneration. The mucous coat of the colon and ileum with dotted red patches and granular deposit. A spiritdrinker. Cirrhosis, 344. 472
208. Anasarca with ascites. Urine of low density and generally albuminous. Died comatose. Kidneys small, with cysts and excess of cortical portion. Cirrhosis. Thrice admitted, 345. . . . 472
209. Febrile symptoms, followed by anasarca, ascites, and dysenteric symptoms. Urine of low density and albuminous. Death by coma. The kidneys in a state of yellow granular degeneration. The mucous membrane of the large intestine ulcerated, and with granular exudation, 346. 474
210. Vesicular emphysema of both lungs. Displacement of the heart. Dilatation and hypertrophy of the ventricles. Athe-

romatous deposit, with ulceration, in the aorta. Granular degeneration of the kidneys. Urine once noted, albuminous. Dropsy, 348. . . Page 474
211. Admitted in an advanced state of disease. Hepatisation of both lungs. Circumscribed pleuritic effusion of the right side. Kidneys enlarged, and in a state of yellow granular degeneration. Urine not tested, 349. . . . 475
212. The subject of intermittent fever, followed by bronchitis, and slight anasarca. Urine of low density, and very albuminous, 351. 476
213. Febrile symptoms and dropsy after exposure to cold and wet. Traces of albumen in the urine, slight throughout, finally disappeared. Addicted to the occasional use of spirits and opium. Finally sunk under increasing asthenia. Granular degeneration of the kidneys, 352. 476
214. Dropsical symptoms with diarrhœa, following exposure to cold and wet. Urine very albuminous. Drowsiness coexisting with sinking pulse, removed by stimulants, did not recur. Death by exhaustion. Kidneys large and granular. Spirit-drinking not admitted, 353. 477
215. Syphilis, primary and secondary. Mercurial influence. Slight dropsy. Albuminous urine, pain of loins, dysentery. Fatal. Bright's disease. Ulceration and granular exudation on intestinal mucous membrane. Cirrhosis. A cretified guinea-worm encysted between the right lung and the pericardium, 354. 478
216. Dysentery. Dropsy. Albuminous urine, with fat globules, in an old spirit-drinker and opium-eater. Fatal. Ulcerated intestines. Kidneys enlarged. Fatty degeneration, 355. . . 479
217. Dropsy. Albuminous urine. Death from dysenteric symptoms. Kidneys enlarged with fatty degeneration. Redness in patches of the intestinal mucous lining. Habits not known, 356. . 480

CHAPTER XX.

ABNORMAL STATES OF THE URINE.

218. Urine thick, white, opaque, coagulating with heat and nitric acid. No improvement under the use of varied remedies. Recovery by attention to the general health, chiefly by change of air, 398. 500
219. Urine thick, white, opaque, coagulating with heat and nitric acid. No improvement from medical treatment. Recovery from change of air, 399. . 501
220. Urine opaque and white, occasionally coagulating spontaneously. Recovery from change of air, 400. Page 501
221. Urine milky, coagulating by heat and nitric acid, becoming clear by addition of sulphuric ether. No improvement from treatment. Change of air recommended. Result not known, 401. 501
222. Chylo-serous urine, removed by change of air. 502
223. Chylo-serous urine, removed twice by change of air. 502
224. Diabetes. Symptoms improved somewhat under the use of creosote and muriate of morphia, 402. . . . 503
225. Diabetes. No improvement from preparations of iron, permanganate of potass, and opium, 403. . . . 504
226. Diabetes. Not improved by treatment, 404. 504
227. Diabetes. No improvement from permanganate of potass, or from creosote alone, but marked benefit from addition of opium, 405. 504

CHAPTER XXI.

PNEUMONIA.

228. Pneumonia extensive of right lung. Grey induration with cavities formed in upper lobe by molecular gangrene, 413. 524
229. Grey, almost cartilaginous, induration of the lower part of the right lung, with several excavations by process of gangrenous molecular softening. The several stages of the process well shown. Bright's disease of the kidney, 414. 525
230. Grey and red induration of the upper lobe of the right lung with gangrenous excavation, 415. 525

CHAPTER XXIV.

PERICARDITIS AND ENDOCARDITIS.

231. Pericarditis. Friction murmur distinct, and then altogether disappearing. He was cured. Eight months afterwards death from cholera. Opaque patches on the surface of the heart. No pericardial adhesions, 448. 573
232. Phthisis pulmonalis. Secondary pericarditis. Friction murmur, distinct for twenty days. Death eighteen months afterwards. Firm pericardial adhesions. Bright's disease of the kidney, 450. 574
233. Asthenic pneumonia, leading to red induration of the upper lobes. In its course, pericarditis and endocarditis of the left ventricle and auricle, causing structural disease of the mitral valve. Not traced to rheumatism. Dilatation of all the cavities of the heart, 461. 576

234. Empyema of the right side of chest. Secondary pericarditis. Friction murmur. Lymph effusions found after death, 462. . . . . . . Page 577
235. Acute arachnitis and pericarditis leading to considerable effusions, coagulating into a jelly-like mass when removed from the body. Friction murmur. In a pregnant female, 463. . 577

CHAPTER XXV.

ORGANIC DISEASE OF THE HEART.

236. Contraction of the orifice of the pulmonary artery, probably congenital. Much hypertrophy, without dilatation of the right ventricle of the heart. No disease of the left side, 236. . . 582
237. Dilatation of both ventricles. Hypertrophy of the left. Disease of aortic valves, and the well-marked results of pericarditis and endocarditis, consecutive on rheumatism, related to syphilis, 464. 583
238. Aneurism of the left ventricle of the heart, consequent on endocarditis and pericarditis, 467. 583
239. Rheumatism, followed by pericarditis and endocarditis. Disease of the mitral valve. Dilatation of the right side of the heart. Dilatation and hypertrophy, with circumscribed aneurism of the left ventricle. Death expedited by acute general peritonitis, 468. . . 584
240. The former subject of rheumatism. Dilatation of the left ventricle. Disease of the mitral valve. Much thickening of the endocardium. An aneurismal sac at the apex. Also the marks of former pericarditis, 471. . . 586
241. Rupture of the heart from fatty degeneration, 479. 587
242. Great dilatation of the ascending aorta and the arch. An aneurismal tumour at the commencement of the descending aorta. There was no external swelling, but the other signs of the disease were very well marked, 494. . . . 588
243. Aneurism of the abdominal aorta. Death by rupture, 493. . . 589
244. Acute rheumatism. Pericarditis and endocarditis. Dilatation of the right side of the heart. Dilatation and hypertrophy of the left ventricle. Ossific state of the mitral valve. Hepatic congestion, 465. 596
245. Aortic and mitral valvular disease. Hypertrophy, with dilatation of the left ventricle. General dropsy. Rapid relief from elaterium. Discharged, 489. . 599

CHAPTER XXVII.

ON DELIRIUM TREMENS.

246. Meningitis. Effusion of lymph and serum in the sub-arachnoid space. Symptoms of delirium tremens, 564. Page 645

CHAPTER XXVIII.

ON CEREBRAL DISEASE AND PARALYSIS.

247. Acute hydrocephalus, 506. . 653
248. Amaurosis of both eyes, headache, fatuity, convulsions, tumour in the brain, with much softening of the cerebral substance, 507. 654
249. Hemiplegia of the right side. Softening of the left corpus striatum, 508. 661
250. Apoplexy. Hemiplegia of the right side. Death. General congestion of the membranes of the brain. Red softening of the left corpus striatum, 509. 661
251. Hemiplegia of the right side. Softening of the left corpus striatum. Disease of the mitral valve, 510. . . 661
252. Symptoms of inflammation of the brain, followed by hemiplegia of the right side, and death by coma. Red softening of the left corpus striatum found after death. 511. . . . 662
253. Hemiplegia of the right side. Meningitis and softening of the anterior and middle lobes of the left cerebral hemisphere. The premonitory symptoms well marked, 512. 662
254. Incomplete paralysis of the left side. Improvement. Disease of heart and valves. Death hastened by diarrhœa. Puriform softening of part of anterior lobe of right cerebral hemisphere, 513. . 662
255. Hemiplegia of the left side. White softening in the right cerebral hemisphere, 514. 663
256. Abscess in the left hemisphere of the brain; for some time general febrile symptoms. Hemiplegia of the right side some days before death, 515. . . 664
257. Apoplexy, followed by hemiplegia of the right side. Gangrene of the left foot and leg, apparently from obstruction of the femoral artery, 516. . 664
258. Hemiplegia of left side, persistent. Facial palsy of the right side, consecutive and transient, 517. . . 665
259. Division of the left half of the spinal cord by a wound. Paralysis and anæsthesia of the left lower extremity, 519. 669
260. Paralysis from arsenical poisoning. Pneumonia also present, 520. . 670

CHAPTER XXIX.

ON TETANUS.

261. Tetanus. Treated with quinine, extract of hemp, wine, and nourishment. Recovered, 521. 686
262. Idiopathic tetanus. Treated with quinine, hemp, wine, and nourishment. Recovery, 522. 686

263. Tetanus in a child. Though fatal, the good effects of treatment with quinine, hemp, and attention to nourishment were very apparent, 523. Page 686
264. Tetanus treated with chloroform. Fatal, 524. 687
265. Tetanus fatal on the 21st day. Whether traumatic or idiopathic doubtful. Treated with quinine, hemp, nourishment, and stimulants. Fatal. Spinal veins congested, 525. . . . 687

CHAPTER XXX.

ON HYDROPHOBIA.

266. Hydrophobia. Three months after the bite, 526. 690
267. Hydrophobia, treated with chloroform, 527. 690
268. Hydrophobia. Chloroform used, but obliged to be discontinued, 528. . 690
269. Hydrophobia in a Parsee boy, 529. 691

CHAPTER XXXI.

ON BLOOD DISEASES.

270. Fever. Several abscesses. Small puriform cysts in lungs. No trace of phlebitis, 535. 694
271. Adynamic fever. Several abscesses. Puriform cysts in the lungs. One in the kidney. Small suppurating wound of heel. No trace of phlebitis, 536. Page 662. 694
272. Adynamic remittent fever. Small abscess on the forehead. Carbuncle on the back. Numerous puriform cysts in the lungs and kidneys, 537. . . 694
273. Many abscesses. Fever. Death by exhaustion. No puriform deposits in the internal viscera, 538. . . 694
274. Adynamic fever. Several abscesses. Recovery, 539. 694
275. Beriberi. Recovery, 549. . . 710
276. Beriberi. Slight discoloration of the gums. Recovery, 550. . . . 710
277. Beriberi. Anasarca. Death. No kidney disease. Liver congested. Cavities of the heart full of thin blood, 551. . 711
278. Beriberi. Anasarca. Gums discoloured. Hydrothorax. Fatal. Cavities of the heart full of fluid blood, 552. . 711
279. A small dog bitten by the Phoorsa snake. Fatal, 553. . . . 717
280. A horse-keeper bitten by the Phoorsa snake. Fatal, 554. . . . 717
281. Parsee woman bitten by Phoorsa snake. Recovery, 555. . . . 718
282. Dog bitten by Phoorsa snake. Fatal. Post mortem examination, 556. . 718

STATISTICAL AND METEOROLOGICAL TABLES.

Table I.—Admissions and Deaths, with Per-centage, from all Diseases, in the European General Hospital at Bombay for the Five Years from July, 1838, to July, 1843 . . . . Page 13

Table II.—Admissions and Deaths, with Per-centage, from all Diseases, in the European General Hospital at Bombay for the Five Years from 1844 to 1848 14

Table III.—Admissions and Deaths, with Per-centage, from all Diseases, in the European General Hospital at Bombay for the Five Years from 1849 to 1853 14

Table IV.—Admissions and Deaths, with Per-centage, from all Diseases, in the Jamsetjee Jejeebhoy Hospital at Bombay, for the Six Years from 1848 to 1853 15

Table V.—Admissions and Deaths, with Per-centage, from Fever of all kinds, in the European General Hospital at Bombay, for the Six Years from July 1838 to July 1843 171

Table VI.—Admissions and Deaths, with Per-centage, from Fever of all kinds, in the European General Hospital at Bombay, for the Five Years from 1844 to 1848 171

Table VII.—Admissions and Deaths, with Per-centage, from Fever of all kinds, in the European General Hospital at Bombay, for the Five Years from 1849 to 1853 172

Table VIII.—Admissions and Deaths, with Per-centage, from Intermittent Fever, in the European General Hospital at Bombay, for the Five Years from July, 1838, to July, 1843 173

Table IX.—Admissions and Deaths, with Per-centage, from Intermittent Fever, in the European General Hospital at Bombay, for the Five Years from 1844 to 1848 173

Table X.—Admissions and Deaths, with Per-centage, from Intermittent Fever, in the European General Hospital at Bombay, for the Five Years from 1849 to 1853 . . . . Page 174

Table XI.—Admissions and Deaths, with Per-centage, from Ephemeral Fever, in the European General Hospital at Bombay, for the Five Years from July, 1838, to June, 1843 174

Table XII.—Admissions and Deaths, with Per-centage, from Remittent and Intermittent Fever, in the Jamsetjee Jejeebhoy Hospital at Bombay, for the Six Years from 1848 to 1853 . . 176

Table XIII.—Admissions and Deaths, with Per-centage, from Intermittent Fever, in the Jamsetjee Jejeebhoy Hospital at Bombay, for the Six Years from 1848 to 1853 177

Table XIV.—Admissions and Deaths, with Per-centage, from Remittent Fever, in the European General Hospital at Bombay, for the Five Years from July, 1838, to June, 1843 178

Table XV.—Admissions and Deaths, with Per-centage, from Remittent Fever, in the European General Hospital at Bombay, for the Five Years from 1844 to 1848 178

Table XVI.—Admissions and Deaths, with Per-centage, from Remittent Fever, in the European General Hospital at Bombay, for the Five Years from 1849 to 1853 179

Table XVII.—Admission and Deaths, with Per-centage, from Remittent Fever, in the Jamsetjee Jejeebhoy Hospital, at Bombay, for the Six Years from 1848 to 1853 180

Table XVIII.—Admission and Deaths, from Intermittent and Remittent Fever, in the Byculla Schools, for the Seventeen Years from 1837 to 1853 . . 181

Table XIX.—Admissions and Deaths, with Per-centage, from Epidemic Cholera, in the European General Hospital at Bombay, for the Six Years from 1838 to 1843 233

TABLE XX.—Admissions and Deaths, with Per-centage, from Epidemic Cholera, in the European General Hospital at Bombay, for the Five Years from 1844 to 1848 . . . . Page 234

TABLE XXI.—Admissions and Deaths, with Per-centage, from Epidemic Cholera, in the European General Hospital at Bombay, for the Five Years from 1849 to 1853 234

TABLE XXII.—Admissions and Deaths, with Per-centage, from Epidemic Cholera, in the Jamsetjee Jejeebhoy Hospital at Bombay, for the Six Years, from 1848 to 1853 235

TABLE XXIII.—Admissions and Deaths, with Per-centage, from Epidemic Cholera in the Byculla Schools, at Bombay, for the Seventeen Years from 1837 to 1853 235

TABLE XXIV.—Admissions and Deaths, with Per-centage, from Dysentery, in the European General Hospital at Bombay, for the Five Years from July, 1838, to June, 1853 318

TABLE XXV.—Admissions and Deaths, with Per-centage, from Dysentery, in the European General Hospital at Bombay, for the Five Years from 1844 to 1848 318

TABLE XXVI.—Admissions and Deaths, with Per-centage, from Dysentery, in the European General Hospital at Bombay, for the Five Years from 1849 to 1853 319

TABLE XXVII.—Admissions and Deaths, with Per-centage, from Dysentery, in the Jamsetjee Jejeebhoy Hospital at Bombay, for the Six Years from 1848 to 1853 319

TABLE XXVIII.—Admissions and Deaths, with Per-centage, from Diarrhœa, in the Jamsetjee Jejeebhoy Hospital, at Bombay, for the Six Years from 1848 to 1853 320

TABLE XXIX.—Admissions and Deaths, with Per-centage, from Diarrhœa and Dysentery, in the Byculla Schools, for the Seventeen Years from 1837 to 1853 320

TABLE XXX.—Admissions and Deaths, with Per-centage, from Hepatitis, Acute and Chronic, in the European General Hospital at Bombay, for the Five Years from 1838 to 1843 418

TABLE XXXI.—Admissions and Deaths, with Per-centage, from Hepatitis, Acute and Chronic, in the European General Hospital at Bombay, for the Five Years from 1844 to 1848 418

TABLE XXXII.—Admissions and Deaths, with Per-centage, from Hepatitis, Acute and Chronic, in the European General Hospital at Bombay, for the Five Years from 1849 to 1853 . . Page 419

TABLE XXXIII.—Admissions and Deaths, with Per-centage, from Acute Hepatic Affections, in the Jamsetjee Jejeebhoy Hospital at Bombay, for the Six Years from 1848 to 1853 419

TABLE XXXIV.—Admissions and Deaths, with Per-centage, from Chronic Hepatic Affections, in the Jamsetjee Jejeebhoy Hospital at Bombay, for the Six Years from 1848 to 1853 420

TABLE XXXV.—Admissions and Deaths, with Per-centage, from Pneumonia, in the Jamsetjee Jejeebhoy Hospital at Bombay, for the Six Years from 1848 to 1853 547

TABLE XXXVI.—Admissions and Deaths, with Per-centage, from Bronchitis, in the Jamsetjee Jejeebhoy Hospital at Bombay, for the Six Years from 1848 to 1853 553

TABLE XXXVII.—Admissions and Deaths, with Per-centage, from Phthisis Pulmonalis, in the Jamsetjee Jejeebhoy Hospital at Bombay, for the Six Years from 1848 to 1853 560

TABLE XXXVIII.—Admissions and Deaths, with Per-centage, from Delirium Tremens, in the European General Hospital at Bombay, for the Five Years from July 1838 to June 1843 646

TABLE XXXIX.—Admissions and Deaths, with Per-centage, from Delirium Tremens, in the European General Hospital at Bombay, for the Five Years from 1844 to 1848 646

TABLE XL.—Admissions and Deaths, with Per-centage, from Delirium Tremens, in the European General Hospital at Bombay, for the Five Years from 1849 to 1853 647

TABLE XLI.—Admissions and Deaths, with Per-centage, from Paralysis, in the Jamsetjee Jejeebhoy Hospital at Bombay, for the Six Years from 1848 to 1853

TABLE XLII.—Admissions and Deaths, with Per-centage, from Tetanus, in the Jamsetjee Jejeebhoy Hospital at Bombay, for the Six Years from 1848 to 1853 688

TABLE XLIII.—Admissions of Guinea-worm into the Hospital of Her Majesty's 4th Light Dragoons at Kirkee, during Eight Years from 1827 to 1834 . 725

TABLE XLIV.—Admissions and Deaths with Per-centage, from Dracunculus, in the Jamsetjee Jejeebhoy Hospital at

Bombay, for the Six Years from 1848 to 1853 . . . . . Page 725
TABLE XLV. — Admissions from Dracunculus, in the Bombay Army, in the Year 1832 726
TABLE XLVI. — Admissions from Dracunculus, in the Bombay Army, for the Year 1833 727
TABLE I.—Observations on the Temperature at Bombay 743
TABLE II.—Observations with the Wet Bulb Thermometer, at Bombay. Page 744
TABLE III.—Barometric Observations at Bombay 745
TABLE IV.—Observations on the Rainfall and the Direction and Force of the Winds at Bombay 746
TABLE showing the Atmospheric Pressure, the Temperature, the Dryness, the Rainfall, and the Direction of the Winds at Poorundhur 747

INDEX.

A

ABSCESS, HEPATIC.—*Pathology;* formation of, 328; opening into lung or pleural sac, 335; into stomach and intestine, 342; into pericardium, 345; into hepatic duct, 345; into peritoneal sac, 345; fatal without rupture, 329, 380; recovery by absorption, 345; character of contents, 359.—*Causes;* pyæmic theory discussed, 365.—*Symptoms* of, 370. 384; pointing towards diaphragm, 380; opening into lung, brick-red sputa, 382. 384.—*Treatment* of, 384; question of puncture fully considered, 393; hepatic abscess not uncommon with cirrhosis, 424.

ANTIMONY—*potassio-tartrate*, use of, in intermittent fever, 28. 53; remittent fever, 110. 118; ardent continued fever, 166; pneumonia, 537; delirium tremens with opiates, 631; cerebral disease, 649.

AORTA—aneurism of, 587.

APOPLEXY—cerebral, 650.

ARSENIC—acute gastritis from, 458; liquor in intermittent fever, 32; paralysis from, 670.

ASTHMA—relation to malaria, 55; to emphysema, 553.

ASTRINGENTS—in cholera, 223; in chronic dysentery, 304. 308. For particulars see these.

AUSCULTATION—importance of, in fevers in India, 532, *note;* in rheumatism, 562.

B.

BARBIERS—alluded to, 669.

BEEBEERINE—use in intermittent fever, 34.

BERIBERI—name objected to, 155, *note.*—*Symptoms*, 705; author's views of its *Pathology* explained, 706. *Treatment*, 708. 713.

BILE—defect of so-called torpor of the liver, 441.

BILIARY CALCULI, 433; ducts, inflammation of, 98. 431; compression of by enlarged lymphatic glands as cause of jaundice, 97. 435.

BLISTERS—use of, in remittent fever, 119; 121. 140; dysentery, 308; hepatitis, 391; pneumonia, 541; pericarditis, 578.

BLOOD-LETTING—general and local, in intermittent fever, 28; cold stage of, 124; remittent fever, 110. 112. 114. 115. 118. 122; continued fever, 166; cholera epidemic, 225. 229; dysentery, 293; hepatitis, 385. 386; pneumonia, 534. 536; pericarditis, 578; cerebral disease, 649.

BRAIN—affections of, 648; congestion of, and determination to, in remittent fever, 70. 81. 118; serous effusion on, 90.

BRIGHT'S disease. See Kidneys.

BRONCHITIS—complicating, intermittent, fever, 52; idiopathic, 552; tabular statements of, in the Jamsetjee Jejeebhoy Hospital, 553.

C.

CALCULUS—urinary, 505.

CALOMEL—cholagogue action in remittent fever, 110; epidemic cholera, 228; in dysentery, 296; hepatitis, 386; abuse in intermittent and remittent fever, 34. 125; Annesley's supposed sedative action of large doses of calomel dissented from, 136.

CANCER—of liver, 429.

CAUSES—of disease, predisposing and exciting, general notice of, 1. 9; of particular diseases, will be found under name of.

CHANGE OF AIR AND OF CLIMATE, in intermittent and remittent fever, 42. 150; dysentery, 312; hepatitis, 414.

CHICKEN POX, 200.

CHILDREN—fevers in, 168; dysentery, 314; hepatitis, 415.

CHOLERA—bilious—not common in numerous classes in India, 214. 440.

Cholera, Epidemic — prevalence of, in Bombay, 202; causes of, 204; symptoms of, 208; different degrees of severity, 209; rate of mortality from, 215; relation of mortality to age, 216; to period of epidemic, 217; to duration on admission, 217.—*Pathology* of, 218.—*Treatment* of preliminary diarrhœa, 221; stage of collapse, 224; of secondary affections, 226; by general blood-letting, 229; hot bath, 229; emetics, 230; hot saline enemata, liniments, injection into veins, inhalation of vapours, 230; galvanism, cold effusion, wet sheet envelope, 231; recapitulation, 232. Statistics of, in European General Hospital and Jamsetjee Jejeebhoy Hospital, Bombay, 233.

Cirrhosis. See Liver.

Colica Pictorium, 456; colique végétale, 455.

D.

Datura poisoning, in Bombay, 641, *note*.

Delirium Tremens — prevalence of, and mortality from, in European General Hospital, Bombay, 624. *Symptoms* and *Treatment*, division into two species, 625; first species, 627; second species, first stage, 628; second stage, 629; cold affusion, 630; tartar emetic and opium, 631; stimulants, 632; importance of food, 633; objections to treatment with free opiates and to expectant method stated, 633. 639; third stage, 635. Remarks on blood-letting, 637; purgatives and emetics, 638; general management, 638. *Pathology*—with remarks on principles of treatment, and diagnosis, 641; complicated with meningitis, 645; in natives of India, 645; statistics of, in European General Hospital at Bombay, 646.

Diabetes—saccharine, 502.

Diaphoretics — in fever, 28. 110; dysentery, 302.

Diarrhœa, 316.

Diathesis—general notice of importance of, 2; great prominence given to it in the etiology of all the diseases treated of.

Diet in remittent fever, 149; dysentery, 311.

Diuresis, 505.

Duodenitis—in remittent fever in relation to jaundice, 98.

Dracunculus—prevalence of, in Bombay Presidency, 720; obscurity of origin, 722; management, 724; statistics, 725.

Dropsy, in Bright's disease, 481; cardiac disease, 593; in scorbutic diathesis Beriberi, 704; in ascites from cirrhosis of liver, 421.

Dysentery—prevalence of, 236.—*Pathology*—general remarks, 237; morbid appearances, change of colour of mucous membrane of large intestine, 239; exudations on free surface and into tissue, 240; implication of follicles and solitary glands, 242; different forms of ulcer, transverse, 245; circular, 253; puriform infiltration, 253; œdema and sloughing erysipelatous, 258; tubular sloughs of mucous membrane, 258; intussuscepted gut, 262; cicatrisation of ulcers, 263; complication of inflammation of mucous membrane of large intestine with peritonitis, 265; adhesions of omentum, 265; tumefaction of region of cœcum or sigmoid flexure, 269; displacement of the colon, 270; complicated with lesions of small intestine and stomach, 271; with enlargement of mesenteric glands, 272; part of intestine chiefly affected, 272; microscopic morbid anatomy of dysentery, 272.—*Etiology of*—preliminary theoretic remarks, 273; importance of noting both predisposing and exciting causes, 273; exciting causes, cold, 273; much importance attached to predisposing causes, 275; common belief that malaria is an exciting cause, dissented from, 276.—*Symptoms*, 280.—*Treatment*—general principles, 288; details of treatment, 291; blood-letting, general and local, 293; cholagogue action of calomel, principle explained, 296; mercurial influence, induction of, condemned, 297; use of ipecacuanha, 298; purgatives, 300; diaphoretics, 302; opium, principles of use explained, 302; chloroform, 304; astringents and tonics, 304; bael fruit, 306; acetate of lead, 306; trisnitrate of bismuth, quinine, sulphate of copper, nitrate of silver, 307; preparations of iron, 307; vegetable astringents, 307; fomentations, blisters, 308; large warm water enemata, principles considered and dissented from, 308; diet, 311; change of air and climate, 312; dysentery in children, 314. Statistical tables, 318.

Dyspepsia—functional notice of, brief, and chiefly inculcating, in reference to etiology and treatment, its character as symptomatic of diathetic states, 462.

E.

Elephantiasis—arabum, 698.

Emetics, use in intermittent and remittent fever, 28. 110. 140; in cholera, 230.

Emphysema of the lungs, 553.

Encephalitis, 604, *note*.

Endocarditis. See Pericarditis.

Erysipelas, 200.

Etiology — considered in reference to each disease, which heads see.

F.

FEBRICULA—162.

FEVER, prevalence of, in India, 16; *Ardent, continued*, 164.—*Symptoms*, 165.—*Pathology* and *Treatment*, 166.

FEVER—*intermittent* types of, 17.—SIMPLE *Symptoms* of, 20.—*Pathology*, 24; mortality, 24.—*Treatment* in different stages, use of quinine, arsenic, bebeerine, muriate of narcotine, mercury condemned, from 28 to 35.—COMPLICATED, with splenic enlargement; *Symptoms* of, 36; abnormal præcordial dulness and cardiac murmur, 36.—*Pathology* of, 38; laceration of spleen, 427, *note*.—*Treatment* of, 40; liability to dysentery and cautions therefrom, 41; use of bromine, iodine, 41; injurious effects of mercury, 41; with hepatic affection—*Pathology*, 44; *Treatment*, 45; with jaundice and affection of stomach and bowels, 47; with cerebral affection, 49; with bronchitis, pneumonia, rheumatism, scorbutus, pericarditis, asthma, 52; relation of asthma to malaria, 55; intermittent fever in children, 168; statistics of, in European General Hospital and Jamsetjee Jejeebhoy Hospital, 174, 176.

FEVER, *Remittent; causes* of, same as of intermittent fever, 56; diagnosis of, from intermittent and ardent continued, 56.—*Symptoms* of ORDINARY remittent, 58; inflammatory, 60; adynamic, 62; congestive, 64; badly developed, 66; unexpected collapse, 67; occasional peculiar symptoms, 69; of COMPLICATED, cerebral, 70; irritability of stomach, 72; gastric and bilious remittent, 73; pneumonia and bronchitis, 73; diagnosis from hectic and symptomatic fever, 74. *Pathology*—mortality from, 75; importance of diathesis or pre-existing structural disease, 76; complicated with cerebral determination, 81; cerebral inflammation, 86; cerebral adynamic, 88; import of cranial serous effusion analysed, 90; gastric irritability, 93; bilious remittent, 93; complicated with affection of bowels, 94; hepatic and splenic affection, 96; jaundice, 97; parotitis, 105; *Treatment*—contrast of principles with those of zymotic continued fever, 105; of ordinary form, 109; inflammatory, 113; congestive, 115; continued and adynamic, 116; badly developed symptoms, 117; of complicated, with cerebral affection, with question of mercurial treatment in, 118, 120; gastric irritability, 121; jaundice, 121; hepatitis, dysentery, 122; remarks on blood-letting, 122; mercurial treatment, author's opinion of, 125; opinion of other writers on, 128; origin and history of, 130; on cold affusion, 137; wet sheet packing, 137; purgatives, 138; emetics, 140; blisters, 140; opiates, use of, dangers from, 140; quinine, 143; question of large doses examined, 146; Warburg's drops, 148, *note*; diet, 149; change of air, use and injudicious application of, 150; question of lunar influence, 154, *note*. *Infectious Adynamic Remittent*—Pali disease, 155; statistics of remittent fever in European General Hospital and Jamsetjee Jejeebhoy Hospital, Bombay, 177, 180; Byculla schools, 181.

FEVER—European relapsing, typhus, unknown as yet in India, 16.

FEVER—typhoid, of occasional occurrence, further research necessary, 160.

FEMALES—hepatitis in, caution in respect to, 415.

G.

GALL-BLADDER—inflammation and distention of, 431.

GANGRENE of lung, 523, *note*.

GASTRITIS—acute, 458; chronic, 460.

GASTRO—enteritis, 316.

GLOSSITIS—efficacy of application of nitrate of silver in, 461.

H.

HEADACHE—paroxysmal, functional, and organic, diagnosis of, 654.

HEART—organic disease of, in natives in the Jamsetjee Jejeebhoy Hospital, 581; dilatation of both ventricles, 581; dilatation and hypertrophy of left ventricle, 581; hypertrophy of right ventricle, 582; aneurism of left ventricle, 583; valvular disease of, 586; previous pericarditis and endocarditis, 586; rupture from fatty degeneration, 587; aortic disease, 587; pulmonary complication, congestion, œdema, hepatisation, emphysema, 589; relation of, to sex, caste, age, occupation, habits of life, season, 590, 591, 592; to pericarditis, endocarditis, Bright's disease, 592; leading *symptoms and signs*, dyspnœa, 593; dropsy, 593; præcordial pain, 593; pain below margin of right ribs, 593; scapular pain, 594; character of pulse, 594; præcordial fulness, 595; increased impulse, 595; præcordial dulness, 595; dulness below right costal margin, 595; character of cardiac murmurs, 595; præcordial thrill, 599. *Treatment*, 599; illustrative cases, 599; heart disease in Europeans in India, 600.

HEMIPLEGIA—in natives, 658; relation to age and caste, 658, 659.—*Pathology* of, 660; illustrative cases, 660; symptoms, 665.

HEPATITIS — anatomical position and relation, important, 321; terms hepatitis and cirrhosis preferred to suppurative and adhesive inflammation, 324. *Pathology* — question of which capillaries affected, considered, 325; inflammation of capsule and substance, 327; turgescence, 327; lymph exudation, 327; formation of abscess, see "ABSCESS;" secondary peritonitis, puriform sacs, 348; secondary pleuritis, general and circumscribed empyema, 352; secondary pericarditis, 352; general secondary peritonitis, 355; relation of secondary serous inflammation with suppuration to cachectic states, 359. *Causes* — not uncommon in natives of India, 323; exciting, cold and heat, 361; special influence of, 363; intemperance not proved, 363; predisposing causes, cachectic states, but not evidence to relate to particular cachexia, 363; relation of hepatic abscess to dysentery considered, 365; primary hepatitis, secondary dysentery, 369; hepatic abscess without intestinal ulceration, cases of, 365; dysentery preceding abscess, 369. —*Symptoms* of acute hepatitis, pain of side, 370; of right shoulder, 371; import of enlargement of liver, 372; tension of right rectus muscle, 373; altered states of biliary secretion, 373; jaundice of no value as a symptom, 373; fever, 374; occasional obscurity, 375; of formation of abscess, see "ABSCESS." —*Treatment* of early stages, 384; general blood-letting, 385; local blood-letting, mercurial and other purgatives, ipecacuanha, 386; caution in regard to relapse, 386; treatment of exudation stage, 388; mercurial influence, principles of, 389; blisters, 391; after abscess formed, see "ABSCESS;" hepatitis in females and children, 415; occasional difficulties in diagnosis, 416; statistics of, in European General Hospital and Jamsetjee Jejeebhoy Hospital at Bombay, 417, 420.

Hepatic phlebitis, 361.

HILL SANITARIA in Deccan—Mahubuleshwur, Pannehgunnee, Porrundhur, Singhur. Principles applicable to all Hill Sanitaria in India, 728—740. 747.

HOOPING COUGH—201.

HYDATIDS—in liver, not common in India, 430.

HYDROCEPHALUS—acute, 652; chronic, 654.

HYDROPHOBIA — as observed in Bombay, illustrative cases, 689.

I.

ILEUS—453.

IPECACUANHA—use of, in dysentery, 298.

IRON — preparations of, in splenic enlargement, 40; dysentery, 307; cachexia of Bright's disease, 494.

J.

JAUNDICE — complicating remitting fever, 73, 97, 121; idiopathic *Pathology*, 433. —*Causes*, 436.—*Treatment*, 438; of no value as a symptom of hepatitis, 373.

K.

KIDNEYS—Bright's disease, prevalence of, in some classes of the native community, 465; want of data in respect to Europeans, 466; summary statement of morbid anatomy of, 467; illustrative cases, 468; dropsical symptoms, 481; secondary head symptoms, believed not to be so common in India, 481; the same statement of secondary cardiac affection, 482; the uræmic theory of the secondary affections discussed, 483; altered relation of albumen in the blood and urine considered, 485; remarks on the proximate cause of albumen in the urine, 486. — *Causes* — Relation to cachectic states, 487; external cold, 490. — *Symptoms* —Relative to the kidney, 491; condition of the urine, 492.—*Treatment*—of the kidney disease, 492; of the secondary affections, dropsical, 493; inflammatory, 495; reference to diagnostic value of epithelial debris, tube casts and oil globules in urine, 492.

L.

LARYNGEAL affections in phthisis pulmonalis, 558.

LEECHES—sizes of, used in Bombay, *note*, 294.

LEPROSY—tubercular and anæsthetic; arrangements for care of lepers in Calcutta, Madras, and Bombay, 695.—*Symptoms*, 696.—*Pathology*, 697.

LIVER—cirrhosis of: *Pathology*, 421.—*Symptoms*, 422.—*Treatment*, 422; illustrative cases, 422; congestion of the liver, 426; cancer and hydatid formations of, 429. 430; fatty degeneration of, 428; lardaceous, 427; so called torpor of, 441; inflammation of. (See *Hepatitis*.)

M.

MALARIA—applied in this work exclusively to the miasmatic cause of intermittent and remittent fever: summary statement of existing knowledge, 4; in relation to intermittent fever, 18. 19, *note;* to remittent fever, 60, *note;* a predisposing cause of dysentery, but not an exciting one, 276, 279; the cause of many obscure derangements, 153; modifying influences on inflammatory symptomatic fever, 278, 374, 327, 576, 542.

Measles—account of in Byculla Schools and elsewhere, 194; mortality rate, 198.

Meningitis—complicating remittent fever, 86; idiopathic, 652.

Mercury—constitutional effect of, injurious in splenic enlargement, 41; use of, in remittent fever fully discussed and condemned, 125 to 136; in dysentery also disapproved, 297; use of, in hepatitis explained, 386, 389; also in pneumonia and in pericarditis, 538, 579.

Meteorology of Bombay, 741; of Deccan Hill Sanitaria, 729, 747.

Mumps, 198.

Myelitis, 667.

O.

Officers, European—diseases of: remittent fever, 75; small-pox, 190; measles, 197; dysentery, 237, *table;* peritonitis, 443; Bright's disease, 466; pneumonia, 508; phthisis pulmonalis, 554; cerebral affections, 650; tetanus, 673.

Opium—use of: in remittent fever, 110, 140; cholera, 222, 225; dysentery, 302; delirium tremens, free and routine use cautioned against, 633.

P.

Paralysis—from arsenic, 670; facial, 671. (See *Hemiplegia* and *Paraplegia.*)

Paraplegia, 668; case of wound of spinal cord, 669.

Pericarditis and Endocarditis—analysis of 25 cases: proportion of pericarditis and endocarditis, 561; result, 563; relation to sex, caste, age, occupation, habits, season, 564 to 567; relation to rheumatism, cachexia, pulmonary inflammation, 567.—*Symptoms and signs*—Pain at margin of left ribs and præcordial region, 568; increased impulse, 568; character of pulse, 569; febrile symptoms, remittent character of, 569, 570; dyspnœa, 570; anxiety of countenance, 570; delirium, 570; increased præcordial dulness, 571; purring tremor, præcordial fulness, friction murmur, 571; duration and causes of friction murmur, 571; jogging movement of heart, 578.—*Treatment*—General and local blood-letting, 578; blisters, 578; mercurial influence, 579; illustrative cases, 573.

Peritonitis.—*Pathology*—Rarity of idiopathic sthenic form, 443; traumatic, 443; sero-puriform, 445; chronic tubercular, 447; chronic form with effusion observed at Aden, 452.

Phthisis Pulmonalis—not unfrequent either in Europeans or natives, 554.—*Causes*—influence of rainy season, question of malarious influence, 554.—*Symptoms,* 556.—*Pathology*—Question of rapidity of course in India, 556; stage in which hospital patients admitted, 557; which side most affected, 557; co-existing pleuritis, 558; pneumonia, 558; laryngeal complication, 558; intestinal ulceration, 558; frequency of diarrhœa, 558; tubercular peritoneum, fatty liver, 559. *Treatment,* 559; statistics of the Jamsetjee Jejeebhoy Hospital, 560.

Pleuritis, 548.—*Symptoms,* 548.—*Causes,* 549.—*Pathology,* 549.—*Treatment,* 551. Question of *Paracentesis of Chest,* 551.

Pneumonia—rare in Europeans, 508; common in asthenic natives, 508; division into primary and complicating remittent fever, considered together, analysis of 103 clinical cases, 509. *Etiology*—relation to sex, age, caste, habits, constitution, season, 509—512. *Pathology*—Preliminary remarks on question, which capillaries affected, 512; rate of mortality, 515; duration of illness before admission, 517; stage of disease, 518; which lung affected, 518; residence in hospital, 520; morbid anatomy, summary of, 521; illustrative cases, 524. *Symptoms.*—Fever, remittent character of, 527; pain of side, 529; pain below margin of right ribs, 529; dyspnœa, 531; cough, 532; delirium, 533; character of the sputa, 533; physical signs, 554.—*Treatment*—Blood-letting, general principles explained, those of some previous writers dissented from, 534; local blood-letting, 536; tartar emetic, 537; mercurial influence, 538; blisters, 541; quinine, utility and principles explained, 542; liquor potassæ, 543; stimulants, 543; concluding remarks on general principles of treatment relative to the use of antiphlogistics and tonics in pneumonia and inflammatory disease generally, 544; statistics of, in Jamsetjee Jejeebhoy Hospital, 547.

Purgatives—use in remittent fever, 138; dysentery, 300; hepatitis, 386; probable injurious effects from, in hepatitis, 366.

Pyæmia, 692, 693; illustrative cases, question of relation to hepatic abscess, 365.

Q.

QUININE—disulphate, use in intermittent and remittent fever, 29, 114, 143; prophylactic use, 149; in pneumonia, both febrile and idiopathic, 542.

R.

RHEUMATISM, 561. 562, *note*, 592. 715.

S.

SCARLATINA—very rare if not unknown in India, 199.

SCURVY—not uncommon in India, 701.

SEA-COAST—Sanitaria, 738. 751.

SMALL-POX — as observed in Jamsetjee Jejeebhoy Hospital, 182; prevalence of, in Bombay, 187; prevention of, 189.

SNAKE-BITE—Phoorsa snake, on Mahubuleshurr Hills, 716.

SPINAL CORD—disease of, 668; wound of, 669.

SPLEEN—inflammation of, rare, 36, *note;* enlargement of, 36;—*Pathology*, 38; *Treatment*, 37; abnormal præcordial dulness from heart, displacement by enlarged spleen, 37; laceration of, by injury, 427, *note.*

STATISTICS—see list of tables; injury to medical science from use of imperfect statistical data, 12, *note;* 311, *note;* 516, *note.*

SUNSTROKE, 603.—*Symptoms*, 606. *Pathology*, 611.—*Etiology*, 614.—*Prevention* and *Treatment*, 619.

T.

TETANUS—prevalence of, 672. *Pathology*, 673. *Causes*, 678. *Symptoms*, 680. *Treatment*, 683; illustrative cases, 686; statistics of, in Jamsetjee Jejeebhoy Hospital, 688.

TONICS—regimen, 10; remedies in dysentery, 304; remarks on general principles, 544.

U.

URINE—imperfect acquaintance with normal standard of, in India, 497; chylo-serous, 498; saccharine, 502; with excess of urates, oxalates, phosphates, 505.

V.

VACCINATION; 189, imperfect in Native Army, 190.

W.

WARBURG'S Fever drops, 148, *note.*

WET SHEET packing, in fever, 137.

THE END.